Pregnancy, 411
Client Need Categories, 420
Authorization to Test, 422
Security Rules, 424
Exam Results, 424
Computerized Adaptive Testing, 425
Medicating the Terminally Ill Patient, 438

 Learning Exercises

Informal Educational Experiences, 2
Self-Evaluation of Sensory Learning Style, 15
Enhance Your Learning, 17
Learning Styles, 19
What Kind of Thinker Are You?, 20
Brain Characteristics, 22
Signs of Possible Adult ADD, 23
Textbook Authority, 24
Phases of Literacy and Comprehension, 24
Self-Test of Time Management, 29
Semester, Weekly, and Daily Planning, 35
Personal Distractions, 43
Your Peers at School, 43
Daydreaming, 43
Active versus Passive Listener, 44
Reading Habit Evaluation, 49
How Well Do You Follow Directions?, 56
Multiple-Choice Items, 57
Checklist—General and Nursing Resources
    and Technology, 61
Nursing Periodicals, 64
Popular Reading, 64
Peer Assistance with Computer/Internet, 70
Using CINAHL® Print Edition, 72
Survey of your Current Level of Critical Thinking, 77
Attitude Evaluation—My Attitude, 80
Nurse Practice Act, 108
Assisting During Planning, 113
Implementing Plan of Care, 118
Evaluating Patient Progress, 119
Communicating with Your Patient, 123
Appropriate Dress Code and Behavior, 125
Self-Evaluation of Personal Characteristics, 126
Cultural Differences, 129
Resolving Conflicts, 135
Making Good Food Choices, 139
Make MyPyramid Work for You, 139
Making Room for Exercise, 140
Your Life Choices and Burnout, 146
Codependency: A Pathological Need, 151
Avoid Negative Stress, 153
Find a Good Role Model, 153

bmoson @ crown college . edu

Make Time for Recreation, 153
Get Enough Sleep, 157
Get to Know the Nursing Team, 168
What Makes You Unique?, 183
Identifying the Roles You Play in Your Life, 183
Who Am I Based on My Roles?, 184
What We Have in Common, 184
Basic Daily Needs, 187
Cultural Patterns: Family, 189
Cultural Patterns: Food, 189
Cultural Patterns: Religion, 189
Cultural Patterns: Time, 190
Cultural Patterns: Communication, 191
Cultural Patterns: Education, 191
Cultural Patterns: Economic Level, 192
Cultural Patterns: Wellness Beliefs and Practices, 193
Cultural Patterns: Pregnancy and Birth Beliefs and
    Practices, 194
Cultural Patterns: Terminal Illness and Death Beliefs and
    Practices, 194
Areas of Cultural Diversity, 194
Your Area's Cultural Groups, 198
Your Personal Spirituality, 207
My Spiritual Practices, 209
Learning About Different Belief Systems, 224
Nonassertive Behavior, 228
Aggressive Behavior, 229
Identify Assertiveness, 231
Identify if Behavior is Passive, Aggressive, or Assertive, 233
Keep a Daily Journal, 236
Celebrate Attaining Your Goals, 237
Review Your Journal, 238
ANA Bill of Rights, 240
Evaluate Protection Against Potential Dangers, 241
Sexual Harassment Policy, 243
Local Health Care Agency, 307
Voluntary Health Care Agencies, 308
Hospitals, 309
Ambulatory Care Providers, 310
Rehabilitation Services, 311
Long-Term Care Facilities, 312
Community Health Services, 313
Adult Day Care Services, 314
Wellness Programs, 314
Develop Your Own Style, 314
How You Support Government Services, 326
Where Is Free Health Care Offered?, 329
How Has Medicare Changed/Evolved?, 330
Identify Changes in the U.S. Health Care System, 333
Identify Restructuring of Health Care in Your Area, 333
Identify Changes in Managed Care, 335
Identify How You Will Stay Current in Your Career, 336
Ethical Issues and Your Nurse Practice Act, 341

Continued on the next page.

SPECIAL FEATURES—cont'd

Procedures and Their Effects, 346
Get Familiar with Your State's Nurse Practice Act, 355
Compact States and the Nurse Practice Act, 358
Interstate Agreement, 358
Malpractice Coverage, 363
Patient's Rights, 369
Maintain Patient Confidentiality, 372
Legal Directives, 375
Terminally Ill Patients, 377
Good Samaritan Act, 378
Consider the Following Questions, 386
Networking for Jobs, 390
Practice Mock Interviews, 391
Seek Critique of Mock Interviews, 391
Pick Your References, 394
Cover Letters, 395
Résumé, 396
Job Application, 398
Impression Counts, 405
Mock Interview, 412
Thank You Letter, 414
Keep the Connections, 414
Letter of Resignation, 415
Practicing in Other States, 418
What Is an Alternate Item Question?, 420
Categories of Patient Care, 421
Fees, 422
Relax!, 426
LPN/LVN Wages, 431
Areas of Interest, 431
Personal Skills and Characteristics, 432
Availability of Leadership Course, 432
Area Job Opportunities, 440

Leadership Activities

Examining Organizational Charts, 249
Determining Your State's Requirements to Assume the
   Position of Practical/Vocational Charge Nurse, 249
Discovering Your Personal Leadership Style, 251
Plotting My Leadership Style Score, 253
Identifying Signs of Stress, 261

Leadership Hints

Communication of the Practical/Vocational Charge
   Nurse, 256
Encouraging Verbal Communication from Nursing
   Assistants, 257

Decision Tree for Problem Solving, 258
Using Unit Mission Statements, 259
Practical/Vocational Charge Nurse Behaviors That
   Encourage Team Building, 259
Life Skills That Help Control Stress, 260
Creating a Less Stressful Work Environment, 260
Avoiding Irrational Thinking, 261
OBRA Provisions That Deal Specifically with Nursing
   Assistants, 263
Applying the Nursing Process to Organize Your Shift, 264
CQI Components That the Practical/Vocational Charge
   Nurse Needs to Incorporate into the Leadership Role, 266
Applying the Nursing Process for Conflict Resolution, 266
Preventing Anger in Nursing Assistants, 268
Personal Anger Management Techniques for the Practical/
   Vocational Charge Nurse, 268
Prevention of Workplace Violence, 268
Providing Feedback to Nursing Assistants, 269
Encouraging Nursing Assistants to Participate in the
   Evaluation Process, 270
Meeting for the Final Evaluation Interview, 270
Strategies to Increase Self-Confidence in Nursing
   Assistants, 271
Strategies to Encourage Personal Growth in Nursing
   Assistants, 271
Sources of Learning Skills for the Practical/Vocational
   Charge Nurse Position, 272

Management Hints

Assigning Tasks, 287
Delegating Duties, 287
Suggestions for Legal Soundness When Delegating, 289
Specific Tasks for Nursing Assistant Assignment, 292
Why Lists of Duties to Delegate Do Not Exist, 294
Examples of Duties Not to Delegate, 294
Communication/Direction Responsibilities of the LPN/LVN
   Charge Nurse When Assigning or Delegating, 297
Supervision and Feedback, 298
Tricia Supervises the Nursing Assistants, 299
Evaluation and Feedback, 299
Reporting to Oncoming Shift, 302

Management Tools

Reviewing LPN/LVN Charge Nurse Job Descriptions, 276
Reviewing Policies and Routines, 280
Reporting Change of Condition to the Physician, 282

When Nursing Assistants Bring Problems from Home, 283

Encouraging Nursing Assistants to Be Accountable for Learning Skills, 283

Interventions to Use for the Demanding/Complaining Family, 284

Reviewing Your Nurse Practice Act for Authority to Delegate, 285

Locating Positions of Nursing Groups and Employer on Delegation Function of LPN/LVN Charge Nurse, 286

Developing Your Personal Form for Collecting Data During Report, 290

Criteria for Delegating Duties, 293

Reviewing Nursing Assistant Job Descriptions, 295

Handling Refusal of Assignment by Nursing Assistants, 295

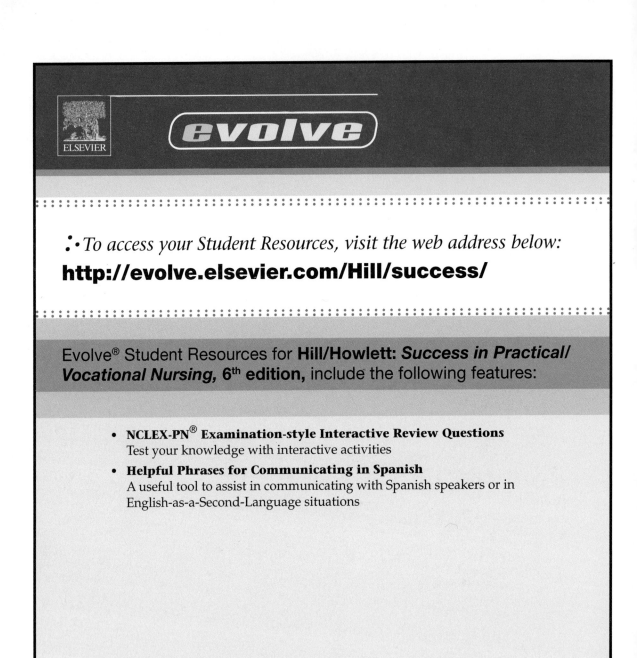

ELSEVIER

evolve

∴ *To access your Student Resources, visit the web address below:*

http://evolve.elsevier.com/Hill/success/

Evolve® Student Resources for **Hill/Howlett:** *Success in Practical/ Vocational Nursing,* **6th edition,** include the following features:

- **NCLEX-PN® Examination-style Interactive Review Questions**
  Test your knowledge with interactive activities
- **Helpful Phrases for Communicating in Spanish**
  A useful tool to assist in communicating with Spanish speakers or in English-as-a-Second-Language situations

SIXTH EDITION

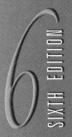

SUCCESS IN PRACTICAL/ VOCATIONAL NURSING

FROM STUDENT TO LEADER

Signe S. Hill, RN, BSN, MA

Formerly Instructor, Practical Nurse Program
Northeast Wisconsin Technical College
Green Bay, Wisconsin

Helen Stephens Howlett, RN, BSN, MS

Formerly Instructor, Practical Nurse Program
Northeast Wisconsin Technical College
Green Bay, Wisconsin

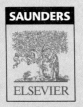

SAUNDERS

ELSEVIER

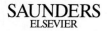

11830 Westline Industrial Drive
St. Louis, Missouri 63146

Success in Practical/Vocational Nursing: From Student to Leader,
Sixth Edition

ISBN: 978-1-4160-5659-1

Notice

Neither the Publisher nor the Authors assume any responsibility for any loss or injury and/or damage to persons or property arising out of or related to any use of the material contained in this book. It is the responsibility of the treating practitioner, relying on independent expertise and knowledge of the patient, to determine the best treatment and method of application for the patient.

The Publisher

NCLEX®, NCLEX-PN® are federally registered trademarks and Service marks of the National Council of State Boards of Nursing, Inc.

Library of Congress Cataloging-in-Publication Data

Hill, Signe S.
  Success in practical/vocational nursing : from student to leader / Signe S. Hill, Helen Stephens Howlett. — 6th ed.
      p. ; cm.
  Includes bibliographical references and index.
  ISBN 978-1-4160-5659-1 (pbk. : alk. paper)
  1. Practical nursing–Vocational guidance.   I. Howlett, Helen A.   II. Title.
  [DNLM: 1. Nursing, Practical. WY 195 H648s 2009]
  RT62.H45 2009
  610.73'0693—dc22

2008016117

Vice President, Publishing Director: Sally Schrefer
Executive Publisher: Thomas Wilhelm
Managing Editor: Robin Levin Richman
Developmental Editor: Mayoor Jaiswal
Book Production Manager: Gayle May
Project Manager: Tracey Schriefer
Senior Designer: Teresa McBryan

Printed in Canada

Last digit is the print number: 9 8 7 6 5 4 3 2 1

This book is dedicated to
Instructors who keep up to date by sifting through mounds
of the latest information and use innovative ways
to involve students in the teaching/learning process
both in the classroom and on clinical.

and

Clinical Nurses who model nursing skills and interaction
with each other, patients, and all professionals
involved in the care of patients.

Acknowledgments

Robin Levin Richman, Managing Editor. We appreciate her steadfast support of our text, *Success in Practical/Vocational Nursing: From Student to Leader,* and us. Robin is always willing to listen and consider our ideas.

Mayoor Jaiswal, Developmental Editor. Mayoor is thorough and meticulous in reviewing the manuscript. She makes reasonable suggestions that make topics easier to comprehend and incorporate into previous knowledge.

Marie Thomas, Editorial Assistant. Marie responds to our sometimes-preposterous requests with promptness, humor, and thoroughness. We would be lost without her organization, wit, and problem solving abilities.

Tracey Schriefer, Project Manager, who promptly answered our questions, responded to our requests, and tied it all together at the end.

Susan C. deWit, a well-known and respected nursing author. We have gained from her friendship, honesty, and willingness to share information sources and materials.

Judith McDowell, Director ADN program at Sheridan College, Sheridan, Wyoming. She graciously took time to introduce us to the unique ADN-RN program and gave permission to include a description of the program in Chapter 23.

Wendy Smith, Marketing and Public Information Director at Sheridan College, Sheridan, Wyoming. Wendy reviewed the material about the ADN-RN program and saw value in including the information in our sixth edition. Wendy also reminded us of the new BSN program partnership with the University of Wyoming.

Dianne Hall, owner of Hall Computer Technology for helping with computer issues. She provided both direct and remote access support.

Jason Gile, President of Computer Works, Green Bay, Wisconsin. He was always on call to promptly answer e-mail questions and provided service.

Cindy Milbach, the local Queen of Clean, for keeping the house so spotless.

Tera, Lenore, Marlene, Sharil, and the five J's … Judy, Jenny, Janet, Julie, and Jane, for their assistance, especially with Chapter 18.

Our husbands, Frank Hill and George Howlett, for cheerfully taking on extra tasks, making trips for cartridges, paper, whatever, as needed.

Michael Hill, MS, CRC, ABDA, ACA, QRC, author of Chapter 21, Finding a Job. Mr. Hill has 25+ years of vocational rehabilitation experience, including job skills training, job placement, labor market/wage surveys, vocational testing, retraining plan development, state and federal workers' compensation, expert testimony, short- and long-term disability plan administration, and Family Medical Leave Act (FMLA) and Americans with Disabilities Act (ADA) consultation.

The staff of Muehl Public Library, Seymour, Wisconsin, for their gracious and timely retrieval of articles.

Robert Yancey, Illustrator, Luxemburg, Wisconsin, who made the original drawing used on the first page of each chapter and the icons for Critical Thinking Exercises, Learning Exercises, Leadership Activities, Leadership Hints, Management Hints, and Management Tools.

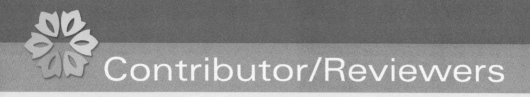

Contributor/Reviewers

CONTRIBUTOR

MICHAEL S. HILL, MS, CRC, ABDA, ACA, QRC
Qualified Rehabilitation Consultant
Employee Development Corporation
New Brighton, Minnesota

REVIEWERS

KORBI KIDD BERRYHILL, RN, BA, CRRN
Instructor, Practical Nursing
South Plains College, Reese
Lubbock, Texas

KATHY LYNN BURLINGAME, MSN, RN, CCRN
Associate Dean of Nursing
Minnesota State Community & Technical College
Detroit Lakes, Minnesota

BRENDA CUCUKOV, BSN, RN, BS, TKB
Instructor, Practical Nurse Program
Vineland Adult Education Center
Vineland, New Jersey

KAREN KATHRYN HAAGENSEN, RNC
Instructor, Vocational Nursing Program
Howard College
San Angelo, Texas

SALLIE NOTO, MSN, RN, MS
Program Director, School of Practical Nursing
Career Technology Center of Lackawanna County
Scranton, Pennsylvania

SHARON M. NOWAK, MSN, RN
Instructor, Practical Nurse Program
Jackson Community College
Jackson, Michigan

RHONDA L. ROLFS, RN, MS
Instructor, Practical Nurse Program
Rochester Community & Technology College
Rochester, Minnesota

SHEILA A. SARVER, RN, MED
Instructor, Practical Nurse Program
Lee County High Tec Center Central
The School District of Lee County
Ft. Myers, Florida

TAMARA D. THELL, BSN, RN, PHN
Instructor, Practical Nurse Program
Anoka Technical College
Anoka, Minnesota

SANDRA WESTHOFF, BSN, RN
Instructor, Washington School of Practical Nursing
Washington, Missouri

To the Instructor

We continue to receive much-appreciated feedback from nursing instructors in practical/vocational nursing programs throughout the United States who use our text, *Success in Practical/Vocational Nursing: From Student to Leader*. From the comments it is clear that practical/vocational nursing programs nationwide continue to be diverse in their structure and curricula. Instructors differ in the order in which they would like to see the text arranged. **Feel free to use chapters in any sequence to fit your curriculum.**

All chapters in the sixth edition have been reviewed and carefully revised to ensure that the information is current at the time of writing. This includes **websites** that have been added to the chapters and Appendix E, and were current at the time of printing of the text. We continue to stress personal responsibility for learning and the need for the student to be actively involved in the learning process.

Instructor comments also indicate that learning needs of practical/vocational nursing students are as diverse as the students themselves. Thanks to orientation by their schools, some instructors indicate no need for content about learning skills or time management, since their students have already developed these skills. Other instructors state that their students need information about the adult learner, learning style, time management, learning skills, and learning resources because their students do not receive this information in orientation.

It was the authors' and editors' decision to update Chapters 1–6 and keep them in *Unit One, Passing the NCLEX-PN® Examination*, since these are basics necessary to understand and retain the information in a practical/vocational nursing program and to develop critical thinking skills to apply that information. Some instructors

find that students are very interested in these chapters when they encounter difficulties in the nursing program.

Chapter 5, Learning During School, for the NCLEX-PN® Examination, and Beyond continues to emphasize what the student needs to know about the learning resource center (LRC) in order to succeed. Students have the responsibility to identify and correct deficiencies. Instructors pointed out the importance of the chapter for students with limited proficiency in English. The role of simulation in nursing programs and etiquette for cell phone, iPod use, and other electronic devices has been added to Chapter 5.

Arab Americans are briefly discussed in *Chapter 12, Cultural Uniqueness, Sensitivity, and Competence*. Although Islam is the predominant influence in most Arabs lives, not all Muslims are Arabs. Islam and the Muslim patient and how religion affects patient care are discussed in *Chapter 13, Spiritual Needs, Spiritual Caring, and Religious Differences*.

Reviewers continue to ask for more information about delegation. **Three scenarios** have been incorporated into *Chapter 16—LPN/LVN Charge Nurse Skills: Management, Including Assignment and Delegation*—to better differentiate and explain the functions of assignment and delegation and help graduates carry out these functions legally and safely.

We include five review items at the end of each chapter. Each item is an example of items included in the NCLEX-PN® Examination. One item is included for each cognitive level tested: knowledge, comprehension, application, and analysis. The fifth item is an example of the alternate format item. The answers to these review items are provided at the end of the textbook.

TEACHING AND LEARNING PACKAGE

We provide a rich, abundant collection of supplemental resources for both instructors and students.

For the Instructor

TEACH Instructor Resources

The new, comprehensive TEACH Instructor Resources Evolve website provides a wealth of material to meet your teaching needs. It includes everything in the Student Resources as well as all the following instructor resources:

- An ExamView Test Bank contains NCLEX-PN® Examination-style questions that include multiple-choice and alternate-format questions.
- PowerPoint Presentations and Lecture Outlines include approximately 1,100 slides with annotations.
- Lesson Plans, which are based on textbook chapter objectives, provide a roadmap to link and integrate all parts of the educational package. These concise and straightforward lesson plans can be modified or combined to meet your scheduling and teaching needs.
- An Open-Book Quiz is provided for each chapter in the textbook.
- Audience Response Questions (iClicker questions) promote interactivity and feedback in the classroom.

For the Student

- Evolve Student Learning Resources include NCLEX-PN® Examination-style interactive review questions that test your knowledge and help you prepare for certification. Helpful Phrases for Communicating in English and Spanish are also provided.

We welcome your comments and suggestions. You can contact us in care of Elsevier, Inc., Nursing Books, 1600 John F. Kennedy Blvd., Suite 1800, Philadelphia, PA 19103. We wish you well in your school year.

SIGNE S. HILL

HELEN STEPHENS HOWLETT

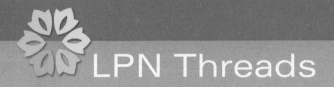
LPN Threads

Success in Practical/Vocational Nursing: From Student to Leader, sixth edition, shares some features and design elements with other LPN titles on the Elsevier list. The purpose of these LPN Threads is to make it easier for students and instructors to use the variety of books required by the relatively brief and demanding LPN curriculum.

The shared features in *Success in Practical/ Vocational Nursing: From Student to Leader,* sixth edition, include the following:

- A **reading level evaluation** performed on every manuscript chapter during the book's development. The purpose is to increase the consistency among chapters and to make the text easy to understand
- Cover and internal **design similarities**. The colorful, student-friendly design encourages the reading and learning of the core content
- Numbered lists of **Objectives** that begin each chapter
- **Key Terms** with phonetic pronunciations and page number references at the beginning of each chapter. The key terms are in color the first time they appear in the chapter
- Bulleted lists of **Key Points** at the end of each chapter

- **References** and **Suggested Readings** at the end of the text
- A **Glossary** at the end of the text

And for instructors…

- An **ExamView Test Bank** with the following categories of information: Topic, Step of the Nursing Process, Objective, Cognitive Level, NCLEX® Category of Client Need, Correct Answer, Rationale, and Text Page Reference
- **Lesson Plans** in the TEACH Instructor Resources on Evolve
- A **PowerPoint slide presentation and Lecture Outline** in the TEACH Instructor Resources on Evolve
- **Open-Book Quizzes** in the TEACH Instructor Resources on the Evolve website
- **Tips for Teaching English-as-a-Second Language (ESL) students** in the TEACH Instructor Resources on Evolve.

In addition to content and design threads, these LPN textbooks benefit from the advice and input of the Elsevier LPN Advisory Board.

LPN Advisory Board

To the Student

It is our privilege to bring you the sixth edition of *Success in Practical/Vocational Nursing: From Student to Leader*. The changes in this edition are based on instructor evaluation of the textbook, student comments, current trends, and new information related to practical/vocational nursing. As always, we attempt to present the most up-to-date information at the time of writing.

Dramatic changes continue to occur in practical/vocational nursing. You are expected to have a working knowledge of four of the five steps of the nursing process and critical thinking. Personally, we are pleased, because all nurses need to share a common language in order to work efficiently and effectively together for the good of the patient. The expectation of your knowledge of nursing process and critical thinking also equalize the significance of the role that the practical/vocational nurse plays as part of the health care team. The message is, finally, "You are equal, but different in what you have to offer in total patient care."

Chapter 6, Critical Thinking and Patient Care, is a primer for beginning to think critically. The process of learning to think critically continues throughout nursing and, combined with *Chapter 8, Nursing Process: Your Role,* makes a powerful tool in planning and evaluating patient care and is good preparation for the NCLEX-PN® Examination. *Chapter 10, Personal Health Promotion,* is included to address the stress that is a part of everyday nursing care. All nurses need to take care of themselves in order to effectively take care of their patients.

Many of the suggestions offered also work in the care of patients.

All end-of-chapter questions reflect the four cognitive levels (knowledge, comprehension, application, and analysis) of questions you will be tested on in the NCLEX-PN® Examination. Also included are alternate-item format questions. You will find an explanation of all cognitive levels in the chapter on critical thinking (Chapter 6), and the alternate-item format in Chapter 22.

Chapter 21, Finding a Job, contributed again by Michael Hill, includes a sample job application with questions currently asked by many employers, including a criminal background check. This is in direct response to reviewer requests. The chapter continues to include updated examples of what to say, what to do, and how to write letters to get you started in finding a job. We are pleased to include information by someone who has been in the field for over 25 years and continues to update his information on an ongoing basis.

We have continued to engage you in the teaching–learning process by including Learning Exercises, Critical Thinking Exercises, and numerous realistic examples. Let us know what you think. Write to us in care of Elsevier, Inc., Nursing Books, 1600 John F. Kennedy Blvd., Suite 1800, Philadelphia, PA 19103.

We wish you well in your school year and new career!

SIGNE S. HILL

HELEN STEPHENS HOWLETT

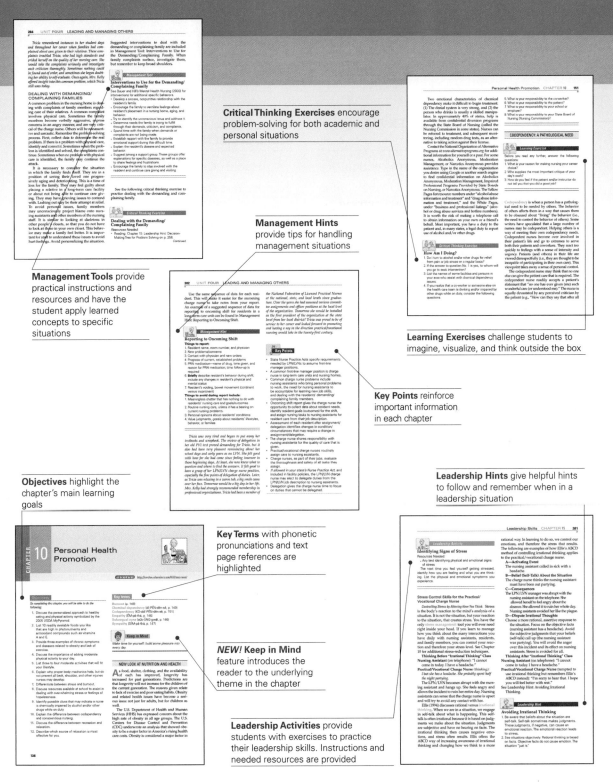

Critical Thinking Exercises encourage problem-solving for both academic and personal situations

Management Hints provide tips for handling management situations

Management Tools provide practical instructions and resources and have the student apply learned concepts to specific situations

Learning Exercises challenge students to imagine, visualize, and think outside the box

Key Points reinforce important information in each chapter

Objectives highlight the chapter's main learning goals

Leadership Hints give helpful hints to follow and remember when in a leadership situation

Key Terms with phonetic pronunciations and text page references are highlighted

NEW! **Keep in Mind** feature introduces the reader to the underlying theme in the chapter

Leadership Activities provide students with exercises to practice their leadership skills. Instructions and needed resources are provided

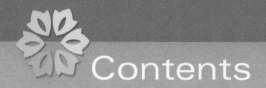

Contents

**UNIT ONE   PASSING THE NCLEX-PN®
EXAMINATION**

1   The Adult Learner and the Practical/
    Vocational Nursing Program, 1

2   Developing a Successful Learning
    Style, 14

3   Time Management: Using a Limited
    Resource Wisely, 28

4   Methods and Skills Used in Learning, 41

5   Learning During School, for the NCLEX-
    PN® Examination, and Beyond, 60

6   Critical Thinking and Patient Care, 75

**UNIT TWO   BUILDING BLOCKS
FOR YOUR CAREER**

7   How Practical/Vocational Nursing
    Evolved, 86

8   Nursing Process: Your Role, 107

9   Straightforward Communication, 122

10 Personal Health Promotion, 138

UNIT THREE   PATIENTS AND COWORKERS

11 The Health Care Team, 159

12 Cultural Uniqueness, Sensitivity,
    and Competence, 180

13 Spiritual Needs, Spiritual Caring,
    and Religious Differences, 205

**UNIT FOUR   LEADING AND MANAGING
OTHERS**

14 Assertiveness: Your Responsibility, 226

15 Leadership Skills, 246

16 LPN/LVN Charge Nurse Skills:
    Management, Including Assignment
    and Delegation, 274

**UNIT FIVE   HEALTH CARE ENVIRONMENT:
BASIC ELEMENTS**

17 Health Care Settings, 304

18 Health Care System: Financing, Issues,
    and Trends, 316

19 Ethics Applied to Nursing, 339

20 Nursing and the Law, 353

UNIT SIX   END AND A NEW BEGINNING

21 Finding a Job, 385

22 The NCLEX-PN® Examination, 417

23 How to Make Your Career Grow, 429

APPENDICES

A   State Boards of Nursing, 451

B   NAPNES Standards of Practice
    and Educational Competencies
    of Graduates of Practical/Vocational
    Nursing Programs, 455

C   NFLPN Nursing Practice Standards
    for the Licensed Practical/Vocational
    Nurse, 458

D   Learning Exercises for Time
    Management, 461

E   Internet Resources, 467

F   The Howlett Style of Nursing
    Leadership, 470

G   Delegation: Concepts and
    Decision-Making Process (NCSBN), 471

Glossary, 474

References and Suggested Readings, 486

Illustration Credits List, 503

Index, 505

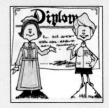

CHAPTER 1

The Adult Learner and the Practical/Vocational Nursing Program

evolve http://evolve.elsevier.com/Hill/success/

Objectives

On completing this chapter, you will be able to do the following:

1. Identify yourself as a traditional adult learner, returning adult learner, or recycled adult learner.
2. Identify personal areas of strength that will help you ensure success in the practical/vocational nursing program.
3. Identify personal areas that could interfere with your success in the practical/vocational nursing program.
4. Explain in your own words three rights of learners.
5. Discuss personal responsibility for learning and active participation in the learning process as learner responsibilities.
6. Identify the purpose of evaluation in the practical/vocational nursing program.
7. Discuss 10 learner responsibilities.

Key Terms

Active learning (p. 7)
Constructive evaluation (kŏn-STRŬK-tivē -VĂL-ū-shūn, p. 9)
Facilitator (fă-SĬL-ĭ-TĀ-tŏr, p. 7)
First Amendment (ă-MĔND-mĕnt, p. 6)
Formal education (p. 2)
Generalization (GĔN-ĕr-ă-lĭ-ZĀ-shūn, p. 2)
Informal education (p. 2)
Paradigm (PĂR-ă-DĪM, p. 7)
Performance evaluation (p. 8)
Positive mental attitude (p. 4)
Recycled adult learner (rē-SĪ-kăld, p. 2)
Referral (rĭ-FŬR-ăl, p. 11)
Returning adult learner (p. 1)
Self-directed learner (p. 3)
Self-evaluation (p. 9)
Teaching (p. 3)

Keep in Mind

Success on NCLEX-PN® and in finding a job begins by assuming personal responsibility for your learning and actively acquiring information and nursing skills. You are accountable for your own success or failure. It starts now, and you are in control!

ADULT LEARNER DEFINED

Adult learners come in all ages and perceive themselves as adults with adult responsibilities. The traditional adult learner comes to an educational program directly from high school or from another program of study. Traditional adult learners grew up in a digital, wireless world and are known as the Net Generation/Millennials (born 1982-1991). They are in transition from late adolescence to young adulthood. In addition to their own developmental tasks, these students are being propelled into situations of responsibility for others. The returning adult learner has been out of school for several years. Many of these learners have not taken any courses since high school. Returning adult learners include Generation Xers, born between 1965 and 1982, Baby Boomers, born between 1946 and 1964, and Matures born before 1946 (Oblinger and Oblinger, 2005).

Returning adult students are experiencing many different life transitions. Perhaps an employer shut down a business or a layoff occurred, resulting in a need for job training. Because of retirement, extra income and health insurance benefits may be needed. Because of valued life and work experiences, returning adult learners have built a strong foundation for the personal commitment and transitions needed in nursing school and practical/vocational nursing.

Adult learners with prior education beyond high school are also an important part of practical/vocational nursing. This learner shares some of the characteristics of both the traditional and the returning adult learners. However, this adult learner might have technical school or college experience or an undergraduate or graduate degree in a discipline other than nursing. Because these adults are starting a new cycle in their lives, we call them recycled adult learners. Reasons for choosing to enroll in the practical/vocational nursing program include the following:
- Desire to change careers,
- Attraction to nursing,
- Desire to acquire new job skills,
- Outlook for a full-time job with benefits is more promising in practical/vocational nursing, and
- Possible lack of jobs in area for which person has a degree.

Regardless of the reason for enrolling in the 9-month to 1-year practical/vocational nursing program, recycled learners find that this program meets their needs in both time and cost. In addition to the characteristics of returning adult learners, the recycled learner brings experience in tackling a challenging educational program, including use of the learning resource center (library). Just as recycling is good for the environment, recycled learners are good for practical/vocational nursing programs. Nursing in general, and practical/vocational nursing in particular, are benefiting from the maturity, focus, and experience of returning and recycled adult learners. These adult learners are also helping to ease the nursing shortage.

Critical Thinking Exercise

Which Type of Adult Learner Am I?

Which type of adult learner are you? Survey your classmates. Determine who consider themselves to be traditional, returning, or recycled adult learners.

FORMAL AND INFORMAL EDUCATIONAL EXPERIENCES

Generalizations can be made about each type of learner. Keep in mind that generalizations are broad, sweeping statements. The characteristics of each type of adult learner are not found in every individual. The traditional adult learner is accustomed to formal education. The practical/vocational nursing program in a vocational-technical school or junior college is an example of a program of formal education. Often, returning adult learners say they are rusty and have not been to school since high school. Only the latter part of this statement is true. They might not have been in a classroom for some time, but they have been learning. They have had informal education experiences every day of their lives. Examples of their informal educational experiences include learning to make a new recipe, using a digital camera, programming a DVD player, filling out a new income tax form, making calls on a new cell phone, and handling a new family problem.

Returning adult learners tend to put more emphasis on formal educational experiences. They underemphasize the value of informal learning experiences. You will find that these experiences can be helpful when you are learning new material. Recycled learners may have recently graduated from college. Some may have entered the practical/vocational nursing program after a career in another field of work. Recycled learners have many formal and informal educational experiences that help them in a practical/vocational nursing program.

Learning Exercise

Informal Educational Experiences

List at least five informal educational experiences you have had since high school.

1.
2.
3.
4.
5.

GEARED FOR SUCCESS

All adult learners have things going for them that allow them to succeed in school. Generally, traditional adult learners are experts at educational routine. They know how to get through registration as painlessly as possible (even online), find the fastest way to get from one class to another, find the best time to get through the cafeteria line, know how to take a test using a computerized answer sheet, have grown up with technology, and are tech-savvy. When traditional adult learners need information, they "Google." When they want to contact a friend, they might instant message or text message. In comparison, some returning adult learners may feel they have used up the last bit of their energy in finding a parking space, and once they do, they may be puzzled about how to find their way to their assigned classroom. When returning adult learners need information, they go to the library or reach for the yellow pages of the telephone directory. To stay connected with friends and family, they might use their landline, cell phone, or email.

 Critical Thinking Exercise

Reasons I Can Succeed

Identify and list three attributes you possess that will help you succeed in the practical/vocational nursing program.

1.
2.
3.

Traditional adult learners have been given the opportunity to develop reading, writing, studying, and test-taking skills. They are at their prime physically, are filled with energy and stamina, and often have fewer out-of-school responsibilities to distract them from their studies.

The returning adult learner is a serious learner who is ready to work. Returning adult learners have had many responsibilities and life experiences that help them relate well to new learning, make sense out of it, and get the point quickly.

They are mature, motivated, and self-directed learners who have set goals for themselves. Many have made economic, personal, and family sacrifices to go back to school.

Recycled learners are also experts in educational routine, and they too have had the opportunity to develop reading, writing, studying, and test-taking skills. They are serious, motivated, and self-directed students. All adult learners are geared for success, and each group has its own strong points. However, each group also has some liabilities—things that could stand in the way of success.

LIABILITIES, PITFALLS, AND HIDDEN DANGERS

HIDDEN DANGER SHARED BY ALL ADULT LEARNERS

One of the greatest liabilities shared by all adult learners is the fear of failure. Fear of anything is a very strong motivator, but in a negative sense. Fear of failure in school is a feeling that usually develops as a result of past negative experiences with learning situations. Perhaps you did not do well in some high school or college classes. Maybe you did not study, studied the wrong way, or allowed yourself to be put down by teachers or professors in the past. Maybe you allowed yourself to underachieve because of peer pressure. Regardless of the cause, you may look at school in a negative, threatening way.

A surprise is in store for you. Your past is history. You have a clean slate ahead of you! Many adult learners with the same history and fears as you have succeeded in their educational programs. You are not a child in grade school. You are an adult in an adult educational experience. You will do yourself a favor if you begin to picture in your mind the rewards of succeeding in the practical/vocational nursing program. Forget the failures and setbacks you may have suffered in high school and other educational experiences. Replace your fear of failure with the desire for success. Keep your thoughts positive, and practice these positive thoughts continuously. Watch the content and tone of your thoughts and words.

Negative thoughts and words can play like a tape. As surely as you learned this negative script, you can learn a positive script. However, it does take time. Replace all your "I can'ts" and "I never coulds" with "I want to," "I can," "I will," and "I'm going to." Avoid dwelling on the past and look to the future. Go all the way with **PMA—positive mental attitude**. If you consistently expect to succeed, and combine this expectation with hard work in your studies, you will succeed. Did you know that your brain believes anything you tell it? If it learned to believe you can fail, it can also learn to believe you can succeed. Start today to engage in positive self-talk.

Sometimes students who have not succeeded in other nursing programs enroll during midterm in the practical/vocational nursing program. Reasons for not making it in prior nursing programs are varied, personal, and confidential. These students may feel the need to be on their guard. They may behave in a defensive manner, especially if there were teacher-student conflicts in the prior nursing program. It is good for these students to remember that the past is history. All that counts is their performance in the present. For them, it is possible to start over with a clean slate.

DANGERS FOR THE TRADITIONAL ADULT LEARNER

The following examples of pitfalls for some traditional adult learners are good examples of generalizations. They may or may not apply to the traditional adult learners you know.

Grade Inflation

A grade of C on a test or for a nursing course surprises some traditional adult students because they always received As in high school. A study by Indiana University found that a majority of U.S. high school students spend 3 hours or less a week preparing for classes yet still manage to get good grades. The same effort will not lead to success in your nursing program (Sanoff, 2005).

Traditional adult learners often have fewer outside responsibilities to distract them from their studies. Some traditional adult students lack time-management skills or motivation when it comes to studying. Some may still be in a habit from high school. Study time required to master content in a practical/vocational nursing program is personal to each student. However, if you are accustomed to receiving A's in high school for minimal effort, you will not experience this reward in the practical/vocational nursing program.

Social Activities

Some traditional adult learners may allow social activities to compete with school and study time. A party mentality is a serious interference with school responsibilities. Parties used to be special occasions for celebrating and getting together. They were well-earned and provided a much-needed break from work and everyday routine responsibilities. Today, work and everyday responsibilities in life and at school sometimes get in the way of some traditional adult learners' party habits. Not all traditional adult learners have a party habit, but some may spend valuable study time "hanging out," surfing the Internet, or enjoying their favorite television programs.

Employment

The amount of time occupied by employment outside of school hours may be another interference for some traditional adult learners. Ask yourself, "How much of the time that I am employed outside of school is necessary for food, shelter, and other realistic expenses?"

Many explanations can be given for the pitfalls listed here for traditional adult learners. Some traditional adult learners may still be working at developing an awareness of who they are and what life is all about for them. Some may lack a sense of direction and have no clear goal or idea of what they really want to do in life. Some may lack inner motivation to be a practical/vocational nurse. These learners can succeed by taking responsibility to make decisions about priorities and personal use of time that will help them meet the goals they have established for themselves.

DANGERS FOR THE RETURNING ADULT LEARNER

Physical

Returning adult learners may experience difficulties with academic behavior. Their reading, writing, test-taking, and study skills may be rusty. Computer and other skills for an electronic information society may be lacking. Physical changes occur as adults age and can affect learning. The senses of vision and hearing are at their peak in the adolescent years and decline very gradually through the adult years. As the decades go by, these adults may notice the need for more illumination when they read. They also may experience problems with reading small print. Some returning adults note that they are not as energetic as they once were.

Social Responsibilities

Returning adult learners have many roles to play outside of school. They may be husbands, wives, mothers, fathers, daughters, sons, grandparents, employees, and/or volunteers. Generally they are very busy people. Returning to school may result in feelings of guilt because they know it will affect their relationships and routines outside of school.

Because of their many roles, returning adult learners have more demands placed on them. Some families may not support their mothers' or fathers' choice to continue their formal education. Spouses may object to the extra demands placed on them. In many cases the returning adult learner must struggle with learning how to juggle the worlds of learner and head of the family.

Despite these demands, returning adult learners, like traditional and recycled adult learners, need to learn how to manage their time. They need to learn how to concentrate when time for concentration is made available. Sometimes, returning adult learners set unrealistic goals for themselves and have to readjust their game plan. Although past experience can be an asset, returning adult learners may have to rethink and possibly unlearn some things they have learned in the past. They might have allowed some of these things to become habits.

When faced with obstacles, some adults may decide to throw in the towel and write off school as a bad idea. This book can help you avoid this negative way of thinking and go on to succeed.

DANGERS FOR THE RECYCLED ADULT LEARNER

The recycled adult learner shares the same pitfalls as do traditional and returning adult learners. Depending on their age and personal responsibilities, recycled adult learners may feel an energy crisis as they pursue their academic life.

Attitude

Some recycled adult learners may have an attitude that because they earned a degree or have some college experience, the practical/vocational nursing program will be a breeze to get through. It is good to remember the difference between obtaining a college degree and obtaining a technical college education. In college a student might have no practical experience with his or her major subject until junior or senior year or after graduation, when hired for the first job in the chosen field. In the practical/vocational nursing program in a technical college the application of current learning is stressed continuously. Students need to apply theory continuously to the clinical area. What you learn on Monday will be used in the clinical area on Tuesday. And you will be expected to consistently apply learning from past nursing classes. Perhaps poor time management resulted in cramming for examinations. Cramming is an ineffective strategy for long-term learning. This measure will be useless in the practical/vocational nursing program because of the consistent expectation of application of theory to the clinical area.

 Critical Thinking Exercise

Personal Pitfalls

Identify and list three things that could stand in your way of success in the practical/vocational nursing program.

1.
2.
3.

SPECIAL CHALLENGES FOR PRACTICAL/VOCATIONAL NURSING STUDENTS

No matter what type of adult learner you are, some learners have special challenges to success in practical/vocational nursing. Learners with a spouse/significant other at home may be extremely busy with school and family affairs. Single parents may feel overwhelmed when the learner role is assumed in addition to all their other roles. It may be good for learners with spouses to imagine what it would be like to be a learner without a spouse to offer support.

Occasionally, practical/vocational nursing learners who speak English as their first language complain about the difficulty of schoolwork and the amount of time it takes to complete assignments. It may be insightful for these learners to imagine being responsible for the same amount of schoolwork when English is their second or even third or fourth language. Learners who speak English as a second or additional language need to strive continually to understand content presented in a language different from their native tongue. Reading assignments need to be translated by these students to their native language to be understood. Taking a test requires extra effort, as these students need to translate test directions and items to their native language for understanding before answering an item. This is comparable to presenting English-speaking learners with textbooks and tests written in Spanish or Russian with the need to translate both to English.

We have met many learners facing the above challenges and commend them for the good job they have done, against great odds, in the practical/vocational nursing program. They are a testimonial that success is within your reach, even if you are faced with these special challenges.

LEARNERS HAVE RIGHTS

As an American citizen, you need to start thinking about some fundamental rights that you have been granted through the U.S. Constitution that will affect you as a learner. The First Amendment gives you freedom of expression, as long as what you want to express does not disrupt class or infringe on the rights of your peers. So when your instructor asks you to join in a discussion, do not be afraid to do so. Instructors want your input in a class session. They have no intention of holding your comments against you. The Fourteenth Amendment assures you due process. Due process means that if you are charged with a violation of policies or rules, you will be presented with evidence of your misconduct and will be entitled to state your position. So relax. The institution in which you are enrolled cannot terminate you at whim, nor does it want to. It exists to help you succeed. A more detailed account of these two rights can probably be found in your school's student handbook. You did not get one? You lost yours? Hurry to the student services department and get a copy today or, if available, download an online copy.

An important learner's right is the right to have an organized curriculum and a responsible instructor who is prepared to teach it. You have the right to know the requirements of each course and how you will be graded for each course. Although your tuition and fees do not pay for all the services you receive at school, you are the most important person on campus. You are the reason the instructor was hired. You do not interfere with the instructor's work—you are the focus of it.

RESPONSIBILITIES OF LEARNERS

The first responsibility of learners is to learn. The authors of this book want you to test your knowledge about the process of learning before you read any further. Read the following four statements and decide if they are true or false. As the chapter continues, these statements will be discussed. You will be expected to check the accuracy of your responses. Remember, your answers are for your eyes only.

Responsibilities of Learners

Read the following four statements and answer "true" or "false" to them.
1. The instructor has the responsibility for my learning.
2. If I fail, it is the responsibility of the instructor.
3. If I succeed, the credit for my success should go to the instructor.
4. My instructor has the responsibility to pass on to me all the information I will need to know in my career as a practical/vocational nurse.

TEACHING VERSUS LEARNING

Years ago a wonderful thing happened in the area of adult education. Teachers were exposed to the difference between teaching and learning. Great emphasis was placed on the role of the learner. Changing emphasis from teaching to learning is called a paradigm (a way of thinking) shift. Learners need to be aware of the exciting world of learning and the roles of teaching and learning in that process. In doing so you will know what is expected of you as an adult learner.

Passive Learners

Many of us (and this includes the authors and some of your instructors) have had educational experiences in the past that encouraged dependency and passivity on the part of the learner. Think back to the educational experiences you have had. Did they involve sitting in classes in which the teacher did most of the talking and you just took notes? Did you view the teacher as someone who possessed knowledge and somehow was going to pass it on to you? And, if you did not pass, did you say, "The teacher flunked me"? When you think about it, these situations are characterized by the adjectives dependent and passive.

The last time you were dependent from necessity was when you were an infant. Even then you were far from passive. When you became a toddler,

you became very independent and began to learn about the world in earnest. You very actively pursued your learning—that is, the acquiring of new knowledge and skills. And you did it with gusto! Now you are an adult learner. How unfair of an instructor to expect you to become dependent and passive in your learning. This is especially true because studies have proved that people learn best when they are actively involved in their own learning and have an interdependent relationship with the instructor.

Instructors—Facilitators of Learning

You have already learned that it is the instructor's responsibility to set up a curriculum. Your state's board of nursing dictates the content of the curriculum in a school of nursing. It is then up to the faculty of your school to decide how that content will be included in the nursing program. Some practical/vocational programs might use the general structure of the NCLEX-PN® examination in developing a curriculum. Instructors are facilitators because they are responsible for creating a learning environment in which learning can take place. They do this by arranging for a variety of activities and experiences. Part of that learning environment involves being available to you when you encounter questions and problems you cannot solve. Instructors also have the responsibility to evaluate learning. They do so by testing and observing learners.

Active Learning

To learn is to acquire knowledge and skills. The verb *acquire* means to obtain or gain by your own effort. As a learner in a practical/vocational nursing program, you need to be your own agent of knowledge and skill acquisition. You have the personal responsibility to acquire the knowledge and skills needed to be a practical/vocational nurse. Active learning is not a passive activity. As a learner, you must open yourself up, reach out, and stretch to gain knowledge and skills. To be successful, you must be personally involved in your learning. It is impossible for instructors to pour knowledge and skills into your head. You need to become self-directed and curious in your learning. You need to use critical thinking skills to help you comprehend what you read in texts and journals, view on videotapes and CDs, and hear in classroom discussions. Instructors will not hover over you and guide your every step. Instructors are there to help you along when needed.

Do not expect the instructor to assume your skill for you, be your medical dictionary, or re-teach Chapter 2 in Anatomy and Physiology because you did not have time to study. Instead, expect your instructor to observe you while you are trying to work through a difficult skill. The instructor will make suggestions and demonstrate a point here and there to help you along. If you are having trouble, expect your instructor to assist you to put a definition of a medical term in your own words. Expect the instructor to answer specific questions you may have about Chapter 2 in Anatomy and Physiology. These are the roles of teacher and learner and examples of their interdependency. If you are to learn and succeed in practical/vocational nursing, you need to become actively involved in your own learning. You say you are too old to learn? You say you cannot teach an old dog new tricks? Much study has been done in this area. To date, studies of adult learning clearly indicate that the basic ability to learn remains essentially unimpaired throughout the life span. Now review the answers to your true/false questions on p. 7. Are there any answers you want to change before looking at the key?

1. *False.* You have the responsibility for your own learning. You must become actively involved in the learning process.
2. *False.* If you fail, it is your own fault. Adult educational programs are geared for success. You are geared for success. Although you could list many reasons why you might not succeed, the teacher flunking you is not one of them. Learners sometimes allow themselves to flunk.
3. *False.* When you succeed (and you are perfectly capable of doing so), only you can take credit for the success. You were the person who assumed responsibility for your own learning. You became actively involved in the learning process.

4. *False.* Instructors have had much experience in nursing. They do not know all the experiences you will have in your career as a practical/vocational nurse. Even if they did, there would be no time or way to transfer this knowledge to you. Instructors help learners learn how to learn. This is important in an ever-changing field such as nursing. Your instructors will encourage you to develop critical-thinking and problem-solving skills, which will enable you to handle new situations as they arise in your nursing career.

If you had no wrong answers, you should be an expert on learning. Now put your expertise to work for you. If you had one wrong answer or more, the authors suggest you reread the "Teaching versus Learning" section in this chapter. The remaining chapters in Unit 1 will help you to become an active learner and a critical thinker and be successful in the practical/vocational nursing program, on NCLEX-PN®, and as a candidate for a LPN/LVN nursing position.

ROLE OF EVALUATION

The second responsibility of learners is to receive and participate in evaluation. Evaluation plays an important role in your education in the practical/vocational nursing program and throughout your career. You have set a goal to become a practical/vocational nurse. As the year goes on, your instructors will evaluate you in several different ways to determine whether you are progressing in the achievement of that goal. When you graduate, you will be evaluated periodically while on the job, sometimes as a means of determining whether you are to receive a salary increase. At other times you will be evaluated to see if you are functioning well enough to keep your job. Evaluation in the practical/vocational nursing program generally occurs in two areas: (1) written tests that measure your knowledge of theory, and (2) performance evaluations that measure your ability to apply your knowledge in the clinical area. Evaluation in these areas is a learning experience in itself.

Theory Tests

Learners and instructors look at test results very differently. Learners focus on the number of items they answered correctly. They need to identify what they did right on a test so they can apply the process of getting the right answer to future tests and apply this information in the clinical area. Instructors focus on the specific items the learner got wrong. Wrong items indicate critical knowledge the learner does not have. Do not just ask for your grades. Try to arrange time with your instructors to review your tests. It is inaccurate to say that grades do not count. You must earn the minimum grade established by your nursing program. But consider this: If you got 80% on a test, it means you did not answer 20% of the questions correctly. Now place yourself in the patient's slippers. What about the 20% of the test questions your nurse got wrong? Was it something the nurse should have known to care for you safely? For this reason, try to look at tests as learning experiences. Be as interested in your wrong answers as you are in your correct answers. Take time to look at your tests with the goal of understanding why the correct answers are correct and why the wrong answers you gave are wrong.

Clinical Performance Evaluations

The most meaningful evaluations you will receive during the year will be the performance evaluations given while you are in the clinical area. Because these evaluations give you an opportunity for career and personal growth, it is important to understand this form of evaluation and the responsibilities you have with regard to it. Clinical performance evaluations also provide an example of how to evaluate others in your expanded role.

In the clinical area, instructors will be observing you as you go about caring for patients. They are observing you to discover the positive things you are doing to reach your goal of becoming a practical/vocational nurse. These behaviors are to be encouraged. They indicate that learning has taken place, you are applying your knowledge, and you are growing and progressing toward your goal. Instructors are also observing you to discover behaviors that stand in the way of reaching your goal. These behaviors are to be discouraged. Your instructor will update you daily on your progress in a verbal or written manner. At the end of a clinical rotation you will receive a written performance evaluation during a conference with your clinical instructor.

From the start you need to look at performance evaluations as a two-sided coin. The instructor is on one side, and you are on the other. As part of their job, instructors have the responsibility of evaluating your performance. As a learner, you have the responsibility of being aware of your clinical behaviors. You are responsible for self-evaluation. Practical/vocational nursing students, at the time of graduation, should be able to look at their nursing actions and be aware of their strong behaviors and behaviors that need improvement. Development of the ability to be aware of one's behaviors begins with day 1 in the practical/vocational nursing program, including the skills laboratory. Objective awareness of one's own behaviors is an important skill to have as an employee. A learner does not automatically have this skill. Learners must consistently work at viewing themselves objectively. Instructors will help in this area. For example, when learning how to make a bed, ask yourself, "Is the finished product as good as I had intended it to be when I started?" Do not wait for the instructor to identify areas of success or areas of needed improvement.

Think back to when you received comments from your teachers and parents about your behavior in grade school and high school. How did you feel when you received these comments? Many people grow up with bad feelings about these episodes of criticism and even about the word itself. Criticism means evaluation. Some people attach a negative meaning to criticism and view it as a put-down.

The phrase "constructive criticism" may evoke negative feelings. The phrase constructive evaluation is frequently used instead. This choice of words may help you look at evaluation of your behaviors in a positive way. It is important to distinguish what is being evaluated. You must separate your behaviors or actions from yourself, the person.

Constructive evaluation directed toward your behaviors has no bearing on your value as a person. Look at your behaviors either as being positive and helping you reach your goal or as needing improvement. Behaviors that need improvement must be modified so that you can reach your goal of being a practical/vocational nurse.

As you progress in the nursing program, you will learn about a systematic way of conducting patient care called the nursing process (see Chapter 8). An important part of the nursing process is evaluation of patient goals while giving patient care. If your actions are not helping patients reach their goals, they need to be modified. Knowledge of the nursing process will help you develop your ability to look at your actions and evaluate them. Comments from instructors will help your self-awareness. Remain open with yourself. **The comments you receive are directed toward your behaviors and not you as a person.**

A good way to start learning self-evaluation is to look at yourself in everyday life. Ask yourself how you look through the eyes of others:
- How would you like to be your own spouse?
- How would you like to have yourself as a learner?
- How would you like to be your own mother or father?
- How would you like to be your own nurse?

If you would not like to be any of these people, identify the reasons why. Another good exercise is to make two lists. On one list note your assets or strong points. On the other list note your liabilities or areas that need improvement. When asked to evaluate themselves, learners traditionally rate themselves more negatively. They tend to neglect their strong points. Identifying strong points is not proud or vain behavior. It is dealing with yourself honestly and openly. After you have identified assets and liabilities, review your assets periodically. Make an effort to continue these strong points while modifying your liabilities.

Work on one liability at a time. If you do so, your assets list will grow and your liabilities list will shrink.

A good place to start self-evaluation in nursing is in the skills lab of your basic nursing course. Practice becoming very observant of the results of your actions. Is the top sheet centered when you are making an unoccupied bed? Are you using the bath blanket as a drape to avoid chilling and invading the patient's privacy? Are you aware of the effect of the tone of your voice on your instructors and peers?

Evaluation is an ever-present reality in any career. Getting into the practice of self-evaluation early in your program of study will help you develop a skill you will use daily in your career and personal life.

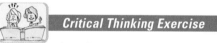 **Critical Thinking Exercise**

Self-Evaluation

List one of your strong areas that you have identified as a new practical/vocational nursing learner. (Review your answers to Critical Thinking Exercise: Reasons I Can Succeed on p. 3.)

_____

List one area needing improvement that you have identified as a practical/vocational nursing learner. (Review your answers to the Critical Thinking Exercise: Personal Pitfalls on p. 5.)

_____

 Critical Thinking Exercise

Plan to Eliminate My Pitfall

Write a plan that will help you eliminate your personal pitfall that needs improvement. How can you convert it to a strong area?

_____

_____

_____

_____

DEALING WITH REFERRALS

If you are evaluated by your instructor as having areas that need improvement, the instructor might refer you to a counselor at school. Examples of areas that require referral are a grade below passing in a major test and frequent absences from class. Counselors at technical colleges and junior colleges are academic counselors who have expertise in helping students identify reasons for academic problem areas. A referral to a counselor is an attempt to help you succeed. These counselors can help students set up a plan of action to remedy the problem. We have seen some students resist going to the counselor because they think it is a waste of time.

 Critical Thinking Exercise

Referral to Counselor

- What could be one reason for thinking that an appointment with the counselor is a waste of time?
- How could keeping an appointment with the counselor be helpful to a student?

OTHER RESPONSIBILITIES OF LEARNERS

In addition to assuming responsibility for your own learning, becoming actively involved in the learning process, and receiving and participating in evaluation, it is necessary to be aware of some other responsibilities you have as a learner.

1. Be aware of the rules and policies of your school and the practical/vocational nursing program. Abide by them.
2. When problems do develop, follow the recognized channels of communication both at school and in the clinical area. The rule is: Go to the source. Avoid "saving up" gripes. Instead, pursue them as they come up. Deal with them in an assertive manner (see Chapter 14).
3. Be prepared in advance for classes and clinical experiences. You expect teachers to be prepared. They expect the same of you. When you are unprepared for classes, you waste the time of the instructor, your peers, and yourself. When you are unprepared for clinical experiences, you are violating an important safety factor in patient care. When you are scheduled for the clinical area, your state board of nursing expects you to function as a licensed practical/vocational nurse would function under your state's nurse practice act.
4. Prepare your own assignments. In post-conference use your peers and the experiences and knowledge they have and learn from each other.
5. Seek out learning experiences at school and in the clinical area. Set your goals higher than the minimum.
6. Seek out resources beyond the required readings. Examples of these resources can be the learning resource center, information from past classes, and the Internet.
7. Assume responsibility for your own thoughts, communication, and behavior. Avoid giving in to pressure from your peers. BYOB—be your own boss.
8. Be present and on time for classes and clinical experiences. Follow school and program policies for reporting absences. Getting into this habit will prepare you to be a favored employee.
9. Enter into discussion when asked to do so in class.
10. Treat those with whom you come into daily contact with respect. Be mindful of their rights as individuals.
11. Seek out your instructor when you are having difficulties in class or the clinical area. Often instructors can tell when students are having problems. More important are the times when they cannot tell, and only the student knows a problem exists. Do not be afraid to approach your instructors. They are there to help you.

12. Keep a record of your grades as a course proceeds. At the beginning of a course the instructor will explain the method of calculating your final grade. You are responsible for knowing how you stand grade-wise in a course at any point in time.

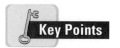

Key Points

- Adult learners can be classified as traditional adult learners, returning adult learners, or recycled adult learners.

- Each category of adult learner possesses characteristics that can help the learner succeed in the practical/vocational nursing program.
- Each group of adult learner also possesses characteristics that can prevent success.
- Liabilities occur in areas in which learners have control over their solutions. They do not stand in the way of success.
- Although learners have rights, they also have responsibilities. The most important of their responsibilities are the personal responsibility for learning, taking an active part in the learning process, and participating in the evaluation of their learning and growth.

REVIEW ITEMS

1. Select the appropriate behavior for the student practical/vocational nurse.
   1. To accept responsibility for personal success, including grades, in the nursing program.
   2. To be as passive a learner as you can possibly be both in classes and the clinical area.
   3. To learn everything from the nursing instructors that is needed to function as a PN/VN nurse.
   4. To blame the nursing instructor for any failures that occur in class or the clinical area.

2. A practical/vocational nursing learner has been referred to the counselor because of a failing grade on the last test in Basic Nursing. Which of the following learner responses indicates the student understands the purpose of the referral?
   1. "The instructor does not like me and wants me to quit the program."
   2. "This is a warning that I will be asked to withdraw from the program."
   3. "The purpose of a referral is to help me identify problems to avoid failure."
   4. "A psychologist will evaluate me for psychological problems interfering with success."

3. A practical/vocational nursing learner has just received the end-of-course clinical evaluation. Which of the following attitudes is most appropriate regarding the role of evaluation of learners in the clinical area?
   1. Instructors and SPN/SVN learners have the responsibility to identify positive behaviors and those that need improvement.
   2. It is the job of the instructor only, to identify positive clinical behaviors and behaviors that need improvement.
   3. When SPN/SVN learners identify positive behaviors, it indicates that they are proud and vain individuals.
   4. When behaviors that need improvement are identified, clinical evaluation may destroy self-esteem in the SPN/SVN learner.

4. Four practical/vocational nursing learners were absent the day tests were returned and reviewed in a pediatric course. Which of the following learners has a plan that will benefit the learner in future testing and clinical situations?
   1. The learner who, next class day, will ask the instructor for the grade on the test, for personal records.
   2. The learner who, next clinical day, asks the instructor to schedule time to go over test items that were correct.
   3. The learner who thinks that because the test is history, it is unnecessary to review test items, since the grade is final.
   4. The learner who asks when there is time to go over all test items, so that reasons for wrong answers can be identified.

ALTERNATE FORMAT ITEM

Which of the following students is not demonstrating behavior for success in the practical/vocational nursing program? *(Select all that apply.)*

1. A recent high school graduate who expects the instructor to teach her everything she needs to know.

2. A student who is a mother of four and spends time in the library each afternoon reviewing class notes.

3. A student who has not been in school for 20 years and seeks out the instructor when content is not understood.

4. A student with college experience who works part-time and joins a group that crams before each examination.

5. A student who speaks English as a second language and studies every night in preparation for class and clinical.

Developing a Successful Learning Style

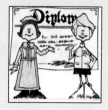

evolve http://evolve.elsevier.com/Hill/success/

Objectives

On completing this chapter, you will be able to do the following:

1. List two differences in the development of the male and female brain.
2. Explain how extroversion and introversion affect learning preference.
3. Discuss three perceptual learning styles.
4. Describe four secondary learning styles.
5. Identify your personal learning preferences.
6. Describe "empathizing," "systemizing," and "balanced brain types."
7. Explain how racial bias in textbooks influences your perception of the topic you are studying.
8. Identify the stages of learning how to read and how they are related to illiteracy.

Key Terms

Adult ADD (p. 22)
Auditory learner (ĂW-dĭ-TO-rē, p. 16)
Balanced brain (p. 21)
Bodily/kinesthetic learner (KĬN-ĕs-THĔT-ĭk, p. 18)
Emotional mind (p. 19)
Empathizer (p. 21)
Extroverts (p. 14)
Fight-flight mind (p. 19)
Hard wiring (p. 19)
Illiteracy (ĭ-LĬT-ĕr-ă-sē, p. 23)
Interpersonal learner (ĬN-tĕr-PĔR-sŏn-ăl, p. 18)
Intrapersonal learner (ĬN-tră-PĔR-sŏn-ăl, p. 19)
Introverts (p. 15)
Kinesthetic/tactual learner (TĂK-chū-ăl, p. 16)
Left brained (p. 20)
Linguistic learner (lĭng-GWĬS-tĭk, p. 18)
Logical learner (LŎG-ĭ-kăl, p. 18)
Musical learner (p. 18)

Perceptual learning style (p. 15)
Right brained (p. 20)
Spatial learner (SPĀ-shăl, p. 18)
Systemizer (p. 21)
Thinking mind (p. 19)
Visual learner (VĬS-ū-ăl, p. 16)

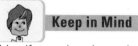 **Keep in Mind**

Identify your learning style: make it work for you in learning, retaining, and applying information in the care of patients.

*E*veryone learns differently. Some practical/vocational nursing students take voluminous notes. Some just listen. Others learn when they have an opportunity to practice what is being presented. You may even hear the latter say, "I'll understand this better when I practice it." All students can be equally successful. There are many theories about what affects learning style. We will review some of them.

PERSONALITY PATTERNS AFFECT LEARNING

Your personality pattern plays an important part in determining learning style(s). Learning about extroversion versus introversion (part of the Myers-Briggs Type Indicator) will aid in understanding a way that a personality pattern affects individual learning needs.

EXTROVERSION

Extroverts find energy in people and things. They prefer action with others and are described as "on-the-fly" thinkers. They talk more than listen and learn by teaching others. Extroverts often begin spontaneously "teaching" others and realize they do not really understand the topic. Suggestions for learning include:

- Group work in class (collaborative projects)
- Out-of-class group projects
- Explaining information to other people helps to identify what is not clear.

Extroverts may be seen as, "Ready, fire, aim."

INTROVERSION

Introverts find energy in the inner world of ideas, concepts, and abstractions. They listen more than talk. They can be sociable, but need quiet to recharge their batteries. Introverts are concentrators and reflective thinkers who want to understand the world. Disconnected "chunks" of information are not considered knowledge. The following are suggestions for learning:

- Lecture-type classes work well.
- Learn how to develop a framework to integrate and connect information, i.e., "see the whole picture."
- Use explaining as a way to interconnect information.

Introverts may be seen as "Ready, aim, aim."

For additional information on the total Myers-Briggs Indicator, check out the website at: *http://www.nwlink.com/~donclark/hrd/learning/styles.html.*

LEARNING STYLES

Learning takes place in different ways. It is important not to pigeon hole anyone, including yourself. Everyone is capable of learning with any learning style and will use another style to reinforce learning.

PERCEPTUAL LEARNING STYLES

Perceptual learning style refers to our three main sensory receivers: Vision (learn primarily with their eyes), Auditory (learn primarily by listening), and Kinesthetic/tactual (learn primarily by hands-on tasks), and is one way to determine

preference in learning style. Before going on to read about each perceptual style, we encourage you to do the following exercise. This exercise will provide an overall view of each sensory receiver style and assist you in planning ways to study successfully.

Learning Exercise

Self-Evaluation of Sensory Learning Style

Directions: Underline the symbol that is most accurate for each statement.

	Yes	Sometimes	No
Prefers to talk rather than read.	●	△	□
Likes to touch, hug, and shake hands.	△	□	●
Prefers verbal directions.	●	△	□
Uses finger spelling as a way of learning words.	△	□	●
Prefers written directions better than verbal directions.	□	●	△
Reads to self by moving lips.	●	△	□
Likes to take notes for studying.	□	●	△
Remembers best by doing.	△	□	●
Likes or makes charts and graphs.	□	●	△
Learns from listening to lectures and tapes.	●	△	□
Likes to work with tools.	△	□	●
Might say, "I don't see what you mean."	□	●	△
Good at jigsaw puzzles.	□	●	△
Has a good listening skill.	●	△	□
Presses pencil down hard when writing.	△	□	●
Learns theory best by reading the textbook.	□	●	△
Asks to have printed directions explained.	●	△	□
Chews gum or smokes almost continuously.	△	□	●

Continued

Scoring

Count all of the • Δ ☐ symbols. The highest number indicates the sensory learning preference(s).

Key

☐ = Visual; • = auditory; Δ = kinesthetic/tactual.

Adapted from and used with the permission of Jeffrey Barsch, EdD. Complete copies of the test may be obtained by writing directly to: Jeffrey Barsch, EdD, Ventura College, 4667 Telegraph Road, Ventura, CA 93003.

 Critical Thinking Exercise

Summarizing Your Learning Style(s)

After you have completed the Self-Evaluation of Sensory Learning Style(s) exercise, make two columns on a piece of paper. Label the columns "A" and "B." Write down the statements that you answered as "yes" in column A. Write down the statements you answered as "sometimes" in column B. You have identified your sensory learning style. In the following segment you will find out how the information can be helpful in your studying.

PERCEPTUAL LEARNING-STYLE PREFERENCE

People think differently. They think in the system corresponding to the sense of vision, hearing, or kinesthetic.

- **Observers:** There are two subchannels for visual learners: visual-linguistic and visual-spatial. Visual-linguistic learners learn best through reading and writing. They tend to remember what they read. They like to write down directions and pay better attention to lectures if they watch them. Visual-spatial learners do less well with reading generally, and learn best through charts, demonstrations, video, and other visual materials. They can easily visualize faces and places and seldom get lost in new surroundings. Observers tend to say, "I see what you mean" or "I think you mean…."

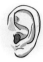

- **Listeners:** Auditory learners think in terms of hearing, talk to themselves, or hear sounds. They may move their lips and read out loud. They learn best by hearing and tend to have difficulty with reading and writing assignments. Listeners tend to say, "I hear what you are saying."

- **Doers:** There are two subchannels for kinesthetic/tactual learners: movement and touch. They tend to lose interest during class if there is no movement or external stimulation. Kinesthetic learners experience feelings in regard to what is being thought about. They learn best by moving, doing, touching, experiencing, or experimenting.

Being identified as a specific type of learner does not mean that a learner thinks exclusively in any one of these overall systems. What it means is that most people think more in one system than another. There are ways to enhance learning by supporting the overall system.

No learning preference is better than another. It is usually easier to feel connected to someone who shares a similar learning preference: "We think in the same language." A learning preference is just that, and there are ways to make it work for you.

Visual Learner

If you are a visual learner, you learn best by watching a demonstration first. Make this preference work for you by using the following techniques:

- Sit in front of the class.
- Stay focused on the teacher's facial expression and body language.

- Make notes in class and highlight, color code, and use mind maps to process and learn content (see Chapter 4).
- Rewrite notes in your own words as a form of studying (e.g., write notes or draw pictures in the margin of your book).
- Use index cards for review or memorization.
- Review films or videos.
- Look for reference books that contain pictures, graphs, or charts, or draw your own.
- Request demonstrations and observational experiences before practicing a new skill.
- "Picture" a procedure rather than memorizing steps.

Auditory Learner

If you are an auditory learner, you learn best by hearing. Make this preference work for you by using the following techniques:

- Listen carefully if the instructor summarizes what you will be learning, points out what is important to remember, and summarizes what has been covered during class.
- Read aloud or mouth the words. Concentrate on hearing the words, especially when reading test questions.
- Read important information into a tape recorder, and then play it back.
- Do well with traditional lecture or any lengthy presentation. Listen to the words instead of taking notes during class. Tape the presentation and discussion, if the instructor and students grant permission. Play the tapes back several times.
- Find a "study buddy" or group with whom to discuss class content. Compare notes and verbalize the information to aid in learning the material.
- Request permission to make audiotapes or oral reports (instead of written reports) for credit.
- Make up silly rhymes or songs (mnemonic clues) to remember key points.
- Request verbal explanations of illustrations, graphs, and diagrams.

Kinesthetic/Tactual Learner

If you are a kinesthetic learner, you learn best by touching, moving, or hands-on tasks. Traditional lectures, in which one is required to sit, read, or listen for long periods of time, may be difficult. It is a problem to process both visual and auditory input. Make this preference work for you by using the following techniques:

- Handle the equipment before you practice a nursing procedure.
- Move while reading or reciting facts (e.g., rocking, pacing, or using a StairMaster or stationary bike).
- Change study positions often. During lectures, you may want to sit in back in order to stand up and take notes without being too obvious.
- Use background music of your choice when studying at home.
- Take short breaks and do something active during that time.
- Offer to do a project as a way of enhancing a required classroom presentation. For example, if you have been asked to explain how oxygen gets out of the capillary and carbon dioxide gets in, develop a project to use as the basis of your explanation.
- Use arrows to show relationship when taking notes. Use flash cards, games, mnemonic clues, and other game-like activities to reinforce content of long reading assignments.
- Draw boxes, pictures, and circles around key concepts, make diagrams and doodles.

(Adapted from: *http://www.nwlink.com/~donclark/hrd/learning/ styles.html*.)

Learning Exercise

Enhance Your Learning

List suggestions that you think will help enhance your learning.

_____

_____

_____

_____

CATEGORIES OF MULTIPLE INTELLIGENCES

Gardner (1999) described what he termed "multiple intelligences" as being more accurate than the single measure of intelligence quotient (IQ) that most people are familiar with. The seven identified intelligences include the following:

1. Linguistic
2. Logical/mathematical
3. Spatial
4. Musical
5. Bodily/kinesthetic
6. Interpersonal
7. Intrapersonal

This knowledge provides additional information that will further enhance your learning.

LINGUISTIC LEARNER (THE WORD PLAYER)

If you are a linguistic learner, you learn best by saying, hearing, and seeing words. You like to read, write, and tell stories. You are good at memorizing names, places, dates, and trivia. Make this preference work for you by using the following techniques:

- Take notes when you read this text and reduce the number of words you have included in the notes.
- Use these notes as your study source. Your love of words and vocabulary may cause you to become distracted from the key points.
- Review all written work before handing it in. Delete extra words and phrases that are not directly related to the topic.

LOGICAL/MATHEMATICAL LEARNER (THE QUESTIONER)

If you are a logical learner as well, you learn best by using an organized method that involves categorizing, classifying, and working with abstract patterns and relationships. You are good at reasoning, math, and problem solving. Make this preference work for you by using the following techniques:

- Take the time to organize a method of study that fits you personally.
- Redo your notes to fit your study method, categorizing the material under titles.
- Study in an orderly area.

SPATIAL LEARNER (THE VISUALIZER)

If you are a spatial learner, you learn best by visualizing, dreaming, working with colors and pictures, and studying diagrams, boxes, and special lists in the text. You are good at imagining things, sensing changes, puzzles, and charts. Make this learning preference work for you by using the following techniques:

- Make your own diagrams, boxes, or lists when they are not available in the book.
- Redo your notes using key concepts only.
- Box key information in the text.

MUSICAL LEARNER (THE MUSIC LOVER)

If you are a musical learner, you learn best by humming, singing, or playing an instrument. You are good at remembering melodies, rhythms, and keeping time. Make this preference work for you by using the following techniques:

- Play your favorite music or hum while studying. Remind yourself which music relates to the content you are studying.
- Play an instrument while reviewing information in your head.

BODILY/KINESTHETIC LEARNER (THE MOVER)

If you are a bodily/kinesthetic learner, you learn best by touching, moving, and processing knowledge through bodily sensations. You are good at physical activities and crafts. Make this preference work for you by using the following techniques:

- Move around when studying. If you work out on a treadmill, stationary bike, or StairMaster, it becomes a good time to read or review notes.
- Dance or act out concepts you are studying to experience the sensations involved.

INTERPERSONAL LEARNER (THE SOCIALIZER)

If you are an interpersonal learner, you learn best by sharing, comparing, cooperating, and interviewing. You are good at understanding people, leading others, organizing, communicating, and mediating. Make this preference work for you by using the following techniques:

- Organize and/or participate in a study group.
- Compare your understanding of material with that of other students.

INTRAPERSONAL LEARNER (THE INDIVIDUAL)

If you are an intrapersonal learner, you learn best by working alone, self-paced instruction, and having your own space. You are good at pursuing interests and goals, following instincts, understanding yourself, and being original. Make this learning preference work for you by using the following techniques:

- Work on individualized projects.
- Trust your instincts in regard to study needs.

(Adapted from Gardner & Hatch, 1990; Miller & Babcock, 1996.)

Be aware of the type of learner you are, but do not limit yourself to those styles. Try out suggestions listed under other preferences. Some of them will further enhance your learning.

 Learning Exercise

Learning Styles

Check out the following website: *http://www.engr. ncsu.edu/learningstyles/ilsweb*. If interested in additional information on personal learning preferences, fill out the "Index of Learning Styles Questionnaire." There is no fee involved. Learning style results arrive quickly and explanations of the styles are available by following directions provided on the results form.

 Critical Thinking Exercise

Implementing Suggestions

Make a realistic plan involving learning styles that you think will work for you. Include observable, desired outcomes, a plan of action, and dates by which you will accomplish this plan. Remember that dates are an educated guess by you, based on intimate knowledge

of how you function. Be sure you note how you will determine progress toward a behavioral change. Use a format that works for you: columns, clustering, doodling, pictures, etc.

BRAIN DEVELOPMENT AND LEARNING

The battle of biology (hard-wiring) versus socialization (how you are raised) in brain development is finally backed by sound scientific evidence. Originally biology alone was credited for male/female differences in areas such as learning and behavior. For a number of years, until the late 1980s, the importance of socialization became the focus. It was thought that men and women became what they are based on their specific socialization. Looking back, it has not worked out this way, and both boys and girls have paid dearly for this singular emphasis.

FIGHT-FLIGHT, EMOTIONAL, AND THINKING MINDS

Paul MacLean, MD, a brain researcher, suggested that the brain has three minds, and each can affect learning. When you feel threatened, intimidated, or criticized, the fight-flight mind becomes active and you begin to defend yourself. It is hard to learn to cut through the negative feelings you are experiencing, because you are in survival mode. The emotional mind is the site of positive feelings, such as love, caring, kindness, and compassion. When more positive feelings are experienced, the emotional brain switches into gear and alerts the thinking mind. Most of your schoolwork, including creativity, reasoning, and analytical thinking, occurs in this part of the brain (i.e., your thinking cap).

If you become anxious over tests, class, or learning situations, this anxiety can trigger the fight-or-flight brain. Your memory can be affected, which can interfere with your test results, learning, and performance. Activate the more positive, emotional side of your brain and your thinking cap will be activated. This results in better learning and success in school.

RIGHT AND LEFT HEMISPHERES OF THE CEREBRUM

It is accepted that the left brain's hemisphere is verbal; the right brain is not. The left hemisphere processes in sequence; the right hemisphere processes spatially (how parts fit together). Confining the activity of creativity to the right hemisphere lacks scientific evidence (Springer and Deutsch, 1997, pp. 292, 297).

The two sides of the brain are designed to form a partnership. Experienced musicians process music in their left hemisphere, not the right, as a novice would. Among left-handed learners, nearly half use the right hemisphere of their brains for language. Higher-level mathematicians, problem solvers, and chess players have more right hemisphere activation during these tasks, whereas beginners in those activities usually are active in the left hemisphere. The right hemisphere recognizes negative emotions faster, whereas the left hemisphere is more active while experiencing positive emotions (Jensen, 1998, p. 8). In the activity of speech, for example, the left side of the brain, being very verbal and fluent, would cause us to talk in computer-like patterns if the right side were not available to add tone and inflection to our voice. The right side of the brain helps us recognize a face in the crowd quickly, even if the person has shaved off his beard, whereas the left side would puzzle over this missing part. In school the left side of the brain helps us break down new information into bits and pieces so that we can master it.

The right side of the brain gives us the total picture of our learning. Unfortunately, we usually limit ourselves to using approximately 1% of 1% of the brain's projected processing capacity (Table 2-1).

Learning Exercise

What Kind of Thinker Are You?

Check out the quiz, "Are You a Right-Brain Thinker? at: *http://www.chatterbean.com/right_brain_thinker/1/*.

RIGHT-BRAINED INDIVIDUALS

Primarily right-brained individuals tend to be intuitive, imaginative, and impulsive. They prefer to start out with a broad idea and then pursue supporting information. They learn best by:

- Seeing and doing in an informal, busy, somewhat unstructured environment.
- Simulations, group discussion, panels, and activity-based learning.

LEFT-BRAINED INDIVIDUALS

Left-brained learners tend to be analytical, rational, and objective. They learn best by:

- Putting together many facts to arrive at a general understanding.
- Having traditional lectures, demonstrations, and assigned readings.

Table 2-1 | *Right and Left Hemispheres of the Cerebrum*

RIGHT HEMISPHERE	LEFT HEMISPHERE
Processes spatially	Processes in sequence
Beginning music students	Trained musicians
Among left-handed people, nearly half use right hemisphere for language	Verbal/fluent side
Adds tone and inflection to our voice	Robot-like speech
Higher-level mathematicians	Beginners in these tasks
Chess players, problem solvers have more activation during tasks	More active during positive emotion
Recognizes negative emotions faster	Puzzles over missing part, such as a shaven beard
Recognizes face in a crowd, even if beard is shaved off	Breaks down new information into bits and pieces so that it can be mastered
Gives a total picture of our learning	

DEVELOPMENTAL DIFFERENCES

This brief review of brain development will be limited to developmental issues that affect learning in the classroom and clinical area.

- The male brain is approximately 10% to 15% larger than the female brain. The reason for, and use of, the additional space has not been clearly identified. Size alone is not proof of intelligence in humans any more than it is in other animals.
- In utero (fetal life) the female brain develops earlier than the male brain. The left half of the brain, which controls thinking, develops somewhat later than the right brain, which is related to spatial relationships. Brain development is even slower for the male. When the right side of the male brain is ready to connect with the left side by sending over connecting fibers (corpus callosum), the proper cells for the connection do not exist. Consequently, the fibers go back and form connections within the right side. This is why the male brain ends up with enriched connections within the right hemisphere (spatial capability). The ability often shows up early in the male child; for example, moving blocks around to see how they use up space, using Legos to create structures, etc.
- The female brain develops faster and is able to develop a larger system of connecting fibers (corpus callosum) between the left and right hemispheres of the brain. There is more communication between both sides of the brain. Being able to draw on both hemispheres benefits the female in reading skills, for example (Gurian, 1997, pp. 13-19).

EMPATHIZING (E), SYSTEMIZING (S), AND BALANCED BRAIN (B)

The E-S theory of brain development is that the female brain is predominantly hard-wired for empathy and the male brain is primarily hard-wired for understanding and building systems. It is called the empathizing-systemizing (E-S) theory.

Empathizer Brain (E)

The empathizer intuitively figures out how people are feeling and how to treat them with sensitivity. The researchers call this type "E." Although the "E" type is known as the female brain, it is not limited to females. They caution that sex alone does not determine brain type.

Systemizing Brain (S)

The systemizer analyzes and explores a system to discover underlying rules that govern and drive the system. The "S" type, as it is known, intuitively figures out how things work and what underlying rules control the system. Systems include anything with input and output (e.g., vehicles, computers, math questions, a nursing unit). The "S" brain is known as the male brain, but is not limited to males.

Balanced Brain (B)

The balanced brain is a balance of empathizing and systematizing. This is known as type "B." If you are interested in additional information on these brain types and where you fit in, check the website for a short test: *http://www.guardian.co.uk/ life/feature/story/0,13026,937913,00.html*.

With the help of imaging techniques, such as magnetic resonance imaging (MRI), more specific information is beginning to emerge on how the brain functions and differs in males and females. For example, results of a recent study show that men listen with the left side of the brain, whereas most women listen with both sides, but predominantly with the left side. The significance of this finding is unknown and does not indicate that one way is better than another.

The driving force for a lot of the brain research is to attempt to learn how men and women recover from brain tumors and strokes. It may also guide surgeons to avoid certain areas of the brain if the patient is male or female.

PRACTICAL APPLICATION OF INFORMATION

In the following chart we will look at specific characteristics related to brain development. Individual differences can always apply in nature. Socialization also enters into expanding the original work of both hemispheres of the brain.

Learning Exercise

Brain Characteristics

Personalize the following chart by marking characteristics that apply to you.
Check all that apply.

☐ Better at sensory data (hear, smell, touch, taste, and see minute detail).
☐ Hear better in one ear. Visual is best sense: Interpret best from left eye.
☐ Differentiate background sounds readily.
☐ Do less well in picking up background noises; may not "hear" someone speaking to me.
☐ Satisfied with limited space. Processes data in sequence.
☐ Increased focus on spatial relationships and activities. Tend to use more space. Like video and computer games and participate in activities that fill more space, such as football, baseball, and so on.
☐ Easy to express myself verbally.
☐ Not so easy to express myself verbally.
☐ Do less well with abstraction skills.
☐ Good abstraction skills. Test out better at math (abstract spatial construction of right hemisphere).
☐ Reading is easy.
☐ Reading takes more time.
☐ Multitask: I can work on several tasks at one time.
☐ Focus on one task at a time. Irritated by interruptions.
☐ Handle issues involving emotions readily.
☐ Difficulty in identifying and expressing emotions.
☐ Detect emotions easily.
☐ Have difficulty detecting emotions in another's face.
☐ Process information or think about things all the time.
☐ Brain shuts down with overload or fatigue.
☐ Rarely aggressive.
☐ Tend to be aggressive.

Critical Thinking Exercise

Making the Brain Work for Me

Read the Learning Exercise: Brain Characteristics. Write down the characteristics that are not working for you. Make a plan for each characteristic on how to modify the characteristic and make it work for you. Develop specific outcomes and timelines for modifying the characteristics you identified.

HOW WE LEARN

Scientists are not exactly sure how the brain can rewire itself with each new stimulation, experience, or behavior and cause learning. Their idea is that a stimulus occurs and is processed by the brain on several different levels. Neural pathways (traces) become more and more efficient when a learning exercise, such as reviewing notes, is repeated. This is done through myelination (coating) of the neurons. Stimulation occurs when you learn something new. The mental or motor stimulation lights up the brain in several areas, producing even greater beneficial electrical energy; for example, you receive a new assignment or have a new clinical experience.

The brain gets its energy for learning primarily from blood—about 8 gallons per hour. Remember to keep up the water intake. "Dehydration is a common problem in school classrooms, leading to lethargy and impaired learning" (Jensen, 1998, pp. 10, 12).

UNDEPENDABLE MEMORY AND LEARNING SYSTEM

There are average and above-average individuals with potential and talent who embrace failure messages and low self-worth. Some of these individuals are part of a population that continues to live with an untreated attention deficit disorder (ADD) as adults. Among the characteristics of adult ADD is an undependable memory and learning system. Take time right now to review the following learning exercise. You may be able to help yourself or a friend find a road to successful studying.

Learning Exercise

Signs of Possible Adult ADD

Read the statements in the following list. See if any of the statements apply to you or someone you know who might benefit from the information. *Check the statements that apply.*

☐ Trouble keeping a steady job.

☐ Difficulty getting assignments in on time; late in filing taxes or renewing driver's license.

☐ Supervisor or instructor complains that you do not do your share of the work.

☐ Feel others are responsible for what happens to you.

☐ Impulse buyer: I need, I want, I must have. Credit cards frequently "maxed" out.

☐ Thrill-seeking impulsive behavior: Live for the moment without considering consequences.

☐ Use alcohol, tobacco, and caffeine to pick you up or calm you down.

☐ Overreact to everyday situations: very happy, very sad, very angry or irritable, grumpy, pessimistic.

☐ Short attention span: easily distracted.

☐ Super-focused: difficulty detaching from task at hand.

☐ Normal noise, sight, or sound causes feelings of intense anxiety or irritation.

☐ Protective of own physical space, but will invade others' space without forethought.

☐ Experiences shame after unexplained explosive outbursts.

☐ Fatigued: seen as a night person but often stays up until exhausted because of nightmares and disturbed sleep patterns.

☐ Has problem with organizing activities of daily living.

☐ Uses charm and humor to manipulate.

☐ More comfortable with monologue than with dialogue.

If you recognize several of these traits, check with your school counselor for further information. We also recommend the book, *You Mean I'm Not Lazy, Stupid or Crazy?!* (Kelly and Ramundo, 1993).

SOME SUGGESTIONS FOR THE STUDENT WITH ADULT ADD

- Identify your learning preference from the categories presented in this chapter. Practice the suggestions offered.

- Use relaxation exercises to quiet your mind and reduce anxiety.
- Use background music (not TV) to shut off background noises.
- Schedule study time for when you feel most alert and fresh.
- Use color to help focus your attention. A color transparency over the page you are reading or large, color poster boards on the desk where you work help draw your attention.
- Use physical activity to enhance study. Play study tapes while walking, or ride a stationary bike while reviewing notes.
- Invent your own comfortable ways of studying.

Critical Thinking Exercise

Help for Adult ADD

Write the statements that apply from the Learning Exercise, Signs of Possible Adult ADD. Write down the suggestions that may be useful. Indicate what you will do with the information. A serious problem may need medical attention for diagnosis. Some schools provide assistance in learning at a school learning skills' center.

MORE BARRIERS TO LEARNING

Barriers may or may not be of your own making. Regardless of the reason for their existence, they belong to you now. It is up to you to identify if the barriers exist, and if they affect your learning. It is also up to you to seek help in dealing with the barriers, if needed. Two such barriers are racial bias in textbooks and a type of illiteracy that involves the ability to comprehend the content of what you have read. Recognizing and reading words with fluency (speed and accuracy) is not the issue.

RACIAL BIAS IN TEXTBOOKS

Textbook content is based on the authors' interpretation of resources used as the basis of their research for writing. Multicultural resources may or may not have been a part of the preparation, even when desirable for a particular topic. A lack of multicultural information in areas such as cultural differences and spiritual practices may give the reader a one-sided viewpoint, especially when the information is presented as being factual; for example, "This race (culture, religion) always...."

According to Byrne (2001) six categories of bias in textbooks include the following:

1. **Invisibility:** The majority culture is used as the only example in the narrative and in all illustrations. This may result in the student of a nondominant culture feeling less significant culturally.
2. **Stereotyping:** The writing preference oversimplifies the behaviors and traits, such as physical appearance, intelligence, personality characteristics, social roles, and ambition. A sense of being misunderstood and undervalued is common.
3. **Imbalance and selectivity:** The majority culture's viewpoint is presented as the only "truth."
4. **Unreality:** Unpleasant realities and topics are avoided, which can promote racial tension by not providing the opportunity to openly discuss cultural practices and behaviors that differ.
5. **Fragmentation and isolation:** Information on non-dominant cultures is separated from mainstream content, supporting feelings of insignificance.
6. **Linguistic bias:** Cultural and ethnic groups are presented as being exotic or primitive.

Learning Exercise

Textbook Authority

Briefly summarize a time you questioned textbook authority.

_____

_____

_____

Critical Thinking Exercise

Textbook Authority

Identify which of the six categories triggered the concerns that lead to the prior question. What did you do with your concern? Did the outcome of the experience influence the way you looked at yourself as a member of a cultural group? If so, how? What would you do differently if you were given the opportunity to repeat the experience?

_____

_____

The authors of this textbook encourage you to question textbook authority whenever you are sincerely concerned. One way to do this is to check out the authors' list of references and suggested readings. The references provide a listing of the materials used in preparation for writing each chapter.

INABILITY TO COMPREHEND CONTENT (ILLITERACY)

Illiteracy, according to the old definition, means not being able to recognize words and read them. This type of illiteracy is rare in the United States. Almost everyone in the United States can read words, but not everyone in the United States has learned to read for content. In fact, Finland is the only country to beat the United States in 4th grade reading scores. (What does this have to do with comprehension?) Educators have noted a fourth-year slump in the United States in reading performance, especially for minority students in less-privileged schools. Years ago, a reading researcher identified several phases we all must go through to become literate. These stages are still considered valid.

Learning Exercise

Phases of Literacy and Comprehension

As you read each of the descriptions that follow, write down which phases you have mastered and which ones you need to develop.

• Before a child starts grade school, the foundation for reading and language has been laid. By being read to, a child learns what books are for and how they are used.

- In grades 1 and 2, a child learns to translate written symbols into sounds and words.
- In grades 3 and 4, the school-age child develops speed and accuracy in reading (fluency). At this time the child has not learned to read for content. The child has not yet learned to comprehend what is being read.
- In grades 4 to 8, the school-age child masters vocabulary and learns how to pick out the main points while reading. This is the beginning of reading for content.
- In high school, students learn to weigh evidence in passages they are reading and evaluate and make judgments about what they read. These behaviors demonstrate the ability to read for content and comprehend what is being read.
- By the end of high school, adolescents have reached the stage in which they are able to manage their own learning process, choosing what to read and knowing how to use what they have learned in areas of interest.
- Many people in the United States have not reached this level.

(Source: Clinton P. Sept/Oct, 2002, p. L6.)

Critical Thinking Exercise

Increase Your Reading Score

Go to the study skills center and check the result of your entrance test reading score. Ask a counselor to interpret the meaning of the score. If the score is close to just passing, request that the counselor assist you in making a plan to increase your reading level. Use the description of the nursing process phases to develop a meaningful and worthwhile plan (see Chapter 8). The phases can be reversed into intelligent questions that you need answered by the counselor.

PUTTING IT TOGETHER

It is not unusual to read information and then say, "But of course this doesn't apply to me." This information does apply. Quality education encourages you to explore and apply alternative thinking, multiple answers, and creative insights.

You become a self-directed learner by using the following techniques:

- Practice critical thinking.
- Identify your major and specific learning preferences. Studying becomes easier.
- Understand basic right- and left-brain functions and how they work together. It helps you appreciate your capacity for learning.
- Do your part to prevent dehydration when studying and participating in classes. Water is a major ingredient of the blood, which motivates the brain.
- Behave in a successful manner. Success reinforces this attitude.
- Set realistic goals and evaluate the results to see whether these goals are being met.

It is an obstacle to learning to think that learning can take place without effort.

- Remember that established preferences of learning may not be working for you. Learning styles can be changed or modified as needed. It is also worth it to try suggestions from other styles to see if the suggestions enhance your learning.
- Tie in new learning to previous lessons and experiences. This gives the material meaning and makes it easier to remember.
- Seek help when it is needed. Sometimes being alone is best; sometimes it is best to study with others. Beginning studies, problems with studies, and the need to be with someone are reasons for seeking out others.
- Identify your reading level and make sure you reach your potential.
- Learn beyond the point necessary for doing or performing the skill. Keep reviewing and practicing the skills you learned. Practice. Practice. Practice.
- Fit your new information into what you already know.
- Question what you do not understand, and question the source of information when you have reason to believe it is incorrect.

- Remember that whatever your learning style is, the best memory aid is **writing it down**.

According to a Chinese proverb, *the weakest ink lasts longer than the strongest memory*!

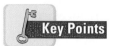
Key Points

- People who are extroverts or introverts learn in different ways.
- People think in different representational systems; the way they think determines their perceptual learning style.
- Some people think in pictures (visual learners). Some hear sounds or talk to themselves (auditory learners). Some experience a feeling in regard to what they are thinking about and learn best by doing (kinesthetic/tactual learners). Each learning style can be enhanced.
- Multiple intelligences also translate into learning styles. Identifying whether you are a linguistic learner (likes words and new vocabulary), a logical learner (organized and consistent), a spatial learner (prefers boxes and diagrams to words), a musical learner (likes to hum, sing, or play instruments), a bodily/kinesthetic learner (likes touching and moving), an interpersonal learner (likes sharing, comparing, and cooperating), or an intrapersonal learner (likes working alone, self-paced instruction) further enhances your learning ability.
- Each side of the brain processes things separately. Based on experimental evidence, it is accepted that the left hemisphere is more verbal and processes things in parts or sequences. The right hemisphere is nonverbal and sees the total picture. A connection between the right brain and music has been established.
- Male and female brains develop differently, which accounts for some different characteristics. Sex alone does not determine the brain type.
- The E-S theory suggests that female brains are hard-wired for empathizing and male brains are hard-wired for understanding and building systems.
- Personal attitude toward learning also influences the learning process. Attitude is closely related to whether you are a reactive learner who expects to be taught or an active learner who takes charge of his or her own education.
- Biases in textbooks may influence a student's perception about others, themselves, and the world they live in.
- Almost everyone in the United States can recognize words and read with accuracy and fluency. The most common form of illiteracy is related to the inability to comprehend what is read.
- Adult ADD often goes unrecognized and continues to make those individuals feel that they are not as capable.
- Most schools of higher learning have a study skills center that is willing and able to assist with adjusting or modifying a learning preference that may not be working for you.

REVIEW ITEMS

1. What does the term kinesthetic learner mean?
   1. Experiences feelings about what is being thought.
   2. Good at reasoning, mathematics, and problem solving.
   3. Good at imagining things, sensing changes, puzzles, and charts.
   4. Learns best by watching a hands-on demonstration first.

2. How do you determine if you process information primarily on the left side of the brain?
   1. When learning a new procedure, you pay more attention to what the total information is rather than focusing on the steps.
   2. You break the information down into smaller units and work to understand each step before proceeding to the next step.
   3. There is a tendency to give up on reading and/or absorbing the new information because it feels like too much of an overload.
   4. You would rather talk the procedure through to yourself rather than having someone else show you how the procedure is done.

3. The instructor is involving all of the students in the teaching/learning process. You will work in groups of four. Your group decides to divide the responsibility based on each student's major learning preference. Which student will be responsible for preparing the demonstration materials?
   1. Dan is a visual learner.
   2. Nan is an auditory learner.
   3. Tom is a tactual learner.
   4. Jill is a logical/mathematical learner.

4. You find yourself discussing the new definition of illiteracy that you have just learned. Your friend does not believe you are correct and challenges you to give him an example. Which of the following statements would be most appropriate in this situation?
   1. The new definition of illiteracy has to do with the inability to understand the meaning of words. Your inability to understand me is a perfect example of illiteracy.
   2. The new definition of illiteracy relates primarily to the kind of teaching that is taking place in the less privileged and minority schools throughout the lesser-developed sections of the United States.
   3. The new definition really is not that important in practical/vocational nursing. We are not responsible for decision making. That is why the RNs get the big bucks.
   4. The new definition of illiteracy recognizes the focus on learning to read and develop fluency in reading during the first 4 years of school. The next step is comprehension.

ALTERNATE FORMAT ITEM

Which of the following statements is not true regarding racial bias in textbooks? *(Select all that apply.)*

1. It toughens the student up for the real world.

2. It creates a sense of feeling culturally insignificant.

3. It presents minority cultures as being significant.

4. It avoids discussion of unpleasant realities and topics.

Time Management: Using a Limited Resource Wisely

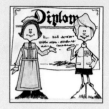

evolve http://evolve.elsevier.com/Hill/success/

Objectives

On completing this chapter, you will be able to do the following:

1. Discuss three benefits of time management for an adult student.
2. Using the four phases of the nursing process as a guide, develop a personal time-management plan to be used as a student practical/vocational nurse.
   a. List the activities of the various roles you fill in daily life.
   b. Arrange the list of various roles according to whether they are high priority or low priority.
   c. Keep at least a 1-day activity log to determine the present use of your time.
   d. Devise a semester schedule and a weekly schedule to reflect present commitments.
   e. Make a daily "to do" list.
   f. Carry out weekly and daily schedules for 2 weeks.
   g. Evaluate the effectiveness of your personal time-management plan and modify it, if necessary.
3. Identify right brain techniques to use in time management.

Key Terms

Data collection (p. 31)
Delegate (DĔL-ĭ-GĀTE, p. 33)
Effectiveness (ĕ-FĔK-tĭv-nĕss, p. 30)
Efficiency (ĕ-FĬSH-ĕn-sē, p. 30)
Evaluation (p. 39)
Habit (p. 30)
Implementation (ĬM-plĕ-mĕn-TĀ-shŭn, p. 36)
Long-term goal (p. 30)
Minitask (p. 37)
Planning (p. 32)

Priorities (prī-ŎR-ĭ-tēz, p. 30)
Procrastination (prĕ-KRĂS-tĭ-NĀ-shŭn, p. 37)
Short-term goal (p. 30)
Support system (p. 33)

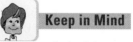

Keep in Mind

Invest your limited time carefully in the fast-paced PN/VN program. Not only will you be preparing for a successful NCLEX-PN® experience, you will also have some time to enjoy during your student year.

Have you noticed at school and in your personal life that some people seem to get more done than others? Worse yet, some of the busiest people are the ones getting the most done. To add insult to injury, all of us are given the same amount of time, 168 hours a week, in which to get the job done. How can some individuals get the job done and some not? The answer does not lie in the fact that some people have fewer responsibilities and less to do in a week's time. The answer lies in their ability to manage their own time.

WHY CAN'T I GET ORGANIZED?

There are several explanations for being disorganized and managing time poorly. These traits can be related to a trauma in your personal life. Organizing may be the last thing on the mind of a person who has been through a divorce or a death in the family. A state of disorganization may be the result of a disorganized upbringing. Disorganization can be the style you grew up with. You might continue this style as a source of comfort. Other disorganized persons may not have committed themselves to something they really want to do. They may use disorganization as a symptom of their discontent. Regardless of the reason for disorganization, millions of dollars are spent annually to hire time management experts to help people get organized. Millions more are spent on gadgets and devices that promise the same organization. This chapter contains free information and tips that can help you get organized and manage your time more efficiently and effectively. If you follow the suggestions, they will help make a challenging year more tolerable for you.

SELF-TEST OF TIME MANAGEMENT

Time management is a major skill that contributes to learner success. It is also a necessary skill for practical/vocational nurses to better manage their time in the clinical area to meet patient outcomes. To start this chapter, it is necessary for you to take a self-test of time management, so you will know how you stand with regard to this important skill. If you are going to be responsible for managing clinical time, you must be able to manage personal time.

The answers to the self-test are the ones suggested by time-management experts. Although different time-management techniques work for different people, these suggested answers reflect basic techniques that could help you succeed in the practical/vocational nursing program.

Learning Exercise

Self-Test of Time Management

Answer "yes" or "no" as you read each of the statements and apply them to your personal use of time.
1. I keep a semester or course calendar to reflect requirements and due dates of work for all my classes.
2. I keep a written weekly plan of everything that must be done at school and in my personal life.
3. I keep a written daily list of things I must do at school and in my personal life.

4. Daily I list and rank in importance my priorities for using school and personal time.
5. After listing and ranking my daily priorities for school and personal life, I stick to the list.
6. I use my best working time during the day for doing high-priority schoolwork.
7. I plan to do lower-priority schoolwork before higher-priority schoolwork.
8. I start school tasks before thinking them through.
9. I stop a school task before I have completed it.
10. I spend the few minutes before class talking to my classmates about anything other than the class.
11. I have trouble starting a major task for school.
12. I become bored with the subject I am studying.
13. I have a hard time getting started when I sit down to study.
14. Sometimes I avoid important school tasks.
15. I find myself easily distracted when I study.
16. I always try to get everything done in my personal life that must be done.
17. I frequently watch television instead of doing schoolwork.
18. I manage to turn a short coffee break into a long coffee break.
19. I study nightly for my classes.
20. I frequently have to cram for examinations.

The following are the suggested answers to the self-test:

1. Yes		11. No	
2. Yes		12. No	
3. Yes		13. No	
4. Yes		14. No	
5. Yes		15. No	
6. Yes		16. No	
7. No		17. No	
8. No		18. No	
9. No		19. Yes	
10. No		20. No	

Count the number of statements you disagree with and plug yourself into one of the following categories:

1-5 Disagree With — You deserve the *Alan Lakein** award.

6-10 Disagree With — Hang in there! With a little guidance you will get on the right track.

Continued

11-20 Disagree With   We know you must be exhausted, but keep on reading, quickly!

---

*Alan Lakein is a famous time-management expert. In 1973 he first published a very readable book entitled, *How to Get Control of Your Time and Your Life.* The key to using time wisely has not changed since his first edition was published.

BENEFITS OF TIME MANAGEMENT

Time management is a technique designed to help you do not only the things you have to get done, but also the things you want to finish in a definite time period. Time management can put you in control of your life rather than making you a slave to it. You will have to give up some of the things you were accustomed to doing before you became a practical/vocational nursing student. Time-management techniques can help you gain some personal time for your family and yourself, so you will not feel that there is time only for school. Time management can help you work smarter, not harder. It will not give you more hours in the week but will help you use what hours you do have more efficiently and effectively. Efficiency will help you get things done as quickly as possible. Time management does not deal solely with efficiency, as did the efficiency experts of the 1950s. The efficiency of the 1950s can bring images of robotlike individuals working to get every task done in the shortest time possible in a machinelike manner. Efficiency needs to be balanced with effectiveness. Effectiveness involves setting priorities among the tasks that need to be done and doing them the best way possible. Efficiency involves doing things as quickly as possible. Effectiveness involves choosing the most important task to do and doing it the right way.

REVIEW OF PERSONAL GOALS

How did you score on the time management self-test? If you are a typical adult, you are probably reading quickly right now to find out how to improve your time management. Take heart, very few of us get the Alan Lakein award. Most of us could stand to learn how to use our time more efficiently and effectively. Ineffective use of personal time is learned behavior, better known as a habit. Any behavior that is learned can be unlearned if you work at it, and new habits can be acquired.

If you have set a goal to be a practical/vocational nurse, you are already on the right track in time management, no matter what you scored. This is your long-term goal and the bull's eye to which you will direct your efforts for the next year. It would be beneficial to write that goal on an index card and place it where you will see it often, such as your car visor, the bathroom mirror, or the refrigerator door. Be specific when you write your goal. Be sure to include the date of your graduation. There will be some tough days in the months ahead, and the visibility of your long-term goal can keep you going. Use all your senses to experience what reaching your goal will be like (e.g., the weather, how you will feel, celebrations that may be planned).

To realize this long-term goal, you must break it down into smaller, more manageable goals. These are called your short-term goals. An example of short-term goals is passing each of the courses you must take to graduate from the practical/vocational nursing program. These short-term goals can be broken down even further to include the individual requirements for each of the courses you must take. For example, for one of your nursing courses, you might have to meet the following requirements to pass the course:

1. Earn a minimum grade on each of a certain number of major tests.
2. Give two oral reports.
3. Write a four-page paper on a selected topic.

Fulfilling each of the requirements will eventually lead to passing the course. When you pass each of the required courses, you will graduate from the program. While keeping your eye on your long-term goal, you will fulfill requirement after requirement until that goal is reached.

Now, start learning how to manage your time.

GETTING ORGANIZED WITH THE NURSING PROCESS

At all levels nursing has a special way of getting organized, called the nursing process. Chapter 8 discusses the nursing process and your role in using it as a practical/vocational nurse. The nursing process and its four components, data collection (assessment), planning, implementation, and evaluation, will be used to help you get organized as a student and in your personal life.

DATA COLLECTION

Data collection in time management involves two important areas: (1) discovering what roles you fill in your daily life, and (2) collecting data on how you actually spend your time.

Enrollment in a vocational-technical program, whether you are single, divorced, widowed, or married, requires some degree of change in the activities in which you were involved before entering the program. Regardless of your state in life, all the roles you fill can be classified into any of five general categories: school, job, family, community, and recreation.

The activities involved in going to school are very structured. You must get there, attend classes and clinical programs at a specific time, and get home. When you are enrolled in a vocational-technical program such as practical/vocational nursing, your school day is chock full. Seldom do you even have the choice of when you will take a specific course. The same structure is not evident in the other four roles. In your other roles you might be involved in some activities that you either did not plan to do, do not enjoy doing, do not have time to do, or feel do not need to be done.

Your Roles and Activities

You are encouraged to complete the Learning Exercise: My Personal Roles and Activities on p. 462 of Appendix D to collect data about your personal roles and activities for the data collection portion of time management. A sample exercise, Time Management: Sample Personal Roles and Activities, and explanation are on p. 461 of Appendix D.

Your Personal Time Use

You are now ready to document how you actually use your personal time. Ideally, a time log should be kept for approximately 1 week to document how you use your personal time. Because time is marching on, a 1-day time log for a class day can give you a general idea of how you use your time at present. Page 463 of Appendix D explains the exercise, Use of Personal Time. On p. 464 of Appendix D you will find a blank page on which you will complete the Learning Exercise: Personal Time and Activity Log.

Supply one more piece of information and your data collection will be complete. Following this paragraph, list one activity you wish you had time for. The activity could have been listed under your roles, but maybe it was not listed at all. Remember, the sky's the limit as long as your wish is something that is really important to you.

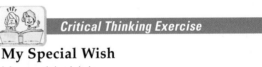

Critical Thinking Exercise

My Special Wish

My special wish is…

_____

_____

_____

_____

BEFORE YOU CONTINUE

How students use their time is partly a result of which side of the brain is dominant. Chapter 2 discusses the difference between right- and left-brain dominance. You may note personal brain dominance in your behavior. Chapter 2 gives you the opportunity to assess your specific dominance on p. 20. Time-management systems generally reflect the left-brain thinking style. This style is linear (prefers a step-by-step, methodical approach), compared with right-brain thinkers who are non-linear (see and do in an unstructured environment). Traditional tools of time management are directed to left-brain thinkers because they process information in sequence. Right-brain thinkers look at the picture as a whole. Right-brain thinkers prefer their own tools/ideas for time management and are good at devising them. Neither system of thinking is good or bad. Both sides of the brain work together and complement each other.

The challenge of time management for practical/vocational nursing students is to find the side of your brain in which the dominance lies. Use the strengths of this side. However, strive to use the resources of both sides of your brain. We will provide some right-brain strategies in the planning stage. Right-brain thinkers will be able to develop tools with which they are more comfortable.

PLANNING

When you have completed the data collection exercises in Appendix D, you will be ready to proceed to the planning stage. The planning phase of time management will result in a blueprint for action. In this phase you will learn how to plan the use of your precious 168 hours a week. Planning involves thinking about setting priorities (most important tasks), but these thoughts need to be written down to be successful. You need to devise a written plan for yourself so that you can program your time on a monthly, weekly, and daily basis. The plan should include the activities that are part of all the roles you fill, and not just your role as a student. Your plan should reflect the total of your activities. The Learning Exercise: Semester, Weekly, and Daily Planning on p. 35 will give you some suggestions for planning your daily, weekly, and semester time.

A plan helps keep you honest. It reflects the classes you must attend and the studying you must do to reach your long-term goal. With a plan you will avoid the roller coaster phenomenon all too familiar to students—falling behind in school and then trying to catch up. Planning helps you include time for friends and family. It helps you avoid overlooking an important part of your well-being—recreation. And, planning helps you avoid the pitfall of allowing extracurricular activities to come before schoolwork, which is the major reason for failure in postsecondary educational programs.

Arguments Against Planning

At this point some individuals will say they do not have time to plan and will pass off the suggestion about planning their time. Individuals who are too busy to plan are the very persons who should be planning. They cannot afford not to plan. If you do not plan, you will overlook priorities and possibly miss some available free time. For the small amount of time planning takes, the benefits are great. Some persons who say they do not have time to plan really do not want to find time to get priority work done. They may use lack of time as an excuse. Some individuals look at planning as leading to inflexibility and loss of freedom. They want to "hang loose" and go in different directions as the opportunities arise. Flexibility of this sort can result in disorganization and the accomplishment of few if any important tasks. As imposed deadlines near, guilt, frustration, and anxiety appear. These individuals wind up being a slave to time instead of being its master. A plan written in accordance with the principles of time management will help you be a master of time. The plan will be written with flexibility in mind, and you will be able to trade time with yourself when unexpected events come up.

Old Habits Die Hard

Unlearning old habits and learning new habits are not easy tasks. Although it takes work in the form of self-discipline and determination to drop old, comfortable ways, it is possible. Studies have revealed that it takes at least 21 days of consistently repeating a new habit to break an old habit. Be sure to practice the new habit whenever the opportunity presents itself. In doing this the new habit will eventually become a part of you. Ah! You say you slipped up and reverted to old habits. Do not give up! Reinstate your plan and try again. An article by Skloot in *O: The Oprah Magazine* describing how to unlearn old habits and learn new ones can be accessed at *www.nasw.org/users/skloot/ChangeStory.pdf*.

Scheduling Time

The only special equipment you need for planning is some form of calendar. Ideally, you need a device that has blank spaces for each date so that you can list activities. These calendars should be available at your school's bookstore. Some school bookstores provide a semester calendar for students. You can also make your own monthly calendar by copying a current calendar. Examples of other methods used for planning include the following:

1. Index cards or Post-it notes for each activity. Use one color card or note for roles and another color for activities. Pile the cards or stick the notes on a wall. This method also helps put activities in appropriate categories or roles.
2. A time line for planning, instead of a calendar.
3. A calendar on your personal computer.
4. A personal digital assistant (PDA). About $400 could buy you a hand-held device with lots of memory to hold your daily plan, to-do lists, calendar, and anything else to keep you organized. However, the other suggestions work just as well!

Setting Priorities

To plan your time, you need to be able to set priorities and delegate activities. In Appendix D the Learning Exercise, Setting Personal Priorities (p. 465), helps you decide which of your activities are most important and which activities need to come first. When setting priorities, remember that there is a difference between importance and urgency. Not everything that is urgent is important. A good example is a ringing telephone during mealtimes. A table to help you differentiate between what is urgent and important regarding priorities can be found at *www.couns.uiuc.edu/brochures/time. html*.

To have a successful year in the practical/vocational nursing program, teamwork is important. Identify the people in your life who make up your team. This is your support system. Inform them of the goals and priorities you have set for yourself for this school year.

Critical Thinking Exercise

My Personal Support System

List the people in your personal support system, using the following blank lines, a piece of paper, index cards, or Post-it notes.

_____

_____

_____

Delegating Activities

Some of your activities can be delegated to specific persons on your team. Box 3-1 lists examples of tasks that can be delegated in this manner. Taking growth and development into consideration, the tasks listed for children are excellent ways for them to learn responsibility.

Delegating to Children. As in the study of growth and development, these suggested activities apply to the typical child of each age group. The suggestions may or may not apply to your children. Do not underestimate your children, however. You will be able to come up with some ideas that do fit your children and can be added to the list. At first it may take some time to instruct your children, but in the long run it will be worthwhile. Have you ever heard the saying, "You have to spend money to make money?" Well, in time management sometimes it takes time initially to teach the people near you what is expected of them. In the long run it will pay off handsomely in time saved. In addition, your child benefits by learning responsibility, skills, and independence.

The same principle will be used in patient care. It may take time to teach patients how to master a skill for themselves. Once they learn the skill, it will save you time, and as a bonus, the patients gain independence. These suggestions are a wonderful way to help a child become independent and develop lifelong skills.

Dealing with a Spouse/Significant Other. Are you having trouble getting your spouse to cooperate? Avoid interpreting stubbornness as laziness or lack of love. Chances are that your spouse grew up in an environment in which household chores were divided by sexual orientation. The spouse

Box 3-1 | *Tasks That May Be Delegated*

SPOUSE/SIGNIFICANT OTHER
- Pay bills
- Help clean
- Take charge of car maintenance
- Mow the lawn
- Paint
- Do small repairs
- Prepare meals
- Start laundry
- Transfer laundry to dryer
- Shovel snow

PRESCHOOL AND EARLY SCHOOL AGE (4 TO 8 YEARS)
- Put dirty clothes in designated area
- Fold laundry
- Make clean laundry piles
- Deliver laundry to correct room
- Clear dishes from table (not best china!)
- Make own bed (avoid criticizing outcome of efforts)

SCHOOL AGE (9 TO 12 YEARS)
- Cook simple meals
- Wash dishes
- Dry dishes
- Put dishes away
- Start laundry
- Shop for a few food items as indicated on list
- Dust
- Run vacuum
- Pack own lunches
- Water plants
- Weed
- Shovel snow
- Make own bed
- Sweep

ADOLESCENTS (13 TO 18 YEARS)
- Run errands with family car if they have a license
- Wash car
- Plan menus
- Prepare grocery list within budget

- Put away groceries
- Mow the lawn
- Paint
- Make own bed
- Clean
- Wash clothes
- Iron if necessary or desired
- Sew on missing buttons

FRIENDS
- Substitute for you at bowling the night before a big examination
- Feed you occasionally

RELATIVES
- Substitute for mom or dad at scout meetings, PTA meetings, or school activities
- Spend time with children
- Holiday baking or shopping

RATIONALE FOR ACTIVITIES CHOSEN FOR
Preschool and early school age. Children in these age groups are experiencing muscle development and noticing their psychomotor development; they want to try new things. Make-believe rides high with these kids, and they love to play house. Capitalize on this.

School age. These children are adults-in-training. Muscles continue to develop, and psychomotor skills are increasing. They need tasks of the real world to engage in and should be encouraged to carry them through to completion.

Adolescents. Sometime during adolescence the ability to think as an adult will develop, allowing this age group to budget and apply principles of basic nutrition to everyday life. One of the tasks of adolescence is to become independent. Encourage its development by delegating meaningful activity to this age group.

School-age children and adolescents can also do activities in the column preceding their column, but would probably prefer the specific activities listed for their age group.

may feel that assuming new tasks jeopardizes his masculinity or her femininity. Gather your thoughts and decide on the areas in which you think your spouse could be most helpful during this hectic time of your life. The answer lies in communication. Talk with your spouse (only you know the best time and situation for this).

Hopefully, you both agree that you should be going to school and have identified the positive features of this endeavor for both of you. Review these positive features. If you have not identified them, do so together. Then collaborate on solutions to ease your lack of time. While you are at it, establish some precious "spouse/significant other only" time to be honored during your hectic year at school. You do not want to create in your spouse the feeling of being left out during this whole experience.

You can find the Learning Exercise, Delegating Activities, on p. 465 in Appendix D. This exercise will help you decide the personal roles and activities that can be delegated, which you can indicate on your paper, index cards, or Post-it notes.

 Learning Exercise

Semester, Weekly, and Daily Planning

SEMESTER PLANNING

Time Involved: Approximately 10 minutes

On your planning calendar/system, list the things that must be done during this time frame. The following are examples of activities to include:

- Your class/clinical schedule
- Dates of major examinations
- Dates papers are due
- Dates of doctors' appointments
- Dates of club meetings
- Dates for haircuts, etc.

Include activities that are delegated. Indicate them by circling the activity on your calendar/planning system. Write the name of the person who is responsible for it. Post these sheets, one month at a time, on your refrigerator for you, your family, or your roommate or significant other to see. The semester schedule needs to be done only once, in pencil. Additions or corrections are made as needed. This is also a way of communicating your new life to those with whom you live. Keep in mind that if you do live with other people, your new schedule is something to which they must get accustomed.

WEEKLY PLANNING

Time Involved: Approximately 10 minutes

The weekly plan is for your peace of mind. A blank form, Time Management: Weekly Schedule can be found on p. 466 of Appendix D. You can copy this sheet on loose-leaf paper or use index cards or Post-it notes. A weekly calendar can also be downloaded at *www.bucks.edu/ %7especpop/weekly-sch.htm*. Fill in all your classes and other fixed activities for the week, or paste/tape your cards or Post-it notes here. Photocopy as many sheets as there are weeks in the semester or time period of your current classes. Use some time each weekend to plan your week. Be sure to include in your planning the time you spend before and after classes. As assignments are

made, add them to your weekly plan. Your weekly plan not only will reflect study time, but will also specify what needs to be studied and when. The following are some suggestions to keep in mind when planning your week:

1. Plan studying for your prime time. Prime time is the time at which you are most effective in doing a task. High-priority courses need to be studied during personal prime time.

2. Plan blocks of time for studying by identifying your personal attention span for various school activities. For example, when reading, note the time you start reading and when you begin to lose your concentration. Note the amount of time that has passed. Do this for several sessions of studying. You will begin to see patterns in your attention span. Take a 3- to 5-minute break at this point in your studying. Vary your activity. For example, throw in a load of laundry.

3. Some people may find they have a 20-minute attention span, whereas others may have an attention span of 1 hour. The important thing is to not let your break extend beyond a few minutes. Condition yourself to get right back to work, without the need for start-up time.

4. It is impossible to tell you exactly how much time you will need for studying for each of your classes. This will vary from student to student and from class to class. Does the class meet daily? If so, you will have a daily assignment. The old suggestion of 2 hours of study for each hour of class will be just right for some classes, too much for others, and not enough for the rest.

5. Identify small blocks of time and make them work for you. They are important sources of time. These minutes can add up quickly to large time losses. These small blocks of time usually occur between classes. Try doing the following during these small blocks of time:

   – Get up.
   – Stretch.
   – Take deep breaths if staying in the same classroom.
   – Walk briskly while taking deep breaths to get to your next class.
   – Review in your mind the class you just attended. These activities will force more oxygen into your bloodstream and help it circulate to your brain. This results in better thinking and a fresher state of mind. One of the worst things to do is to grab a soda or a cigarette. The soda, if nondiet, will quickly elevate your blood sugar level and encourage insulin to be

Continued

deposited in the blood. The insulin will quickly lower the sugar content of your blood, leaving you with a tired, dragged-out feeling. Smoking constricts your blood vessels and decreases the amount of oxygen carried to your brain. Your brain needs oxygen to help you think and to keep you alert.

6. While waiting for your next class, select one of the following activities:
   – Review your notes from the class you just finished. This will allow you to fill in any gaps you may have in your notes. You will aid your retention and understanding of the material by reviewing it in this way.
   – Mentally prepare for your next class. If it is a lecture or discussion class, review your assignment. If it is an autotutorial class, review your plan of activities for the class.
   – Discuss an assignment with a peer. School is a social activity, but do not waste time by fooling around during all of your small blocks of free time. The more you get done at school, the less you will have to do at home.

7. Include only what is essential on your plan. Details take too much time to write down and are a real turn-off.

8. Plan for three meals a day with appropriate snacks, based on what you have learned in your nutrition course. Eating properly and keeping up your fluid intake will help avoid tiredness and irritability. With a busy schedule, you need to avoid being tired and irritable at all costs.

9. Plan for adequate sleep. Individuals have personal sleep patterns. Try to get in tune with yours. Do you ever wake up before your alarm? Next time you do, calculate how many hours of sleep you have had. Odds are your hours of sleep are some multiple of 1.5 hours. Brain research has shown that you will function better if you get up after 6 or 7.5 hours of sleep rather than after 7 or 8 hours. Apparently, we repeat a sleep cycle every 1.5 hours. If you get up a half hour into your next cycle, you could be very sluggish. Think of this when you set your alarm. When the alarm goes off, resist the temptation to reset the alarm on snooze.

10. Remember, although some sacrifices must be made, your life is more than just school. Review "My Special Wish" on p. 31 of this chapter and include it on your weekly schedule.

DAILY PLANNING

Time Involved: Approximately 5 minutes.

This schedule could prove to be the most important one as far as getting things done. Alan Lakein calls the daily plan a "to do" list. He states that both successful and unsuccessful persons know about to do lists. Successful persons use such a list every day to make better use of their time. Unsuccessful people do not (Lakein, 1973, p. 64). This is the simplest schedule to make.

1. Use a 3 × 5-inch card and head it "To Do." List the items you plan to accomplish, either directly on the card or on Post-it notes that you attach to the card. Be sure to include the high-priority activities for school and your personal life that you identified on p. 462 of Appendix D. Refer to your weekly calendar/planning system to refresh your memory about your assignments and their due dates. Rank (prioritize) your activities so that you can handle first things first. Use numbers, highlighters, or colored Post-it notes to indicate priority.

2. Map a "to do" list. See Chapter 4 for an explanation of mapping.

Decide for yourself the best time of day for preparing your to do list. Some people like to prepare this list while eating breakfast, as a way to get into the activities of the day. Some people like to prepare the list right before they go to bed. These people may be getting an extra benefit that they are not aware of. Their subconscious will be able to go over the "to do" list while they peacefully sleep and renew themselves. Carry your list with you. Stick to the activities and priorities you have listed. Cross off/tear off the activities when you have completed them. Ah, what a feeling!

Planning takes so little time. It can be fun and not a chore. Just think of all the benefits that come out of taking 10 minutes to plan each month, 10 minutes to plan each week, and 5 minutes to plan each day. What great returns for so little effort! And, by writing your plans and lists, you have freed your brain from one more source of clutter and saved it for all the learning you need to do.

IMPLEMENTATION

Implementation is the part of your time-management program in which your plans become action. The only value of a plan lies in its being used. Thanks to the planning you have done, you now have an incentive to get started because you already know exactly where you have to be and what you have to do. Now for some hints on how to follow that plan.

General Hints

As you begin to follow your personal plan, you may notice that some of your peers at school are not planning their time. They may even give you static for attempting to plan yours. Even if it means leaving some peers in the shuffle, have the intestinal fortitude to follow your schedule. You paid your tuition and have your own personal time problems to contend with to get full mileage out of that tuition. There may be some students who put their efforts into games instead of scholastic pursuits. They might think they will look better if others do not succeed. You will recognize these students when they tell you straight out that your efforts will make them look bad. Whose problem is that, anyhow? Make sure you never miss a class, regardless of peer pressure or any reason other than an emergency. When you miss a class, you spend more time trying to obtain the missed information than if you would have attended the class. You may never capture all of it.

Critical Thinking Exercise

Return on Your Investment

Write a few sentences about what *your* tuition is buying for *you.*

_____

_____

_____

In actually carrying out your schedule, be aware of a pitfall that can occur when you assign a specific time to a task. Sometimes the time it takes to do a task, whether for home or school, can stretch out to fill whatever time you have assigned to it. Therefore practice setting realistic time limits in which to complete tasks so you do not fall into this trap.

Procrastination

You know what you have to do and when it must be done, but do you ever find yourself putting off high-priority tasks to some time in the future?

Critical Thinking Exercise

High-Priority Task That I Have Put Off

List one high-priority task that you have put off this week.

_____

_____

How did you feel about postponing this task? Such action usually leads to tension. Fear of failure may cause students to put off things to the last minute. Putting off provides the student with an excuse for not doing well. What is causing your reluctance?

Re-evaluate the task you have been avoiding. Is it really a high-priority task? Remember, your planning needs to be flexible. The priority status of tasks can realistically change. Be careful if you find yourself using this explanation too often. Besides fear of failure, other causes for putting off what is important are ill health (you do not have the energy), laziness (you do not have the motivation), and past successful episodes of procrastination (if you did not do it, someone else did or nobody cared). Regardless of the cause, we all procrastinate to some degree. Some people make more of a habit of it than others do.

Minitasking

If you look truthfully at the tasks you keep postponing, odds are they are unpleasant, difficult, or time consuming. It seems we never postpone things that are fun or simple to do. In fact, sometimes we avoid high-priority tasks and do a bunch of low-priority ones. This action gives us an immediate yet false feeling of accomplishment.

A sure way to finish those unpleasant, difficult, and time-consuming tasks is to reduce the entire task to a series of minitasks. There are two rules for doing this. First, the minitask must be simple to do and take no more than 5 minutes of your time. Second, for best results the minitasks need to be written and carried in your pocket for quick reference. Many students fear upcoming major tests and put off studying for them. Some examples of minitasks for this situation could include the following:

1. Before and after each class, review your current class notes and related material covered previously.
2. Write the more difficult information you must know for the test on index cards. For example, write a term on one side of the card and its definition on the other. List causes of, consequences of, prevention of, and differences between items of class content, and have these cards handy for quick reference whenever you have a spare minute. One of us studied vocabulary for a German final in this way while undergoing a root canal procedure.
3. Follow the same procedure as in minitask No. 2 for items you got wrong on quizzes.
4. Talk to a peer about course content.

Refer to Chapter 2 for information on identifying your personal learning style preference. Now write some minitasks for the high-priority task you identified in the Critical Thinking Exercise, High-Priority Task That I Have Put Off.

Critical Thinking Exercise

Minitasks for High-Priority Task

1.
2.
3.

_____

_____

These minitasks will get you involved in starting the task in a less painful way. Just starting a task, even in a minimal way, is a positive force. Getting started takes more effort than keeping momentum.

Whatever the cause of your procrastination, to be behind in work is to be behind in success. Most times it takes more time and energy to escape the task than to do it in the first place. Start today to keep life in the present. Avoid deferring life and all its opportunities to the future.

Hints for Handling the Home or Apartment

No matter how much you delegate, if you are a spouse and parent, a single parent, or a single adult, you must realize that your house or apartment is not going to be as spic and span as usual while you are a student. A few hints may help ease the transition. Some of these hints are also helpful for persons who are helping out while the other goes to school and for single adults who are living on their own for the first time.

- Your grandmother always told you to tidy up to make it look like you really cleaned. Pick up papers and magazines as you pass through a room.
- If you do not have time to wash dishes, rinse and stack them, to be done later rather than just collecting them on the kitchen counter. If you have a dishwasher, rinse briefly and stack.
- Make your bed each morning when you first get up. It only takes a minute and improves the appearance of the bedroom dramatically. In fact, you can teach yourself to smooth out the top covers before you get out of bed and then slither out.
- Place dirty clothes in a laundry basket in your bedroom or bathroom instead of just heaping them on the floor. Hang up other clothing instead of just draping it over furniture.
- Clean the tub or shower after use by soaping up your washcloth and washing the sides of the tub or shower walls while they are still warm, then rinsing. (Be sure to put your washcloth in the laundry and get out a clean one.) Or while it is still wet, you may spray the shower with a product that eliminates the need for later scrubbing.
- Put away any hair dryer, cool curling iron, or similar devices after use, or collect them in a basket to reduce clutter.
- If you live in a two-story home, put a box at the top of the stairs and another one at the bottom for objects that need to go upstairs or be brought downstairs. There is always something coming or going, and this will save extra trips.
- Having trouble with the family remembering their assigned chores? One idea is to draw the shape of a house on

cardboard, draw 31 windows on the house, and number them in sequence. Cut three of the four sides of each window so that it opens up. Place the cardboard over a piece of shelf paper and write in names and chores for each day on the paper. Paste this chore sheet in place and tape up the windows. The first month takes the most time, but the chore list is a snap after that. Be sure to include a surprise or treat occasionally.

- A fun and fast way for an adult or child to dust is to wear a washed garden glove. Briefly spray the glove with furniture polish and go to it.

The sky's the limit as far as creative ideas for saving time at school and in your personal life. You will come up with some ideas out of sheer necessity as the year goes by. When you do, be sure to share them with your peers and authors (care of Elsevier Health Sciences).

EVALUATION

Evaluation of your time-management program will take place continuously from the minute you start implementing your plan. Evaluation involves determining how well your plan is working and how you are progressing toward meeting your short-term goals and long-term goal. It is a crucial part of time management. Why continue with a plan if it is not helping you reach your goals?

If the plan is not working, modify it. Ask yourself, "What changes should I make in my plan so that it will help me reach my goals?" The best gauge you have for evaluating your plan is your test grades. Grades will tell you if you are devoting as much time as needed to make the grade in a course.

How is your daily participation in class? Do you have assignments completed when they are due? Are you even aware that you had an assignment? Did you forget the test was on Thursday because you didn't mark it on your weekly calendar/planning system? Are you lapsing into the habit of procrastination? Not only will evaluation help you see how well you are progressing toward your goal, but it will also help you develop the evaluation and modification skills you will need as a practical/vocational nurse.

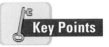
Key Points

- Time management is the efficient and effective use of personal time to meet goals.
- Techniques of time management can help you gain control over your life rather than being a slave to it, and can help you work smarter, not harder.
- Most systems of time management are geared to the left-brain style of thinking. Students with a right-brain thinking style need to adapt time-management systems to styles that reflect their interests and strengths.
- By using elements of the nursing process, you can set up time-management techniques to fit your personal life and style.
- Data collection includes the activities in the various roles you fill and collecting data about present personal time use.
- Planning involves composing semester, weekly, and daily plans to include high-priority activities.
- Implementation involves carrying out your plan.
- Evaluation involves deciding whether your plan is helping you meet your short-term goals and long-term goal of completing the practical/vocational nursing program and modifying your plan accordingly.

REVIEW ITEMS

1. Developing an action blueprint of time use is an example of which stage of time management?

   1. Planning
   2. Evaluation
   3. Implementation
   4. Data collection

2. Which of the following statements most appropriately describes the benefits of time management for the practical/vocational nursing student?

   1. Time management reduces the need to give up any activities in a student's personal life while in school.
   2. Time management helps students manage classroom responsibilities and manage time with patients on clinical.
   3. Time management requires students to get responsibilities at school and at home completed as quickly as possible.
   4. Time management eliminates the need to develop short-term and long-term goals for class and clinical rotation.

3. A practical/vocational nurse failed the first two major tests in the nursing program. The student claims there is no time for study and admits that personal responsibilities are overwhelming. To set up a time-management program, select the intervention this student needs to adopt initially.

   1. Write a plan to show how time will be spent in the next month at school.
   2. Follow the personal plan for use of time while in school and in clinical.
   3. Review personal daily responsibilities and document present use of time.
   4. Determine how much progress is being made to reach the goal of graduation.

4. Choose which of the following behaviors is a priority of effectiveness in time management?

   1. Finish low-priority tasks on personal to do list as quickly as possible, and then study.
   2. Complete your reading assignment for tomorrow's practical/vocational class.
   3. Start a low-priority task you love to do before beginning to work on a class paper.
   4. Before studying for a test on Friday, complete a two-page paper that is due next month.

ALTERNATE FORMAT ITEM

Which of the following practical/vocational nursing students used principles of the planning stage of time management during their student year? *(Select all that apply.)*

1. Matt arranged for his mother-in-law to take his three children for their physicals so they can participate in sports.

2. Holly had the family reunion at her home as a means of taking her mind off the fact that she is flunking everything.

3. Elizabeth took time to teach 3-year-old Alexander how to fold his laundry when it comes out of the dryer.

4. Dominic contacted all the people in his support system and told them about his priorities for this year.

5. Because of the system she developed using Post-It notes, Ruby did not miss a class assignment all year.

4 Methods and Skills Used in Learning

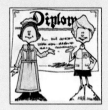

evolve http://evolve.elsevier.com/Hill/success/

Passive listener (p. 44)
PQRST method (p. 49)
Stem (p. 57)
Understanding (p. 47)

Objectives

On completing this chapter, you will be able to do the following:

1. Use techniques in learning situations that will:
   a. Increase your degree of concentration.
   b. Improve your listening skills.
   c. Enhance your comprehension of information needed for critical thinking as a practical/vocational nurse.
      1) Use each step in the PQRST method of textbook study.
      2) Use visual strategies.
   d. Develop your ability to store information in long-term memory.
      1) Form neural traces to store information for recall.
2. Use hints for successful test taking when taking tests in the practical/vocational nursing program and NCLEX-PN® examination.

Key Terms

Active listener (p. 44)
Clustering (p. 45)
Comprehension (KĂM-prĭ-HĔN-shŭn, p. 47)
Distracters (dĭ-STRĂK-tĕrz, p. 57)
External distractions (p. 42)
Idea sketches (p. 52)
Internal distractions (p. 42)
Key concepts (p. 45)
Mapping (p. 45)
Mental imagery (p. 52)
Mnemonic devices (nĭ-MŎN-ĭc, p. 54)
Options (p. 57)
Outlining method (p. 45)

Keep in Mind

Prove research wrong. Spruce up your study skills and sail through test days at school stress free. This includes NCLEX-PN®. After this biggest of tests you will say, "That wasn't so bad after all!"

Many vocational schools and junior colleges offer courses in how to study before learners enter a program, and have departments that offer study skill services after a learner is enrolled. There are millions of Internet sites that provide information about study skills. Despite these resources, lack of study skills, including test-taking skills, is a major factor for failure in nursing school (Kinser, 2005). Learners who need these services are not always aware that they need them. Learners cannot assume they have the study skills necessary to succeed in the practical/vocational nursing program because they have attended high school or college. It takes time and effort to comprehend, store, and recall the knowledge and skills needed for critical thinking in your chosen career. Returning adults and any learner with many responsibilities outside of school will benefit from improvement of study skills.

GENERAL HINTS FOR LEARNERS

CONCENTRATION

Concentration is the ability to keep your mind completely on the task at hand. The major enemy of concentration is distraction. Many distractions in a learner's life compete with the need to buckle down to school assignments. These distractions can be summarized as two types: (1) those that come from outside yourself (external distractions) and (2) those that come from inside yourself (internal distractions).

External Distractions

External distractions occur in your physical and social environments. An obvious distraction is hunger. Be sure you have met hunger needs before settling in to study. Nutritious snacks can provide reason for needed breaks.

Personal Study Area. Your physical environment is a potential enemy of concentration. Locate one or two realistic areas for studying. These chosen areas should be associated with learning, not with daydreaming or napping. If your school has a learning resource center, it can be used between classes and after school. Many times study rooms can be reserved. Another area can be a place in your home or apartment. This could be the kitchen, a corner of your bedroom, or part of the basement. The place you choose needs to be away from family or roommates. A writing surface, a lamp, and a chair are necessary. Have on hand a supply of pens, sharpened pencils, highlighters, loose-leaf paper, scrap paper, index cards, a calendar, an English dictionary, a thesaurus, a medical or nursing dictionary, and add additional tools that help you learn. Keep these items organized and readily available. You will save time and aggravation by not having to look for your study tools each time you sit down to study. Choose a chair you feel comfortable in, but not one that you associate with snoozing. Avoid studying in bed.

Lighting. The light you choose for studying is almost more important than your chair. Many students have a table lamp. This is fine as long as the bulb is shaded and your writing surface is light enough to reflect light. It is important to eliminate glare. The shade and light surface will help in this matter. Try using a "soft white" light bulb to further reduce glare. Be sure that the bulb is screwed into its socket to ensure a tight connection and reduce flicker. If a ceiling light is also available, turn this on in addition to your table lamp to reduce shadows. There are reading lamps available that advertise natural white light and a light grid to reduce eye-tiring glare.

Eyestrain can occur if lighting allows glare, shadows, or flicker to exist in your study area. If you have tried to eliminate these three unwanted lighting conditions and still experience symptoms of eyestrain, such as headaches, dizziness, tiredness, or blurred vision while reading, it is time to have an eye examination to rule out the need for corrective lenses. Some learners discover that they need glasses only after they enroll in an educational program that demands much reading, such as the practical/vocational nursing program.

Background Noise. Keep in mind that research studies on learning styles show that some learners concentrate better with background sounds (e.g., music, voices). Other learners require quiet surroundings. Honestly identify the type of environment that allows you to get the most out of your study time. Your grades will be the criteria by which you can judge whether your environment is helping or hurting. Strive for a study environment that meets your learning style preference (see Chapter 2). If you require a quiet environment, sometimes home does not provide this. Past learners have told us they were successful in disciplining themselves to ignore noise at home and concentrate on studying. Television, stereos, and iPods are considered background noise. Despite learning style preferences, some learners state that they study best in the presence of these external distractions. If these habits are a carryover from high school and are interfering with your concentration, establish new habits to help you with your more difficult subjects. High school and college study habits do not automatically guarantee success in the practical/vocational nursing program.

Learning Exercise

Personal Distractions

List any external distractions that are affecting your concentration.

_____

_____

What can you do to eliminate these distractions?

_____

_____

_____

_____

Internet. The Internet offers a vast amount of resources for all your classes. You may have assignments that need to be completed by using the Internet. Much can be learned and discovered on the World Wide Web. Watch your time when you are online because hours can slip by before you know it. It is easy to get distracted by the information available on the Internet.

Your Peers. Have you considered your peers as a possible external distraction? The energy devoted to any of the activities in the following exercise can seriously deplete the energy needed to achieve success in the practical/vocational nursing program. These behaviors can also create unneeded stress and frustration.

Learning Exercise

Your Peers at School

Answer the following questions about your peers in the practical/vocational nursing program.

1. Are the persons you associate with at school encouraging your progress in the practical/vocational nursing program?
2. Do you and your peers support and encourage each other?
3. Do you pick a special person to sit with in class so you can privately chat while others are talking?
4. Do you seek out other students who have negative attitudes? If so, what are the conversations you engage in during a supposedly relaxing coffee break?

5. Do the people you associate with love to belittle, complain, and tear down the instructor, the course, and various students in your group?
6. Does your anxiety level increase when you carpool with certain students on test days?

_____

Internal Distractions

You can have the perfect desk, lighting, chair, noise level, equipment, and peers for studying but still not be able to keep your mind on the task at hand. The culprit may be distractions arising from inside you. The following two paragraphs contain common examples of internal distractions and suggestions for overcoming them.

Complaints of Mental Fatigue. Some learners confuse boredom with fatigue. In setting up a study schedule, make sure you do not study one subject so long that you get bored with it. Keep up your physical self with proper food, sleep, and exercise. At the first sign of getting tired, take a short break (not a snooze) and come back to new material so that you can get your mental second wind.

Daydreaming. Daydreaming can be a creative adventure or wasted time. Every time you find your mind wandering from the topic at hand, try putting a check mark on a piece of paper that you keep at your side. This may remind you that you are drifting off and need to get back to work. Students who use this technique find that the number of check marks decreases dramatically with time.

Learning Exercise

Daydreaming

List four topics that you daydream about when studying.

_____

_____

_____

_____

_____

Other Techniques for Improving Concentration

To improve their concentration, learners have used the following techniques successfully. Try them to see whether they can help you.

Using simple tools such as a pencil or highlighter will keep you active in your learning. Underlining or highlighting main ideas, writing in the margins, or diagramming what you are studying, and so on will keep you active and your concentration at its peak. Remember the hints related to your personal learning style (see Chapter 2).

LISTENING

The Active and Passive Listener

The human voice takes up much of class time. Whether you are involved in a minilecture class, discussion, or activity, or are viewing videotapes and CD-ROMs as part of course assignments, you are going to miss a lot if your mind wanders. Listening is much more than the mechanical process of hearing. There are two kinds of listeners. Which type are you?

- The passive listener receives sounds with little recognition or personal involvement. This listener may be doodling, staring out the window, or even staring at the instructor, but thinking about having to change the oil in the car or deciding what to cook for dinner.
- The active listener is always thinking, not just hearing the words. Active listeners listen with full attention, are open-minded and curious, and are always asking themselves questions about the content. The active listener, who really listens to hear, is searching for relevant information and strives to understand it, and is always trying to figure out how content fits into the big picture. Active listeners realize that listening is an important method of gathering information, and they work at developing this skill. The active listener looks for ways in which the speaker's words can be put to practical use regardless of the student's level of interest in, or degree of, fondness for the instructor or the instructor's dress or mannerisms. Box 4-1 gives you hints to become an active listener.

Box 4-1 | *Hints for Active Listening*

- Be well rested for class.
- Complete assignments, extra readings, and exercises before class.
- Focus on what is happening with the lesson. Listen for key information, central ideas, examples, and study hints, not facts.
- Ask questions before, during, and after class.
- Make eye contact with the speaker.
- Listen when other students are speaking.
- Seek help when a difficult concept is not understood.

 Learning Exercise

Active Versus Passive Listener

Identify and list behaviors that indicate you are an active or passive listener.

My active listening behaviors:

_____

_____

My passive listening behaviors:

_____

_____

_____

Note Making Versus Note Taking

An important part of listening is remembering what you have listened to. Some students say that taking notes interferes with their listening skills. They are correct if they are in the business of taking notes. Research has shown that a student remembers only 50% of a 10-minute lecture when tested immediately afterward and only 25% of that lecture when tested 2 days later. You can improve those percentages to as much as 80% to 90%. The secret is to engage in note making whenever you are listening. Because teachers derive test questions from minilectures, discussions, activities, videotapes, CD-ROMs, and readings, that 80% to 90% of a specific learning activity could translate into a comparable test score. Note making will help you to pay attention, concentrate, and organize your ideas.

Suggestions for Note Making. Never try to capture every word the speaker says. This is *note taking* and is impossible. A speaker can put out 100 to 125 words or more per minute. Time yourself to find how many words you can write per minute. Ask a peer to read for 1 minute while you try to write everything down. The number of words you wrote will shock you. Besides not being able to get every word down, you will also not be able to capture the meaning of what was said. Instead, strive for *note making*, formulating condensations of what is said in a telegram-like manner. Actively listen for the main ideas. Capture them in a way that reflects your personal learning style or styles. You are recording ideas or key concepts that you will later add to, correct, and study. Your goal is to understand the information, *not* memorize it.

One 8.5 × 11-inch loose-leaf notebook with dividers is suggested to be used for all your courses. Spiral notebooks have the disadvantage of not allowing handouts to be included easily with daily notes. With the loose-leaf system the notebook can be left at home and a supply of paper taken to school daily. Make sure your name, address, and telephone number are on your papers and in the notebook in case you misplace them.

Avoid taking notes in shorthand. Shorthand notes have to be transcribed after class, another poor time-management technique. Develop your own personal symbols, abbreviations, and shorthand of sorts to help you capture the main ideas, yet retain readability without having to transcribe the notes. Use abbreviations as presented in your charting classes. Make your notes in pen so they don't smudge. When a mistake is made, cross out the error. Erasing is time consuming. Avoid typing or rewriting your class notes word for word. Instead, use this time to think about what is important in the notes and condense as you rewrite. This is especially helpful for visual learners. At first your notes may seem to be a disaster, but remember that you are not competing for a penmanship award. With practice, they will improve. Your goal is a set of notes you can use today, next week, and at the end of the program for review for the NCLEX-PN® examination.

Two Methods for Making and Reviewing Notes

Outlining Method. The first method is the outlining method, which has been used for ages. Outlining is especially popular with left-brain dominant individuals. Outlining with some adaptations can result in a format that encourages active learning and critical thinking. It involves adapting normal loose-leaf paper so that you have room to take notes, summarize content, and test yourself on your notes. This method can be used to prepare yourself continuously for testing of the material. This method is also useful for making notes when reading textbooks, viewing videotapes, and other audiovisual materials. Figure 4-1 is an example of traditional note making, used to summarize this chapter so far.

The actual form used can be adapted to your preference. Suggestions for note making using the outlining method can be found in Box 4-2. Some students think that writing material in note form alone will help them retain the material. Active and frequent review of your notes is an important step in retention of material so that you can recall it at a later time.

Mapping (concept map). Brain researchers have suggested an alternative to the linear method of note making. It encourages using the right side of the brain, with its emphasis on images. Color and drawings are processed by the right side of the brain and are important components in mapping. Information presented in a linear manner, as in traditional note making, is not as easily understood as information presented by key concepts. The use of key concepts is the primary way in which the brain processes information. The brain takes these key concepts and integrates them in relationships. So, if the brain does not work in lines or lists, the method of note making called mapping can enhance your ability to understand, review, and recall this information. Mapping is a method in which information is organized graphically so that it is seen in a visual pattern of relationships. Mapping is most meaningful to the person who draws the map. Box 4-3 gives hints for note making, using the mapping method. Figure 4-2 is an example of a summary of this chapter so far using clustering, a basic form of mapping that helps simplify topics. Clustering is especially helpful for visual learners.

	Assig.	*5-17-09*
	Test p. 200-220	*510-863*
	Be ready to discuss	
	Objectives 2 & 3 *Note Making*	
Benefits of Note Making	*1. Improve rate of remembering*	
(I'll understand the	*2. Pay attention*	
material)	*3. Therefore, concentrate*	
	4. Organize ideas	
Definition of Note Taking	*• Note Taking:*	
	* — capture every word*	
	* — speak 110-160 wpm*	
	* — time self in dictation*	
	* — don't get any meaning*	
Definition of Note Making	*• Note Making:*	
	* — condensation of what said*	
	* * like telegram*	
Hints for N.M.	* — actively listen for main ideas*	
	* — use loose-leaf notebook*	
	* — divisions for each class*	
	• Identify each division	
	* — never tape-record—poor T.M.—3 for 1?*	
	* — don't use shorthand*	
	* * time to transcribe—poor T.M.*	
Why pen?	* * develop own abbreviations and symbols*	
	* * use med. abbrev.*	
	* * use pen*	
	* * cross out errors*	
Methods of Note Making	*• 2 Methods of Note Making*	
How to... ⓛ Brain	*1. Standard linear tool (top: date, course #, assignment)*	
	* — ⓛ—extend margins 1"*	
	* — Ⓡ—notes*	
	* Bottom 1"—summary of page.*	
	After class—ⓛ margin—write cues as key words. Write in questions	
	or comments. Gives visual organization, (ⓛ) brain emphasis)	
How to... Ⓡ Brain	*2. Mapping—info organized graphically, (Ⓡ brain). Info adds relationships*	
Color would be good	*in visual patterns, understanding, review, recall.*	
here.	* — Put key concept in center and circle it*	
	* — Arrange key concepts around this*	
	* — Connect these ideas to main key concept with lines*	
	* — Clustering—an unstructured map*	
	Can't just listen to lecture. Must make notes. Listen actively and make	
	condensations of key concepts/main ideas. Use standard linear method or	
	try mapping.	
	Benefits: concentration and understanding, improves test scores.	
	REVIEW NOTES AFTER CLASS!	

FIGURE **4-1** Traditional note making.

Regardless of the side of your brain dominance, you can benefit by using each of the aforementioned methods of note making. Some nursing programs have found mapping helpful in developing critical thinking skills by having learners use this format to develop nursing care plans as concept maps, instead of the traditional column format.

Hints for Note Making: Outlining Method

- Use the margin at the top of the page to write the date and course number and any assignments that are given.
- Extend the left margin another inch. Take your notes in your personal learning style to the right of this line.
- After class, in the area at the left of the page, record key words or phrases that serve as cues for the class activity on the right. Also use this area as a space for questions or comments. These will be used to clarify your understanding of content.
- The bottom inch of each page should be left blank. A summary of the content of the notes on that page, in your own words, can be made in this section. This summary forces you to think about and come to grips with the ideas in your notes. You are critically thinking about the information, not passively copying it to be memorized later.

Hints for Note Making: Mapping Method

- Start with your note paper in a horizontal position.
- Draw a small circle in the middle of the paper.
- Put the main topic of the activity in the circle.
- Add branches off the circle for important ideas or subtopics. Arrange these branches like spokes of a wheel. Use a different colored pen for each of the branches. Draw more branches off branches, as needed for each topic.
- Draw a picture to go with each key topic or idea. Artistic ability does not count here. What is important is that the picture gives meaning to you.

HOW TO UNDERSTAND (COMPREHEND) INFORMATION

READING ASSIGNMENTS

"I read the material four times and got a D. My friend read the material once and got an A. It isn't fair." The learner who is speaking is correct. It takes a lot of time to read material four times for a test. The missing ingredient is lack of understanding (comprehension) of information that is read. To think critically in nursing, you must have information. To acquire information, you must be able to read with understanding. Reading with understanding makes possible retention of the information. Retention ensures recall. Earning only a D by merely reading words is a poor return on your time investment. Did you ever drive somewhere without remembering how you got there? That is the same as reading the text four times or getting to the end of a page and not knowing what you read. These readers have zoned out and have mindless reading. As they read, their minds will be somewhere else. They may be hungry, thirsty, tired, need to go to the restroom, or thinking about other things. Their comprehension of the information is low to absent and test scores will suffer (Feller, 2006).

To think critically you must have information. To acquire information you must be able to read with understanding. Because you are responsible for large amounts of reading in the practical/vocational nursing program, the ability to read with understanding (comprehension) is a necessary skill. Most of us are able to read printed words on a page. However, the reading demanded of a learner and future employee requires understanding of the meaning of words we read. Reading to learn and understand involves a rate of speed and degree of understanding that are effective.

You probably had to take a reading test as part of your pre-entrance tests for the practical/vocational nursing program. Generally these tests are brief. If you scored low, you were referred for help with this skill. Perhaps you were one of those who achieved an acceptable score on these short-reading tests, but could use some hints on how to increase your reading efficiency. Evaluate your reading habits by answering "yes" or "no" to the questions in the following learning exercise.

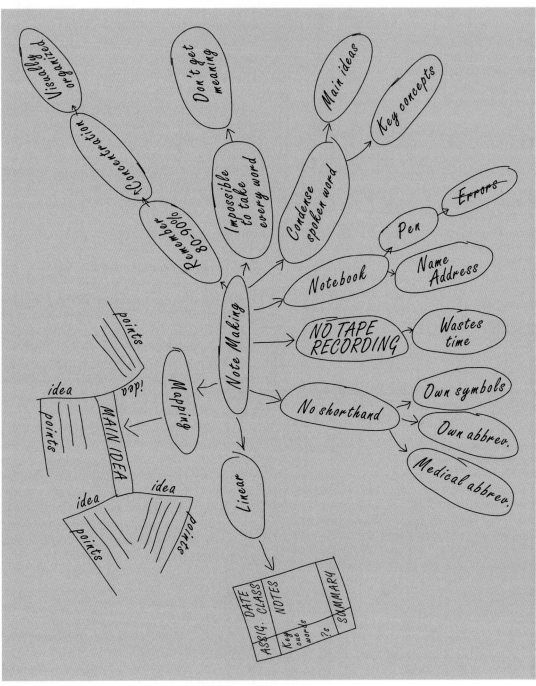

FIGURE **4-2** Clustering.

Learning Exercise

Reading Habit Evaluation

Circle the reading habits that apply to you.

1. Do you ever reread a sentence before you come to the end?
2. Do you ever have trouble figuring out the main point of an author?
3. Do you stop reading every time you come across a word you cannot define, and look up the word immediately?
4. Do you read novels, popular magazines, newspapers, and textbooks at the same speed?
5. Do you ever have trouble remembering what you read?
6. Do you have trouble understanding what you have read?
7. Do you ever think of other things while you read?
8. Do you read every word of a sentence individually?
9. Do you focus on details when you read?
10. Do you tire quickly when reading?
11. Do you skip uncommon words when you read?

If you answered yes to any of the previous questions, you could benefit from help with your reading. A trip to your school's study skill center (if you have one), or consulting with your instructor for assistance with reading, can help improve skill in reading more efficiently and effectively.

PQRST Method of Textbook Study

The experts in study skills have come up with a variety of study systems for using textbooks and related reading materials. We have chosen the PQRST method as described by Staton (1959) in *How to Study*, which is still available today. The PQRST method is a critical-thinking approach to reading and mastering content. It increases comprehension of material by ensuring that information is stored in long-term memory. Each letter of the PQRST method stands for a step in the study method: Preview, Question, Read, State, and Test. *Regardless of the length of time available for studying, studies have shown that learners who use each step of this method consistently scored higher on tests.* Each of the five steps in the method needs to be used. Learners have reported that the

system is easier to use than they thought it would be. Each of the five steps will be discussed by identifying the meaning and benefits of each step, describing how to carry out the steps, and why they work.

P = Preview

What It Means. Preview is an overview or survey of what the material is about. It gives you the general big picture of what the author wants to accomplish, not the fine details.

Benefits. Previewing helps you look for and recognize important points or main ideas of the reading material.

Why It Works. The Preview step makes you reflect or think about the material. It also increases your concentration level. You become active in your reading. These are important elements in the storage of information in long-term memory.

How to Do It

1. When you first buy your textbooks, look at their table of contents to get a general sense of the organization of the books.
2. Read the Preface to find out the author's purpose for writing the book, the organization of the material, letter to the Instructor, letter to the student, and suggestions for reading the book.
3. Before reading each assignment:
   a. Read each of the topics and headings.
   b. Read the summary.
   c. Read the first and last sentences of each paragraph.
   d. Using the general hints listed for reading, read the assignment.

Q = Question

What It Means. As you preview the reading material, ask yourself questions that may be answered when you read.

Benefits. Formulating your own questions, as well as using the author's questions, will give you pointers about what details to look for in your reading. These questions will help you prepare for examinations.

Why It Works. By providing you with clues, this step points out what to look for in your reading. The Question step also makes you reflect on your reading and increase your concentration level. You become active in your reading.

How to Do It

1. Look at the chapter title and each heading.
2. Turn titles and headings into questions.
3. If questions are included at the end of a chapter, read these questions before going on to the next step.
4. Most authors include learning objectives at the beginning of each chapter. Use these objectives to keep your mind inquisitive and to seek ends to these objectives.

R = Read

What It Means. In this stage you actually read the material. You are now gathering information to be stored in your long-term memory. Look carefully at pictures and charts. They may contain new information or clarify what you have read.

Benefits. You will accumulate information and facts and be able to store them in long-term memory.

Why It Works. Being an active reader by seeking answers to the questions you have formulated will keep up your level of concentration. This allows you to store information in your brain's long-term memory.

How to Do It

1. Review the Hints to Reading Effectively on page 51.
2. Practice these hints so you can remain active during this step. You are seeking the answers to the questions you formulated.
3. If you own the text, underline key phrases as you read.
4. If you own the text, write notes in the margin of the text.

S = State

What It Means. To state means to repeat, in your own words, what you have read.

Benefits. You will understand the organization of the material you are reading and the relationship of the facts to each other. By increasing comprehension, you will be able to apply the information in the clinical area. Rote memory fails when it comes time to apply information on tests, and in the clinical area. Stating content in your own words will help you evaluate whether you did indeed store the information.

Why it Works. Stating something aloud involves another sense (hearing). This provides an additional channel for information to be stored. Stating facts in your own words indicates understanding of the material.

How to Do It

1. At the end of each paragraph, look away from your book.
2. Ask yourself the main ideas that were covered in the paragraph.
3. State the ideas aloud and in your own words. This is the key to the success of this step. As you become more proficient in this step, you will find that you are able to read more than one paragraph and still state the main ideas and the answers to the questions you have formulated.
4. Review your marginal notes.
5. Try to go into detail about your marginal notes.

T = Test

What It Means. This final step occurs several times after your first study session and involves testing yourself on what you remember.

Benefits. Because the testing step is ongoing, it will indicate your weak areas. This gives you time to remedy them before an examination. Better grades are sure to follow.

Why It Works. This stage settles once and for all whether the information is in your long-term memory. It also indicates your comprehension of the material. When you identify your weak spots, you can review them and make sure they are retained in your long-term memory. You will be covering the information in small doses, but more often. This activity is the best way to encourage the brain to remember.

How to Do It

1. The testing stage is really a review stage.
2. Review your marginal notes.
3. Restate the main ideas presented in the chapter.
4. Review your class notes.
   a. Relate class notes to the information in the textbook.

b. Write the information you are having trouble with on index cards, to be carried with you so you can test yourself while on the run.

PQRST Method Tips. To be effective, experts suggest that nearly half your study time be devoted to the Preview and Read steps. The other half should be devoted to the Question, State, and Test steps. These steps require critical thinking (reflective thinking), use of your memory, and organization of ideas through your own efforts. The strength of this system lies in the State step. The reflective thinking required in this step takes work. Resist the temptation to skip over the State step.

 Critical Thinking Exercise

Improving Reading Habits

Write your plan to increase reading efficiency and effectiveness. Note how you will determine progress.

Reading Effectively

1. Read in phrases, a few words at a time, rather than word by word. Although the brain can view only one word at a time, it understands only when words are in phrases. For better understanding you should read as you speak (i.e., in phrases).
2. Move your lips while reading. Vocalization, whether aloud or to yourself, is a tool used by the auditory learner to increase understanding. For some learners reading aloud, word by word, can decrease speed and comprehension.
3. Put expression into your reading. You do not speak in a monotone, so why read that way? Musical learners can benefit by singing what they read. Try it. It may work for you.
4. Be aware of your reading assignments that are technical or scientific in nature and vary your reading speed accordingly. The more recreational your reading material (e.g., novel or newspaper), the faster you can read. For more technical or scientific material you must slow down. As you

become accustomed to this type of reading you will find yourself increasing your speed. Regardless of your learning style, when the going gets tough in a paragraph of assigned reading, reading the difficult material aloud may help clear up more challenging information.

5. Underline unfamiliar words as you read. When you are finished reading, copy the words on an index card and look them up in the appropriate dictionary. Most of the unfamiliar words you come across will be medical terms, which can be found in the medical dictionary. At first you will think these words are Greek, and you are right. Quite a few of them are derived from the Greek language. The rest are derived from Latin.
6. Write the definition on the other side of the card. Break down the word with vertical slashes into its prefix (the word beginning), root (core word), and suffix (word ending), so that you begin making associations with other words that have the same prefix, root, or suffix. If your medical dictionary does not include this information with each word, the information can be found in medical terminology texts or as part of a computer program in your learning resource center.
7. Nursing involves learning a new language. If possible, include your own drawing to represent the definitions of these words with the verbal definition. This can help you recall the meaning of the word. Using index cards allows your language development to progress because you can take the cards wherever you go. Learning can occur whenever you have a few minutes to spare.
8. Underline key phrases and write in the margin. We assume you own your textbooks. Underlining will keep you active and result in the identification of key concepts for study and review.

Remember, an important part of any textbook is the index found in the back of the book. The subject index includes an alphabetical list of topics. Page numbers are included for information discussed. This index will help you locate information quickly.

VISUAL STRATEGIES TO ENHANCE UNDERSTANDING

Your scholastic world is bombarded with words, sentences, and paragraphs. One of the most beneficial techniques to comprehend and remember all new information is to balance this verbal mixture with visual strategies. Each of the following visual strategies will help you understand and ultimately remember information better. They deal with the right side of the brain. You will be tapping a resource that possibly you have not used often. If you have right-brain dominance, your understanding will be improved by adopting left-brain strategies of organizing information, as discussed in Chapter 2. If you have left-brain dominance, your understanding will be improved by adopting right-brain strategies of organizing information. These strategies include improving the general organization of material and writing and restating new information in your own words.

Draw Idea Sketches

These drawings will probably be comprehensible only to you. The emphasis of idea sketches is not on the quality of the drawing, but on the process you must go through to take a verbal concept and represent it graphically, without words. To go through this process you must understand the verbal concept. You can even set it up as a cartoon. Use stick figures and describe the concept verbally. Figure 4-3 is an idea sketch illustrating the function of the drug Lanoxin (digoxin), which is used to slow and strengthen the heartbeat.

Use Color in Whatever Form of Note Making You Use

Use highlighters, crayons, colored pencils, or felt-tip pens. Avoid merely underlining or highlighting the sentences. Use the different colors to help capture and direct your attention to information that fits in different categories. The different colors will help your brain organize and retrieve information.

Make Your Own Diagrams as You Read

If you commit ideas to memory by using words only, you are using only half of your brain's resources, those of the left side. If you also produce a sketch of that idea, you will have brought the right side of your brain into use. Using both sides of the brain encourages the storage and retrieval of information. Those who rely solely on pictures of ideas, benefit by also using words.

Engage in Mental Imagery

Engaging in mental imagery will help you remember material because it demands that you understand the information. When you use mental imagery, you become the idea that you are having difficulty understanding. The right side of your brain generates pictures of the idea, and the left

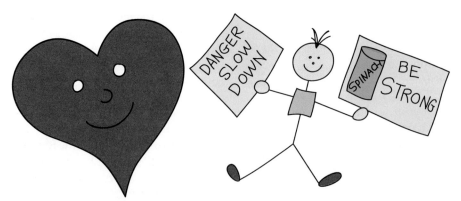

FIGURE **4-3** Idea sketch: Action of Lanoxin (digoxin).

side supplies the script to explain what is going on in the pictures (and always in your own words).

Box 4-4 provides an example of a mental image developed by a practical nursing student to give herself a simple understanding of the function of insulin, a hypoglycemic agent that increases glucose transport across muscle and fat cell membranes. Notice how she uses the senses of hearing and feeling and also body movement to help achieve understanding. She also uses a metaphor, equating something she knows about with something she is trying to learn. The student recites this image to herself while she closes her eyes and visualizes it. First, she had her roommate read the story while she visualized the scenario.

Perhaps a physiologist would wince at this description. However, it is nothing to be ashamed of if it helps you understand a concept. Plus, mental imagery can be fun!

Critical Thinking Exercise

Increasing Understanding of Concepts

Choose a concept you are having trouble with in one of your nursing classes or text readings and try to increase understanding by using the following:
1. Draw an idea sketch.
2. Use mental imagery.

REMEMBERING AND FORGETTING

We all can recall things from the past, indicating that our brains have the ability to store information. But how many times have you said, "I forgot," or "I can't remember"? Possible causes of forgetting include the following:

- A *negative attitude* toward the subject, which interferes with the motivation to remember,
- *New knowledge*, which interferes with the recall of old learning, and
- *Old knowledge*, which interferes with the recall of new learning.

Valid as these causes of forgetting may be, perhaps the most common reason why students cannot remember is that they never understood and stored the information in the first place. They really did not internalize the information and comprehend it to begin with. Perhaps they did not listen actively, or they just read words and created a mental blur.

FROM TEMPORARY TO PERMANENT MEMORY BY WAY OF A NEURAL TRACE

To store information in your long-term memory, a neural trace or record of the information must be laid down. Psychologists have found that it takes 4 to 5 seconds for information to move from the temporary, or short-term, memory to the permanent, or long-term, memory. To form a long-term memory of information, you must strive to understand that information. In doing so, you will give your brain the chance to lay down a neural trace. Presto! You have created a memory of that information. Short but frequent study periods with concentration will help you

---

Box 4-4 | *Mental Image—I Am Insulin*

I am insulin—a job description. I am insulin, and I am shaped like a canoe. In fact, I am a canoe, a green one. My job is to make the sugar or glucose in the blood available to most of the cells of the body for energy. I like my job. I like things that are sweet but not too sweet, so normal blood sugar is just my thing. Sometime after the person who owns the pancreas where I am stored in my canoe rack eats a meal, a whistle blows, and I know this is a signal for me to launch myself into the bloodstream. As I ride the currents of the blood, I rock gently back and forth and the sugar in the bloodstream jumps right in to be a passenger in the canoe. Blood sugar likes me. I think this is because I am green, but I might be wrong. When I am pretty full, but not full enough to swamp, I pass through the blood vessels, paddle through the sea of tissue fluid (boy, it smells salty) around the cells, and pass through the cell membrane. Then I deposit the sugar by making these molecules jump out of the green canoe and into the fluid inside the cell. I feel pretty important in my job. Without me the blood sugar molecules would be unable to pass through the cell membranes. Because of this, I am given the official job title of hypoglycemic agent. I lower the level of sugar in the blood.

Excuse me. There goes the whistle!

understand information and store it in your long-term memory. Then it is ready for recall.

Remember that positive mental attitude is a factor in learning, allowing you to understand and remember. Remind yourself that all the basic courses in which you are enrolled are essential. They are the building blocks for all the remaining courses you will take in the practical/vocational nursing program. You have already started your career. The following techniques help increase understanding of your studies by allowing neural traces to be recorded in your brain.

- *As you listen or read, seek out key concepts, basic principles, and key ideas. Be selective and learn to sift out and reject unnecessary details.* You cannot memorize everything. If you could, you would not have an understanding of anything. The student who memorizes has difficulty in applying course information and solving problems in the clinical area. The activity of being selective helps you lay down neural traces. Emphasize accuracy, not speed. You want correct information to make a clear neural trace. It is difficult to unlearn wrong information and replace it with correct information.

- *Short study periods followed by short rest periods are better than long study marathons.* This type of study will re-energize you and allow neural learning to continue during rest periods. Those seemingly wasted 10 minutes between classes or standing in the cafeteria line can be used to your advantage. It seems that cramming for examinations is treated like a rite of passage among some students. Brain research has shown that short but frequent study periods help you store information in long-term memory. This will make the information available for testing and later for application in the clinical area.

- *Use as many body senses and as much body movement as possible when trying to learn new information.* Recite the information aloud as you read, using your own words. If you can explain it, you must understand it and will know it. Hearing yourself say the information aloud is an additional channel that allows neural traces to be recorded. Write down the information in your own words. This muscle action will help you clarify ideas and improve thinking. *Do not copy word by word from a book.*

The following techniques of using body senses and body movement are all elements of tactual learning discussed in Chapter 2. They help lay down a neural trace. Try them—they may work for you. Adopt the suggestions that help you understand the material in your classes. They will increase your long-term memory of that information.

- Vary your body position while studying. Lean against a wall. Sit on the floor. Pace. You will keep alert and awake.

- Using your muscles by gesturing can help improve memory of information by matching a gesture to information that needs to be remembered. When the gesture and word are associated in your mind, performing the gesture can retrieve the word.

- Physical motion can jog memory and promote recall. You should see some of the motions students go through during an examination! If it works, don't knock it.

MEMORY AIDS

Mnemonic devices are examples of memory aids. You know what they are. Some examples include the following:

- *Rhymes*
  Thirty days hath September…
  I before e except after c…
  In fourteen hundred and ninety-two…

- *Acronyms*
  Every good boy does fine (to remember the line notes of the treble clef in music)
  There are also devices in nursing that can help you remember information. For example:

- *CMTSP* (for assessment of the nerve and blood supply to an extremity)
  C = color
  M = motion
  T = temperature
  S = sensation
  P = pulse

- *PERRLA* (for assessment of the pupils)
  P = pupils
  E = equal in size
  R = round
  R = regular in shape
  L = react to light
  A = accommodation (pupils constrict)

Memorizing these acronyms can help the practical/vocational nurse remember a series of information. They do not take the place of or help you to understand the information.

HINTS FOR SUCCESSFUL TEST TAKING

Focus on remaining an active learner in all your classes. Set a goal to understand the information you are learning with an eye to application of that learning. The majority of items on the NCLEX-PN® examination are written at the application or analysis levels of cognitive abilities. (Test plan for the National Council licensure examination for licensed practical/vocational nurses, effective April 2008.) You can anticipate application or higher type of questions as part of theory tests in the practical/vocational nursing program.

Test-taking skills are divided into two general areas: (1) preparing for the test, and (2) actually taking the test. The following sections address these areas.

PREPARATION FOR THE TEST
Preparation for Test Taking Begins the First Day of Class

Preparation includes: (1) your system of note making for class and assignments, and (2) your goal of understanding information as a preparation for tests and for clinical performance, and the focus on application and analysis for these activities.

Clarify Content to Be Covered on the Test and the Form of the Test

Avoid asking what will be on the test. You already know what will be on the test. The instructor will be measuring your understanding and application of understanding of all the objectives that the test covers. Clarify the types of questions that will be asked on the tests. For example, will the test be multiple choice and/or short answer? Specific hints for taking multiple-choice and short-answer tests are included in this chapter.

Periodically Review the Material You Have Already Studied

This hint is necessary to get the information into your long-term memory. Use the Test step of the PQRST method often, and the audible recitation suggested. Make index cards of the material you are having difficulty understanding. Cramming—last-minute studying of new material for a test—sometimes results in short-term memory of material that might help you pass a test. However, because you did not engage in repetitions spaced over days, storage in long-term memory will not occur and application of the material to the clinical area will be difficult. Cramming for an examination is like packing your suitcase for a vacation at the last minute. You will wind up with a suitcase filled with things you do not need and a whole list of things you forgot to bring.

Use Time-Management Techniques to Help You Organize Your Time Before the Test

Make a schedule to help identify study times to do a grand review for each test. Do not reread the textbook. You have already completed your reading with understanding. Because you have studied the material periodically since the last test and used study-skill techniques, all you must do at this point is focus on your summaries, margin writings, underlinings, and index cards to check your understanding and retention of the information. The night before the test, do a review early in the evening, do something you find relaxing, and go to bed at your usual time.

TAKING THE TEST

Arrive at the classroom with plenty of time to get your favorite seat, arrange your pencils, and so on. Beware of peers who may try to get you nervous by saying, "You didn't study *that*, did you?" or "You mean you *didn't* study that?" It may be best for some students to arrive just in time for the test so they do not have to listen to all that chatter. You organized your time and systematically reviewed for this test. Keep a positive mental attitude. Silently rehearse your facts to keep out distractions. Take slow, deep breaths to reduce tension. It is almost test time and you are ready!

Would you believe that some people who have organized their notes and their time, systematically reviewed, and understood the material have nevertheless done poorly in tests? The main reason for this could be that they did not follow the directions on the test. How well do you follow directions? Take out a blank sheet of paper and test yourself on the following exercise.

Learning Exercise

How Well Do You Follow Directions?

Directions: Read the following directions carefully. You will have 1 minute to do the exercise after reading the directions. Be sure to write legibly. When you have finished, check your answers against the directions before handing in the paper. Be sure to read the entire exercise before beginning.

1. On a sheet of paper, print your name in the upper left-hand corner, last name first.
2. Under your name, write the last four digits of your Social Security number.
3. In the upper right-hand corner, write the name and number of the course for which you are taking this exercise.
4. In the lower left-hand corner of the paper, write today's date.
5. In the lower right-hand corner, write your instructor's name, last name first.
6. Fold your paper in half lengthwise.
7. Number the left half of your paper 1 to 6, skipping three lines between each number.
8. Number the right half of your paper 7 to 12, skipping three lines between each number.
9. Now that you have read all of the exercise, do only No. 1 of the exercise and hand your paper to the instructor.

How did you do? If you did not follow the directions, do you feel tricked? You were not. The directions were clear, and you simply did not follow them. Listen meticulously to oral directions

and read the written directions completely before each test. To those of you who did follow the directions for this exercise: Keep up the good work! If directions are ever unclear, ask the instructor before proceeding. Clarify the time limit of the examination. Now you are ready to begin. The following hints will come in handy for test taking.

- Quickly skim the entire examination to set up an overall picture of the types of questions on the test, so you will be able to figure out the amount of time you can devote to each section. Then answer the questions you know well. This will boost your confidence level.
- Avoid spending large amounts of time on difficult questions and do not get upset about them. Both these activities waste time and do not earn points. Go on to the next question and return to the skipped item later. However, be aware that on the NCLEX-PN® examination, you will not be able to skip items and then go back to them. For the NCLEX-PN® examination, you need to answer each item as it comes up on the test.
- Take the full time for the test. If you finish early, try to answer the questions you skipped. This brings up the point of guessing at answers. If you are not penalized for guessing, answer all the questions. However, if the test will be graded by subtracting the number of wrong answers from the number of right answers, generally speaking, do not guess.
- Make sure you have not missed an item or group of items.
- If it is a multiple-choice examination, make sure your answers match up with the proper slot on the answer sheet. The instructor cannot possibly know you put the answer to number 37 in the slot for number 36.
- Should you change an answer? Although research has shown that test scores are generally improved by changing answers, we have seen many learners decrease their test scores by the same action. If you have given the item further thought and feel it should be changed, change it. Test by test,

keep tabs on your test scores to see whether changing answers is helping your final score and modify your behavior accordingly.

- If you are using a separate answer sheet that will be machine corrected, be sure you erase your first answer completely if you change answers.

REVIEWING YOUR TESTS

Chapter 1 discussed tests as a learning tool. When the examination is corrected and returned to you, do the following:

1. Read the items you missed. Why are they wrong? Did you make a careless mistake? Did you know the material? Can you correct the item without looking in your textbook or notes? If not, look up the answer.
2. Read the items you answered correctly. What did you do right to get credit for these items?
3. Decide which of your study skills and test-taking techniques are and are not working to your benefit. Modify your test-taking strategies accordingly.

HINTS FOR SPECIFIC TESTS

The types of tests you will be taking in the practical/vocational nursing program, including the NCLEX-PN® examination, are achievement tests. They measure how much you have learned. Achievement tests are of two types: objective and subjective.

Objective Tests–Multiple Choice

Objective achievement tests include multiple-choice questions, which are called items. Each multiple-choice item includes a stem, three distracters, and a key. The stem is the first line of an item. It defines the situation for which the learner must pick out the correct answer. The stem is presented as a sentence or a question. Four statements, called options, follow the stem. Three of the options are incorrect answers and are called distracters. One of the options is the correct answer and is called the key. The format of the NCLEX-PN® examination is multiple-choice items most of which measure application or higher levels of nursing knowledge. Box 4-5 gives general hints for taking multiple-choice tests.

Box 4-5 | ***Multiple-Choice Test Hints***

- Read over all the options given before making any decision.
- Eliminate the options you know are definitely wrong.
- When a number is involved, consider the number in the mid-range.
- Remember the course subject matter for which you are being tested.
- Eliminate options that are not related to the subject matter.

Subjective Tests–Short-Answer Items

Subjective achievement tests include short-answer items. In short-answer items you are given a statement that requires you to (1) complete the statement with one word, (2) fill in a blank or two, or (3) provide an answer in one or two sentences. Box 4-6 gives hints for taking short-answer tests. Samples of these two test forms are included here to help you understand them.

Box 4-6 | ***Hints for Short-Answer Tests***

- Think before you write.
- Be sure to give the information that the statement asks for.
- If sentences are required, watch the verbs in these items, and do what they ask you to do. For example, list means to record a series of things; compare and contrast requires identifying how things are alike and different.
- Give objective, concrete answers.
- Write complete sentences.
- Concentrate on packing information into your answer if sentences are requested.

Learning Exercise

Multiple-Choice Items

Choose the appropriate option (the key) for the following multiple-choice statements. There is only one answer to each multiple-choice statement.

1. Multiple-choice items are examples of:
   1. Sentences for which one-word answers are required.
   2. Questions or sentences with four options for answers.
   3. Two vertical columns that must be matched item by item.
   4. Statements that require a sentence on the answer sheet.
2. When answering multiple-choice options, it is not necessary to:
   1. Read all of the directions.
   2. Eliminate wrong options
   3. Read each of the options.
   4. Ignore any negative words.

Answers to Multiple-Choice Statements

1. Key = 2. A question or sentence is given with four options. Only one option, the key, is correct. The rest of the options are distracters; that is, options that are there to test whether you really have learned the material and can apply it. Option 1 describes fill-in-the-blank items, option 3 describes matching tests, and option 4 describes short-answer items.
2. Key = 4. This multiple-choice item contains a negative word in the stem that can complicate things. Read the stem without the negative word to get some meaning out of it, and then read the options. One option should not fit in with the others. Now reread the original stem with the negative word and see whether the option you have already isolated fits in. Items with negative words in the stem are sometimes accused of being more of a reading test than a test of understanding of content. Although the test begins with directions, there may be additional directions before individual multiple-choice items. These directions may ask you to select one best answer or select what is most important of four correct answers. A new type of item on the NCLEX-PN® examination may ask you to select all options that apply. *Remember, do not stop reading when you think you have the correct answer.* There may be a better option yet to come. Incidentally, options 1, 2, and 3 are true.

Multiple-choice items are not "multiple-guess" items. Think through each response thoroughly before choosing your answer. Should you ever guess? To be able to make a decision about guessing, you must know whether you will be penalized for wrong answers. Even if you are penalized, figure out the odds. If you can eliminate one distracter for certain, you have a better chance of answering correctly. Can you eliminate two out of four distracters? Your chances are now even better. You make the decision. Remember, on the NCLEX-PN® examination you will have to answer every item as it comes.

Answers to Short-Answer Items

1. In a short-answer item, you are given a simple command to complete an incomplete statement, fill in the blank, or provide an answer in one or two sentences on your answer sheet.
2. Seven hints for answering short-answer items include:
   a. Think before you write.
   b. Be sure to give the information that the statement asks for.
   c. Watch the verbs in these items, and do what they ask you to do.
   d. Give objective, concrete answers.
   e. Write in complete sentences.
   f. Concentrate on packing information into your answer.
   g. If you must fill-in-the-blank, place only one word per blank.

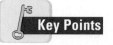 **Key Points**

- Learning how to learn is important because study skills enable the SPN/SVN to understand and store in long-term memory the theory and skills required to be a practical/vocational nurse.
- When theory and skills are stored in long-term memory, they can be retrieved or recalled as the basis for critical thinking.
- Perhaps your most important skill for success in the practical/vocational nursing program is your reading skill.
- The PQRST method of reading a textbook is an effective technique for storing information in your

long-term memory, so that it is available to recall for tests and can be applied in the clinical area.
- There is no easy way to learn information.
- Techniques that have been proved effective in increasing your level of concentration are creating a personal study area, controlling background sounds, evaluating the influence of peers, and decreasing daydreaming.

- Improving your listening skills requires you to be an active, rather than a passive, listener.
- Effective note making and visual strategies may enhance your ability to understand information.
- Using the suggestions in this chapter, including hints for test taking, can help you succeed in the practical/vocational nursing program.

REVIEW ITEMS

1. Select the type of test that presents the student with a stem and several options from which to choose the correct answer.

   1. Matching
   2. Essay exam
   3. Short answer
   4. Multiple choice

2. Which of the following statements describes the "S" step of the PQRST method of textbook study?

   1. Repeat, in your own words, the main points.
   2. Survey all of the material in the assignment.
   3. Periodically check to see what you remember.
   4. Carefully read charts, tables, figures, and boxes.

3. A student in the practical/vocational nursing program frequently daydreams during classes that use lecture as a learning strategy. What is the most important behavior for this student to improve listening skills?

   1. Doodle to focus on what is being said.
   2. Stare at the instructor while lecturing.
   3. Listen with attention to the instructor.
   4. Focus on instructor mannerisms to stay alert.

4. Which of the following strategies is most effective to increase reading comprehension?

   1. Put concepts in the form of a drawing.
   2. Avoid writing notes in shorthand form.
   3. Make a time line of important concepts.
   4. Use textbook terms to explain concepts.

ALTERNATE FORMAT ITEM

Understanding information that is read in the practical/vocational nursing program is necessary to save that information in long-term memory so that it can be retrieved when needed for critical thinking. Which of the following students are using strategies that help in accomplishing this task? *(Select all that apply.)*

1. Cole, while previewing a reading assignment, formulates questions from chapter titles that he can answer while reading the assignment.

2. James takes a concept that he is having difficulty understanding and creates a story in his own words while visualizing the story.

3. Cheyenne repeats what she reads in her own words after completing the assignment and again several times after the initial reading.

4. Levi takes a verbal concept that he is having difficulty understanding and without using words, draws a picture to explain the concept.

Learning During School, for the NCLEX-PN® Examination, and Beyond

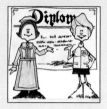

evolve http://evolve.elsevier.com/Hill/success/

On completing this chapter, you will be able to do the following:

1. Identify your knowledge of your school's learning resource center, including:
   a. Resources
   b. Technology
   c. Procedures to obtain resources
   d. How to use technology to obtain resources
2. Discuss the value of reading assignments in periodicals.
3. Use a periodical index; locate an article related to nursing.
4. Discuss six hints used to gain full value from lectures.
5. Discuss your responsibilities for each of the following course learning strategies:
   a. Minilecture, discussion
   b. Cooperative learning
   c. Distance learning
   d. Technology use during learning activities
6. Discuss the purpose of the following resources in your personal learning:
   a. Syllabus or course outline
   b. Nursing skills lab
   c. Study skills lab
   d. Audiovisual materials
   e. Internet
   f. Computer-assisted instruction (CAI)
   g. Simulation
      1) Case scenarios
         a) Paper
         b) Computer
   2) Static mannequins
   3) Electronic mannequins
   4) Virtual clinical excursion
7. Describe how the following resources help you stay current in practical/vocational nursing:
   a. Internet
   b. Periodical indexes
   c. CD-ROMs
   d. Nursing organizations
   e. Community resources
   f. Guest speakers

Key Terms

Audiovisual (AV) materials (ĂW-dē-ō VĬZH-ū-ăl, p. 69)
Bucket theory (p. 64)
Call number (p. 63)
Case scenario (p. 71)
CD-ROM (p. 73)
Community resources (p. 73)
Computer-aided instruction (p. 70)
Computer simulation (SĬM-ū-LĀ-shun, p. 71)
Cooperative learning (kō-OP-ĕr-ă-TĬV, p. 66)
Copyright laws (p. 64)
Course outlines (p. 68)
Database (p. 73)
Discussion buddy (p. 65)
Distance learning (p. 66)
Electronic (p. 64)
Guest speakers (p. 73)
Interlibrary loan services (p. 64)
Internet (p. 63)
Learning resource center (LRC) (p. 61)
Lecture-discussion strategy (p. 66)

Librarian (p. 63)
Nursing organizations (p. 73)
Nursing skills lab (p. 68)
Online catalog (p. 63)
Periodical indexes (p. 71)
Periodicals (PĬR-ē-ŏd-ĭ-kăls, p. 64)
Reference materials (p. 63)
Simulation (p. 71)
Stacks (p. 63)
Study group (p. 68)
Study skills lab (p. 69)
Tutoring (p. 68)
Virtual (p. 63)

 Keep in Mind

Knowing where and how to access nursing information makes keeping up-to-date and passing NCLEX-PN® less stressful. It will protect your nursing license, too.

The focus of this chapter is to provide information about additional resources for information used in practical/vocational nursing. Because you are never done learning, suggestions are given to help you stay up-to-date in nursing for clinical and NCLEX-PN®. Even if you have past experience in an educational program of study, you will find information in this chapter that will help you adjust to and succeed in the practical/vocational nursing program with less stress and frustration.

YOUR SCHOOL'S LEARNING RESOURCE CENTER (LRC)

If you are a returning adult student, you know the learning resource center as the library. *LRC* merely reflects the increased scope of the library in the twenty-first century. The center consists of a lot more than books. How do you feel when you find out you must use the learning resource center? If you have some negative feelings, perhaps it is because you are unfamiliar with the sources of information contained in this resource, their location, and how to use them.

DIFFERENT STUDENT SKILL LEVELS AND DIFFERENT RESOURCES OF THE LRC

All LRCs have similar resources or access to these resources. However, not all LRCs are equal in the areas of resources and technology. The LRC is a large item in any school budget. States faced huge budget deficits in the recent past, and deficits continue. These budget deficits may affect which technology and resources your LRC contains. Some of you are skilled at using the LRC and its resources (Box 5-1). We recognize your ability. If you are skilled in this area, be aware that some of your peers may not be as skilled in using the LRC and its general resources and technology. They will find the hints in this chapter helpful. Because of the differences in your LRC, compared to the LRC of other programs and student differences in skill level, this chapter will focus on what tasks you need to be able to do as a practical/vocational nursing (SPN/SVN) student in your LRC to obtain nursing information for class and clinical (Box 5-2).

- Box 5-1 includes a checklist of tasks you need to carry out to fully use the **general** resources and technology of your LRC for your student year and as a graduate.
- Box 5-2 includes a checklist of tasks you need to carry out to fully use the **nursing** resources and technology of your LRC.

Despite prior LRC experience, you need to identify and correct any deficiencies in regard to using nursing resources and technology in your school's LRC. Knowing how to carry through the tasks will save you time and frustration.

Learning Exercise

Checklist—General and Nursing Resources and Technology

On index cards, list the general and nursing LRC tasks from Boxes 5-1 and 5-2 for which you are not familiar.

Box 5-1 *Checklist of Tasks Needed to Fully Use LRC General Resources and Technology*

Identify which of the following tasks you are able to carry out in your LRC by writing "Yes" next to them. Write "No" next to the tasks you are unable to carry out.

- How does my LRC classify all of its holdings (books, videotapes, periodicals, CD-ROMs, etc.)?
- How can I find the call number of a specific item?
- Once I have the call number, how can I locate a specific item?
- Where do I check out a specific item for home use?
- Can I access resources in our LRC from my home computer?
- How do I check out AV equipment for home use?
- How can I obtain needed resources that are not in my LRC?
- Where are reference materials located (e.g., English dictionary, medical and nursing dictionaries, encyclopedias, almanacs, yearbooks, atlases, handbooks, and other similar categories of books)?
- Can I access learning resources in other schools' LRCs?
- Where is the circulation desk?
- Where are the duplicating machines?
- Are there computers for personal use? Do they have Internet access? Are word processors available?
- Where can I study in the LRC?
- How can I reserve a room for group study?
- Where are pamphlets located?
- Does my school's LRC have a virtual reference program?
- Is there a WiFi hot spot for personal laptop or wireless use?

Box 5-2 *Checklist of Tasks Needed to Fully Use LRC Nursing Resources and Technology*

Identify which of the following tasks you are able to carry out in your LRC and write "Yes" next to them. Write "No" next to the tasks you are unable to carry out.

- Where are the periodical listings located?
- Where are periodical indexes for nursing and general topics located?
- Where are current nursing journals and periodicals located?
- Where are back issues of nursing journals and periodicals stored?
- How can I view back issues of nursing journals and periodicals?
- How can I obtain a copy of articles in back issues of nursing journals and periodicals?
- How can I obtain a copy of an article in a nursing journal or periodical if my LRC does not subscribe to the publication?
- Does my LRC have CD-ROM databases for nursing and general information?
- Where are the nursing texts located in the stacks?
- What is the procedure for accessing nursing materials that have been put on reserve for nursing classes?
- Are personal digital assistants (PDAs) available for use in the clinical area? If so, what nursing information is available for use with a PDA?
- Are portable media players, for example, iPods available for class/clinical use?
- Are nursing clips available for use with personal media players?
- Are earphones supplied?

WHERE TO START

Investigate your learning resource center. Ask for an informational brochure so that you have an idea of the LRC's general hours of operation and physical layout. You will find that your LRC contains a wealth of services that will help make your time in the practical/vocational nursing program easier and less stressful. Ask the librarian the best way for you to find the answers to items on your checklists with which you are unfamiliar. Some LRCs have self-guided tours on audio tape. An hour spent touring the LRC can save you many wasted hours and much frustration later in the school year. LRC staff may offer a personal tour and answer questions. Because the LRC is a learning area, you need to help to keep it a quiet environment. A simple "please" and "thank you" for staff efforts will be appreciated.

Filling in Gaps in My LRC Knowledge

On the index cards you used for the previous learning exercise (Boxes 5-1 and 5-2), list the solutions to the tasks you could not carry out but found by investigating the LRC. To save time when using the LRC, refer to these cards as needed.

General Information About Resources of the Library

Librarian. This is perhaps the best resource in the whole school. The librarian is a college-educated specialist who knows what the library has to offer in the area of information and where that information can be found. Look at the librarian as a professional educator about information for learning and as a person who is always ready to assist you. When you do go for assistance, be sure to watch the process the librarian uses to obtain the information you need. Next time you will be able to help yourself.

Virtual Reference Program. If you have a computer and Internet access at home or at school, you will benefit if your school participates in a virtual reference program network. This type of program allows users to find books, videos, or other library materials via the Internet, within the network of libraries that participate in the program. You can obtain this information by accessing their websites in the network. The same program may allow users to access information, sometimes 24 hours a day, by asking questions of library staff or the reference librarian by means of the Internet and getting responses via email and chat rooms. If answers to questions or materials cannot be found, these inquiries can be forwarded to other libraries nationally or internationally.

Circulation Desk. The circulation desk is the area where library materials are checked out and returned. Materials reserved by your instructor will probably be found here and can be checked out for short periods, along with audiovisual equipment to use with the material, if needed. Some reserve materials may be on electronic reserve.

Online Catalog. You can obtain a lot of information about your LRC by yourself once you understand the cataloging system. Most LRCs have converted their card catalogs to an online (computerized) catalog. All books found in your LRC, but not magazines and newspapers, are indexed in this computerized system. In addition to books, cataloged materials also include **audiovisual materials** (audiotapes, videotapes, CD-ROMs, etc.). You can search for desired materials by subject, title, or author. If the LRC does not have the material you are searching for, but another LRC on the online system does, this information might also be included.

At a moment's notice students can determine the availability of a source miles away. In some systems students are able to access the online catalog from home via computer. This system of cataloging can save students valuable time and energy.

LOCATING YOUR MATERIAL

Libraries may choose to use either of two systems to classify materials so they are easy to locate: (1) the Dewey decimal system and (2) the Library of Congress classification system. Regardless of the system your library uses, the call number shown on the author, title, or subject screens is the same number as that on the material itself. Get in the habit of copying, in order, all the letters and numbers in the call number.

The Stacks

Armed with the call number, you can proceed to the stacks—the place where the majority of materials that can be checked out are located. The books are placed in call-number order according to academic disciplines. When you do find the material you are looking for, note that materials covering the same subject are shelved in the same area. You might find additional useful material on the same shelf.

Reference Material

Reference materials include dictionaries and other similar categories of books, including medical and nursing dictionaries, almanacs, yearbooks, atlases, encyclopedias, and handbooks. You will find up-to-date information on any subject in this area. Reference material generally does not circulate. Information from reference materials may be copied on a copy machine if the book cannot be checked out.

Interlibrary Loan Services

Interlibrary loan services allow your LRC to borrow materials you need that are not in your library's holdings. Books and audiovisual materials are available through this service. If your LRC does not have the periodical in which an article you need is located, a photocopy of the article, free of charge, might be obtained from a library that does have the periodical.

Vertical File (Pamphlet File)

The vertical file contains pamphlets of various subjects arranged in alphabetical order by topic.

Professional Journals

Practical/vocational nurses need to be aware of sources that will provide up-to-date information on nursing topics. Professional journal articles give you the opportunity to stay on top of the latest research in nursing, and its application. In addition to articles that are assigned reading, practical/vocational nurses need to be self-directed in finding and using articles that pertain to selected nursing topics and nursing problems occurring in the clinical area. Professional journals of interest to practical/vocational nurses include, but are not limited to, the following: *The Journal of Practical Nursing; Advance for LPNs; LPN 2008* (the year changes with each calendar year); *Men in Nursing; RN; Nursing;* and *The American Journal of Nursing.*

Learning Exercise

Nursing Periodicals

Identify the location of the aforementioned nursing journals in your learning resource center. Determine which of them will help you keep up-to-date in nursing. Identify the location of other nursing periodicals.

Articles

All learners are looking for the perfect textbook, the one that is complete and self-contained. It does not exist! Specific journal articles may be assigned to give you up-to-date information to supplement the readings in your textbooks. Use the same PQRST method and hints for reading textbooks when reading these articles.

Copyright laws prohibit the instructor from copying an article for each of you. For this reason the required reading articles are available on a reserve basis in the LRC by photocopy or electronic format. You can make notes from these articles. Because copyright laws allow you to have one copy of an article, photocopy or print the reserve article for your own use. Underline, highlight, and write in the margins of your photocopy. Remember, the instructor knows you are busy. Articles are not busy work, but are a necessary part of any career education to keep current in your discipline.

Magazines and Newspapers

Include newspapers and popular magazines as sources of information on health-related topics. Magazine articles never replace professional journal reading, but they do provide information that your patients read. As one practical/vocational nursing student said, "I had better be up-to-date and understand what my patients are reading." Be aware of the author's expertise. This will help you evaluate the accuracy of the information on the topic.

Learning Exercise

Popular Reading

List two newspapers or popular magazines that you read.

_____

_____

_____

CLASSROOM LEARNING STRATEGIES

LECTURES

Some of your teachers may have been taught using the "bucket theory" of education. The bucket theory suggests that merely by lecturing, a teacher can transfer knowledge from the teacher's mind to the mind of the student. This teaching method evolved from Aristotle's day. The teacher was considered the source and the vehicle of transmission of information—similar to a sage on the stage. Of course the printing press had yet to be invented!

Research has shown that students learn best from methods other than traditional lecture. Although traditional lecturing is an outmoded form of instruction, *brief lectures* (minilectures) can be valuable as a means of enhancing your assigned readings and clarifying information. A minilecture situation is a brief episode, taking no more than 30% of class time. Minilectures are intended to enhance your reading assignment, not replace it. A minilecture reflects the fact that the teacher spent time searching, reading, selecting, and organizing information for your benefit. The instructor has done all the work and has become smarter in the process. However, minilectures are passive learning experiences that do not actively involve you in the learning process. During minilectures you have the responsibility to apply all active learning suggestions found in Chapter 4. You need to remain especially alert and actively involved.

The instructor may introduce various techniques to keep you actively involved during minilectures. Box 5-3 shows an example of a learning strategy called **discussion buddy**.

What goes on in the classroom is just as important as what goes on in a reading assignment. There is, however, one great difference between the two. *You can repeat a reading assignment, but you can never repeat a missed class.* Here are some hints to help you learn from any class situation.

1. *Before taping a class activity, clarify if taping is allowed.*
2. *Never skip a class unless you are faced with an emergency.* Some students skip class to get another hour's sleep, use the time to prepare for another class or an examination, or get in their legal number of cuts (if legal cuts are in your school's policies). When an emergency does make it necessary for you to miss class, photocopying notes is not the answer to catch up on what you missed. Ask a peer to go over his or her notes and tell you about the class. Recall what you learned in Chapter 2 about personal learning styles.
3. *Come to class prepared.* By having the assignment completed before class, key terms and concepts will be familiar to you. You will be ready to participate in learning activities. You will save yourself embarrassment by avoiding questions that are answered easily by the readings. Come to class in time to get a seat close to the instructor and the blackboard. Heading for the last row is heading for distractions and lower grades. Have a pen and papers pertaining to the assignment ready to go.
4. *Listen for verbal cues that will inform you of key points during minilectures* (Box 5-4). Keep

Box 5-3 *Learning Strategy: Discussion Buddy*

1. You may be assigned to a discussion buddy before class.
2. The two of you will be given a discussion task.
3. Focus carefully on the minilecture so you will be able to formulate an answer to the discussion task.
4. After the minilecture, discussion buddies share their answers with each other. A new answer is formulated from both your responses.
5. The instructor will choose students at random to share their newly composed answers with the class.

Box 5-4 *Verbal Cues for Key Ideas in Minilectures and Discussion Activities*

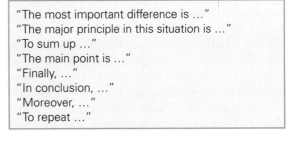

"The most important difference is ..."
"The major principle in this situation is ..."
"To sum up ..."
"The main point is ..."
"Finally, ..."
"In conclusion, ..."
"Moreover, ..."
"To repeat ..."

vigilant for nonverbal cues given by the instructor that will also inform you of key ideas. Examples are raising the hands, a long dramatic pause, raising or lowering the voice, and leaning toward the class. Be sure to copy everything that is written on the blackboard.

5. *The instructor speaks at a much slower rate than you are capable of thinking.* The fact that you can think faster than the instructor can speak allows you to relate this new information to information you have learned in the past, and to formulate questions when you do not understand. Ask these questions in class, or seek out the instructor after class. It is your responsibility to question what you do not understand.

6. *Look over your notes as soon after class as possible.* Use the hints given in Chapter 4. Follow these techniques to comprehend the information you learned in class and place it into your long-term memory.

7. *Be present while in class.* Avoid using class time to work on other projects. Be an active listener.

LECTURE-DISCUSSION

In the lecture-discussion strategy the instructor shares several ideas with the class and then stops to let the class discuss the ideas. Sometimes the instructor may say that the next class will be nothing but discussion of the assignment. The instructor then acts as a discussion leader. The instructor has developed several learning strategies to help keep the discussion focused on course objectives. Box 5-5 gives you some hints for participating in discussions and related activities.

COOPERATIVE LEARNING

Cooperative learning is a technique that emphasizes individual accountability for learning a specific academic task while working in small groups. Cooperative learning encourages you to (1) be actively involved in your learning, (2) develop critical-thinking skills, and (3) develop positive relationships with your peers. Besides helping you learn the course content, cooperative learning helps you develop traits you will need in your future job. Cooperative learning encourages the development of teamwork. The ability to

| Box 5-5 | *Hints for a Discussion Class* |

- Be prepared to participate in the discussion by completing your assignment before class. This will allow you to be an active participant.
- Be sure you have made a list of questions about the assignment. Discussions are the perfect time to clear up questions.
- While other learners are speaking, listen to what they have to say. Some learners make the mistake of using other learners' speaking time to formulate their own comments.
- You may disagree with others during a discussion. Do so assertively and firmly. Avoid yelling matches at all costs. It enriches your world to listen to another's point of view before responding.

work in a team situation is what an employer is looking for in an employee. Use the suggestions listed under the previous Lecture-discussion section to help you get full mileage out of this learning strategy.

DISTANCE LEARNING

Perhaps some of the courses in your practical/vocational nursing program or parts of courses are available through distance learning. In this learning strategy the student and teacher are separated by physical distance. The course could take part in "real time" in which all students in the course and the instructor participate simultaneously by means of interactive TV. A popular alternative is the type of instruction in which students can choose when and where they will attend class. This type of distance learning is carried out, for example, by resources received through the mail or seen on TV, such as videotapes and audiotapes, and web-based courses. The following hints will help you succeed in this type of distance learning.

1. Have the equipment needed, *or access to* equipment needed, to complete course assignments. Depending on the distance learning course, the equipment list *could* include any of the following:

a. Computer with adequate hard disk space
b. Word processor
c. Modem
d. Fax machine
e. Internet service provider—dial-up or broadband
f. Telephone line—preferably two if you do not have broadband—which allows you to stay online while seeking assistance from technical staff via telephone
g. Cable TV hook-up
h. VCR
i. CD/DVD player

2. Time-management skills, self-discipline, and motivation are important tools for success. The time-management information in Chapter 3 will help you establish a weekly class and study schedule and stick to it. The nature of the course requires you to have access to email and check your emails daily for messages from instructors and fellow students. You also may be required to post items as class assignments.

3. Study skills are a must. Chapter 4 emphasizes the need for the proper study skills, including study environment. Because distance learning courses require much reading, Chapter 4 and its emphasis on the PQRST method of study will be beneficial. The ability to understand ideas by means of the written word is important. Chapter 2 helps you determine your personal learning style and can help you decide if distance learning is right for you.

4. Because distance learning requires you to communicate by methods such as videotape, writing, email, and fax, Chapter 9 will help you organize your thoughts so that you can present them in a concise manner and communicate your intended message. These hints will be especially useful if you are taking an Internet course sponsored by a school that participates in real-time discussion or postings by students and teachers on electronic bulletin boards and in chat rooms.

Distance learning has proved to be at least as effective as traditional methods of instruction. Positive features include the fact that students become more active in personal learning and

---

Box 5-6 | *Technology Courtesy for Learning Activities*

- Check school policy for use of cell phone, Blackberry, iPod, and laptop.
- If cell phones allowed, turn off ringer and put on vibrate.
- If it is necessary to return a call, leave the immediate area, quietly make your call, and quickly complete it.
- Avoid emailing, text and instant messaging, and playing games during class activities.
- Avoid surfing the Internet during class activities.
- Avoid listening to music on your iPod during class activities.

---

have more involvement in and control over the learning process.

TECHNOLOGY USE DURING LEARNING ACTIVITIES

Class time requires active listening and participation in learning activities. Avoid using class time for snoozing, talking to friends, or any of the activities in Box 5-6. Your time in the practical/vocational nursing program gives you the opportunity to sharpen (bring to an excellent level) professional behavior that is appropriate for your job as a practical/vocational nurse.

In a 24/7, 365 wired/wireless world, you may seem to be accessible at all times to friends and family. Set limits by sharing your class and clinical schedules with friends and family and restrict being contacted to emergencies only at those times.

OTHER LEARNING RESOURCES

SYLLABUS AND COURSE OUTLINES

A **syllabus** is an up-to-date course document given to you at the beginning of a course. At a minimum that syllabus includes a course description, course objectives, course requirements for a passing grade, required textbooks, grading scale, instructor information (office location, office phone number, office hours), course policies, and testing policies.

Some schools of practical/vocational nursing also use course outlines for each course. These outlines are a great help to an adult learner. They contain unit-by-unit course objectives and content areas, which indicate what the learner must know to pass the course. Each objective begins with a verb. Watch the verb carefully because it tells you the level of understanding you must achieve to meet the objective. If an objective states you must *list* something, that task is quite different from having to *compare* and *contrast* the same information. Instructors develop their test questions from the course objectives and course content. The course outline will include a list of resources indicating where the information to answer the objectives is found. Supplementary material in the form of worksheets, charts, activities, and additional reading may be included to round out your learning.

STUDY GROUPS

Do you have a desire to achieve better grades? Do you need to study more effectively? Do you need a little support? Joining a study group could be the strategy for you. Students usually form their own study groups out of need. Studies have shown that despite each person's preferred learning style, *actively* participating in a study group can improve academic performance. Notice we said *actively* participating. Sometimes students join a study group thinking that the group will help them pass, and they avoid active participation; these students are similar to freeloaders. Study groups work when students use them to become actively involved in their own learning. The group provides an outlet for oral rehearsal of material, which promotes retention. Active study group members usually develop questioning and reasoning skills on a higher level.

TUTORING

Tutoring is a very select study group. For best results, the student arranges tutoring through a special department by means of instructor referral or self-referral. The purpose of tutoring is to help a student understand the material better and pass the course. We guarantee one thing in tutoring: The tutor will probably get an A. Students who need tutoring *sometimes* have learning disabilities. In these situations, because of an excellent attitude on the part of these students and their active participation in the tutoring process, tutoring can be beneficial. Students without learning disabilities who actively participate in the tutoring process also are successful in passing courses.

We are concerned about students at risk for failure who expect the tutor to "learn for them." These students do not actively participate in the tutoring process. We have also seen some privately arranged tutoring situations fail because the tutor felt that the student at risk needed to "be saved." Please note: Students cannot be saved. Nothing can replace active participation on the part of the learner. If you want to pass a course, you must become actively involved in your own learning. There are also students who need tutoring but say they do not have time for it. Comment on this response.

NURSING SKILLS LAB

The nursing skills lab is a resource that will allow you to practice and develop your physical nursing skills. It is to be used throughout your nursing program. This lab contains the physical items needed to make the practice area as similar to the workplace as possible. *Skills must be practiced.* Reading about skills, watching a film, and watching other students practice are only the first steps in developing a physical skill. Practice until you are proficient in each skill, so that you will feel comfortable performing these tasks in the clinical area. Remember that you recall 10% of what you hear, 20% of what you see, 50% of what you read, and 90% of what you do, so do all you can. The Teton Lakota Indians have a proverb that summarizes how practical/vocational student nurses need to approach the skills component of their nursing program: "Tell me and I'll listen. Show me and I'll understand. Involve me and I'll learn."

You will be required to make appointments to give a return demonstration of skills. This routine will give you an opportunity to organize your time. This is what is expected of the practical/vocational nurse as part of patient care. When you make an appointment with the skills lab, you are entering into an agreement with the lab personnel. Your responsibility is to practice the skill until you can perform it in the time frame of your appointment. If you are unable to keep your appointment, inform the lab personnel. This will allow them to schedule other students into lab time for skills testing.

STUDY SKILLS LAB

If your school has a study skills lab, it is available to help you with academic problem areas. Examples of areas in which help is available are study skills, time management, reading (including vocabulary and comprehension), listening skills, math skills, test-taking skills (especially situation tests), note making, writing, and any other academic problem you may have. You can go to the skills lab on your own or by referral of your instructor or counselor.

 Critical Thinking Exercise

No Time for the Skills Center

Some students who need the study skills center state they do not have time to go for help. Comment about this response.

AUDIOVISUAL MATERIALS

In addition to lectures, discussions/activities, textbooks, and articles, the instructor may have included films, videotapes, or CD-ROMs as part of your assignment. Audiovisual (AV) materials are not considered extra or additional assignments. They are a significant part of all areas of learning. These learning resources give faith to the saying, "A picture is worth a thousand words." AV materials provide an additional sensory channel for learning, compared with reading. In some nursing courses, especially autotutorial skills courses, the AV medium is the course. The student progresses independently,

attending periodic lecture-discussion classes and seeking out the instructor when questions arise. Approach the AV material as you do a class. Realize that you have the option of repeating all or part of the presentation when you do not understand it. Remember television, especially the cable network, can be a source of information for topics related to your coursework.

INTERNET

The Internet offers unlimited resources on many subjects. The Internet is the physical infrastructure that allows the electronic circulation of vast amounts of information to Internet-ready computer users. An Internet provider charges a monthly fee and is a computer user's link to the Internet. Provider services can be either dial-up modems or dedicated service lines (DSL), meaning that you have instant access when your computer is turned on.

When people are linked to the Internet, they are said to be online. An example of a provider service is instant access RoadRunner. Local service providers also provide Internet access and are usually a dial-up service. The World Wide Web (www) is the most effective means of providing access to the vast amount of information available on the Internet. Everything on the Internet has an address (called a URL) that helps in locating a specific site. Most addresses begin with http://www, followed by a dot. The next letters in the address are specific to the site you wish to access; for example, www.nclex will provide access to the site that provides info about the LPN/LVN licensing exam. This is followed by three letters, called a domain name, which denote the site's source. The following are common domain names and their meanings:

- com—for-profit sites
- gov—the U.S. federal government
- edu—4-year degree granting colleges and universities
- org—usually reserved for nonprofit organizations
- net—network infrastructure machines and organizations

Search engines are programs that can help students zero in on the exact information for which they are looking. Search engines periodically scan the web and index it. Therefore search engines are like the telephone book. A popular search engine is Google.com. Appendix E contains some suggestions of Internet sites that can be used by practical/vocational nursing students as learning resources and for patient teaching resources. Box 5-7 contains guidelines for gathering Internet information for your use or to share with patients.

 Learning Exercise

Peer Assistance with Computer/Internet

If there are students in your class who have computer/Internet experience, ask them for hints for using this technology and information resource.

COMPUTER-AIDED INSTRUCTION

Computer-aided instruction (CAI) is an increasingly used teaching strategy in nursing education. It has the following benefits:
- Allows learners to be actively involved in their learning.
- Encourages problem solving, a skill that employers expect of practical/vocational nurses.
- Provides immediate feedback by quickly evaluating answers and decision-making strategies.
- Provides an opportunity to develop the ability to follow directions.

Learning by CAI is enhanced for students with right-brain dominance. CAI can also be used effectively by any student to master new material. It simplifies concepts and reinforces skills that have been presented previously. If you do not have computer skills and CAI is used in your practical/vocational nursing program, you will be taught the skills necessary to use this type of teaching strategy. The process is simple even if you do not have any computer experience. Many of you will also be using the computer in the clinical area to store and retrieve

Box 5-7 | *Guidelines for Gathering Internet Information*

- The Internet is not regulated in any way. Anyone can publish anything they want on the Internet. When searching the Internet, you can find the most recent and accurate information, as well as the most inaccurate and out-of-date information.
- Let the user beware—people can spend a lot of time on the Internet. To save time, take a few minutes to read the section that gives hints for using a specific site. Stay focused on your purpose. Avoid getting sidetracked.
- Check the professional credentials and qualifications of the author of the information.
- Determine the organization, group, agency, company, and so on that created the site. This will help you evaluate the credibility of the information. The domain name is helpful in evaluating credibility. For example, a site that has a ".gov" domain name may be more credible than a ".com" site that may be promoting a product.
- Check the date the information was created and last modified. This will ensure up-to-date material.
- What are the objectives of the author of the material? Does the author express opinions? Does the author have a personal bias?
- When conducting searches, supply keywords to help the search tool narrow the document results to just the ones you want to see.
  - When using keywords for a search engine, use phrases or single words that are pertinent to your topic, and describe it objectively.
  - Use nouns only and put the most important words that describe your topic first.
  - When searching with a phrase (e.g., study skills), surround the phrase with quotation marks.
  - Plus signs (+) or the word "AND" identify words that must appear in the search (e.g., nursing + practical).
  - Minus signs (–) or the word "NOT" exclude words from the search (e.g., NCLEX-PN, NOT RN).

patient information. And in less than 1 year, all of you will be taking the NCLEX-PN® examination by computer.

SIMULATION

Simulation is a learning activity that makes use of imaginary patient situations that mimic the reality of the clinical environment. The learner has the opportunity to think like a nurse and gather data, set priorities, plan, and evaluate care in a virtual (reproduced/replicated by a computer) patient situation without risk to the patient. Simulation encourages decision-making and critical thinking.

Simulation can take many forms. Case scenarios can be accessed in a printed format or by computer. In each type, an imaginary patient story will bring reality to theory in the form of a clinical situation. Both forms may be used when the patient census is inadequate for patient assignments, when a desired patient situation is unavailable, or when enhanced learning of specific concepts is desirable.

Computer simulation can be a learning situation on a floppy disk or CD that is inserted into a computer. The computer-patient simulation changes, as it would in the clinical area. This requires the student to evaluate the situation and plan new assessments (data collection) and interventions. Review of available software reveals few computer simulations that are intended specifically for practical/vocational nursing students. Your instructors can suggest modifications of existing simulations for your use.

Static and electronic simulations allow students to practice patient care before reaching the clinical area. Static mannequins are full-size body models or models of specific parts of the body made to be realistic. These mannequins are used for practicing skills and returning demonstrations of procedures, for example, urinary catheterization, insertion of intravenous solutions, and application of colostomy bags. Electronic mannequins are a high-tech, pricier simulation model that can be programmed to set up different patient situations and allow practice of nursing procedures and data collection (assessment).

Virtual clinical excursions are computer programs that electronically (controlled by a computer) provide a virtual hospital floor and patients. This experience provides a patient record, Kardex, medication administration record, drug guide, medical dictionary, and text books learners can access to collect data, set priorities for care, administer medications, manage patient care problems, and document care. These excursions encourage students to critically think and problem-solve in a safe and secure environment (deWit, 2006).

STAYING CURRENT IN PRACTICAL/ VOCATIONAL NURSING

PERIODICALS

Because nursing magazines are published weekly, monthly, and quarterly (i.e., periodically), they are often called periodicals. They are also referred to as journals—publications that contain news or material of current interest to a particular discipline. Professional journals contain articles that include the most recent information available on a specific subject and subjects that are too new to be included in texts. This is the reason periodicals are important resources for a learner in a field changing as quickly as nursing and health care. The titles and authors of various articles cannot possibly be included in the online catalog of the LRC. These can be found instead in two sources: bound books called periodical indexes and CD-ROM databases.

Bound Periodical Indexes

Entries in periodical indexes are listed by author, title, and subject. The following are two periodical indexes that are of special value to practical/vocational nursing students.
1. *Reader's Guide to Periodical Literature*. This comprehensive index to more than 200 popular American nontechnical magazines includes articles published between the dates printed on its cover. This guide is useful for recreational reading on specific topics, such as setting up a workshop, decorating with stenciling, and learning about the Internet.

The *Reader's Guide*, or green book, is valuable for practical/vocational nursing students because technical data on health topics are presented in understandable language for the general public.

2. *Cumulative Index to Nursing and Allied Health Literature* (CINAHL®). This comprehensive and authoritative periodical index contains current listings for nursing and allied health fields and for others interested in health care issues, including biomedicine, consumer health, and alternative medicine. About 1800 nursing, allied health, and related journals are reviewed and indexed for over 11,000 topics. A videotape and CD-ROM are available to provide instruction on how to use the print index. Figure 5-1 illustrates the information found in a typical entry in the CINAHL® print edition. Some schools have access to online CINAHL® databases.

Your LRC will have a periodical listing. The listing includes the professional journals and magazines and the dates of the issues that are found in your library. If the article you need is in a journal or magazine that is not held in your library, see the librarian. The librarian can track down the article in another library and arrange for you to receive a photocopy by interlibrary loan. If your library has the date and issue you need, go to the section of the library that contains the periodicals.

If the issue you need is not there, inquire how back issues are accessed.

Understanding how to use a periodical index is still a necessary skill. How well do you understand the information found in a print periodical index entry? The beginning of each CINAHL® book contains directions for using the source. Use the following CINAHL® print entry to test your understanding of CINAHL® citing. Answer the questions found underneath the entry. Refer to Figure 5-1 if you need help in reading the CINAHL® citation.

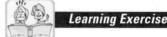

Learning Exercise

Using CINAHL® Print Edition

Using the following citation, supply the information requested.

Smoke Out Lung Cancer (Edmondson, D.) (ceu exam questions) LPN 2008 Jan./Feb. 4:1 38-49 (5 ref.)

Author:
Title of article:
Volume and number of periodical:
Name of periodical:
Date of article:
Pages:
Additional information found in article:
Are there references in the article?
If so, how many?

```
1-Cardiovascular
  2- Taking valve disorders to heart 3- Quigley, P.
4- (tables/charts) 5- LPN 2008 6- Jan/Feb 2008; 7- 4(1)
8-26-37 9- (4 ref)
```

Key: 1. Subject. 2. Title of the article. 3. Author of the article. 4. Additional information found in article. 5. Periodical in which the article appears. If the periodical is abbreviated, the periodical index in the front of the book will have a list of periodical abbreviations and the full name of the journal for which those abbreviations stand. 6. Date of publication. 7. Volume and number of periodical. 8. Page numbers of article. 9. Number of references used.

FIGURE **5-1** Explanation of an entry from Cumulative Index to Nursing and Allied Health.

CD-ROMs

Public and school libraries have these valuable sources of information. The audio CDs you use at home play music. The CD-ROM in the library plays "information." CD-ROM systems differ in the subjects and the level of coverage they offer.

CD-ROMs are a source of textbook type of information for practical/vocational nursing students. Examples of information that can be found on CD-ROMs include encyclopedias, textbooks, and drug books. Some texts have a separate CD-ROM edition. Some of these resources provide audio pronunciation of terms, heart and breath sounds and generally enhance learning. Some texts provide a CD-ROM with a test bank of questions to allow you to test your learning.

CD-ROM Databases. Because of computer technology, the process of keeping "up-to-date" has been simplified, as far as finding information is concerned. CD-ROM databases are expensive sources of information. If your LRC has this technology available for student use, be sure to use it. The systems are user friendly. Combined with a helpful LRC staff, you cannot lose! Because CD-ROM databases are costly, some schools of practical/vocational nursing may share a computer system with a health care institution. Student use of these databases may be restricted.

NURSING ORGANIZATIONS

Nursing organizations often organize speakers, seminars, and workshops on up-to-the-minute nursing topics and related health care topics. These programs are frequently made available to students. Specific nursing organizations are discussed in Chapter 23.

COMMUNITY RESOURCES

The city library and museums sometimes sponsor programs and exhibits on topics of interest and use to practical/vocational nursing students. Additional community resources are health care facilities, such as hospitals and clinics, which offer lecture series.

GUEST SPEAKERS

Nurses and other health professionals are sometimes invited to visit nursing classes as guest speakers or make presentations via video. These speakers donate their time to present current information on their areas of expertise and updates on specific nursing topics. Often their employers released them to visit nursing classes or to make a videotape for class use. Regardless of the method of presentation, students need to treat these speakers with attention and respect.

Key Points

- The hints for using learning strategies and resources found in this chapter will help you obtain the information you need to get better grades on tests and achieve your goal of becoming a practical/vocational nurse.
- The LRC may be your most valuable resource for learning as a student and for keeping up-to-date as a graduate.
- In addition to textbooks, minilecture, lecture-discussions, and cooperative learning are specific course-learning strategies that will most probably be used by the practical/vocational nursing student.
- Methods of delivering instruction, such as distance learning, make learning more student-oriented.
- Additional learning resources include articles from periodicals, the syllabus, course outlines, study groups, tutoring, audiovisual materials, the Internet, computer-aided instruction, and simulation.
- Staying current in practical/vocational nursing is made possible by using periodical indexes, CD-ROM databases, the Internet, skills lab, nursing organizations, community resources, and guest speakers.
- After learning the information you need to be a practical/vocational nurse, you must demonstrate that learning has taken place by your performance in the clinical area and on tests.

REVIEW ITEMS

1. Select the activity that is the least-suggested learning strategy in an SPN/SVN program.

   1. Distance learning
   2. Lecture-discussion
   3. Instant messaging
   4. Nursing skills lab

2. A nursing instructor suggests that a practical/vocational nursing student receive help with study skills at the school's Skills Center. Which student response most accurately indicates that the student understands the purpose of the Skills Center?

   1. "I cannot afford the fee to attend study programs in the Skills Center at my school."
   2. "In high school, only students with learning disabilities attended the Skills Center."
   3. "It will take too much time out of my limited study time to go for help with studying."
   4. "Even a few visits to the Skills Center can help me get more out of my study sessions."

3. Classes in a practical/vocational nursing program may be conducted in a lecture-discussion format. Select the student behavior that is least effective for this learning strategy.

   1. When time is needed to study for a test in a different class, arrange for a peer to take notes for you in your absence.
   2. Complete all assignments before going to class and prepare questions you have about parts of readings that are unclear.
   3. If you disagree with a student during a discussion, assertively present your point of view after the student finishes speaking.
   4. Listen while instructors and students are speaking; avoid using this time to prepare your comments to add to the discussion.

4. Four practical/vocational nursing students are commenting at break time about the personal/vocational assignment to take a tour of the LRC. Select the statement that indicates understanding of the purpose for this assignment.

   1. "Knowing the location of nursing journals in the LRC will save me time and frustration when they are assigned."
   2. "I know a library's resources and how they are organized because I took business courses in college last year."
   3. "Because taxpayer money funds the learning resource center and its holdings, nursing faculty need to encourage its use."
   4. "I have a part-time job and a family, and I do not have time in my schedule to tour the learning resource center."

ALTERNATE FORMAT ITEM

A variety of learning resources and strategies are used in a practical/vocational nursing program. Which of the following students are using these resources and strategies to their advantage? *(Select all that apply.)*

1. Devin joined a study group that meets every day after school to review and discuss class notes.

2. Colin frequently skips lectures to study for a test in another class and to play video games for relaxation.

3. Instead of watching assigned videotapes, Julia borrows notes of the tapes from friends who viewed them.

4. Because of a long commute, Duncan signed up for a distance learning class to save more study time.

Critical Thinking and Patient Care

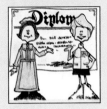

evolve http://evolve.elsevier.com/Hill/success/

Objectives

On completing this chapter, you will be able to do the following:

1. Discuss the difference between nonfocused and directed thinking.
2. Explain what makes critical thinking an advanced way of thinking.
3. Use techniques that enhance the understanding of information needed to be a practical/vocational nurse.
4. Differentiate among the terms knowledge, comprehension, application, and analysis.
5. Evaluate your personal need for help in comprehending information.
6. Identify two new suggestions for increasing reading effectiveness that you will begin to apply immediately.
7. Develop a plan using critical thinking to increase your ability to think critically.

Key Terms

Analysis (ă-NĂL-1-sĭs, p. 83)
Application (ĂP-lĭ-KĂ-shŭn, p. 83)
Attitude (p. 80)
Capability (KĂ-pă-BĬL-ĭ-tĕ, p. 82)
Cognitive levels (KŎG-nĭ-tĭv, p. 82)
Comprehension (KŎM-prĕ-HĔN-shŭn, p. 82)
Critical thinking (p. 76)
Directed (or focused) thinking (p. 77)
Knowledge (p. 82)
Problem-oriented thinking (p. 77)
Reflective thinking (rĕ-FLĔK-tĭv, p. 84)

 Keep in Mind

Become an active learner and critical thinker, and be successful in the practical/vocational nursing program, on NCLEX-PN®, and as a candidate for a job you love as an LPN/LVN.

OVERVIEW OF CRITICAL THINKING

The following are the *Top 10 Reasons to Improve Thinking,* adapted for practical/vocational nurses:*

10. Things are not what they used to be, or what they will be, in this changing health care system.
9. Licensed practical/vocational nurses (LPN/LVNs) frequently care for patients who are not yet stabilized and have multiple problems.
8. More patients and their families are involved in health care decisions.
7. LPN/LVNs must be able to move from one health care setting to another.
6. Rapid change and information explosion requires LPN/LVNs to develop new learning and workplace skills.
5. Patients, families, and insurance companies demand to see evidence of benefits, efficiency, and results of care given.

*Adapted with permission from Alfaro-Lefevre R. (2009). *Critical thinking and clinical judgment: a practical approach* (4th ed.). Philadelphia: WB Saunders, inside cover.

4. Today's progress often creates new problems that cannot be solved by old ways of thinking (e.g., ethical and legal issues involved in end-of-life decisions, questions regarding stem-cell research, who is entitled to receive expensive medical care, and so on).

3. Redesigning care delivery and education programs is useless if students and nurses do not have the thinking skills required to deal with today's world.

2. Learning how to improve your thinking skills does not have to be difficult.

1. **Your ability to focus your thinking on how to get the results you need can make the difference between whether you succeed or fail in the fast-paced health care system.**

Years ago nurses saw themselves as doers, not thinkers. Nurses were primarily directed what to do, and they carried out the orders. Certainly there were exceptions, such as Florence Nightingale and Mary Seacole, to name two historical pioneers in nursing.

By 1996 the National Council of State Boards of Nursing (NCSBN) included four phases of the nursing process (no diagnosis) in the NCLEX-PN Examination. Questions were at the cognitive level of knowledge, comprehension, and application (NCSBN, 1995). In 1999 the four phases were integrated throughout the test plan (NCSBN 1998). **By 2002 the NCSBN integrated all phases of the nursing process, as well as critical thinking, into the NCLEX-PN® Examination**. The cognitive level of analysis was added to NCLEX-PN® Examination questions (NCSBN, 2001). The expectation was that both nursing process and critical thinking would be taught to the practical/vocational nursing student (SPN/SVN). Critical thinking is an integral part of the nursing process. To do the nursing process, the work of nursing, is to have to think critically. Today nurses who cannot think critically become one of the problems, rather than the solution, in nursing.

WAYS OF THINKING

DEFINITION OF APPLIED CRITICAL THINKING

Just what is critical thinking, and how does it relate to the nursing decisions you will make at school and during your career? Alfaro-Lefevre (2003) provides a definition of critical thinking and clinical judgment in nursing.

Critical thinking and clinical judgment in nursing, adapted for practical/vocational nursing,* is defined as the following:

• Entails purposeful, informed, outcome-focused (results-oriented) thinking that requires careful identification of the problems, issues, and risks involved (e.g., deciding whether a patient needs one or more staff to move from bed to chair in a manner that is safe for both patient and staff).

• Is driven by patient, family, and community needs. The practical/vocational nurse must be able to use knowledge to tailor approaches based on circumstances.

• Is based on the principles of the nursing process and on scientific methods; for example, making judgments based on evidence (facts), rather than guesswork. This is a major difference between LPN/LVNs and unlicensed assistive personnel (UAPs).

• Uses both logic and intuition, based on knowledge, skills, and experience of the LPN/LVN.

• Is guided by professional standards, such as those developed for the LPN/LVN by the National Association for Practical Nurse Education and Services (NAPNES), the National Federation of Licensed Practical Nurses (NFLPN), and the practical/vocational nursing code of ethics.

---

* Adapted for practical/vocational nurses with permission from Alfaro-Lefevre R. (2006). *Evidence-based critical thinking indicators.* Available at: www.AlfaroTeachSmart.com.

- Calls for strategies that make the most of human potential (e.g., using individual strengths) and compensates for problems created by human nature (e.g., overcoming the powerful influence of personal beliefs, values, and prejudices).
- Is constantly reevaluating, self-correcting, and striving to improve (e.g., practicing skills, learning new skills, attending classes, and workshops).

Thinking is divided into nonfocused thinking and directed thinking. At one time or another, most of us have used the following examples of thinking:

- **Nonfocused thinking**: You engaged your brain out of habit without much conscious thought.
- **Habitual thinking**: We get up to go to the bathroom, shower, dress, etc. This type of thinking involves any routine we do that is important, but that does not require us to think hard about how to do it (automatic pilot).
- **Random thoughts**: Multiple short scenes and thoughts come and go through the mind and have no particular purpose or goal (mental channel surfing).
- **Ruminative thinking**: The same situation or scene is replayed in the mind over and over, without reaching an outcome (instant replay).
- **All-or-none thinking**: The mind is made up, and no additional facts will be considered (black-and-white thinking with no grays in between).
- **Negative thinking**: The mind is stuck on negative thoughts and blocks worthwhile thinking (emotional sabotage).
- **Directed (or focused) thinking**: Purposeful and outcome oriented.
- **Problem-oriented thinking**: Focus on a particular problem to find a solution (e.g., planning your school, work, and home schedule). This could involve collecting information on school and work schedules, and schedules of family members who rely on you. It might include delegating tasks,

requesting help, making your goals known, and listening for input from those involved in the immediate situation, etc. (see Chapter 3). Once the schedule is developed, no further attention is given to the situation until another problem emerges (problem solving).

- **Critical thinking**: Critical thinking is an advanced way of thinking; a problem-solving method, and more. It is used to resolve problems and to find ways to improve a situation even when no problem exists. It answers the question, "How can we do this better?"

Learning Exercise

Survey of your Current Level of Critical Thinking

Based on a scale of 0-10 (with 0 as least and 10 as highest), rate each statement about thinking as it applies to you. Afterward list the items you rated as lowest.

___I identify the purpose of my thinking.
___My thinking is goal (or outcome) directed.
___I have an organized method of thinking.
___I question what I do not understand.
___I continually question: What does this mean? Is this useful? Is it fact?
___I question the reliability of sources and information available.
___I keep an open mind.
___My judgments are based on fact (evidence).

_____

_____

Critical Thinking Exercise

Make a Personal Plan

1. Prioritize the critical thinking items you need to work on from the previous learning exercise. Choose the items you think are most important to work on first.
2. Make a schedule and estimate the amount of time it will take to see progress. (We all need to work on critical thinking throughout our lives.)
3. Identify how you will determine what progress is being made.

_____

CRITICAL THINKING AND PRACTICAL/ VOCATIONAL NURSING

Critical thinking involves questioning with meaning. This type of thinking involves examining personal thinking and the thinking of others. Judgments are made on facts (evidence), not assumptions. The critical thinker avoids criticizing just for the sake of having his or her own way. Decisions are based on the right thing to do rather than emotions or a need to save face. New ideas and alternatives are offered in a constructive way. The thinker is willing to consider other ideas and recognizes that there may be more than one right way to do something. The thinker realizes that there may not be a perfect solution.

Critical thinking is at its best when you have your brain purposefully engaged; for example, while you listen to a minilecture, view a video, play a CD-ROM, participate in a discussion or study group, or are being tutored. A critical thinker is paying attention to what the speaker is saying.
- Do I understand it?
- What does it all mean?
- Where does it all fit in?

You are examining your thinking and the thinking of others. Critical thinking is based on science and scientific principles. The principles include the following:
- Collecting data in an organized way
- Verifying the data in an organized way
- Arranging the data in an organized way
- Looking for gaps in information
- Analyzing the data
- Testing it out (Is the data purposeful and outcome/goal oriented?)

These scientific principles align with the nursing process, as you will learn in Chapter 8. A major difference for the scientist is that a problem is identified and then data is collected. The nurse using nursing process collects data first and then determines the nature of the problem (Ignatavicius D. *Medical-surgical nursing* (5th ed.), p. 11). The critical thinker should routinely ask the following questions about the subject of the

thinking task at hand. "Critical Thinking: 10 Key Questions," has been adapted, as follows, for practical/vocational nurses (from Alfaro-Lefevre R, 2009):
1. What major outcomes (observable beneficial results) do you expect to achieve (e.g., when working with the RN to develop a care plan for a newly admitted patient)?
2. What problems, issues, or risks must be addressed to achieve the major outcome (e.g., the hospital unit you are working on is short-staffed)?
3. What is the circumstance or context (e.g., the LPN/LVN is working in the patient's home, where equipment will have to be improvised)?
4. What knowledge is required (e.g., in an area such as mental health, in which you did not have a clinical experience)?
5. How much room is there for error (e.g., the patient is positioned properly after surgery and begs to turn over)?
6. How much time do we have (e.g., the patient who was just admitted is bleeding profusely)?
7. What human and professional resources can help me/us (e.g., the patient is acutely ill and refuses care because of lack of insurance or adequate personal funds)?
8. What perspectives must be considered (e.g., the patient has refused to be examined because of religious beliefs)?
9. What is influencing my thinking (e.g., you are against abortion and do not want to take care of a patient hospitalized because of self-induced abortion)?
10. What must we do to prevent, manage, or eliminate the problems, issues, and risks identified with Question 2?

For each element the thinker, in this case the practical/vocational nurse must be able to reflect on the 10 key critical thinking questions that shed light on the effectiveness of his or her thinking. In other words, is the thinking solving the problem or finding the answer for which you are looking? Critical thinking is an essential part of nursing. The overall purpose of nursing is to assist people to: (1) stay well or (2) regain their maximum state of health as quickly as possible. Both purposes are to be achieved in a cost-effective manner, and in a manner that fits with their belief system. Nurses make decisions that affect both purposes. Nursing decisions must be accurate and based on sound thinking and data. As a nurse your critical thinking skill will vary according to your education and clinical experience. Box 6-1 lists suggestions to increase your critical thinking.

Box 6-1 | *Ways to Challenge You to Think Critically*

- Anticipate questions that the patient or instructor might ask.
- Ask for clarification of what you do not understand.
- Ask yourself if there is more that you can do.
- Reword in your own words what you have read or been told (e.g., stating a nursing diagnosis as a nursing problem).
- Make comparisons with something similar to help you understand.
- Organize information in more than one way to see if you have missed anything important. This is to avoid being impressed when the "facts" fall into place, but you have missed the obvious.
- Ask your instructor to check out your conclusions.
- Strive for objectivity. Keep an open mind and avoid drawing conclusions in advance.
- Review all your data again, especially after a period of time. It may look different, and you may reach a different conclusion.
- Get used to saying, "I don't know, but I will find out."
- Learn from your mistakes. Fix them if you can. Do not hide an error. Someone's life may be at stake, and others can learn from your error.
- Think about what you are reading about while you are reading it. Ask your instructor or peer to challenge you to think critically while you are on the clinical area.

WHAT YOU NEED TO THINK CRITICALLY

For the practical/vocational nurse to think critically, it will be necessary to do the following:
1. *Access information.*
2. *Comprehend information.*
3. *Store comprehended information in long-term memory. This includes having strategies to move information to long-term memory.*
4. *Recall the comprehended information when needed.* (You will need to have the most important information in your head for patient care on clinical.)
5. *Know what to do when information is not in long-term memory.*

As a practical/vocational nursing student you will be exposed to a great deal of new knowledge during the year in the practical/vocational/nursing program. You will gain knowledge, as stated in the course objectives. Your real test as a practical/vocational nurse will be your ability to access information, understand that information, recall it, and use it as the basis for critical thinking in the clinical area.

Critical Thinking Exercise

Critical Thinking Case Scenario

A couple in their twenties had a 2-year-old child. The child became very ill. The baby sitter said to the parents that the child seemed feverish, was extra fussy, and was not eating or drinking his usual amounts. He was admitted to the hospital on the evening of the third day with a fever of 105°F. As his physical condition improved, nurses noted that he was unable to do the things his parents said he could do prior to the illness. Testing showed that the child had suffered brain damage. The parents were alarmed that their normal baby was going to need a great deal of physical care—probably for the rest of his life. The father was in his second year of medical school. His wife had just graduated from college and started a good job that would help him finish medical school. Their physician indicated that an alternative would be to place their child in a home for mentally handicapped children.

Continued

Using critical thinking as described in this chapter, what would your decision be if you were one of the parents, and what is your rationale for the decision?

FACTORS THAT INFLUENCE CRITICAL THINKING

Your current critical thinking status is influenced by the following personal and situational factors:

- **Upbringing and culture**. Having family and teacher support and opportunities to learn to read well and understand the meaning of what you read; beginning to make simple, limited choices at an early age, which become more complex with consequences as you grow.
- **Motivation**. Whether you learned early to rely on others for motivation, or whether you decided you would learn in spite of the lack of external motivators, motivation determines in part the progress you have made in problem solving and critical thinking. You have the ability to think critically if you choose to do so. It is a preference on your part. Remember that the brain is like a muscle: The more you exercise it, the better it works.
- **Attitude influences thinking**. Critical thinkers are humble and recognize that they do not have all the answers and may be influenced by their beliefs and values. While in the process of patient care, it makes a critical difference in whether a problem is recognized, missed, or ignored. Take time to collect some data on your attitude by completing the following learning exercise.

Learning Exercise

Attitude Evaluation—My Attitude

Directions: On a scale of 0-10 (with 10 as the best), rate your attitude.
___I am aware of the limitations of my knowledge.
___I am aware that my dislikes, biases, and prejudices may influence my decisions.

___I try to be fair-minded.
___I am interested in understanding other people's thoughts and feelings.
___I check to find out if my statements are clear.
___I can be influenced by another person's conclusions, if based on fact.
___I question other people's sources of information.
___I acknowledge that what I have been thinking can be incorrect.
___I question the availability of additional alternatives.
___I listen to my intuition and compare it with my reasoning.
___I am aware that perfect solutions are not always available.
___I am willing to work as a team member.
___I try to anticipate problems before they occur.
___I am continually looking for ways to improve my thinking.

These items describe your strong attitudes for the development of critical thinking. The items are attitudes you need to improve to increase critical thinking. Box 6-2 lists characteristics and attitudes of critical thinkers.

Critical Thinking Exercise

Attitudes to Work on

Prioritize the attitudes you choose to work on first, to help increase your critical thinking. How will you recognize improvement in each item you listed?

ADDITIONAL FACTORS THAT INFLUENCE CRITICAL THINKING

Alfaro-Lefevre (2009) discusses the following personal factors that also influence critical thinking. These are summarized with some additional thoughts for practical/vocational nurses.

1. **Effective Reading**
   a. Effective reading, as you have learned, is more than reading with speed.
   b. It means that you are able to identify the significance and potential application of what you are reading.

Box 6-2 | *Characteristics/Attitudes of Critical Thinkers*

- Self-confident: Expresses ability to think through problems and find solutions
- Inquisitive: Seeks reasons, explanations, and new information
- Honest and upright: Speaks and seeks the truth, even if the truth sheds unwanted light
- Alert to context: Looks for changes in circumstances that may warrant a need to modify thinking or approaches
- Open and fair-minded: Shows tolerance for different viewpoints; questions how own viewpoints are influencing thinking
- Analytical and insightful: Identifies relationships; shows deep understanding
- Logical and intuitive: Draws reasonable conclusions (if this is so, then it follows that … because…); uses intuition as a guide to search for evidence
- Reflective and self-corrective: Carefully considers meaning of data and interpersonal interactions; corrects own thinking; observant for mistakes; identifies ways to prevent mistakes
- Sensitive to diversity: Expresses appreciation of human differences related to values, culture, personality, or learning style preferences; adapts to preferences when feasible

Reproduced with permission from Alfaro-Lafevre R. (2006). *Evidence-based critical thinking indicators.*™ Available at www.AlfaroTeachSmart.com.

   c. An effective learning skill means that you are able to organize the data you have so you can access it efficiently.

   d. Chapter 4 provides suggestions to make studying, note making, etc., work for you. Remember that employers need more than someone with random-access memory.

2. **Maturity**

   a. Maturity most often comes with age.

   b. Maturity provides past opportunities to have worked through problems. It becomes easier to see problems through someone else's eyes.

   c. Do you work to understand others before expecting them to understand you?

3. **Problem Solving and the Nursing Process**

   a. Knowledge of problem solving and of the nursing process is based on many of the same principles as is critical thinking.

   b. Do you use the problem-solving steps to work out problems now? Understanding and applying the problem-solving steps gives you a head start in thinking critically.

4. **Communication Skills**

   a. Communicating effectively means being aware of the message you are sending verbally, in writing and through body language. Are you willing to listen and consider ideas and views different from your own? Do you express yourself well in writing? Communication is discussed more fully in Chapter 9.

5. **Self-Confidence**

   a. Self-confidence is often the personal characteristic that is the least available to a student.

   b. Without self-confidence the student is wasting a lot of energy worrying that they will not "get it."

   c. It may help to remember that no one can give you self-confidence. You develop self-confidence as you succeed in your endeavors. This is where the saying "self-confidence is earned not learned" comes from.

   d. Overconfidence may cause the individual to assume that they are correct even before there is data to back up what they believe to be correct. Do you acknowledge the limits of your knowledge and skills?

6. **Moral Development**

   a. Moral development creates fair-mindedness, a strong sense of what is right and wrong and just. Have you examined your values, and can you separate them from the values held by others?

7. **Capability in Nursing**
   a. Capability in nursing is essential. You must have nursing knowledge and skills to do the work of nursing and know how to access the resources.
   b. Nursing instructors have an enormous amount of factual information that they expect to introduce to their nursing students. The amount is often overwhelming to both the instructor and the student.
   c. Determining what is absolutely necessary to know, from what is nice to know, is no easy task. The tendency is to hang onto what is fun to know and old information, just in case someone asks or it is in a test somewhere.
   d. With the knowledge explosion instructors can no longer infuse their students with all they need to know.
   e. What are needed are the tools for how to locate information and comprehend information, how to store information in long-term memory, and how to recall the comprehended information when needed.

8. **Collaboration**
   a. Students and instructors still tend to work alone rather than collaborate with each other in the learning/studying process.
   b. A collaborative effort has been shown to promote critical-thinking skills; for example, a small student group could work together on a significant learning project. First, it would entail presenting the instructor with a well-thought-out plan (including observable, project outcomes/goals).
   c. We have had a student now and again come to class and be angry to find out that lecture was not the primary way of teaching. A student who was an auditory learner (learns by listening) expressed her anger because she had never before had to read her text and be prepared for a discussion. Being prepared to discuss would have showed that she really understood the information. She had been able to memorize enough just by listening to pass her tests because testing for knowledge was common in the past.

9. **Anxiety**
   a. When anxiety overwhelms, it effectively stops critical thinking.
   b. The same is true with a high level of fatigue. This is why we are including a new chapter on personal health promotion (see Chapter 10).

10. **Mentors and Experience in Nursing**
    a. Time limitations are a real problem in doing the work of nursing. They make a big difference in which area you have chosen to work.
    b. Work experience and the guidance of nursing mentors, starting with your instructor, will assist you in learning to identify priorities in nursing care.
    c. Depending on the work area, patients may be there to seek help for a few hours or days (emergency or treatment), or for the rest of their life (nursing home).

CRITICAL THINKING AND NCLEX-PN®

NCLEX-PN®, the national licensing examination for practical/vocational nurses, includes items that require various levels of thinking to answer a test item. These various levels are called cognitive levels. The cognitive levels used on the NCLEX-PN® examination are knowledge, comprehension, application, and analysis. The following definitions will help you comprehend the meaning of the words *knowledge* (knowing), *comprehension, application,* and *analysis.*

1. Knowledge refers to the ability to recall and repeat information you have memorized. *Memorizing is not the same as understanding a concept.* Knowledge is the lowest level of learning. Defining a concept as stated in a dictionary is an example of knowledge level.

2. Comprehension refers to the ability to very basically understand information, recall it,

and identify examples of that information. To comprehend is to *grasp the meaning* of the material. Comprehension is the lowest level of understanding. An example of the comprehension level is the ability to repeat information in your own words. This indicates that you understand the information.

3. Application means being able to *use learned material in new situations.* For example, you apply what is learned in class to your clinical work. Application involves being able to prioritize or determine what is most important, what comes first. Application is a higher level of understanding. *You must be able to use knowledge to tailor approaches depending on circumstances.*

4. Analysis means to be able to *break down complex information into its basic parts,* and relate those parts to the whole picture. An example of analysis is the ability to *organize and prioritize* (what is most important, most urgent) two or more pieces of information in a patient situation to *process a safe response.* Analysis is a higher level of application. To be able to choose the most important symptoms that are all present in a patient with a specific problem is an example of analysis.

Comprehension, application, and analysis are what employers expect of a practical/vocational nurse on the job. Your instructors will also expect this level of competence in the clinical area as you continue to develop your critical thinking skills. Past students with college degrees have told us that the consistent requirement to apply and analyze both prior and newly learned information is the major point about practical/vocational nursing that differs most from their college experience.

The review items for each chapter in this text will include five items. Four items will be in multiple-choice format, the same as in the NCLEX-PN® examination. These multiple-choice items will test you at the knowledge, comprehension, application, and analysis level. They will help you understand the four cognitive levels and help you prepare for testing. Most important, they will keep your focus on understanding information to be able to continue the development of your critical-thinking skills.

In April 2005 the National Council revised new item formats on NCLEX® examinations (first introduced in 2003). Called *alternate format items,* these items may include: (1) multiple response, (2) fill-in-the-blank (e.g., calculation, ordered response), and (3) hotspot (e.g., the place on a diagram that answers the question). All item formats may have charts, tables, or graphic images. The fifth review item we are including with each chapter is an alternate-format, multiple-choice item that requires you to select more than one response. The 2005 NCLEX-PN® examination required the application of all levels of cognitive ability. The majority of items were written at the application or higher levels of cognitive abilities (2005 NCLEX-PN® test plan). Currently, test items are written at the application and analysis levels (2008 NCLEX-PN® test plan). Your instructor has access to more NCLEX-PN® type questions in Evolve and the Instructor Resource Manual and Test Bank. The *Saunders Q&A Review for NCLEX-PN® Examination* by L. Silvestri (2007) has 3000 practice questions including alternate format question and an 85-question comprehensive examination.

Storing information in long-term memory and being able to recall the comprehended information when needed is dealt with in Chapter 4. We stress the importance of learning this information thoroughly. Your effort will make a difference in all of your studies and in being prepared for the NCLEX-PN® examination.

MAKING IT WORK FOR YOU

This is a good time for you to be reminded that we all have special, although different, abilities in the area of thinking. The trick is to discover what those abilities are, embrace them, and make them work for you. You can choose whether to make the most of your abilities. You can also choose to not make a decision about your abilities. However, not deciding is also a decision.

There is also the tendency to be impressed by someone who begins to speak immediately to an issue as though they have the facts, when in truth their style of processing is outside of themselves. Perhaps your way is to process internally and not speak out until you have all the words in place. The one who processes externally may ask the questions you wish you had asked. This difference is related to their personality. Their verbalization sounds impressive and tends to frighten the person who processes internally before speaking. Both types can be equally effective in their ability to think critically. Each way is different: A difference in personality is all it has to be unless you allow yourself to begin thinking negatively about your abilities.

WHERE TO GO FROM HERE

This chapter has been written as a critical thinking primer, and is limited to need-to-know information. The questions and suggestions offered are those that are within the scope of the LPN/LVN and the nursing program. Reflective (critical) thinking will assist you in determining if you need outside assistance from your school's study skills center or the instructor in setting up realistic observable goals/outcomes. You may even decide that the awareness of personal and situational characteristics is enough to get you started on your own. The critical thinking exercises provide you with a practical framework for increasing your critical-thinking ability.

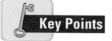

Key Points

- Thinking is divided into nonfocused thinking and directed thinking.
- Critical-thinking answers the question, "How can we do this better?"
- Critical thinking is the basis for learning and applying the nursing process.
- To think critically, it is necessary to (1) access information, (2) comprehend information, (3) store comprehended information in long-term memory, and (4) recall the comprehended information when needed.
- Comprehension, application, and analysis are what employers will expect from LPN/LVNs on the job.
- The cognitive levels used in the NCLEX-PN® examination are knowledge, comprehension, application, and analysis. Most questions are written at the application or higher level of cognitive thinking.
- The ability to read with understanding is the cornerstone of critical thinking.
- Both personal and situational factors influence critical thinking.
- The decision is yours whether to use the abilities you already possess to enhance your critical-thinking ability.

REVIEW ITEMS

1. When was the nursing process and critical thinking mandated as part of SPN/SVN education?

   1. 1990
   2. 1992
   3. 1997
   4. 2002

2. What is a major difference between knowledge, comprehension, application, and analysis?

   1. Knowledge is the ability to understand and give examples of what you have learned.
   2. Comprehension is the ability to explain or summarize information you have read.
   3. Application is the ability to break down information into its component parts.
   4. Analysis is the ability to use principles and general ideas in concrete situations.

3. Which pattern shows the use of critical thinking?

   1. During report, you learned that the new patient is short tempered. You decide you will humor her, do what is necessary, and give her plenty of space the rest of the time.
   2. Mr. Fodor has to have six small feedings each day, and although he can feed himself, you have decided to increase the intake by sitting on the bed and feeding him.
   3. Mrs. Still is crying when you arrive to give her a bath. She tells you her baby died after birth. You cheer her up by telling her, "That's nothing. I lost two babies."
   4. Charlie was admitted as an emergency admission. You are asked to hold him in position for a spinal tap. Hold him firmly in position and speak softly and reassuringly.

4. Which of the following is a negative example of thinking?

   1. The brain grasps information in phrases.
   2. Negative thinking works as a conscience.
   3. Critical thinking looks beyond the obvious.
   4. Habitual thinking is useful in our life.

ALTERNATE FORMAT ITEM

Which of the following statements do not reflect reasons for thinking critically? *(Select all that apply.)*

1. Time would be better spent on developing an up-to-date curriculum for students.

2. The way nursing has always been done is the best it can be for nurses and patients.

3. Rapid change and information explosion creates a need for new learning and skills.

4. Focused thinking in every area may make a difference between success and failure.

How Practical/Vocational Nursing Evolved

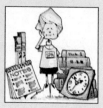

evolve http://evolve.elsevier.com/Hill/success/

Objectives

On completing this chapter, you will be able to do the following:

1. Describe the role of self-defined practical nurses throughout history.
2. Discuss four major events that influenced changes in practical nursing.
3. Identify the year and place the first school of practical nursing was founded.
4. Name the year in which licensing for practical nursing first began.
5. Present the rationale for your personal stand on entry into nursing practice.

Key Terms

Almshouses (p. 92)
Attendant nurses (p. 98)
Barton, Clara (p. 98)
Dix, Dorothea Lynde (p. 97)
Gamp, Sairey (p. 93)
Mississippi, 1914 (p. 100)
Nightingale, Florence (p. 94)
Phoebe (fē-bē, p. 92)
Prig, Betsy (p. 93)
Seacole, Mary (p. 95)
Self-proclaimed nurse (prō-KLĀM, p. 86)
Semmelweis, Ignaz Philipp (p. 93)
Sisters of Charity (p. 92)
Wald, Lillian (p. 99)

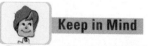

Keep in Mind

The first nurses were practical nurses and you are part of that proud heritage.

The length of the course for the modern practical (or vocational) nurse is approximately 9 months to 1 year in most states. There is some variation in the actual number of weeks. Historically speaking, all nurses had less educational preparation for their work than do current licensed practical/vocational nurses (LPN/LVNs).

SELF-PROCLAIMED NURSE

Practical nurses have a varied and colorful evolution. In this narrative, practical nurses are referred to in a broad sense as those who, from the beginning of time, chose (or were appointed) to care for individuals who were ill, injured, dying, or having babies. Names used to designate this person have included attendant, wet nurse, self-proclaimed nurse, midwife, trained nurse, and practical nurse. Most often the individual doing this work was someone who seemed to have a "gift" or "touch" for helping others during a medical crisis. Some "nurses" learned from others in an apprenticeship setting, and others extended their "mothering" skills to the care of the sick. The practical nurse was the original home health nurse and visiting nurse. Much of the care was offered in the home, and these nurses were on call for the needy.

EARLY PRACTICAL NURSE TRAINING PROGRAMS

Early practical nurse training programs carefully limited teaching to those things that would be known by a good homemaker or a competent maid. Training included information that would in no way compete with that of the physicians of the time. Physicians themselves had limited knowledge and training. It is interesting to realize that nursing history did not parallel medical history. When medicine advanced, nursing did not. When medical advances slowed down, nursing progressed.

MODERN PRACTICAL NURSES

Nursing has experienced many changes throughout its history. The changes continue. Two major changes that have occurred in practical nursing are a gradual increase in the required formal knowledge base and a requirement for licensing to practice practical nursing. Unlike the historically untrained or poorly trained practical nurse, who had unlimited and unsupervised freedom to practice, the present practical nurse is now often a hybrid. Today's practical/vocational nursing student (SPN/SVN) is being taught basic skills during the educational program. After licensing, the LPN/LVN is permitted to perform complex nursing skills, as delegated by the registered nurse (RN) and allowed by their state's nurse practice act. Delegation is allowed as long as the following requirements are met:

- An RN is willing to teach the skill.
- An RN observes the return demonstration.
- An RN documents the teaching or learning process for the LPN/LVNs file in the place of employment.

In addition, most nurse practice acts call for direct supervision by RNs for all complex nursing tasks delegated by them. See Chapter 16 for information on delegation.

WHY LEARN ABOUT NURSING HISTORY?

Reading nursing history helps you see your place among the many centuries of women and men who have given care, relief, and support to the sick. This chapter provides a broad overview of the role of nursing during different periods of history. If you know about the changes that occurred in nursing, you will be ready to better understand and adapt to changes in the future (Table 7-1). Currently you are the future of nursing. Years from now you will be part of nursing's rich and varied history.

Table 7-1 | *Practical Nursing Milestones*

PERIOD IN HISTORY	EVENT
Ancient Egypt	Midwives delivered babies
	Untrained attendants assisted priests in caring for the ill
Ancient Hebrews	Wet nurses and attendants nursed the sick and acted as companions
Ancient Greece (fifth century BC)	Household nursing and child care were done by domestics and servants
Age of Christianity (first to fifth centuries)	Both men and women were nurses; each cared for members of own sex
	Phoebe—The first visiting nurse
Dark Ages (476-1000)	Monks and nuns continued to do practical nursing
	Knights Hospitalers—A military order trained to fight as well as to tend the sick and wounded
Middle Ages (1000-1475)	Time of epidemics. Highborn women renounced their heritage to care for the sick
	Alexian Brothers founded—A nursing brotherhood that still exists in a dual religious and nursing role

Continued

Table 7-1 | *Practical Nursing Milestones—cont'd*

PERIOD IN HISTORY	EVENT
	At the end of the Middle Ages, religious orders no longer assumed as much responsibility for care of the sick
Renaissance (1400-1600)	Scientific methods of the Greeks were employed again, but nursing declined until the nineteenth century
Age of Industrialization (eighteenth and nineteenth centuries)	Deplorable, unsanitary conditions
	Untrained care givers
	Semmelweis—Developed antiseptic methods (1847)
Seventeenth and eighteenth centuries (American Colonies)	Almshouses and pesthouses
	Nursing done by untrained persons
Nineteenth-century America	Nursing considered an inferior, undesirable occupation. Care given by untrained lay people often drawn from the criminal population
	Charles Dickens' novel *Martin Chuzzlewit* (1849) introduced Sairey Gamp and Betsy Prig as the nurse prototypes of that period
1836	First real school of nursing, in Kaiserswerth, Germany. Florence Nightingale attended for 3 months
	Eighteen years later, after start of Crimean War, she nursed wounded with 38 self-identified (untrained) nurses
1860	Florence Nightingale established a school of nursing in England. She wrote several books. The most famous was *Notes on Nursing*
Civil War (1861-1865)	In the South: Most nursing done by infantrymen assigned to the task. Southern women volunteered services
	In the North: Dorothea Lynde Dix, a teacher, was appointed Superintendent of Nurses and organized a corps of female nurses (untrained)
1864	Clara Barton, a teacher, collected supplies for soldiers. This led to her appointment as Superintendent of the Department of Nurses for the Army
1881	Clara Barton established the first chapter of the American Red Cross in Danville, New York
1892	First class for formal training of practical nursing: YWCA, Brooklyn, New York
1893	Nightingale Pledge written by Canada-born Lystra Gretter, principal of Farrand Training School in Detroit
	Henry Street Settlement founded by Lillian Wald, a social worker who graduated from a nursing program
	Practical nurses pioneered in this new public health movement. They went into homes and taught the basics of cleanliness and control of communicable diseases to families in New York slums
1897	Ballard School for Practical Nursing opened in New York
1907	Thompson School for Practical Nursing opened in Brattleboro, Vermont
1914	Mississippi is the first state to pass a law to license practical nurses
1917	Standardization of nursing requirements for practical nursing by National League of Nursing Education (now the National League for Nursing [NLN])

Table 7-1 | *Practical Nursing Milestones—cont'd*

PERIOD IN HISTORY	EVENT
World War I	Shortage of practical nurses. Army School of Nursing established.
	Smith Hughes Act of 1917 provided money for developing additional schools of practical nursing
1920s	Acute shortage of practical nurses
	Many did not return to nursing after the war
1920-1940	Most practical nursing limited to public health agencies and visiting nurse associations
1938	New York only state to have mandatory licensure
World War II	Shortage of RNs created need for LPNs. At home, practical nurses worked in clinics, health departments, industries, and hospitals. In the war, they ventured into hardship tours in Europe, North Africa, and the Pacific.
1940	The number of practical nurses peaked in 1940 at 159,009
1941	NAPNES (National Association of Practical Nurse Education and Service), the nation's professional organization dedicated exclusively to practical nursing, was founded
1944	Comprehensive study of practical nursing by U.S. Department of Vocational Education. This was the first time that tasks of practical nursing were agreed upon
End of World War II	Nursing shortage saw movement of practical nurses into hospitals and gradually increasing responsibilities
1949	NFLPN (National Federation of Licensed Practical Nurses) was founded to provide structure nationwide through which LPNs could promote better patient care and act on behalf of LPNs. The NFLPN organized Joint Committee on Practical Nurses and Auxiliary Workers in Nursing Services recommended use of the title licensed practical nurse and differentiated between tasks of registered nurses and LPNs
1951	*Journal of Practical Nursing* published by NAPNES (now *Practical Nursing Today*)
1952	Approximately 60% of the nurse work force was made up of practical nurses
1955	All states had licensure laws for practical/vocational nurses
1957	NLN established a Council of Practical Nursing Programs
1960	By 1960 every state had a nurse licensure law
1961	NLN began offering accrediting services for practical nursing programs
1965	ANA (American Nurses Association) first moves toward two distinct levels in nursing—professional and technical
1975	1315 state-approved PN programs. More than 45,000 PN graduates. After 1975, number of PN programs and graduates declined.
1979	NLN published first list of competencies for practical/vocational nursing programs
1980s	Resurgence of ANA moves toward two distinct levels of nursing. This resulted in some states adopting two levels of nursing and then rescinding their decision because of the nursing shortage. By late 1980s, RN salaries were considerably higher than LPNs. Many RNs replaced LPNs.

Continued

Table 7-1 *Practical Nursing Milestones—cont'd*

PERIOD IN HISTORY	EVENT
1984	Creation of ALPNA (American Licensed Practical Nurses Association)
1989	The American Medical Association (AMA) initiated and subsequently dropped the registered care technician (RCT) proposal
1990s	Unlicensed personnel are used for client care. The number of hospital jobs has decreased. The primary employment site has moved into the community.
1994	First computerized adaptive test (NCLEX-PN®) available to practical/vocational nursing graduates
1995	Full-time nursing positions in hospitals decreased. Patient/nurse ratios increased. Primary employment in community continues
1996	Long-term care certification examinations for LPNs/LVNs by National Council of State Boards of Nursing with the National Association for Licensed Practical Nurse Education and Service
2000	Increased demand for LPNs/LVNs in nursing homes and extended care; demand down in hospitals
2007	Nursing shortage: Fewer students are entering nursing programs

ANCIENT CULTURES

Nursing history has been recorded for approximately 150 years. It is interesting to speculate about nursing history before then. For example, primitive cultures looked on illness as a direct reflection of a personal relationship with the gods. Ill fortune, as it applied to health, was regarded as a sign of disfavor because of behavior that was not pleasing to the gods. Among these cultures there was generally a wise person (medicine man) who possessed magical powers. This allowed him to get in touch with, and deal with, the angered gods. For example, some pagan cultures had a shaman (holy man) who would go into a trance. While in the trance he would "slip into a crack in the earth" to travel down the river to the "valley of the dead." There he would bargain with the gods to find out what was needed from the one who was ill, or if indeed the ill person would die. Stories of these customs were passed on through song. Few women assisted the medicine man. Women primarily attended women during childbirth.

ANCIENT EGYPT

No direct evidence exists of nursing in Egypt. However, written records of procedures used in ancient Egypt were probably those of the male attendants (nurses), who assisted the priests in caring for the ill. Temples became sanitariums where diseased people were treated. It is believed that 4000 years ago Egyptian physicians and attendants had an extensive list of treatments for specific illnesses, which differed remarkably from medicines used today. Interesting evidence was found in the tomb of an eleventh-dynasty queen. Her tomb included a medicine chest complete with vases, spoons, medicines, and herbs. "Lizard's blood, swine's ears and teeth, putrid meat and fat, tortoise brains, old books boiled in oil, milk of a lying-in woman, water of a chaste woman, lice and excreta of men, donkeys, dogs, lions, and cats are examples of some of the ingredients that were used" (Kalish and Kalish, 1995).

Egyptian physicians were considered skillful at treating fractures. The custom of embalming enabled the Egyptians to become well acquainted with organs of the body. From clinical observation they learned to recognize some 250 different diseases. To treat them they developed a number of drugs and procedures, such as surgery (Deloughery, 1998). There is evidence of detailed instructions for daily nursing care, which included recording the pulse, using splints, dressing wounds, feeding patients, and using hollow reeds for urinary catheters.

BABYLONIANS

Ancient Babylonians were intellectually, socially, and scientifically well developed. Many wars brought them misery, illness, and injury. There is evidence of some kind of medical and nursing service. The men dominated women and men did the primary care of those who were sick and injured.

ANCIENT HEBREWS

Illness and misfortune were blamed on God's wrath according to the *Old Testament* and *Talmud*. People depended on God to restore health. The ancient Hebrews had houses for the sick and homes for the aged, and began many practices of personal hygiene and public sanitation. They combined health and dietary practices according to religious beliefs. Ancient Hebrews had also adopted hygienic practices learned while captors of the Babylonians. They burned infested garments, isolated ill persons, and scrubbed homes of those who were infected. Close association between religion and medicine was seen, as priests functioned in the role of major health officer.

The *Talmud* mentions nurses as persons caring for the sick at home. The *Old Testament* has many passages that refer to wet nurses, and to those who nursed the sick or acted as companions.

ANCIENT GREECE

The greatest civilization of its time, ancient Greece (fifth century BC), gave the world Hippocrates, Socrates, Plato, and Aristotle, and a system of logical thought. This paved the way for the rational treatment of illness rather than people accepting illness as god-inflicted.

Hippocrates, the "father of modern medicine," translated teachings that were once the secrets of priests into a textbook of medicine. He introduced patient-centered care, medical ethics, a method of assessment, and a system of observing symptoms and applying carefully reasoned principles to care. These observations replaced the superstitions and illogical concepts of primitive medicine. Temples were built for restoration of health. They were more like our health spas of today. Priestesses served as attendants to care for the sick. Pregnant women and individuals considered incurable were not admitted. Writings by Hippocrates refer to procedures that today would be undertaken in modern hospitals by nurses. Hippocrates labeled the health care provider a physician. Physicians and physicians' assistants carried out the Hippocratic nursing procedures. Many of Hippocrates' teachings were discarded because of previously established beliefs. Today the Hippocratic Oath continues to be the ethical code of modern medical practice.

Aristotle provided additional knowledge about the heart and blood vessels. Because it was forbidden to touch the dead, his knowledge was not widely used. Women in Greece occupied a low position and were not considered worthy to be trained in medicine and nursing. Domestics and servants provided household nursing and child care.

 Critical Thinking Exercise

Hippocratic Oath

Obtain a copy of the Hippocratic oath. Note that Hippocrates referred to all health care workers as physicians. Does the oath apply to the work you will do as an LPN?

EARLY AND MIDDLE AGES

AGE OF CHRISTIANITY (FIRST TO FIFTH CENTURIES AD)

Greece's power and prestige declined. The Roman Empire was the dominant power at the time of Christ's birth. Rome established military hospitals; relatives and friends did much of the practical nursing of the day. Much of the knowledge of medicine and nursing gained in the Greek era of power was lost. Few could read and understand the works of Hippocrates and other great thinkers of his time.

As Christianity grew, nursing developed as a form of Christian charity. Christian nurses, including both men and women, cared for members of their own sex. St. Paul, of Biblical fame, introduced a woman named Phoebe (about 60 AD), an ordained deaconess, to Rome approximately 30 years after Jesus was crucified. Phoebe, a practical nurse, is known as the *first visiting nurse*.

Fabiola, another Roman woman, spent her wealth nursing the sick and poor. She provided a free hospital in Rome in about 370 AD.

DARK AGES AND MIDDLE AGES (476–1000 AD AND 1000–1475 AD)

When the power of the Roman Empire declined, invading tribes brought violence and chaos to Europe. The period from 476 to 1000 AD has been called the Dark Ages, to reflect the loss of widespread education and learning in Europe. Ongoing battles between the church and state hindered care of the sick and poor. The Christian church retreated behind the walls of convents and monasteries. Learning was kept alive within these walls. In the Middle Ages both men and women were involved in nursing: Female religious orders took care of the sick and poor and male orders served on the battlefield. The *Knights Hospitalers* was an interesting group of monks, a military order trained to fight, as well as to tend the sick and wounded.

One of the nursing brotherhoods founded during this time was the *Alexian Brothers*. It exists today in a dual religious and nursing role. The history of nursing during this period includes stories of highborn women who renounced their heritage to care for the sick. Someone needed to do the nursing because the Middle Ages was a time of horrible epidemics, such as that of the infamous bubonic plague, which killed millions of people. At the end of the Middle Ages, Europe seemed to be old and worn out. Religious fervor

was replaced by cynicism and despair. Religious orders no longer assumed as much responsibility for care of the sick.

THE RENAISSANCE (1400-1600 AD)

The Renaissance was a time for rebirth of learning. The information of the ancient Greeks and Romans was sought and put to use. The scientific method of the Greeks was employed again. The disciplines of anatomy, physiology, and scientific healing were developed.

Nursing declined and was all but forgotten until the nineteenth century. The religious Reformation, in which the church split into Catholic and Protestant factions, contributed to the decline in organized nursing. Monasticism nearly ended in Protestant countries such as England and Germany, and with its end, nursing. Greater personal freedom may have been achieved during the Renaissance; with it the tradition of unselfish service to humanity almost disappeared. It was a cruel age marked by neglect of the poor, homeless, and ill. St. Vincent de Paul almost single-handedly organized the Sisters of Charity in France to care for the poor and to nurse the sick.

SEVENTEENTH AND EIGHTEENTH CENTURIES

Hospital care did not exist in the North American colonies during the seventeenth and early eighteenth centuries. Family members cared for those who became ill. What did exist were almshouses for the poor and pest houses for those with contagious diseases. Motivation for building the pest houses was to protect the public, not to treat the sick.

Medicine in America was less developed than that in Europe. Colonial physicians were poorly trained. Exceptions were the few who obtained their education in England. Untrained persons, and those in a few religious orders whose mission was to care for the sick, did nursing.

The first real hospital in America was built in the mid-1700s in Philadelphia, at the urging of Benjamin Franklin. All the early American hospitals emulated French and English hospitals.

Hospitalization was made available to the poor for a small fee.

Hospitals obtained medical services by permitting teaching on the wards. Medical advances were slow. The treatment of choice for many diseases was brandy, whiskey, emetics, purgatives, and bleeding. The illustrations in this chapter depict historical nursing settings.

AGE OF INDUSTRIALIZATION

Industrialization became more widespread in the eighteenth century, as did problems with disease. The movement of people to cities, the unhealthy working conditions, child labor, and overcrowding had an impact on health care during the Industrial Revolution. They grew in number, as did their mortality rates. Many patients shared the same bed amid unsanitary conditions. The practice of asepsis had not yet become a part of medical and nursing knowledge. Once inside the hospital, patients often contracted additional diseases. Home care continued without benefit of training. Chances for survival were probably better in the home than in the hospital. During this time in Vienna, women in labor begged to be allowed to deliver in the street rather than in the hospital. To be admitted meant sure death because the mortality rate was 100% at times.

Not until 1847 were *antiseptic methods* first developed and used. Ignaz Philipp Semmelweis, a Hungarian obstetrician, began to study what was called *childbed fever*. A physician friend died after he cut his finger during an autopsy. Semmelweis recognized that his friend had died from essentially the same disease that killed women who had babies. He identified the cause of childbed (puerperal) fever as septic material carried to the mothers (on the hands of medical students), directly from the autopsy room. He insisted medical students and physicians wash their hands in a solution of *chloride of lime* before entering the obstetric ward. Antisepsis soon included the instruments and utensils used in the ward. As a result, the rate of death from childbed fever dropped dramatically in that ward.

NINETEENTH CENTURY

Early nineteenth-century American hospitals were places of confinement where one picked up additional diseases. The hospital wards were overcrowded, dirty, unventilated, and filled with patients with discharging wounds and lacking trained help. Perfume was used to cover-up offensive odors. Nurses of that time used snuff as a way of trying to make their work conditions bearable. Pain, hemorrhage, infections, and gangrene were the order of the day. Nursing was considered an inferior, undesirable occupation. Lay people, often drawn from the criminal population, replaced religious attendants (nurses). They exploited and abused patients. Supervision was nonexistent. There was little or no nursing service at night, unless a delivery or a death was expected. A "watcher" was hired in these cases.

Nurses were often widows with large families. Drinking on duty and accepting bribes from patients and families were commonplace. Nurses often drank the stimulants intended for the sick and were seen drunk and fighting over the dead. "Vice was rampant among these women, who sometimes aided the dying by removing pillows and bed clothes and by performing other morbid activities to hasten the end" (Kalish and Kalish, 1995). They were paid by undertakers to provide additional bodies.

In Europe, nursing in secular institutions had become nonexistent. This was especially true in Protestant countries, where the services of the Sisters of Charity were not available. Typical of the hospital nurse at the time were ignorant, gin-soaked nurse midwives, such as Sairey Gamp and Betsy Prig, in Charles Dickens' 1849 novel, *Martin Chuzzlewit.*

Nursing care in America was every bit as bad as the situation in Europe. An excerpt describing the cholera epidemic in the Philadelphia General Hospital in 1833 painted a picture of overcrowding and demands for increased wages. Finally, an appeal was made to the Bishop for the services of the Sisters of Charity. They came, restored order, and nursed the sick.

FIRST SCHOOL OF NURSING (1836)

The *first real school of nursing* was founded by the Lutheran Order of Deaconesses under the supervision of a German pastor, Theodor Fleidner, in Kaiserswerth, Germany. The year was 1836. The purpose of the program was to teach principles of nursing care to the Lutheran Order of Deaconesses. Many of the graduates of Kaiserswerth Deaconess Institute settled in other parts of the world and established similar programs. The school's most famous pupil was the Englishwoman, Florence Nightingale, founder of modern nursing. She attended the school for 3 months and studied under Caroline Fliedner.

FLORENCE NIGHTINGALE (1820-1910)

Florence Nightingale (Fig. 7-1) was born in Florence, Italy. Her parents named her after the city and called her "Flo." Nightingale's parents were wealthy, influential, and accepted in society. Florence was presented at court and was expected to follow the social pattern of other women of her day. Women were considered intellectually inferior to men. Education for middle- and upper class women often consisted of lessons in etiquette, dancing, music, deportment, embroidery, painting, and modern languages. Instead of being tutored by governesses or in a private school, Nightingale's father tutored her in modern and ancient languages, history, composition, philosophy, and mathematics, including statistics. He was strict; she was an eager student (LeVasseur, 1998).

Nightingale turned down a proposal of marriage—a man her sister later married. Early on, Nightingale knew she had a purpose in life to fulfill. She begged her parents to permit her to go into the nurses' training program in Kaiserswerth, Germany. Her parents were not pleased since nursing was seen as a job suitable only for the Sairey Gamp type of woman. As we know, Nightingale got her way. Upon graduation, she became superintendent for The Institution for the Care of Sick Gentlewomen in Distressed

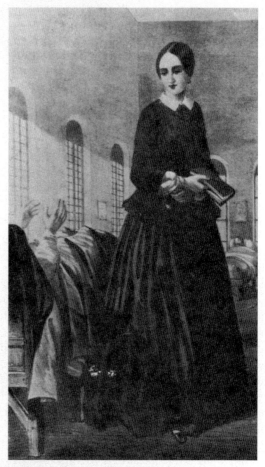

FIGURE **7-1** Florence Nightingale carrying out the "nursing process." (Nursing Mirror photograph.)

Circumstances, now the Harley Street Nursing Home in London (Romanoff, 2006). As you might guess, she began to take steps to make the work of nurses who served the gentlewomen easier. Dumbwaiters were installed, so the nurses did not have to carry heavy trays up and down stairs. Nightingale also developed a system of call bells that could be seen in hallways to identify which person was summoning. Because the institution discriminated against Catholics and Jews, she dropped religion as a requirement for admission. Some of the governing board members were not happy with her changes.

The following year as Nightingale was planning to become superintendent of King's College Hospital in London, the Crimean war broke out. She sent a letter to the Secretary of War offering her services. She did not know that he had also sent a letter to her requesting assistance.

CRIMEAN WAR

Shortly after the start of the 1853 Crimean War (in which Britain, France, Turkey, and Sardinia fought Russia for control of access to the Mediterranean from the Black Sea), information about the neglect and poor care of casualties began to reach England. A correspondent for London's *Times* newspaper wrote vivid accounts of the deplorable conditions and lack of medical and nursing care for the British troops. The Sisters of Mercy tended Russian troops, the Sisters of Charity tended the French, and the wounded of England were almost completely neglected. The correspondent's charges were so persistent that a commission was sent to investigate. As a result, the Secretary of War decided that England, too, should have a group of women nurses to tend the war casualties.

The Secretary of War contacted Florence Nightingale and explained the situation to her. Because she had both nursing and administrative experience, the Secretary perceived her as the one nurse in England capable of organizing and supervising care in a foreign land.

Being appointed to the task of organization and supervision of nurses during the Crimean War gave Nightingale an unexpected opportunity for achievement. She left for Crimea, taking with her 38 self-proclaimed nurses of limited experience, 24 of whom were nuns. On arrival, they found overcrowded, filthy hospitals with no beds, no furniture, no eating utensils, no medical supplies, no blankets, no soap, no linens, and no lamps. Wounded soldiers lay on the floor in their battle uniforms, in filth. Soldiers were more likely to die from infected wounds than the wound itself. Nightingale took charge. Using the supplies she brought, and raising funds, she purchased supplies that doctors could not obtain for the army. Nightingale hired people to clean up the "hospitals" and established laundries to wash linens and uniforms and prepare nutritious meals. She expected a great deal of herself and those who worked with her. It was not an easy task. A major prejudice that had to be overcome was that of medical officers, who considered the nurses intruders. The hours were long and difficult for Nightingale and her nurses. An additional concern was that sometimes nurses became more involved in converting patients to their particular faith than in giving general care. Nightingale hired tutors to teach convalescing soldiers how to read and write. Many soldiers had family following them, and recreation rooms were set up for their use. She believed that the best nurses were those of good character, experienced a sense of calling, and were well trained to meet the physical needs of patients. The barracks, a 4-mile labyrinth of cots meant for 1700 patients, packed in 3000 to 4000 patients. She did not want her nurses on the wards after dark and could often be seen after hours making additional rounds with her lamp to check on patients. The soldiers fondly referred to her as "Birdie." These extra efforts earned her the title, "The Lady with the Lamp" as immortalized in Longfellow's poem, "Santa Filomena."

MARY SEACOLE; HONORED FOR HER WORK

Nightingale had help during many of those nights. Mary Seacole, a nurse from Jamaica, also played an important role in the history of nursing. She used her own money to build a lodging house and turned the second floor of it into a hospital. Seacole was especially knowledgeable about tropical medicine and used herbs and natural plant medicines to treat patients with cholera, yellow fever, malaria, and diarrhea. At the end of her day she would go to the barracks hospital and offer her help to Nightingale. They worked side by side caring for the soldiers. Both Seacole's government and the British Commonwealth honored her for the lives she saved (Cherry and Jacob, 1999).

DEATH RATE DROPS; NIGHTINGALE DECORATED

By the end of 6 months it was obvious that the efforts of Nightingale and her nurses were paying off. The death rate among the wounded dropped from 420 deaths per 1000 casualties to 22 per 1000. She stayed through the war and was the last to leave. Many of her nurses had become ill during the war and were sent home to recover. Nightingale became ill with Crimean fever, probably typhus, and almost died. When she returned home, Queen Victoria decorated her for her efforts in the war.

NIGHTINGALE ESTABLISHES FIRST SCHOOL OF NURSING IN ENGLAND

One of Florence Nightingale's major goals was to establish a school of nursing in England. An overwhelming number of physicians opposed such a school. Their opposition was that "because nurses occupied much the same positions as housemaids, they needed little instruction beyond poultice making, the enforcement of cleanliness, and attention to their patients' personal needs" (Kalish and Kalish, 1995).

In 1860 Nightingale established the Nightingale Training School at St. Thomas Hospital in England. It was a 1-year program. She chose this site because of the hospital's reputation for progressive medical care. The school was independent from the hospital and financially independent as well. She believed nurses should work only in hospitals, not in private duty. Nightingale had strict admission standards that emphasized high moral character and intelligence. She was strict with her nursing students. They were locked up at night as a way to assure the middle-class parents that their daughters were safe against harassment. Upon graduation, she gave the nurses gifts of books and invited them to tea. When her graduates went to work in far-off places, she sent flowers to welcome them to their new home (Romanoff, 2006).

Her personal and nursing decisions showed the influence of works by Plato and Hippocrates. Examples include her decision to remain single, sense of mission, concern with patient environment, focus on the whole patient, and the need for keen observation and assisting nature to heal the patient (LeVasseur, 1998). Nightingale wrote over 200 publications, the most famous of which is *Notes on Nursing*. Although she was reclusive, she was influential in matters of military and public health policy, because she kept such precise notes, which included statistics. She even advised the American Secretary of War how to set up hospitals for the wounded during the Civil War.

NIGHTINGALE'S CORE BELIEF ABOUT NURSING

The core of Nightingale's spirituality was a belief in perfection. To her, nursing was a sacred calling, a commitment to work for mankind, not a business. Other Victorian women like her shared the sense of the sacredness of time and belief that wasting time was a sin. Nursing became a way for Florence Nightingale to work toward the perfection of mankind and her personal salvation. She was against licensure. To her it was too much like nurses being in a union. Her major contributions were the following:

- Elimination of prejudice against a better class of women entering nursing, and
- Creating a push toward development of nursing as a respectable vocation.

She was intelligent, well educated, and skeptical. This combination made her the foremost critical thinker, in nursing, of the meaning of nursing and the nursing role.

Nightingale continued to be involved in health policy well into her eighties. She was the first woman to receive the Order of Merit from the King of England. She died in her sleep of old age and heart failure at age 90. The government offered to bury her at Westminster Abby, but according to her wishes, she was buried in the family plot at East Wellow, Hampshire. The marker reads: F.N. Born 12 May 1820. Died 13 August 1910.

Lystra Gretter, principal of Farrand Training School in Detroit, wrote the Nightingale pledge in 1893. It continues to be recited in many schools during graduation, primarily because of the mistaken belief that Nightingale wrote it.

Critical Thinking Exercise

Nightingale Pledge and Nursing

Review the Nightingale pledge. Does it apply to the practical/vocational nurse in the twenty-first century?

NIGHTINGALE MUSEUM ON THE SITE OF HER SCHOOL OF NURSING

In the spring of 1989 the Florence Nightingale Museum opened in London. It is on the grounds of St. Thomas Hospital, the site of the Nightingale School of Nursing. The museum is a tribute to this nursing leader, despite the fact that she wrote before her death: "I do not wish to be remembered when I am gone" (quote from Nightingale's journal, as found in the museum). Despite her great and courageous contributions to nursing, Florence Nightingale saw only her own faults and her failures.

Critical Thinking Exercise

Nursing—Vocation or Profession?

What would Florence Nightingale say to nurse applicants today who say they are entering nursing to "help" people, to get a job, or to make money? Have we matured as a vocation or as a profession? What do you think?

EARLY TRAINING SCHOOLS IN AMERICA

Nurses in America were scarce and poorly trained. In 1849, Pastor Fliedner of Germany, who helped establish the first hospital and nursing school in Europe, came to America with four of his highly trained deaconesses. While Pastor Fliedner was involved with establishing the first protestant hospital in America, the deaconesses started the first formal training program for nurses in the United States. The hospital, known as the Pittsburgh Infirmary, still exists in Pennsylvania as the Passavant Hospital. The training program was separate from the hospital with the intent being to educate nurses.

As the nursing shortage continued, hospital-based schools of nursing emerged as a cost-effective (i.e., free) labor force for the hospitals. Living conditions and working long hours required a great deal of physical and emotional endurance of the students (Fig. 7-2).

CIVIL WAR (1861-1865)

There was a great deal of prejudice about women working in hospitals, especially in the South. There was general male opposition but especially opposition from the medical profession. As a southern woman put it, "It seems strange that what the aristocratic women of Great Britain have done with honor is a disgrace for their sisters on this side of the Atlantic to do" (Kalish and Kalish, 1995).

Casualties were high on both sides during the Civil War. Many soldiers died right on the field. Others died because of a poorly trained medical corps. Southern women offered their services as volunteers, but most of the nursing was done by infantrymen assigned to do a task they did not want to do. It was many months before the Confederate government recognized southern women for their contribution.

In the North during the Civil War, women offered their services as nurses to the government. One hundred women were selected to take a short training course from doctors in New York. Dorothea Lynde Dix, a teacher by profession, was appointed Superintendent of Nurses. Her task was to organize a corps of female nurses. She requested women younger than age 30 who were plain looking, wearing simple brown or black dresses, without bows, curls, jewelry, or hoop skirts. Women who did not meet the criteria nursed anyway, but without official recognition or pay from the government.

In evaluating the nursing of the Civil War, doctors decided that the nursing system was defective. They did not approve of the women. However, it was a success in the eyes of the wounded soldiers.

A long-time advocate for better conditions for the mentally ill, Dix went on to establish the first hospital for the mentally ill.

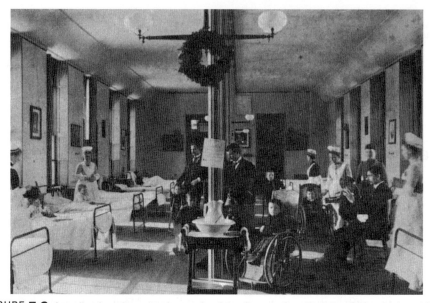

FIGURE **7-2** A pediatric unit under the aegis of the Connecticut Training School (circa 1878). Note that there are two faculty members supervising three students.

CLARA BARTON

Clara Barton, a teacher by profession, was one of the first civilians in the Civil War to round up army supplies. She rented a warehouse, filled market baskets, and encouraged friends to send food, blankets, etc., for the soldiers. Her efforts resulted in her being appointed Superintendent of the Department of Nurses for the Army in 1864. Clara Barton's efforts frequently found her on the front lines, and she nearly lost her life on two occasions. After the war, President Andrew Johnson commissioned her to do what she wanted to do—find missing prisoners of war. Later, while visiting in Europe for health reasons, she met J. Henri Dunant, founder of the *International Red Cross*. He asked for her help in introducing the Red Cross to America. Through Barton's efforts the first chapter of the *American Red Cross* (1881) was established in Danville, New York.

FORMAL TRAINING: PRACTICAL NURSING

In 1892, the Ballard School under the auspices of the YWCA opened the first formal practical nurse program in Brooklyn, NY. It was three months in duration and focused on home health care for the chronically ill, invalids, children, and the elderly. It included cooking, nutrition, basic sciences, and basic nursing procedures. The graduates were referred to as attendant nurses. Other similar schools include the Thompson School for Practical Nursing in Brattleboro, VT, in 1907. The Thompson School of Practical Nursing still operates and is accredited by the NLN. The Household Nursing Association School of Attendant Nursing opened in Boston in 1918. The name was later changed to Shepard-Gill School of Practical Nursing. The focus continued to be home nursing and light housekeeping duties. Hospital experience was not a part of the early programs. Before 1940, there were few controls, little education, planning, and minimal supervision.

NURSING IN THE HOME

Until World War I most nursing done by practical nurses was home nursing, primarily because most people were cared for in the home. Even operations were performed in the home. There is some truth in the way that old Western movies portrayed surgery on the kitchen table. The nurse's 24-hour schedule included such procedures as cupping and applying leeches; preparing stupes for relief of abdominal distention, mustard plasters for relief of congestion, and poultices for drawing out pus from infections; and administering enemas. These were often nutritive enemas that contained eggnog with brandy or chicken broth. Remember there were no intravenous solutions then. Some practical nurses also assumed the then-accepted role of midwife. They taught new mothers the basics of cleanliness, diet, and care of children (Fig. 7-3). Approximately 1700 midwives attended 30% of all births in New York in 1919.

FROM HOME TO PUBLIC HEALTH NURSING

By the end of the nineteenth century there was renewed interest in charitable work and concern

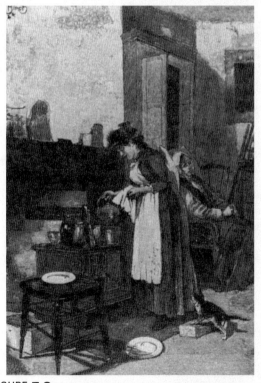

FIGURE **7-3** Caring for a sick person in a tenement house.

for the sick. Practical nursing began to expand from home nursing to public health nursing, care of patients in the slums, school nursing, industrial nursing, and well-baby care. Once again, practical nurses pioneered in this new public health movement.

One of the best-known centers in 1893 was the *Henry Street Settlement* in New York. Lillian Wald, a social worker, graduated from nursing school and intended to become a doctor. Wald taught home nursing to immigrants, and was so impressed by their need for medical care that she left medical school to begin a nursing service, the Henry Street Settlement. Practical nurses who were members of the Henry Street Settlement taught families in New York slums the basics of cleanliness and control of communicable diseases. There was a decrease in school absenteeism because the spread of childhood illness was reduced. School nurses visited schools and new mothers and their babies. They taught mothers the basics of preventing the summertime killer of infants—cholera infantum. It was estimated that their efforts resulted in survival of 1200 more babies than usual during the summer heat wave. Another original contribution of the nurses was the development of "Little Mother Leagues" in the slums, in which all girls older than age 8 were taught how to take care of their younger siblings, including the infants.

TWENTIETH CENTURY

Practical nursing evolved to meet the nursing shortage and to make better use of nursing personnel. By 1903 states began to take steps that ultimately led to monitoring of practical nursing. During this period, nursing organizations were developed. *The National League of Nursing Education* (now the National League for Nursing, or NLN) took the most influential step. In 1917 the league developed a nationwide system of standardization of nursing requirements for practical nursing.

MISSISSIPPI: FIRST TO LICENSE PRACTICAL NURSES

In 1914 Mississippi was the first state to pass a law licensing practical nurses. This was an important event because the public had no way of knowing who was providing nursing care. Remember that for centuries self-proclaimed nurses were responsible for the majority of the nursing that was done. Licensing, however, was not mandatory, and by 1938 New York was the *only state to have mandatory licensure.*

 Critical Thinking Exercise

State License

Does your state have mandatory licensure? What year did it begin?

WORLD WAR I NURSES

At the onset of World War I there were few practical nurses and few schools of practical nursing. Hurriedly "trained" nurses were rushed to the battlefront. An army and navy school of nursing was established to combat the severe nursing shortage and improve the overall quality of care. Supply could not meet demand and nurses and women looking for glamour and excitement volunteered their service and instead found superhuman demands made of them during the war.

SMITH HUGHES ACT OF 1917

The homefront was facing a battle of its own in 1917-1918, with a major epidemic of pneumonia in 1917 and a worldwide epidemic of Spanish influenza in 1918. The mortality rate was high, especially in 1918. The *Smith Hughes Act of 1917* provided money for developing additional schools of practical nursing. The first high-school vocational practical nursing program opened at the Minneapolis Girls Vocational High School in 1919. However, the new schools could not supply nurses quickly enough to meet the severe shortage in the United States.

NURSES RETURN HOME: ACUTE NURSING SHORTAGE FOLLOWS WORLD WAR I

After the war many nurses did not continue nursing. There was an acute shortage of nurses in the 1920s. Many more hospitals opened schools of nursing. Their real purpose was to provide staffing. Hospitals without schools were staffed heavily with untrained help.

In the period between the two world wars, 1920-1940, six states made laws licensing practical nurses, but there were few practical nursing schools throughout the country. Much of the nurse's work continued to be in public health agencies and visiting nurse associations.

DEPRESSION OF THE THIRTIES

During the Depression of the 1930s many nurses lost their jobs or worked in hospitals for room and board rather than a salary. When it became fairly obvious that America was becoming involved in World War II, nursing leaders began to prepare for the need for all levels of nurses. They did not want to face the nursing shortage experienced during World War I. This was a monumental task because nursing had decreased in popularity as a vocation.

WORLD WAR II

Practical nurses played a significant role both at home and in World War II. At home, practical nurses worked in clinics, health departments, industry, and hospitals. At the battlefields, nurses could be found in Europe, North Africa, and the Pacific (Fig. 7-4). One of the most widespread diseases they fought was malaria in the East Indies, the Philippines, and southern Asiatic countries. The number of practical nurses in America peaked at 159,009 in 1940. By 1944 practical nursing was already experiencing a decline.

PRACTICAL NURSING RESPONSIBILITIES INCREASE AFTER WORLD WAR II

The end of World War II saw a continuing shortage of nurses. This shortage helped practical nurses play an important part in hospital nursing. Most

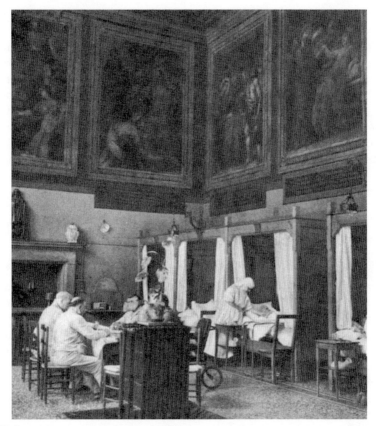

FIGURE **7-4** A Sister at the Hotel Dieu in Beaune, Burgundy, France, giving care to a patient in a room compartment. Ambulatory patients enjoy meals at the table in the center. Note the works of art.

hospitals gradually increased the responsibilities designated for the practical nurse. By the 1940s there were nearly 50 approved practical nursing programs in the United States.

PRACTICAL NURSING DUTIES OUTLINED

In 1944 the U.S. Department of Vocational Education made a comprehensive study of practical nursing. This marked the first time that tasks of practical nursing were agreed on. Extensive specific duties were outlined, with an emphasis on maintaining aseptic technique. The terms "to judge," "to appraise," "to recognize," and "to determine" were often used to describe the scope of the practical nurse's job.

RN AND LPN TASKS DIFFERENTIATED

Other important changes followed. In 1949 the Joint Committee on Practical Nurses and Auxiliary Workers in Nursing Services recommended use of the title "licensed practical nurse." Furthermore, the committee differentiated between the tasks of the RN and the LPN. They saw the LPN as being under the supervision of the RN. The committee also suggested that practical nurses organize to make decisions on their salary, working conditions, and employment standards.

Because of the work of the Joint Committee, many practical nursing programs were strengthened with regard to content. They focused for the first time on the preparation of practical nursing instructors. Up to this point any graduate nurse was eligible to teach practical nursing. During the 1950s the number of programs continued to increase and programs were extended to 9-, 12-, and 18-month programs.

RNs REACT

By 1952 nearly 60% of the nursing workforce was made up of practical nurses. In many instances RNs expressed bitterness because hospitals, clinics, and other agencies were hiring practical nurses for less money, and assigning tasks to them beyond their educational level. RNs also expressed concern that the public was unable to differentiate between the levels of nurses. Both wore the same type of white uniforms, caps, and pins. Many practical nurses quickly stopped wearing the practical nursing insignia, which was meant to identify the practical nurse. In many agencies, pay continued to be poor. For less compensation practical nurses alternately performed tasks belonging to the RN one day and those belonging to nursing aides on other days. Many practical nurses felt trapped in such situations because of their need for employment.

PUBLIC LAW 911

In 1956 Public Law 911 provided for millions of dollars to expand and improve practical nursing programs. By 1975 there were 1337 programs, which graduated a total of 46,080 practical nurses. Approximately two thirds of the practical nurses were employed in hospitals, 17.3% in nursing homes, 7.5% in private duty, and 6.5% in doctors' offices, clinics, and dental offices. Admission standards in most schools increased, as did the difficulty of the curriculum. Levels of nursing temporarily gained momentum.

ANA MOVEMENT TOWARD TWO LEVELS OF NURSING

In 1965, the American Nurses Association (ANA) presented a position paper outlining how to solve the issues of levels of nursing. They recommended that all RNs graduate from a 4-year collegiate program and all LPNs graduate from a 2-year technical program. Many

hospital-based RN programs closed during that time. In the 1980s a resurgence of the ANA 1965 movement toward establishing two levels of nursing temporarily gained momentum. Some states worked toward adopting the ANA recommendations. North Dakota made the change to a 2-year practical nursing program and a 4-year BSN professional nursing program. Because a serious nursing shortage developed in the late 1980s, the ANA movement stalled in other states.

AMA MOVES TO EASE NURSING SHORTAGE

With the goal of easing the nursing shortage, the American Medical Association (AMA), in the summer of 1989, proposed a new health care worker—the registered care technologist (RCT). The RCT was to be trained in 1- and 2-year programs. Because this new level of health care worker correlated with existing personnel, the practical nurse and the associate-degree nurse, the RCT proposal was not successful. **This event is a gentle reminder for practical/vocational nurses to be strong, organized, and vigilant as a group.** Changes in the health care system are occurring daily, as are opportunities for LPN/LVNs.

UAPs

During the 1990s unlicensed assistive personnel (UAP) were hired to give patient care. A major concern for LPN/LVNs and RNs was their legal responsibility for the care given by the unlicensed caregivers. Meanwhile, primary employment for nurses, especially for the LPN/LVNs, moved out of hospitals and into the community.

FIRST COMPUTERIZED TESTING: NCLEX-PN®

In 1994 the first computerized adaptive testing (NCLEX-PN® examination) became available for the practical/vocational nursing graduate. The computer format provided an individualized test for each graduate, based on the answer to the previous question. It also excluded questions that were not within the nurse's role, according to their state's Nurse Practice Act.

LONG-TERM CERTIFICATION

In 1996 long-term care certification became available to LPN/LVNs in some states. Since that time other certifications have become available for LPN/LVNs in some states (see Chapter 23).

TWENTY-FIRST CENTURY

Nursing organizations continue to define the responsibilities of the different levels of nursing. More remains to be resolved. Nursing shortages have created changes in nursing programs. Approximately 50 years ago, AD nursing programs were set up in technical schools and they have flourished. Approximately 60% of the current RN work force is AD RNs. One of the goals of AD programs was to move nursing education out of hospital-based programs and the other, to help ease the shortage by shortening the amount of time to become an RN. However, the AD graduate, hospital-program graduate and baccalaureate graduate all take the same licensing examination to become an RN. It was and continues to be confusing for those doing the hiring at a facility, since all RNs regardless of their education, can legally assume the same responsibilities. Finances are always a major concern for health facilities. Years ago, when LPN/LVN earned much less than RNs, more LPN/LVNs were hired. When salaries were narrowed and the difference in salary was considerably less, more RNs were hired.

Nursing organizations continue to work on resolving the issue of nursing levels and present new recommendations and position papers. Nursing shortages continue periodically and currently there is a serious shortage of nurses. Changes in how health facilities are reimbursed for patient care has had major impact on patient acuity, staffing ratio, overtime, patient care loads, and patient safety. Some nurses are leaving nursing because of the heavy workload and high levels of stress. Counselors report that fewer young people are going into nursing. Some students judge nursing as, "too demanding, too undervalued, and too unrewarding" (Gosnell, 2002). The average age of the nurse work force continues to increase.

Historically a nursing shortage has provided a notable opportunity for well-educated LPN/LVNs, and is doing so again. Take advantage of the learning available to you at this time and seriously consider pursuing certifications that will be available to you after graduation.

IMPORTANT INFLUENCES IN NURSING HISTORY

Many RNs influenced the course of nursing and practical nursing history. Table 7-2 identifies some of those registered nurses and events in nursing history.

Table 7-2 | *Some Persons/Events in Nursing History*

Mary Robinson	1859	First visiting nurse
Linda Richards	1873	America's first professionally trained nurse (1 year program); organized other training schools; developed a system of written records and orders
Euphemia Van Rensselaer	1876	Introduced first uniform—apron and cap (Bellevue Training School for Nurses)
Mary E. P. Mahoney	1879	First African-American graduate nurse
Clara Barton	1881	Established the American Red Cross
Elizabeth Weston	1888	First American Indian nurse. Graduate of Training School of the University of Pennsylvania. Came from Lincoln School for Indian girls in Philadelphia. After graduation returned to care for her people on a Sioux reservation in North Dakota

Continued

Table 7-2 *Some Persons/Events in Nursing History—cont'd*

Emily L. Loveridge	1890	Graduate of Bellevue Training School for Nurses. Went west to establish first school of nursing in the Northwest at Good Samaritan Hospital, Portland, Oregon
Mabel Staupers	1890-1989	First executive director and last president of the National Association of Colored Graduate Nurses. Credited with integration of African American nurses into ANA and other nursing organizations. Wrote *No Time for Prejudice*
Isabel Hampton Robb	1893	Wrote first substantial nursing text: *Nursing: Its Principles and Practice for Hospital and Private Use.* Promoted nurses' rights, 3-year training program, 8-hour day, and licensure
Lillian Wald and Mary Brewster	1893	First visiting nurse service for the poor: Nurses Settlement House in slum section, lower East Side, New York City. Later moved to Henry Street and name changed to Henry Street Settlement House
Lavinia L. Dock	1896	First president of forerunner of ANA (Nurses Associated Alumnae of the United States and Canada). Wrote four-volume *History of Nursing* with Adelaide Nutting. Outlined principles on which ANA was founded
Dita H. Kinney	1901	First Superintendent of Nurses of the Army Nurse Corps
Mrs. Bedford Fenwick (Great Britain)	1901	First president of International Council of Nurses. Proposed state registration of nurses
Adelaid Nutting	1907	First graduate of Johns Hopkins Training School for Nurses. First nurse in the world to hold professorship in a university (Columbia). In 1917, Chair of Committee to Develop National Curriculum
Lillian Wald, Ella Phillips Crandall, Mary Beard, Mary Lent, Edna Foley, Lystra Greiter, Elizabeth G. Fox	1912	Formed National Organization of Public Health Nurses. Lillian Wald, first president
Margaret Sanger	1916	A public health nurse, she spearheaded the birth control movement as a response to high maternal and child mortality. Opened first birth control clinic in America
Annie W. Goodrich	1918	President of ANA. Became Chief Inspecting Nurse for army hospitals at home and abroad. Supported formation of Army School of Nursing, became dean of school
	1924	U.S. Indian Bureau Nursing Service founded
Mary Breckenridge	1925	Organized Frontier Nursing Service of Kentucky
Sage Memorial Hospital School, Ganado, Arizona	1930	First school of nursing for American Indians
Lucile Petry	1943	Director of U.S. Cadet Nurses Corps
Esther Lucille Brown, Ph.D., a researcher	1948	"Brown" study: Advocated movement of nursing education to collegiate setting
Mildred L. Montag	1952	Appointed as first Associate Degree Nursing Program Project Coordinator. Project based on Montag's doctoral thesis, "Education of Nursing Technicians." Project located at Queen's College, New York

YOU HAVE COME A LONG WAY

As a final note it may be interesting to compare present practical/vocational nursing tasks with those that you would have been expected to perform in 1887. Practical/vocational nursing has indeed come a long way.

The job description in Box 7-1 was given to floor nurses by a hospital in 1887 (author unknown).

Box 7-1 | *Hospital Nursing 1887*

In addition to caring for your 50 patients, each nurse will follow these regulations:
- Daily sweep and mop the floors of your ward, dust the patient's furniture and window sills. Maintain an even temperature in your ward by bringing in a scuttle of coal for the day's business.
- Light is important to observe the patient's condition. Therefore each day fill kerosene lamps, clean chimneys, and trim wicks. Wash the lamp windows once a week.
- The nurse's notes are important in aiding the physician's work. Make your pens carefully; you may whittle nibs to your individual taste.
- Each nurse on day duty will report every day at 7 AM and leave at 8 PM, except on the Sabbath, on which day you will be off from noon to 2 PM.

- Graduate nurses in good standing with the director of nurses will be given an evening off each week for courting purposes or two evenings a week if you go regularly to church.
- Each nurse should lay aside from each payday a goodly sum of her earnings for her benefits during her declining years so that she will not become a burden. For example, if you earn $30 a month, you should set aside $15.
- Any nurse who smokes, uses liquor in any form, gets her hair done at a beauty shop, or frequents dance halls will give the director of nurses good reason to suspect her worth, intentions, and integrity.
- The nurse who performs her labors and serves her patients and doctors without fault for 5 years will be given an increase of 5 cents a day, providing there are no hospital debts outstanding.

Key Points

- Varied and colorful evolution of practical nursing is described with limited reference to roles played by RNs in the course of nursing history.
- Accounts show practical/vocational nursing students that their vocation began to develop in ancient times and is not an appendage of professional nursing.
- Duties have changed according to the needs present at various times in history.
- Currently, practical/vocational nurses are taught basic skills during their educational program.
- According to some states' nurse practice acts; LPN/LVNs are allowed to perform complex skills delegated by an RN. An RN must teach complex skills involved, be satisfied with the LPN/LVNs performance, and document this in the LPN/LVN's file. Direct supervision by an RN is required for performance of complex nursing tasks in most states.
- Historical figures in nursing include (1) Florence Nightingale, founder of modern nursing, (2) Clara Barton, founder of the American Red Cross, (3) Lillian Wald, founder of public health nursing, and (4) Dorothea Lynde Dix, advocate for the mentally ill.
- Practical nurses have always been in the forefront of doing real, down-to-earth nursing tasks—often what no one else dared or cared to do.
- The focus is on figures in nursing history who had limited nursing education, and yet enormous courage to care for patients, most often without glamour or fanfare.

REVIEW ITEMS

1. Which year did licensing for practical/vocational nursing begin?

   1. 1914

   2. 1919

   3. 1938

   4. 1907

2. Which statement relates to Florence Nightingale's contribution to nursing?

   1. She established the first visiting nurse service for the poor in the lower East Side slum section of New York.

   2. She wrote the Nightingale Pledge in 1893 to set guidelines and inspire her nurses on graduation.

   3. She wrote the first substantial nursing text and promoted nursing rights, including the 8-hour day.

   4. She stressed environment, need for careful observation, care of the whole person, and critical thinking.

3. Periodically, various organizations have suggested eliminating practical/vocational programs. Which statement objectively provides a reason for continuing the LPN/LVN programs?

   1. LPN/LVNs possess the same level of skill in patient care as do registered nurses.

   2. RN education is more focused on nursing theory and less on patient bedside care.

   3. LPN/LVN programs evolved to make better use of nursing personnel.

   4. Physicians prefer to work with LPN/LVNs because they follow orders without question.

4. Florence Nightingale provided a positive role model for all nurses. Which of the following historical figures is a negative role model for nursing?

   1. Sairey Gamp, because of her experiences in nurse midwifery.

   2. Phoebe, because of her ministering to Roman women.

   3. Lillian Wald, because of her nursing care of immigrants in the slums.

   4. Mary Seacole, because of her use of herbs and plants to treat disease.

ALTERNATE FORMAT ITEM

Which of the following were not self-proclaimed nurses? *(Select all that apply.)*

1. Well-trained nurses who were licensed by the physicians of the day.

2. Persons with a "gift" or a "touch," who could help during a medical crisis.

3. Persons who provided home care, including "wet-nursing" and delivery of babies.

4. Persons with extended "mothering" skills to care for the ill, injured, and dying.

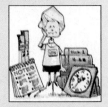

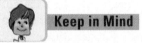 http://evolve.elsevier.com/Hill/success/

Objective information (ŏb-JĔK-tĭv, p. 110)
Outcome (p. 108)
Planning (p. 109)
Subjective information (sŭb-JĔK-tĭv, p. 110)

Objectives

On completing this chapter, you will be able to do the following:

1. Discuss how the nursing process has evolved from the 1950s to now.
2. Define your role in the nursing process according to the nurse practice act of your state, territory, or country.
3. Describe assisting with the four phases of the nursing process for the practical/vocational nurse:
   a. Phase 1: Data Collection
   b. Phase 2: Planning
   c. Phase 3: Implementation
   d. Phase 4: Evaluation
4. Describe nursing diagnosis as the exclusive domain of the registered nurse (RN).
5. Explain why the nursing process and critical thinking are part of the practical/vocational nursing program curriculum.

Key Terms

Data collection (p. 109)
Dependent role (dĕ-PĔN-dĕnt, p. 108)
Desired patient outcome (p. 115)
Evaluation (ĕ-VĂL-ū-Ā-shŭn, p. 109)
Goals (p. 109)
Implementation (Ĭ-plĕ-mĕn-TĀ-shŭn, p. 109)
Independent role (ĬN-dĕ-PĔN-dĕnt, p. 109)
Interdependent (ĬN-tĕr-dĕ-PĔN-dĕnt, p. 109)
NANDA-I (p. 109)
NIC (p. 119)
NOC (p. 119)
Nursing diagnosis (DĪ-ăg-NŌ-sĭs, p. 109)
Nursing process (p. 107)

Keep in Mind

Nursing process is a way nurses communicate with each other to identify what the nurse will do to safely assist the patient reach desired patient outcomes. It provides for continuity of safe care on every shift.

As a student you will develop nursing care plans. Nursing care plans are learning tools for practical/vocational nursing students (SPN/SVN). They are traditionally used in practical/vocational nursing programs to help students learn about patient needs. *A critical thinking exercise is using your role in the nursing process to devise a care plan as a SPN/SVN in preparation for patient care.* Devising a nursing care plan prior to patient care is necessary to ensure safe patient care.

Currently, unlicensed persons are doing the tasks and skills that licensed practical/vocational nurses (LPN/LVNs) perform. It is the nursing process and critical thinking that separate the LPN/LVNs from the unlicensed assistive personnel (UAPs). These distinctions make LPN/LVNs attractive to employers. The modern LPN/LVN uses critical thinking and nursing process to carefully identify patient problems, issues, and risks involved, through focused thinking. Judgments are based on evidence rather than assumptions and minimal training. The LPN/LVN thinks before acting. The RN uses the nursing process and critical thinking, but at a higher skill level based on education, and makes final decisions on **nursing diagnosis** and patient care plans.

NURSING PROCESS: 1950s

The nursing process originated in the 1950s to provide structure for thinking in nursing. *"Nursing process was designed to organize thinking so that the problems encountered by patients could be anticipated and solved quickly"* (Peseit and Herman, 1998). The 1950s *four-step* process was based on the scientific method, which included **data collection**, **planning**, **intervention**, and **evaluation**. A major difference between the scientific method (problem-solving method), and nursing process is that scientific method identifies the problem first and then goes on to gather data, etc. Nursing process gathers data first and then identifies the problem (nursing diagnosis). Initially, nursing did not yet see itself as having something unique to contribute to patient care that was separate and additional to its dependent role to physicians. Consequently, nursing education programs and textbooks focused on patients' medical problems and associated nursing interventions. To add to the confusion, suggested nursing interventions varied in nursing textbooks and at health care agencies. Although the nursing process had been introduced, it still had a long way to go. The most important outcome of the nursing process for nurses was to provide a structure for *thinking before acting*.

NURSING PROCESS: 1970s-1990s

When the American Nurses Association (ANA) published the standards of nursing practice in 1977, it established a *five-step* nursing process for the RN: assessment (data collection), nursing diagnosis (the new step for RNs), planning, intervention, and evaluation. The problem-solving format of the original nursing process was replaced with

a *reasoning* model. It introduced a way for nurses to identify and respond to patient need within the scope of nursing. These included the following needs:

- Physiological needs,
- Psychological needs,
- Social needs, and
- Spiritual needs.

It also gave nurses an organized, unique way of contributing to patient care that was separate and additional to its dependent role to physicians. It involved the following roles:

- Collecting data (assessment),
- Nursing diagnosis (RN responsibility),
- Planning,
- **Implementation**,
- Evaluating nursing care,
- Including the patient in planning, and
- A way to communicate with other nurses and care givers.

Initially SPN/SVNs were not taught the steps of the nursing process or how to think critically. Although nursing diagnosis was, and continues to be, within the RN's legal role, it became clear that LPN/LVNs had an important role in **assisting** the RN in the other steps of the nursing process.

 Learning Exercise

Nurse Practice Act

With the assistance of your instructor, review the nurse practice act of your state, territory, or country. Your role in the nursing process is spelled out in this law. There are variations within the states, territories, and countries. It defines your scope of nursing practice.

In 1996 the National Council of State Boards of Nursing (NCSBN) included four phases of the nursing process (no nursing diagnosis) in the NCLEX-PN® examination. The percentage of test questions in the client needs categories and phases of the nursing process categories were based on the 1994 LPN/LVN job analysis (NCSBN 1995). In 1999 the NCLEX-PN® examination was based on the 1997 job analysis for

LPN/LVNs. Additional concepts and processes were integrated throughout the test plan, representing changes taking place in practical/vocational nursing (NCSBN, 1998).

NURSING PROCESS: 2000 AND BEYOND

In 2002 the NCSBN integrated the nursing process into all areas of the NCLEX-PN® examination. By doing so, the council validated the significance of the nursing process and critical thinking for the LPN/LVN as the way to do the work of nursing.

Definitions of the nursing process for the NCLEX-PN® examination (NCSBN, 2001) are as follows:

- "Data Collection is a systematic gathering and review of information about the patient, which is communicated to appropriate members of the health team
- Planning involves **assisting** the RN in the development of nursing diagnosis, goals, and interventions for a patient's plan of care and maintaining patient safety.
- Implementation is the provision of required nursing care to accomplish established patient goals.
- Evaluation compares the actual outcomes of nursing care to the expected outcomes, which are then communicated to members of the health care team.
- **Definitions** of nursing process remain the same for the 2008 NCLEX-PN examination."

WHAT DIFFERENTIATES YOUR ROLE FROM THE RN ROLE?

Because of the depth of the RNs basic education, the RN functions **independently** in all five steps of the nursing process (including diagnosis). The nursing actions based on nursing diagnosis do not require a physician's order. Both RNs and LPN/LVNS share an interdependent relationship with other health team members. For example, RNs and LPN/LVNs both carry out orders for treatments and medication written by a medical doctor, podiatrist, or dentist.

The LPN/LVN acts in a more dependent role when participating in the planning and evaluation phase of the nursing process. The LPN/LVN acts in a more independent role when participating in the data collection and implementation phases of the nursing process. RNs are taught assessment skills as part of their basic education. The skills include patient interview and physical assessment of all body systems. However, practical/vocational nurses learn to gather data about the patient and the environment during every encounter with the patient (as do RNs and UAPs, according to their knowledge and skill level). Data collection for the SPN/SVN includes taking vital signs, checking therapeutic responses to medications and treatments, collecting data on symptoms of health problems, etc. The focus of data collection is based on the current unit of study for the practical/vocational nurse. With each course SPN/SVNs increase their data collection capabilities. SPN/SVNs continue to hold onto skills they acquire, and add onto these skills as they complete each nursing course. LPN/LVNs may choose to learn more complex skills as part of a postgraduate assessment course.

Some schools offer physical assessment as a course separate from the practical nursing program. Ask your instructor if a physical assessment course is available. It is an excellent way to learn additional interview, observation, and physical assessment skills. Whether you use part or all of these skills at work, the knowledge will improve the care you provide patients.

Nursing diagnosis is a summary, in nursing terms, of actual problems or potential problems that nurses can respond to. The RN uses an established list of current nursing diagnoses developed by the North American Nursing Diagnosis Association International (NANDA-I). NANDA-I was developed as a standardized language that would provide a common language for nurses to communicate with each other. RNs are encouraged to use this approved nursing diagnosis list. NANDA-I is periodically updated to meet current changes and needs.

DEVELOPING YOUR PLAN OF CARE FOR ASSIGNED PATIENTS

Patient care for you as a student is a learning experience. It is necessary to plan for patient care assignments. Legally, your nurse practice act will require you to give care at the level of an LPN/LVN. The nursing diagnosis is the problem the patient presented with, and the RN fits this into the categories established by NANDA-I. Because you do not study the NANDA-I diagnostic categories in most practical/vocational nursing programs, it is helpful (i.e., clearer, more objective, more explanatory, makes more sense to you in the learning situation) if you use the original nursing problem the patient presented with. Turn the nursing diagnosis back to the presenting problem. In this way you clearly understand what you are working with in everyday terms. At this stage you have the benefit of your instructor to help you through the planning process. Planning for patient care becomes easier with each plan. You internalize your role in four phases of the nursing process, and are improving your ability to think critically as a practical/vocational nurse.

PHASES OF THE NURSING PROCESS

DATA COLLECTION: PHASE 1

Data collection includes many aspects.

Systematic Way of Gathering Information

Data collection begins on admission and continues with each patient encounter. The patient is the primary source of information in data collection. After all, patients know themselves and their body better than anyone else. All patient interview questions should be directed to the patient, unless he or she is unable to respond. The RN interviews the patient to obtain the health history and assesses body systems. As part of a practical/vocational nursing program, learning communication skills does not include the formal interview process.

- **Subjective information** is based on the patient's opinion. Some refer to subjective information as symptoms. This usually includes feelings of physical discomfort, anxiety, and mental stress that are more difficult to measure. The nurse cannot experience subjective symptoms.
- **Objective information** includes data that the nurse can verify; it is also known as "signs." A physical assessment provides objective data. The terms *check, observe, monitor, weigh, measure,* and *smell* are cues that you may be involved in objective data collection. Obtaining initial data, such as vital signs, height, and weight, is often assigned to the LPN/LVN. Objective information helps support or cast doubt on subjective information. For example, a patient's subjective statement about feeling feverish can be verified by taking his or her temperature (objective).

Verify the Information

This is an important step in thinking critically. As an SPN/SVN it is very important that you seek the assistance of your instructor to discover what resources are available to you for verification of data. Suggestions in verifying information include the following:

- Verify the data and question any information that is not a match or is unclear.
- Differentiate between subjective and objective data. Remember decisions must be based on fact (evidence), not assumptions.
- Compare findings with the RN and other staff involved with the patient.
- Other staff may help verify when a client has mental limitations.
- Patient or family member may be able to validate information you obtained during data collection (family members with patient permission).
- Document all data and sources, especially when it is not a match.
- Compare data you collected with the medical record.

- Know that what you do for verification will depend on your skill level and whether you are an SPN/SVN or LPN/LVN.
- As a student ask your instructor for guidance on how to verify data and how to determine if there is a relationship between presenting problems.

Communicate Information to Appropriate Health Care Team Members

- **Emergency data** are reported immediately. For example, suppose you learn that the patient with a fracture has diabetes and fell on his way home from a bar, where he goes daily for "just four beers." Does him saying, "I pace myself" reassure you that this is not an immediate issue? Recall that what you have heard is subjective data, but as a student you will not be in a position to verify it further without direction from the RN. Report what you have heard, and any objective data, such as vital signs and observations, to the appropriate person. You have just activated your brain to think critically.
- **Incomplete toolbox:** Subjective data will be charted as "Patient states…" Objective data, such as temperature, pulse, and respiration (TPR), blood pressure (BP), weight, and skin color, will be charted as what you observe and measure, without judging or drawing conclusions. Your involvement in this step depends on your place of employment and your skill level. The LPN/LVN usually has more responsibility in the nursing home, where the patient's condition is more stable. At the conclusion of your practical/vocational program you will have acquired strong, although incomplete, data collection skills: "The toolbox is not complete." An incomplete toolbox is nothing to be ashamed of. For example, you measure the TPR and BP properly. Be proud of your data collection skills. They provide valuable data.

Other Aspects of Data Collection

Data Collection Continues. Data collection starts during the patient's admission. It continues daily at the beginning of the shift for the baseline observations, then periodically during the shift, and right before doing your final documentation and reporting off. The practical/vocational nurse is always collecting data on therapeutic responses to treatments and medications (Box 8-1).

Accuracy in Data Collection. Florence Nightingale said that if you do not observe your patient, you should not be a nurse. With each contact the LPN/LVN must see, hear, smell, and touch the patient

---

Box 8-1 *Examples of Practical/Vocational Nurse Data Collection*

These examples can apply to acute care, nursing home care, long-term care, etc.
- Observing results of a laxative or enema.
- Observing for signs of congestive heart failure for a patient taking furosemide (Lasix) and digoxin (Lanoxin).
- Observing an ulcer on the lower leg of a diabetic: size (measure it), location, appearance, any drainage, etc.
- Observing the ulcer each time the leg is dressed.
- Observing behavior for signs of disorientation or confusion.
- Observing NPO patient drinking water.
- In acute care: observing position in bed. In community: observing gait and posture.
- Observing whether 76-year-old patient is showing signs of ego integrity or despair. (Although the patient should be at ego integrity, he is not capable of being there. Because of his cerebrovascular accident [CVA], he has to be washed, fed, and lifted everywhere. He is incontinent. His needs remind you of an infant. You will work at establishing trust in the patient instead of ego integrity.)
- Observing family interactions.
- Observing the environment for need for safety factors: spills, bed rails, glasses on table, hearing aids, dentures, etc.
- Observing the urine for color, odor, amount, and other characteristics.

when necessary, and use all the senses to gather data about the patient and the environment. Data collection is vital; the patient condition changes throughout the day. This is why accuracy in measuring vital signs, describing vomitus, bleeding, or a skin lesion, and determining level of consciousness, for example, is so important. Has the patient's skin lesion changed since the last time you checked the lesion? How? How much? Sometimes LPN/LVNs do not understand that what they are assigned to do is a vital part of the data collection.

Introduce Yourself. Data collection, whether partial or total, involves courtesy. Introduce yourself to the patient and explain what you are going to do. Address the patient as Mr., Mrs., Miss, or another title, as appropriate. Avoid using a first name unless you have the patient's permission. Remind yourself that this is a *professional,* not a personal, relationship you are building. The most common complaints put forth by patients include, "I don't know which one is the nurse," "I am treated with disrespect," "I am not their grandma," and so on. Familiarity, i.e., acting toward a patient as though he or she is a family member or friend, does not give the patient a sense of confidence in your nursing skill. When in the patient's presence, stand or sit where he or she can see you. Patients often experience fear on being hospitalized or transferred to a new facility. Confusion or lack of skills on the nurse's part serves to increase that fear. The focus of the nurse's job is to serve the patient with the greatest skill possible.

Asking Questions. Avoid asking questions that have been asked before unless you are directed to do so, or your observation based on critical thinking alerts you to do so. Be sure that you have looked at the record before entering the patient's room. Explain why you are asking questions and reassure the patient that he or she has the right to not answer questions that cause discomfort. Be a good listener. Encourage confidence, but do not promise to keep secrets. Request clarification rather than pretending that you understand: "I am not sure that I understand what you mean by that statement." Check out what you think you

understand: "Am I correct in saying that you are worried about the kind of care you will receive here?" Avoid using reassuring promises that you cannot deliver, such as, "Don't worry, everything will be just fine." Also avoid giving approval; for example, "That's right." This statement may make it difficult for a patient to change his or her mind. Nursing responsibility does not involve judging the patient's behavior, values, or decision. Finally, avoid verbalizing disapproval or belittling the patient with statements such as, "You know you shouldn't have done that." Chapter 9 elaborates on communication techniques that will assist you in making the best use of the limited time you have to obtain needed data from the patient.

Barriers in Data Collection

You must be alert to several possible barriers to data collection. Barriers include insufficient time, cultural differences, poor skills in data collection, and communication failure, such as a comatose patient, a patient who presents a language barrier, the presence of distractions, or a patient who is too sick to want to talk. If your personal values get in the way, you may label the patient before the interview is complete, instead of basing decisions on facts. Respectful distancing is necessary if the nurse is to remain objective and use all senses clearly.

PLANNING: PHASE 2

Planning includes assisting the RN to develop nursing diagnoses, outcomes, and interventions.

Assisting the RN to Develop the Nursing Diagnosis

Only the RN can develop the nursing diagnosis, goals, interventions, and plan of care. It is illegal for the LPN/LVN to write the plan and for the RN to initial it. *The LPN/LVN assists the RN to collect and group the data that have been collected in a logical order.* The LPN/LVN assists in determining a significant relationship between data and patient needs or problems. The focus is on patient functions that will benefit from nursing interventions. After the problems are identified and organized, the RN makes the nursing diagnosis.

Learning Exercise

Assisting During Planning

In the planning phase the SPN/SVN takes the nursing diagnosis and states it as a nursing problem the patient presented with. SPN/SVNs state the problem, set outcomes, list interventions, and then list data collection for care plans. This process seems to be reverse that of the RN, but remember that practical/vocational nurses do not have primary responsibility for data collection (phase 1). The SPN/SVN does not study NANDA-I lists and relies on the RN for the final nursing diagnosis. To demonstrate understanding of the nursing diagnosis the practical/vocational nurse states the nursing diagnosis in objective and specific terms as a nursing problem (Table 8-1).

Realistic, Useful Nursing Care Plan. For a nursing care plan to be a useful, realistic tool for the nursing staff, priorities must be established. A care plan will not include all patients' problems. It is unreasonable to think that nurses will be able to respond to all of the patient's needs and problems. The most important problems, those that are potentially life threatening, must be taken care of immediately. Nurses often use Maslow's Hierarchy of Needs to assist in prioritizing patient needs. The lowest level of needs, according to Maslow, is the physiological (survival) level of needs. This means that in prioritizing patient needs, attention is paid first to problems related to food, air, water, temperature, elimination, rest, and pain. (See p. 254 for a review of Maslow's Hierarchy of Needs.)

When working on several problems at the same time, it is not uncommon to find that a relationship exists between problems. Priorities may also change rapidly, depending on the patient's condition. The nurse has to remain flexible and recognize the need to shift priorities according to patient needs. Patients will be far more cooperative with the care plan if they are included in identifying the priorities of care. According to Maslow, regression takes place during illness. The amount of regression depends on the circumstances and severity of the illness. As the patient recovers, he or she advances on Maslow's

Hierarchy. Ideally the patient is able to regain the former level of functioning. Cooperation is much more likely when the nurse understands this and respects it. Whenever a new problem emerges, practical/vocational nurses collect data about the problem because of their data collection skills. They collaborate with the RN, and the RN formulates a new nursing diagnosis.

Critical Thinking Exercise

The Seven Survival Needs

Write an example of a problem for each survival need.
1. Food _____
2. Air _____
3. Water _____
4. Temperature _____
5. Elimination _____
6. Rest _____
7. Pain _____
Possible answers:
1. Not enough or too much food intake
2. Shortness of breath
3. Dehydration, caused by vomiting
4. Temperature above or below normal
5. Diarrhea
6. Sleeping too much or too little
7. Pain that interferes with functioning

Assisting the RN to Develop Outcomes

Think back to phase 1, data collection, and ask yourself the following questions: What did the patient say on admission about expectations, wants, or needs while a patient? Did you also remember to collect data on patient strengths?

Strengths. Strengths are building blocks in developing a realistic plan. Strengths include whatever the patient and family continue to be able to do that will aid patient care. Patient and family are important partners in attaining the goals/outcomes. Building on patient strengths provides a sense of contribution and some control for the patient. The following are sample questions that may help make the question of strengths patient focused:
- Can the patient move from the bed to the chair and back alone?

Table **8-1** *Student Assignment Sheet and Patient Care Plan*

Student_____

Patient initials_____ Room_____ Doctor_____ Allergies_____

Age_____ Marital Status_____ Religion_____ Occupation_____

Admission Date_____ Date of Surgery_____ Diet_____

Medical Diagnosis_____ Surgical Procedure_____

Meaning in Own Words_____ Meaning in Own Words_____

Primary Nursing Problem_____

CATEGORIES OF HUMAN FUNCTION	DATA COLLECTION	NURSING PROBLEMS	OUTCOMES	NURSING INTERVENTION	EVALUATION
Protective (e.g., personal care and hygiene, environment, surgery)	You will: Check, observe, monitor, weigh, and measure. Collect data (1) at beginning of shift for baseline, (2) periodically during shift, and (3) right before reporting off duty.	What is the problem, in your own words? Be specific and objective. Could use nursing diagnosis, but....	The patient will: (Reverse the problem and state positively what patient will do—realistically, measurably, time-referenced).	The nurse will: (Be objective and specific. Care plans in texts rarely are. What the nurse will do to help patient meet outcomes.)	What progress is patient making toward outcomes? Results of data collection in objective terms.

Sensory-perceptual
Comfort, rest, activity, and mobility (e.g., sleep and rest, body alignment)
Nutrition
Growth and development (e.g., identify Erikson's developmental stage)
Fluid-gas transport
Psychosocial cultural (e.g., emotional support, spiritual support, diversion, and recreation)
Elimination (e.g., urinary and gastrointestinal elimination)
Need for community resources

- Does the patient feed himself or herself? Completely? With some assistance?
- Does the patient eat best if someone is present? Alone? During conversation about family?
- Are there any family members who can be instructed in how to act as partners in meeting patient goals?
- Is responsibility for the intervention within the LPN/LVN role?

Goals and Outcomes. Goals state a general intent about what is being accomplished (e.g., "I will learn the medical prefixes, roots, and suffixes by the end of the semester."). Outcome describes a specific result that can be observed at some point (e.g., "I will learn the prefixes, roots, and suffixes well enough by the end of the semester to get an A grade on the final test"). The terms are used interchangeably in some agencies, although the ANA prefers the term outcome. The focus of the outcome is on the patient, not the nurse. An outcome is thought of as, "The patient will...." What is agreed on is that well-written outcomes include patient input, if at all possible, and must have the following characteristics:

1. Realistic (attainable, based on the patient's condition and desire),
2. Measurable (tells how you will know that the outcome has been reached), and
3. Time-referenced (an educated guess on the part of the nurse as to how long it will take to attain the outcome).

It may be easier for an SPN/SVN to use the terms *desired* (or *observable*) *patient outcome*. **The term focuses directly on what the patient will accomplish rather than on what the nurse will do.** For example, the term consists of the following characteristics:

1. It uses the word *patient* as the subject of the statement.
2. It is realistic for the patient and his or her problem.
3. It uses a measurable verb: Is specific for the patient and his or her problem.
4. It includes a time frame for patient reevaluation.

To state an outcome as a student, *reverse the problem and state it in positive terms.*

The statement tells what the patient will do to overcome the problem rather than what the patient will not do, for example:

- Observable outcome: The patient will eat 1500 calories of ground foods and liquids during each 24-hour period.
- Unclear statement: The patient will not miss any feedings during a 24-hour period.

Assisting the RN to Develop Nursing Interventions

Nursing interventions identify specifically what the nurse will do to assist the patient to reach desired patient outcomes. Sometimes this means encouraging the patient to do certain activities, such as self-feeding. (Think back to the patient strengths that were initially identified and additional strengths you have noted since then.) Interventions are also called "nursing approach," "nursing action," or "nursing care." Interventions focus on the "related to" (R/T) portion of the nursing diagnosis. They tell nursing personnel who, what, where, when, and how much. When nursing interventions are clearly written, all nursing staffs, according to their skill level and if within their legal role, will be able to carry out the nursing action. *It needs to be identified on the care plan if the RN, LPN/LVN, or UAP will carry out the intervention.* Check the nursing interventions: Are they objective and specific as written? Interventions you will develop in your care plan as an SPN/SVN are based on courses you have taken, additional reading, and finding information from alternate sources. Interventions do not just come from the top of your head. (See Chapter 5 for information on learning resources.)

Table 8-2 takes you through the process the SPN/SVN can use to plan care for an assigned patient. In the example: (1) The nursing diagnosis, as written by the RN, is shown; (2) The nursing diagnosis is turned back into the problem the patient presented with to make it clearer and more specific; (3) The SPN/SVN wrote the outcome by reversing the problem statement; it states clearly what the patient will do, what the observable outcome

Table 8-2 | *Nursing Diagnosis, Nursing Problem, Outcome, and Interventions*

NURSING DIAGNOSIS	NURSING PROBLEM	OUTCOME
Altered nutrition: less than body requirements. Related to (R/T) decreased calorie intake.	Eats only 5% of each meal. R/T loss of appetite and weakness.	The patient will eat 1500 calories of ground foods and drink 2000 ml of liquids during each 24-hour period. (The problem is reversed and stated positively).

INTERVENTIONS

1. Six small, ground meals at 8 AM, 10 AM, noon, 2 PM, 4 PM, and 6 PM. Patient seated in an easy chair with minimal assistance. Encourage self-feeding. Assist only if needed. Record time, amount, and type of food eaten.
2. Offer 240 ml of liquids at 6 AM, 9 AM, 11 AM, 1 PM, 3 PM, 5 PM, 7 PM, and 9 PM. Vary choices: likes Jell-O, ice cream, 7 UP, chocolate milk, and pineapple juice. Drinks herbal tea with meals. Record time, amount, and liquids taken.

will be; and (4) The nursing interventions identify what the SPN/SVN will do to assist the patient in attaining the desired outcome. After checking the plan with the instructor the SPN/SVN is prepared to begin patient care.

Care Plans Vary. Different kinds of care plans are available. An individualized written care plan has been demonstrated. Some facilities use **standardized care** plans. These plans are based on research of the best possible options for a nursing diagnosis (nursing problem). To individualize a standard plan, cross out interventions that do not apply to the patient and add appropriate interventions that do apply. **Computerized care plans** are popular. Individualized plans can be entered into the computer. More commonly, standardized care plans are used and then individualized to deal with the nursing problem. **Multidisciplinary (collaborative) care plans** work well in settings in which staffs from varied professions and disciplines are involved with the patient. An example is a long-term care or psychiatric setting. More recently, they are being used in medical-surgical and other units. Plans are developed by a multidisciplinary team and reflect specific interventions used by each discipline (e.g., physical therapist, nutritionist, nurse, and physician). Maintaining a separate plan for each profession is considered repetitious. The plan is developed with an interdisciplinary focus for each professional involved. The language must be common to each discipline involved. Therefore the

medical diagnosis is used rather than a nursing diagnosis. A prioritized problem list is developed based on the medical diagnosis, providing a common language for all health team members involved. The plan identifies shared and specific responsibilities for all professions represented. Progress is usually documented on a common form or computer in order to provide easy access for all involved with the plan. A clinical pathway is another type of multidisciplinary plan that schedules clinical interventions over an anticipated time period for a specific type of patient health problem. The clinical pathway is used for high-risk, high-volume, high-cost care. Often care is documented right onto the clinical pathway. A concept map, another type of care plan, is a diagram of a patient's condition, and treatments. It can help the nurse plan interventions and is also a way to monitor patient progress.

Maintaining Patient Safety. All steps of the nursing process are directed toward patient safety. Remember the patient for whom you were collecting admission data? You discovered that he was diabetic, had four beers at the bar, and fell on his way home, which resulted in a fracture. You reported it immediately to the RN, along with a statement about his vitals. Your critical thinking made you alert the RN to a potentially serious safety issue.

Documenting the Care Plan. Documenting (charting) the plan of care is essential. Legally, if it was not charted, it was not done. In a lawsuit a lawyer reviewing the chart may interpret sloppy charting as sloppy nursing care. Where the documentation takes place depends on the facility and the type of care plan used. It may be done on the computer, in longhand in the nurse's notes, on flow sheets, or on the plan itself. Some agencies have a special care plan Kardex, or clipboard, at the patient's bedside. Eventually these become part of the patient's permanent record. Meanwhile the plan is the recipe for meeting the patient's needs.

IMPLEMENTATION: PHASE 3

The key for all your activity, regardless of your position and the agency involved, is to use the care plan as the basis for your nursing actions and reporting. For example, as an SPN/SVN you draw information from the care plan on how to provide individualized patient care. While providing care you continue to collect data based on your knowledge of the patient's strengths and disease conditions. You chart on flow sheets and nurses' notes, following the priorities indicated by the nursing problem, plus any new observations you have made according to the charting system in the agency. You use the care plan as your guideline when reporting to the RN and offer information on any changes you have noted. Specifically you focus on the nursing interventions outlined in the care plan: Do interventions continue to be appropriate? What patient changes, or lack of changes, have you observed? With this information the RN can update the plan of care, and needs only to validate the data.

Implementation includes many aspects, which are discussed in the following sections.

Nursing Action

- Follow the established plan of care. Sit with the patient during meals, encourage eating, and assist minimally, if necessary.
- Participate in the patient care conference and offer input. Report specifically on tasks assigned to you; changes, and progress or lack of progress.
- Review the procedure before preparing the patient. Prepare the patient for procedure.

Ask for help if you are uncertain about what to do.

Maintaining Patient Safety

- Use safe and appropriate techniques during patient care. Check the patient's position before lifting up safety rails to be sure arms do not get caught between the bed and the rail.
- Use precautionary and preventive interventions in providing care to patient. Make sure that wheelchair wheels and bed wheels are locked before moving patient from the chair to the bed and back again.
- Institute nursing interventions to compensate for adverse responses. If the patient gets weak while standing, assist him or her to lie or sit down and place their head between their knees (if not contraindicated by physical condition).
- Initiate life-saving interventions for emergency situations. If the patient begins to choke on food, perform the Heimlich maneuver.
- Monitor care given by unlicensed personnel. As an LPN/LVN charge nurse, you will be involved in this.
- Collect data during every patient contact. Be alert to even minor changes in skin color, breathing, respirations, etc., even though your contact does not occur at a scheduled time (i.e., perhaps you just brought in the lunch tray).

Initiating Teaching That Is Within Your Role and Supports the RN's Teaching

- Encourage patients to follow their plan of care and treatment regimen. Be alert to any deviations from the care plan. Know all staff persons' roles so that you have a basis for your observations.
- Assist patients to maintain or enhance optimal functioning. Passive range of motion is done every morning as part of basic care for the bedridden patient who has been assigned to you.

- Provide an environment conducive to attaining observable patient outcomes. If the room smells of feces, locate the source and deal with it.
- Reinforce teaching of principles, procedures, and techniques for maintenance and promotion of health. For example, the patient has been newly diagnosed as having type 2 diabetes. Reinforce the steps of foot care the RN taught earlier in the morning (you sat in on the session). Be alert to questions that the patient has, based on lack of understanding, and seek answers for the questions as needed. Demonstrate techniques used by the RN, if requested. Check with the instructor if this is something you have not done before.

Reporting and Documenting

- Collect data during every patient contact. If you note the patient is beginning to perspire profusely for no apparent reason, measure vital signs.
- Report observations to relevant members of the health team. Report the aforementioned observation immediately to the RN. Report all daily observations before leaving the unit.
- Document the patient's response to nursing intervention, therapy, or teaching. Document all interventions, responses, and changes. Use the care plan as your guide for documentation and reporting.

 Learning Exercise

Implementing Plan of Care

As an SPN/SVN the next phase is *implementing* the plan of care that you have developed with your instructor's supervision. Did you remember to include the patient strengths you identified during your data collection? *Which interventions are within the LPN/LVN role?*

Does LPN/LVN Responsibility Differ from the SPN/SVN?

As a graduate your responsibility will vary according to the work area in which you are involved, and whether you are functioning in a beginning or expanded role. In an acute care setting your primary responsibility will be to use the care plan as a guideline for providing direct patient care, continuing data collection, making verbal reports to the RN, and charting. In nursing homes and extended-care facilities you may be functioning in the role of an LPN/LVN charge nurse and have responsibility for managing patient care under the supervision of the RN.

EVALUATION: PHASE 4

The evaluation phase includes assisting in determining patient progress and communicating the findings. These two aspects are discussed in the following section.

Assist in Determining Patient Progress Toward Meeting Desired Patient Goals/Outcomes

- Collect data during every patient contact. If the patient outcome is written correctly and the data collection list is complete, evaluation will be the result of your daily data collection. The continual data collection helps make daily evaluation part of the natural flow of good nursing care (Table 8-3).

Table 8-3 | *Data Collection, Outcome, and Evaluation*

DATA COLLECTION LIST	OUTCOME	EVALUATION
Check intake: Amount and type of liquid in milliliters Amount of food taken at each meal	The patient will eat 1500 calories of chopped foods and drink 2000 ml of liquids during each 24-hour period.	By day 2 the patient was able to consume 1500 calories in ground meals and 1600 ml of liquids during a 24-hour period.

- Compare actual outcomes with desired patient outcomes. If progress is being made toward meeting the outcomes, continue as is.
- Assist in determining the patient's response to nursing care. If the patient is not meeting the outcome, check the way the outcome is written. Is it measurable, realistic, and time-referenced? If you cannot evaluate the outcome, the outcome probably is not measurable or realistic. If necessary, change the portion that needs revision or restate the desired outcome.
- Assist in identifying factors that may interfere with the patient's ability to implement the plan of care. Talk with the patient. He or she may be able to tell you why progress is not being made. Review your daily data collection notes. There may be a pattern that emerges. Have the patient's strengths been considered in the plan of care? Are the stated observable outcomes less than or beyond what the patient can accomplish? Are they realistic? Is the focus on evaluating nursing care, as opposed to evaluating patient progress toward meeting desired outcomes? If necessary, revise nursing interventions that are not working. (Refer to the Leadership Hint Decision Tree for Problem Solving on p. 258.)

Communicate Findings

- Document patient's responses to care, therapy, or teaching.
- Report findings to relevant members of the health care team.

Have you noticed how heavily dependent each step of the care plan is on the others, and how the steps are often going on simultaneously? Have you noticed that as desired outcomes are met, other problems emerge? Recall Maslow's Hierarchy: Regression occurs with illness. As observable outcomes are achieved at the lower level (patient begins to improve), higher levels of needs begin to emerge.

 Learning Exercise

Evaluating Patient Progress

The time-referenced portion of the desired outcome states the approximate date by which the patient will attain an observable outcome. It is an educated guess on the part of the RN, based on education and experience. The SPN/SVN makes an educated guess on the assignment care plan regarding the time it will take the patient to meet his or her outcome. As an SPN/SVN your daily data collection assists the RN in evaluating how far the patient has progressed and what difficulties there may be. A complete daily data collection list is essential and, as pointed out, is the basis of your data collection during every patient contact.

WHERE ARE WE NOW IN THE NURSING PROCESS?

Nursing continues to grow as a profession. Nursing research and health industry focus and policy all drive the change from general to specific nursing interventions and measurement of outcomes. Two such well-researched projects are the Nursing Interventions Classification (NIC) and the Nursing Outcomes Classification (NOC) taxonomies.

NIC

NIC standardizes, defines, and assists in choosing the appropriate nursing interventions for nurses, student nurses, administrators, and faculty. It includes these interventions: physical and psychosocial; illness treatment and prevention; health promotion; individual, group, family, and community; indirect and direct care; and independent and collaborative interventions (McCloskey and Bulechek, 2000).

NOC

NOC standardizes the terminology and criteria for measurable or desirable outcomes as a result of nursing interventions. NOC has identified desired outcomes for individual patients and family care givers, as well as family- and community-level outcomes (Johnson, Maas, and Moorhead, 2000).

NANDA-I, NIC, AND NOC

NANDA-I is a source that helps the RN to determine nursing diagnosis. NIC is a source for choosing standardized nursing interventions. NOC identifies desired outcomes as a result of nursing interventions. NIC and NOC can be used alone or linked with nursing diagnosis, using NANDA-I taxonomy (Johnson, Bulechek, Dochterman, et al., 2001). If linked interventions are used in the health care facility where you are working, you will find the information specific and easy to apply. The RN has the final decision on nursing diagnosis, choice of nursing interventions, and measuring desired patient outcomes.

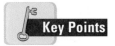

Key Points

- The Nurse Practice Act of your state identifies your legal role in the nursing process as an LPN/LVN. Take time to read it and question what you do not understand.
- Nursing process was originated in the 1950s to provide structure for thinking in nursing. The four-step process included data collection, planning, intervention, and evaluation (thinking model).
- The ANA standards of nursing practice, published in 1997, added nursing diagnosis to

make a five-step nursing process (reasoning model). Nursing diagnosis is the exclusive responsibility of RNs because of their broad, science-based education.
- In 1996 nursing process was included in the NCLEX-PN® for the first time. Nursing process and the practical/vocational role became an important part of nursing education for LPN/LVNs.
- In 2002 nursing process and critical thinking were integrated throughout the NCLEX-PN®. The four phases of nursing process for LPN/LVNs were redefined.
  1. Phase 1: *Data collection* involves gathering patient data and reporting it to appropriate personnel.
  2. Phase 2: *Planning*—the LPN/LVN assists the RN to develop the nursing diagnosis, outcomes, and interventions for the patient's plan of care. This includes maintaining patient safety.
  3. Phase 3: *Implementation*—nursing interventions in the care plan are put into action.
  4. Phase 4: *Evaluation*—actual outcomes of the interventions are compared with desired patient outcomes (emphasis is on patient progress toward meeting outcomes). Results are reported and documented.
- Critical thinking and nursing process is mandated for SPN/SVN education.
- NIC is a way of identifying standardized nursing interventions. NOC is a system for measuring patient outcomes. Trial implementation in select hospitals has shown the value of combining NANDA-I, NIC, and NOC.

REVIEW ITEMS

1. How did origination of nursing process in the 1950s change the course of nursing?

    1. It provided a reasoning model.
    2. It provided a specificity model.
    3. It provided a problem-solution model.
    4. It provided a critical thinking model.

2. Some RNs and instructors have questioned the value of teaching SPN/SVNs nursing process and critical thinking. Which statement provides a valid reason for including both in the SPN/SVN curriculum?

    1. Knowledge of nursing process and critical thinking encourages postgraduate education, so that one day the LPN/LVN can be an RN.
    2. LPN/LVNs and RNs both do the work of nursing: A common language provides an organized way of understanding what is to be done.
    3. Learning nursing process and critical thinking provides the opportunity to be working on both LPN and RN levels of nursing at the same time.
    4. Learning nursing process and critical thinking provides a cookbook method of learning and provides time to deal with job stresses.

3. Which request by the RN will you refuse to do because it is beyond the LPN/LVN scope of practice?

    1. "Do Mr. Frederic's plan of care, and I will initial it as soon I get back from lunch."
    2. "Catheterize Mrs. Jones as soon as you can and report total output to me STAT."
    3. "Check Mr. Neap's pressure sore on his right hip for changes since his admission."
    4. "Assist Sally (RN) by doing an assessment of our new admission on the south wing."

4. Which action is within the LPN/LVN scope of nursing practice when a patient aspirates a piece of meat and you are sitting opposite the patient in the dining room?

    1. Ask someone to get help as you move quickly toward the patient to perform a Heimlich maneuver.
    2. Ask another patient to straighten up the patient while you go to get an RN or other qualified staff member.
    3. Immediately call the patient's doctor for permission to perform the Heimlich and mention you are an SPN/SVN.
    4. Because you do not know if this patient has a do-not-resuscitate order on the chart, send someone to check.

ALTERNATE FORMAT ITEM

Which of the following is not a reason for verifying data? *(Select all that apply.)*

1. Patient and family account of what happened differ.

2. You believe that persons of this culture are dishonest.

3. Patient complains of fever, but the forehead feels cool.

4. You note that the patient's body language and words match.

9 Straightforward Communication

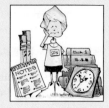

evolve http://evolve.elsevier.com/Hill/success/

Objectives

On completing this chapter, you will be able to do the following:

1. Explain the sender-receiver process in:
   a. One-way communication
   b. Two-way communication
2. Discuss how nonverbal and affective communication can support or cancel the meaning of verbal communication.
3. Provide an example of how you use communication strategies in nursing.
4. Give an example of blocking therapeutic communication.
5. List two common differences in male/female communication that have biological roots.
6. Give an example of a cultural communication difference in the area in which you live.
7. List two common factors related to role change for a hospitalized patient that can create distress.
8. Identify a communication difference for patients in two separate age groups.
9. Explain how common characteristics apply to straightforward communication with all people.
10. Discuss ways to resolve conflict between you and another staff member

Key Terms

Active listening (p. 125)
Affective communication (ă-FĔK-tĭv, p. 123)
Belittling (bĕ-LĬT-lĭng, p. 127)
Chiding (chĭd-ĭng, p. 127)
Closed-ended questions (p. 126)

Commitment (kŏ-MĬT-mĕnt, p. 131)
Communication blocks (p. 127)
Empathy (ĔM-pă-thē, p. 131)
False reassurance (RĒ-ă-shŭr-ĕns, p. 127)
Feedback (p. 123)
Focused questions (p. 126)
Giving advice (p. 127)
Honesty (p. 131)
Humor (p. 131)
Knowledge (NŎL-j, p. 131)
Message (p. 123)
Nonverbal communication (p. 123)
One-way communication (p. 123)
Open-ended questions (p. 126)
Pat answers (p. 127)
Patience (p. 131)
Probing (p. 127)
Purpose (p. 125)
Receiver (p. 123)
Respect (p. 131)
Self-esteem (p. 132)
Sender (p. 123)
Sensitivity (SĔN-sĭ-TĬV-ĭ-tē, p. 131)
Therapeutic communication (THĔR-ă-pū-tĭk, p. 125)
Trust (p. 131)
Two-way communication (p. 123)
Verbal communication (p. 123)

Keep in Mind

Purposeful communication is an integral part of your personal and professional world. Take time to learn, and know that language is never innocent.

COMMUNICATION PROCESS

Sara walked into the patient's room without knocking on the door. "I'm going to measure your blood pressure. Give me your arm," she said. The patient gave her a quizzical look, but he put out his arm. This was Sara's first contact with a patient. When she finally got the cuff on, her face was flushed, and her own heart was beating so hard that she could not hear the patient's heartbeat.

 Learning Exercise

Communicating with Your Patient

1. What kind of communication did Sara engage in with the patient?
2. Who was Sara's focus?
3. What steps did Sara skip that resulted in showing disrespect for the patient?

Sara engaged in one-way communication, in which the sender (Sara) controlled the situation by telling the receiver (patient) what she was going to do (the message). Sara offered no opportunity for feedback (response) from the patient. Feedback would have provided the patient an opportunity to question, agree, or refuse the procedure. Sara was so focused on herself that she omitted common courtesies: a knock on the door, addressing the patient by name, and introducing herself, her position, and reason for being there. The patient's unspoken response may have increased Sara's discomfort.

ONE-WAY VERSUS TWO-WAY COMMUNICATION

One-way communication is used to give a command, as in the military service, or information with no expectation of feedback. Sometimes one-way communication must be changed to two-way communication, in which there is feedback or discussion. During an emergency a doctor may give an order. Take a few seconds to change the order to two-way communication by repeating the order to the doctor so that it is verified for accuracy. Two-way communication is the usual form of conversation. Each person contributes equally, and feedback is both expected and respected.

FACTORS THAT AFFECT COMMUNICATION

Some common factors that can influence communication include the following:

1. Personal characteristics of both the sender and receiver,
2. Cultural characteristics,
3. Situational influences, and
4. Context in which the message is sent and received.

Personal characteristics can include such things as age, gender, income, and marital status. Life experiences, attitude, and personal opinions are other personal characteristics.

Cultural characteristics can involve space and distance, language and dialect, use and meaning of touch, bad or good manners, meaning of gestures, time of day, and season of the year.

Situational influences can include the physical and emotional state of the patient and nurse, room temperature, interruptions, background noises, and body odor.

Context can include the appropriateness or inappropriateness of the communication. "What can I do to make you more comfortable?" is an appropriate question directed to a dying patient. Discussion by the family about who gets what after the patient dies, within earshot of the patient, is inappropriate communication.

TYPES OF COMMUNICATION

Three types of communication are identified: verbal communication (spoken or written word), nonverbal communication (body language), and affective communication (feeling tone). They may or may not all occur together. When they do occur together, all three must mirror each other (be congruent) for the communication to be honest (Fig. 9-1).

VERBAL COMMUNICATION

The spoken word is powerful. A patient may accept what you say as completely as though

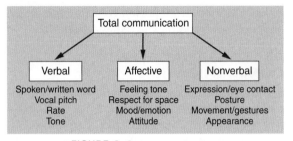

FIGURE **9-1** Communication.

the team leader or doctor had spoken. Know in advance what you can or cannot discuss with a patient. Sometimes your response will be, "I do not know, but I will find someone who does."

Speak as clearly as possible, using proper grammar. Slang is usually not appropriate and may have a different meaning. Depending on age and culture, the patient may not understand slang. Out-of-date slang may also make you come across as unprofessional or silly.

Medical jargon is rarely helpful. If you truly understand the medical terms, you can translate the words into everyday language.

Use of colloquial (common) expressions will be appropriate with some patients. For example, the word urinate may be understood by some as pass water, tinkle, or pee-pee. Use the word that the patient understands. Remember that the patient needs a professional he or she can look up to, and one who will **respect** his or her individual differences; the patient does not need the nurse to be a buddy. Maintain professional boundaries. Interestingly, a patient will respect you and is more likely to follow the directions you are giving, than if you are trying to be "familiar" with him or her. When a nurse at a nursing home was asked why she continued to wear her white uniform and cap instead of wearing scrub type clothes like the rest of the staff, she responded, "The residents take the medications I give them and will follow directions I offer them. They also ask for me by name if they are worried about something or do not understand what is happening to them. They know that they can trust me. Sometimes residents want to know who all these other people are who come into her room! I know

that wearing my uniform plays a big part of the rapport I have with the residents."

Some illnesses also affect a patient's interpretation of verbalization. Patients diagnosed with schizophrenia interpret words concretely (literally). They experience difficulty with abstract (inferred) meanings. For example, after using a stationary bicycle a patient was asked by the nurse, "How do you feel now?" He grabbed his buttocks and responded, "My butt is numb; that's how." The nurse had been trying to determine change in his stress level. Instead, his response was based on literal interpretation of the question.

NONVERBAL COMMUNICATION

Commonly known as body language, nonverbal communication either supports or cancels out verbal communication. Expressions, posture, movements, and gestures, whether they are your own or the patient's, give important clues to the truth of the verbalization. Careful observation of body language may clue you in to patient discomfort, even though pain has been denied verbally. Gathering additional data will help clarify the real issue creating the discomfort.

Verbal communication works both ways. Patients tend to observe you closely, as well, looking for clues regarding the seriousness of their illness. For example, your distressed look may be interpreted as disapproval or serious concern about their health. How are they to know that you brought your personal life worries to work?

Physical appearance is a part of nonverbal communication. The patient's appearance on admission provides signs of personal care plus important clues about the illness. Patients also quickly evaluate you and, based on what you project, even before you speak, draw conclusions about your competence as a nurse. "Clothing communicates a nonverbal message about competence and professionalism to a patient which can influence the nurse-patient relationship" (Arnold & Boggs, 2003). This is a major reason why most nursing schools continue to have a dress code. It is also the reason why your instructors model appropriate dress and behavior for their students.

Appropriate Dress Code and Behavior

What kind of statement do you think you are making by the way you dress and behave at the patient's bedside?

AFFECTIVE COMMUNICATION

Affect refers to mood or emotion. The feeling tone that you pick up on as you approach a person or step into a room is real. For every thought you have there is a physiological response in your body. The same is true for the patient and others that you encounter. We are made up of energy; therefore we emit energy. The tendency may be to ignore this level of communication because we cannot see, hear, or read it. Affective communication is as significant as verbal and nonverbal communication. Truly honest communication integrates verbal, nonverbal, and affective communications so that they all express the same message.

Affective Communication

1. Give an example of a time that you stepped into a room or approached a person, and before anyone spoke, experienced a feeling of excitement, happiness, sadness, anger, or some other emotion. What was the outcome?
2. Think of a time when you were angry and trying to hide the feeling. Did anyone pick up on your feeling tone and ask you if you were angry? How did you deal with the question?
3. Give examples of how you try to be congruent (together) verbally, nonverbally, and affectively in your communication.

COMMUNICATION STRATEGIES

Please do not interpret the term *strategies* (hints) to mean predetermined script, as in telemarketing. In real life this would be awkward, even boring. You might even lose track of where you are in your conversation because of the focus on strategies. Work to understand the meaning of active listening, active listening behaviors, and types of questions discussed.

ACTIVE LISTENING

This is probably the most important part of any therapeutic (health-related) communication. Key factors in active listening include purpose, disciplined attention, and focus. Purpose refers to the health-related reason for gathering data or giving information. *Disciplined attention* means that you do not assume accuracy of information without checking it out. Clarify what you think you understand the patient to say and ask further questions as needed. This applies both to gathering data and giving health-related information. *Focus* means that all your senses are alert to clues that the patient may be communicating. A common mistake in listening is to listen to the words, but not really hear the words (i.e., comprehend the meaning).

ACTIVE LISTENING BEHAVIORS

The most commonly used *active listening behaviors* include restating, clarification, reflection, paraphrasing, minimal encouraging, silence, summarizing, and validation.

Restating refers to repeating in a slightly different way what the patient has said. For example:

Patient: "My chest hurts. I can't sleep at night."

Nurse: "You've been unable to sleep at night because of chest pain."

Clarification is asking a closed-ended question in response to a patient's statement to be sure you understand. For example:

Patient: "My chest hurts."

Nurse: "Exactly where does your chest hurt?"

Reflection is putting into words the information you are receiving from the patient at an affective communication level. For example:

Patient: "I'm sick of seeing doctors and not getting answers."

Nurse: "You are upset with the lack of answers to your health problems."

Paraphrasing refers to expressing in your own words what you think the patient means.

Patient: "I don't think I'm being told the truth about my condition."

Nurse: "You think you may be more ill than what the doctor is telling you."

Minimal encouraging involves using sounds, words, or short phrases to encourage the patient to continue. For example:

Patient: "It just happened so fast…."

Nurse: "Yes … go on … and then what … hmmm … uh huh…."

Silence involves pauses used with skill. The tendency is to fill silence with chatter or your speculation. This may cause the patient to "turn off" or change the story. Maintaining disciplined attention and focus during silence lets patients tell the story in their own way. Avoid making interruptions and doing busy work while the patient is speaking.

Summarizing means briefly stating the main data you have gathered. For example:

Nurse: "This is what I heard you say: Is that correct?"

Validation provides the patient with an opportunity to correct information, if necessary, at the time of summary. For example:

Patient: "That is correct," or "No, you got the part wrong about…." (This allows the patient to correct the information.)

TYPES OF QUESTIONS

Three types of questions are commonly used in **therapeutic communication**. They are open-ended, closed-ended, and focused questions. Open-ended questions permit the patient to respond in a way most meaningful to him or her. The questions often begin with what, where, when, how, or why. For example: "What happened to your leg?" Closed-ended questions require a specific answer. For example: "When did you first notice the pain?" Focused questions provide even more definitive information. For example: "On a scale of 1 to 10, with 10 as the worst possible pain, how do you rate your pain right now?"

NURSE/PATIENT COMMUNICATION EVALUATION

Communication is far more complex than just talking. Some of the many contributing characteristics are listed in this section, with a brief description in the following learning exercise.

Evaluate the characteristics that are working for you and those you need to work on.

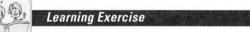
Learning Exercise

Self-Evaluation of Personal Characteristics

Characteristic	Desirable	Self-Evaluation
Eye contact	Usually 3-5 seconds. Cultural variations.	_____
Respect for personal space	Approximately 1.5 feet, except for personal care. Cultural variations.	_____
Appropriate touch	Gentle, but firm. Cultural variations.	_____
Attitude	Nonjudgmental. Practices unconditional love.	_____
Voice/tone	Moderate or according to growth and development needs. Example: Newborns	_____ _____
Rate	Paced according to patient's ability to comprehend	_____
Appearance	Models positive nursing image. Looks healthy.	_____ _____
Posture	Open, without folded arms or hands on hips. Stand or sit tall.	_____
Gestures	Moderate to enhance conversation.	_____
Language	Speaks effectively and at patient's level of understanding. Correct grammar.	_____ _____
Expression	Congruent with topic. Nonjudgmental.	_____

A Plan for Change

List the personal characteristics that are not working for you. Develop a plan for change and measuring improvement, using the phases of the nursing process.

BLOCKS TO COMMUNICATION

It is sometimes easy to slip into communication styles that block communication. Perhaps the patient reminds you of someone you know, or you have had personal dealings with the patient in the past. Sometimes you do not like the patient or are just plain tired. Whatever the reason, it is worth thinking about the possibility in advance. As a nurse you want to continue to give every patient the best care possible, regardless of your personal response. Common communication blocks involve **false reassuring**, **probing**, **chiding**, **belittling**, **giving advice**, and providing **pat answers**.

AVOIDING BLOCKS

False reassurance involves telling the patient, "Everything will be OK," "You'll be just fine," "Don't worry about anything," "We'll see to it that you get well," "This experience will make you stronger," or, "You'll see the good in this some day." There is no way you can guarantee what you have just finished saying to the patient.

Probing means pushing for information beyond what is medically necessary to know. Curiosity takes over and the patient's privacy is no longer respected. Ask yourself about the value of the information and how you will use the information once you have it. Think twice before continuing with statements such as, "Let's get to the bottom of this once and for all."

Chiding (scolding) for behavior such as smoking is of limited value for the patient with severe emphysema or lung cancer (or perhaps the patient never smoked). Your information is hardly an "alert." You can be sure that she or he has heard the message over and over. Without supporting the behavior you can continue to be therapeutic to the patient.

Belittling involves mimicking or making fun of the patient in some way. It may include downplaying the importance of the symptoms. For example: "You could be having heart surgery! This is just wart removal." As a physician pointed out, "If you have a tonsillectomy, it's minor surgery; if I have a tonsillectomy, it's major surgery." It is all a matter of perspective.

Giving advice, when you know what someone else should do, is so tempting. Unsolicited advice is rarely beneficial and closes the door to having the patient problem solve. A more beneficial response, even when the patient asks what you would (or he or she should) do, is to say, "What ideas do you have? I'm sure you've thought of ways you might solve this problem." Listen carefully, summarize what the patient has said, and then ask, "Which one of your ideas do you want to begin with?" After the patient's response, you could say, "When do you think you'll start?"

Pat answers, such as, "Everyone feels this way," come so easily. Patients feel dismissed and misunderstood. They do not really care that everyone else feels this way. As far as they are concerned these feelings are theirs, are different, and need comforting words or touch. If you can, offer something you know you can deliver, such as, "I'll be with you the entire time you are having your bone marrow drawn," or, "I'll be in the room when you return."

MALE/FEMALE DIFFERENCES

Being equal does not mean being the same. Men and women communicate differently for biological reasons. Although there are examples of similarities between the sexes, most males and females follow certain patterns. According to Sieh and Brentin (1997), four areas that relate to nursing communication are conversation patterns, smiling, head movements, and posture.

CONVERSATION

Men tend to approach conversation with an eye to maintaining status and independence, to report or to get information, and to solve problems. They express their ideas more assertively; women do so with less certainty. Therefore male opinions are often valued more highly without validation. Women seek to establish intimacy and develop rapport, share feelings, and establish relationships. Men ask fewer questions, but readily interrupt during conversations without apology. Women use questions to encourage conversation. They wait for a pause to seek clarification and apologize for the interruption. Men apologize for a wrong; women say "I'm sorry" to indicate regret, sympathy, or concern. Men rarely say, "I don't know"; women often phrase ideas as questions, such as "Have you thought of …?" Men make decisions; women are looking for agreement. Men make demands more often, whereas women express preferences with reasons. Men's sentences are shorter and fewer; women create longer, more complex sentences, linking more ideas together. Men make declarations, whereas women often end a statement with a question, such as, "Don't you think so?" (Tannen, 1990).

HEAD MOVEMENTS

Men nod if they are in agreement. Women nod to show they are listening. A man may be surprised to discover that a woman does not agree at all with what he said. Men hold their heads erect while speaking; women frequently assume a lower status position by tilting their head to the side or placing their chin down with eyes gazing upward (Sieh and Brentin, 1997).

SMILING

Smiling by a woman may or may not denote happiness. A smile is also used to mask unhappiness and other emotions. Reactions by others to her smiles may leave her feeling unheard. Others may accept her nonverbal communication and be unable to interpret that she is feeling sad, angry, afraid, etc. Sometimes men will mask their emotion with a smile. Usually men tend not to show an outward reaction when criticized, making them seem strong and in control.

POSTURE

A rounded posture with the chest in and chin down gives an appearance of being threatened. Standing tall, with shoulders back and head held high, speaks of confidence and control.

Looking at differences in the way men and women communicate has important implications in working with patients, staff, and instructors. Smiling and nodding by a woman does not have to mean she understands the instructions. A lack of questions from a male patient may not mean he knows what the surgery entails. Gather all three types of communication data. Ask the patient to tell you what he or she understands, then summarize and validate. *Make use of the skills you are learning.*

CULTURAL DIFFERENCES

Members of subcultures within our cultures embrace and value their beliefs and practices. You have to be respectful of these beliefs and practices and respond therapeutically. Know about cultural differences in communication. We briefly review communication differences for the white American and the four most prominent groups in the United States, according to the 2000 U.S. census: African Americans, Mexican Americans, Hmong Americans, and American Indians. *The differences listed apply generally to groups as a whole.* Individual patient differences need to be identified. Be sure to read Chapter 12 for a more complete understanding of cultural diversity. Mark the chapter and use it as a reference when questions arise.

WHITE AMERICAN

The white American's major language is English. The speech pattern and tone are moderate. Distance is preferred between speakers. Time is highly valued and tends to regulate one's life.

AFRICAN AMERICAN

For the African American the dominant language is English. The use of African American vernacular English may cause misunderstanding between the patient and nurse. Speaking in loud voices may occur among family and friends. Speech may be rapid, and the space during conversation may be close. Touch may be common within the family and extended family. Eye contact conveys respect and is often maintained. Expression of pain may be open or public.

MEXICAN AMERICAN

For the Mexican American everything in their communication flows from respect. The major language is Spanish. Depending on their area of origin in Mexico, their language may have different meaning. Speech is rapid and loud. Personal space is close. Touch is common, especially among members of the same sex. Touching the arm or shoulder when making a point shows **trust** or rapport. However, touch by strangers may convey disrespect. Shaking hands is a common greeting when saying hello or good-bye. The patient may avoid direct eye contact. Pain is open or public. Grief may be overtly expressed.

HMONG AMERICAN

In this part of the American population older individuals speak Hmong and Lao. Younger individuals speak English and Hmong, but may not be proficient in interpreting for their elders. The voice is modulated. They are polite and respectful. Long, direct eye contact may be considered rude. They do not display affection publicly. Touching by a nurse may be accepted. "Yes" does not always mean agreement. Shaking hands is acceptable.

AMERICAN INDIAN

Most American Indians speak English, but there are 150 tribal languages. The tone of their voice is soft. The speech pattern is slow. Examples, anecdotes, and metaphors are used to discuss situations. Long pauses may be used in the process. Do not interrupt the patient. Keep a respectful distance. Expressions of pain are closed and private and may be expressed as being "uncomfortable." American Indians may not ask questions, but expect the health provider to know and direct them in health issues. Eye contact is considered a sign of disrespect.

Learning Exercise

Cultural Differences

List two cultural differences of someone in the area in which you live.

1. _____

2. _____

The characteristics described in the previous section are brief and cover a small number of the cultures within the country. Communication patterns change with time, vary with the situation, and differ in public or private settings. It is important to learn as much as possible about the cultures frequently served where you work. Remember also, that just because you can identify someone's ethnic background, families may have been in this country for generations, and differences may be nonexistent.

ROLE CHANGES FOR THE PATIENT

What happens to patients who find themselves in a dependent position after having been in charge of their lives? The concerns they have go beyond the physical realities into areas we consider in the next section.

Critical Thinking Exercise

Immediate Concerns upon Hospitalization

Imagine yourself being hospitalized. List four immediate concerns you would have.

1. _____

2. _____

3. _____

4. _____

IT BEGINS WITH, "HELLO, MY NAME IS...."

Whatever you communicate verbally, nonverbally, and affectively sets the tone for rapport with the patient. You have some preliminary information (a name), even if the patient is just being admitted. Knock on the door or the door frame; pause briefly to collect data *before* walking in. You begin to pick up nonverbal and affective communication clues. Address the patient as Mr., Mrs., Miss, or Ms., or by professional title if it applies. Extend your hand (unless culturally improper). Give your name; identify yourself as a student practical/vocational nurse, plus the name of the school and your purpose for being in the room.

It may sound like this: "Mrs. Hill, my name is Mr. Fry. I am a student practical nurse from the Middle American Technical College. I am here to measure your blood pressure, pulse, and respiration. It is a part of the admission procedure." The patient may request that you address her by first name, but do not assume this without permission. Some hospitals and other health agencies limit staff use of name to first name only. This will dictate how you introduce yourself. You will never have an opportunity to make a positive first impression with this patient again.

NURSING JARGON

Remember how time-consuming it was to learn all those medical terms and abbreviations? Using the terms may sound impressive to you now and involve a feeling of having arrived. However, use of unknown terminology can serve to increase patient fears and cause misunderstanding. "What does it mean that I will have an IV started, have a WBC stat, and you'll be doing vitals q2h for now?" When you really know something, you can explain words and symbols in terms understood by a layperson. Now *that's* really impressive!

FEAR OF THE UNKNOWN

Patients often have numerous unspoken fears about tests, procedures, and possible outcomes. These include, but are not limited to, pain, sleep, needle sticks, thirst, hunger, and being treated respectfully. A pat answer of "Everything will be OK" shows lack of understanding of the depth of the fears. Patients may not ask questions because of fear of embarrassment: "Silly question," "Everyone is so busy." An open-ended question

from you, such as, "What questions do you have? If I don't know the answer, I'll try to find out for you," can open the way for expression of fears.

PERSONAL FACTORS

A patient's illness rarely affects the patient alone. Thoughts and concerns may extend to family, work, finances, and so on. For example, the mother of a newly hospitalized child was irritable and inattentive when the nurse was explaining the unit rules. Finally the nurse stopped mid-sentence and said to the mother, "Tell me what is troubling you." The mother looked at her and then blurted out that she had a sick child at home, her husband worked nights and slept days, and she had been up most of the last 3 nights. "Where should I be? Both kids need me, and my neighbor can only come in for two hours a day. I'm at my wit's end!" The mother could not begin to focus on the unit rules until there were solutions to the home problems. You may not have a solution, but you can be a catalyst to make needs known to the instructor or team leader. They are aware of additional resources.

ENVIRONMENTAL FACTORS

A health care setting—whether a clinic, hospital, rehabilitation center, or nursing home—is so different from home. There is no true opportunity for privacy. A variety of staff show up at different times throughout a 24-hour period; lights are on day and night; the staff makes more noise than they realize; machinery is humming, buzzing, or beeping; staff check out different parts of your body, picking and poking—you get the picture. The patient may have put the light on because of a need to go to the bathroom now. By the time someone arrives it may be too late, much to the patient's embarrassment.

Advance communication and planning does not take as long as it sounds. You may find out that the patient always has a snack of toast and tea at 9 PM, always gets up to go to the bathroom at 11 PM, always has bran cereal and a banana at 6 AM, etc. Notes of this nature in the patient's care plan assist in continuity of communication and care.

COMMUNICATING WITH INSTRUCTORS AND STAFF

Communication characteristics involve respect, trust, honesty, empathy, sensitivity, humor, knowledge, patience, commitment, and self-esteem. These characteristics are equally important in communicating with patients, instructors, and staff.

RESPECT

Respect involves both self-respect and respect for others. You communicate self-respect by doing your best each day. When you treat yourself with self-respect, it becomes easy to extend respect to your instructors, staff, and patients. Patients quickly pick up on whether they are being respected during conversation and physical care (verbal and nonverbal communication, such as eye signals between staff).

TRUST

Trust begins with confidence in your ability to make decisions. You communicate this to instructors and staff by consistently doing the required preliminary preparation for assignments.

HONESTY

Honesty implies that you will not deliberately deceive in order to present yourself in a more favorable light. Arranging a time with the instructor for you to repeat a procedure for more practice is an example of this characteristic in communication.

EMPATHY

Empathy is the ability to understand and appreciate what someone else is feeling without experiencing the emotion itself. When you are sympathetic, as you would be with a family member or dear friend, you actually experience the emotion. Being empathetic permits you to understand how someone is feeling, why they feel that way, maintain control of your emotions, and think clearly. For example, you might offer to help a staff member who is having a bad day do patient care (a practical intervention), instead of getting pulled into an "isn't it awful" conversation.

SENSITIVITY

Tuning in on nonverbal and affective communication helps you verify verbalization or lack thereof. Picking up at nonverbal and affective levels permits you to check them out with the staff or instructor. "Is there something else I need to know?"

HUMOR

Healthy humor at the patient's level of appreciation can help "lighten up" a situation. Offensive humor and poking fun at the patient or at other cultures or races is unacceptable. The staff sometimes privately gets involved in "gallows humor," which is laughing at something very serious or medically gross. Look for examples in movies and television programs with medical themes.

KNOWLEDGE

The cornerstone of gathering data and other health-related communication is knowledge. Instructors and staff quickly determine your level of knowledge. Instructors communicate the significance of this characteristic by making assignments early enough for you to research the information. You communicate back to the instructor (and staff) by preparing for patient care.

PATIENCE

In this modern world we are often accustomed to instant results and gratification. It is sometimes difficult to provide the time needed to learn, receive explanations from instructors, or follow staff orders. This extends to our work with patients, in whom illness and growth and development levels dictate the need to slow down or repeat directions. The patient (or you) may be tempted to say "I know" when such is not the case. The characteristic of patience takes time to perfect. You may initially feel like you are moving backward in your communication attempts with patients.

COMMITMENT

Commitment means incorporating all the previous characteristics as a part of your nursing communication. Decide that you are in nursing because you really want to be here. Then do the work that needs to be done. It shows, and it pays off. Take time to appreciate the uniqueness of each patient (see Chapter 12).

SELF-ESTEEM, THOUGHTS, AND STRAIGHTFORWARD COMMUNICATION

Self-esteem is earned, not learned. No one can give it to you or take it away! It is that special sense that it is okay to receive credit for something you did well. Self-esteem also gives you permission to recognize that you have something very special to offer in nursing communication— such as being able to communicate effectively with patients and other health workers.

Pause for a few moments. Think about your thoughts. Are they positive or are they negative in regard to you? There are two basic kinds of thought: random and active. Random thoughts just show up. You initiate active thoughts. Random thoughts usually pass through, unless you pick a thought and change it into an active thought. What do the active thoughts say to you about you and the person you are? Do they support your sense of self or do the thoughts tear you down? If your thoughts are not serving you, change them. If you have made a mistake, learn from it and let it go. No need to continue punishing yourself. Everyday, look for what you have done well and give yourself a cheer for a job well done! Thoughts also set the feeling tone for how you communicate with patients and other staff. "How you feel about something creates actions, which bring about results. Actions are the bridge from the inner world to your outer world. Start by changing your inner world" (Fuimano, 2004).

Practice makes your conversation meaningful. Make peace with silence. If you find yourself talking just to fill in the silence, **stop**. Learn to say what you mean. Be direct in your conversation, remembering that language is never innocent. When giving patients information or directions, avoid medical jargon. Being long-winded just means that you do not know how to express yourself clearly. Ask the patient what they think

you said as a way to avoid misunderstanding. If you are on the other end of a long-winded conversation, remember that you can take control. Check out what it is the person really wants you to know and set a time limit if needed: I have to go in __ minutes.

Remembering the affective component of conversation helps you be aware of your and the other person's feelings. It is not unusual that after a conversation, the other person's feelings mirror the feeling you were experiencing. "If you take care of the words you chose, if you take the time to be purposeful and intentional, if you practice, knowing that it takes time to become an effective communicator—you'll become more effective in every area of your life: you'll experience more joy and satisfaction, and you'll achieve the results you want" (Fuimano, 2004).

LIFE SPAN COMMUNICATION

Growth and development levels, male/female differences, and medical conditions all affect communication with patients. Each age group, whether infant, preschool, school age, teenage, adult, or elderly, has somewhat different communication needs.

INFANT

Infants' communication includes crying, cooing, and body language. They act out their feelings with total body language. As their recognition of words grows certain words act to soothe or trigger reaction. Up to that time infants are most influenced by the sound of the voice. As one father pointed out, "I used to put my baby to sleep each night by rocking her and reading the *Wall Street Journal* aloud in a soothing voice." Newborns respond favorably to a high-pitched voice, but that changes by the end of the first month. After that calm, low tones are more soothing.

Parents (caretakers) are the best source for learning the meaning of different cries. They learn quickly to differentiate between wet, hungry, and uncomfortable. Rely on them for specific information on communication style.

PRESCHOOL

We are including toddlers in this category of early preschoolers. They are usually known for magnificent tantrums. Little wonder: They have learned some words, but when frustrated, may not be able to put them together effectively. Hence the body acts out what the words cannot tell. Laughing at or trying to reason with the preschooler is counterproductive.

Removing the child from the immediate situation and audience helps. Once preschoolers are more composed they can communicate by pointing or showing on themselves, or in a picture, what is upsetting them. During procedures explain briefly and simply what is going to happen. Tell them what they can do to help. For example, preschoolers will often assist and cooperate with receiving injections if patiently coached on exactly what to do (e.g., position, what to do with their feet and hands, how long they need to stay still, what to expect during the injection).

SCHOOL AGE

The vocabulary of school-age children has increased considerably. They are ready to be a part of most (but not all) discussions with their parents. Drawings or pictures can be used to explain an illness or procedure. Ask for feedback to avoid misconceptions. "Tell me in your own words what...." The child may not be privy to all information. In that case go to a separate area so that the child will not overhear the conversation or parts of it. Whispering and misinterpretation can evoke new problems. Remember that younger children think well in the afternoon.

TEENAGE

Teenagers are the easiest or the most difficult to communicate with, depending on your perspective. When ill, they need to believe that someone knows more than they do and that someone is in charge. Deal with them with the same courtesy that you extend to adults. Have similar expectations of them. Encourage expression of feelings, fears, and concerns. Their sense that nothing will happen to them has been shaken. Answer questions within your role. Seek out answers as appropriate. Avoid hiding behind nursing jargon. Use of teen slang generally does not work out. Without real knowledge of the meaning, you may end up appearing foolish instead of "hot."

ADULT

Many of the issues discussed in this chapter apply to adult communication. Collecting data at all three levels of communication is essential. Remember to limit your questions to areas that are medically related. Pushing and probing based on curiosity may open Pandora's box (i.e., painful issues that have been suppressed). It does not work to probe and leave the patient to pick up the pieces of what has been revealed to you under pressure.

Patients with diminishing memory seem to have a relatively preserved reading ability. Visual information seems to be more permanent. Verbal information is so transient that the person may not have time to process it completely before it is gone (Banotai, 2007) Writing the information in the size that is easy for the patient to read is worth trying by the health care worker or family member. Written information seems to be more neutral and does not evoke the emotional reaction that words would have.

ELDERLY

What picture do you hold of elderly people in your "mind's eye?" Unresolved parental issues, for example, can get in the way of quality care. If you can see aging as just another part of the life cycle, you may be able to work effectively with elderly patients. "Boys and men take in less sensory or proximal data than girls and women. They smell less, taste less, get less soothing and input from tactile information, hear less and see less" (Gurian, 1997). Most elderly people think more clearly in the morning.

Lower-frequency sounds are easier to hear for both men and women when hearing begins to diminish. As with younger men, check with the elderly man as to which ear has the best hearing. Remember that the left eye, even without loss of vision, has more acuity for a man. It works best for explanations and table games to be focused on the left side. Women see and hear equally well with both eyes and ears. Women also differentiate sounds easier from background noises. There is some evidence that both men and women recall emotional words better when spoken into their left ear. The elderly man may not hear you if you call when the TV is on. The male brain shuts on and off according to load. Part of it must remain functioning to continue vital functions. Men may continue to have reading problems. Read directions aloud for the male patient without visual problems. You will continue to find that many female patients are orderly and satisfied with a smaller amount of space. The male patient is generally the opposite, and you may have to seek additional space for games and puzzles in the day room.

Preparing for discharge begins after admission. The nurse takes advantage of teachable moments to interject information, demonstrate techniques, and have the patient return demonstrations. This includes the patient and any family members or friends who are planning to assist post-hospitalization. Listen carefully when the patient describes what is waiting at home. Will adaptive equipment be necessary? Will other health providers have to be involved in making the transition between this facility and home? The best part of being a student in this situation is that the instructor and RN assigned to the patient are available to assist you.

CONFLICT RESOLUTION

In the health setting, conflict can be related to diversity, English as a second language, differences in gender, generation, and personality. Doctors and nurses often provide information in different formats. "Nurses are taught to communicate through narrative, through a story, to give a lot of background. Physicians are trained to communicate in bullet points. So they have two totally different styles" (Federwische, http://www.nurse.com, 2007). Differences are magnified in high stress situations. It is thought that only about 2% to 3% of

physicians and nurses are truly disruptive, but that creates problems for the rest of the staff. Problems can translate into medication errors, patient safety, and even patient mortality. Some health facilities have set up major programs to teach their staff how to communicate with each other. In general, there are some basic steps to keep in mind.

You will want to focus on a mutually beneficial solution based on shared interests.

1. Accept conflict as a natural part of life. Different points of view, needs, and beliefs are often involved.
2. Shift your own attitude and behavior. Be aware of your initial reaction and take a deep breath. (Your automatic defense system wants to dig in and fight.)
3. Take time to think critically before reacting. For example, had you thought through what you needed to report, or did you come off rambling?
4. Treat conflict as an opportunity to voice your own opinion and listen to the other side of the story. Know that you may have to take the initiative to approach the physician or nurse (or other person), regarding what you are seeing as a conflict. They may not be aware of how you are being affected and ultimately feelings may escalate and patient care will suffer.
5. Choose your approach. A winner takes all: A win-lose approach will only escalate the intensity of the feelings involved. The best choice for a solution depends on the situation. There is no "blanket" correct way.
6. Listen and learn. Conflicts are often based on assumptions and lack of information. If you did happen to be entirely wrong, apologize, and find how to correct your mistake in future incidences. Take your lumps and get on with it!
7. Discover what is important, i.e., the core issue. It can range from hurt feelings to unmet needs. Getting to the root of the problem gets you closer to resolving the conflict.

8. Respect each other. Conflict can be very emotional. Show respect despite the angry and hurt feelings. Stay away from name calling and blaming. Use of genuine "I"-centered statements helps each individual own their own statements.

9. Find common ground to create the highest common denominator. In this case it is generally for the patient's highest good.

Learning Exercise

Resolving Conflicts

Think of a time recently when you experienced a conflict with someone. What was the outcome? Are you still upset with the other person or was the issue resolved in a mutually beneficial way? What part of your behavior are you especially pleased with? What, if anything would you do differently?

ELECTRONIC COMMUNICATION

Use of facsimile (fax) machines, computer patient charting, and electronic mail (email) are all valuable modern methods of communication when used effectively and appropriately. Fax machines, for example, often shorten the time in which information can be sent between agencies and departments. Computer patient charting ideally provides a location where all agency professionals involved in patient care enter the most recent information. Computer charting may be part of your basic education for learning to enter medications and treatments. Each facility may have slightly different protocols. Email is a popular way of communication with administration and other departments. Before getting involved in sending email, it is important to review the basics of email etiquette. According to Lauchman (1999), some people email things they would never write in a memo or say directly to someone. Box 9-1 includes some e-mail essentials, as suggested by Lauchman.

| Box 9-1 | **Email Etiquette** |

- Consider the content of the email message and to whom you are sending it.
- To emphasize a point, let the sentence stand alone. Special effects, such as boldface, may not show up on someone else's screen.
- Keep your sentences and paragraphs short.
- Skip a line to separate topics.
- Send your message to the right person.
- Be especially careful filling in the "subject" line. People read this first to decide whether the message is worth opening.
- Be specific. Avoid useless information.
- Determine whether email is the best way to send your message.
- Be cautious with humor. The person sees only the written word.
- Check your spelling and punctuation. Proofread all messages before sending them.
- Avoid typing an entire email in uppercase. The message "screams" at the recipient.

CELL PHONES AND TEXT MESSAGING

You are sitting in class or watching a demonstration on clinical, when someone's cell phone rings. It certainly disturbs the chain of thought both for the students and the instructor. Although the phone can be set to vibrate, the shuffle to see who called is annoying. Who knows, you may have missed something essential for the care of a future patient.

Text messaging has been integrated into student life with astonishing momentum. Some students continue to text during class, often by holding the phone under the desk. An additional concern is not only the distraction, but that some students are using it as a way to cheat on exams.

Many programs have had to adopt a rule of shutting off cell and text messaging phones during class and clinical. As a matter of etiquette, it is just plain rude to behave in ways disruptive to the instructor and other students.

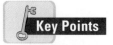
Key Points

- Communication can be one-sided or two-sided. Both forms involve a sender, a receiver, and a message. In one-sided communication the receiver does not have the opportunity to provide feedback. During two-sided communication, feedback is an expectation.
- Communication involves verbal, nonverbal, and affective communication.
- The most important part of therapeutic communication is active listening. It involves purpose, focus, and disciplined attention.
- Common active listening behaviors involve restating, clarification, reflection, paraphrasing, minimal encouraging, silence, summarizing, and validating.
- Common blocks to communication involve false reassuring, probing, chiding, belittling, giving advice, and pat answers.
- Male/female differences do exist. Some differences are "hard wired" biologically. Characteristics can be modified, if desired.
- Cultural differences in communication exist, especially with individuals who are new to the country and/or continue to have strong cultural ties.

- Role changes for the patient during an illness experience can be distressing. Staff attitude, nursing jargon, fear of the unknown, and personal and environmental factors are all involved.
- Communicating with the instructor and staff involves the same characteristics as communicating with a patient. They include trust, honesty, empathy, respect, sensitivity, humor, knowledge, patience, and commitment. Self-worth is earned as your knowledge and skill in application grow.
- Life span communication differences are related to growth and other issues, male/female differences, and medical problems.
- Be alert to what your thoughts are saying and if they help you or hinder you.
- Take your conversation seriously: Practice saying what you mean and know that your thinking affects your feelings and the way you communicate with patients and staff.
- Successful conflict management is based on a mutually beneficial solution.
- Email etiquette is essential for effective and efficient electronic communication.
- Many programs have adopted a no cell or text messaging policy during class or clinical.

REVIEW ITEMS

1. What accounts for basic male/female differences in communication?

   1. Socialization
   2. Environment
   3. Acculturation
   4. Biology

2. What is the sender-receiver-feedback process in one-way communication?

   1. It concludes when the message reaches the receiver.
   2. It uses verbal, nonverbal, and affective communication.
   3. Once feedback has been provided, the message is final.
   4. It is useful, short-hand communication in close friendships.

3. Which is an appropriate response to the patient when you pick up affectively and nonverbally on the patient's anger?

   1. Leave the room and report your observations to the team leader immediately.
   2. Lighten up the situation by sharing some funny email jokes with the patient.
   3. Provide observations of nonverbal behavior and ask the patient what is going on.
   4. Continue what you came in to do silently and leave as soon as you are through.

4. Which statement most accurately reflects a communication difference that is age related?

   1. Speaking in a loud, high voice makes it easier for the elderly patient to hear you.
   2. School-age patients are ready to be included in discussions about their illness.
   3. Distract the toddler with a tantrum by offering a special treat if they cooperate.
   4. Use of medical jargon and current slang gets the teenager to see you as human.

ALTERNATE FORMAT ITEM

Which of the following are the most prominent subcultures in the United States? *(Select all that apply.)*

1. African American
2. Mexican American
3. Hmong American
4. American Indian

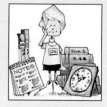

evolve http://evolve.elsevier.com/Hill/success/

Objectives

On completing this chapter, you will be able to do the following:

1. Discuss the personalized approach to healthy eating and physical activity symbolized by the 2005 USDA MyPyramid.

2. List 10 readily available foods you like that are high in phytonutrients and antioxidant compounds such as vitamins A and E.

3. Provide three examples of chronic symptoms and diseases related to obesity and lack of exercise.

4. Discuss the importance of adding moderate physical activity to your day.

5. List three to four moderate activities that will fit your lifestyle.

6. Explain why proper body mechanics help, but do not prevent all back, shoulder, and other injuries nurses may develop.

7. Differentiate between stress and burnout.

8. Discuss resources available at school to assist in dealing with overwhelming stress or feelings of hopelessness.

9. Identify possible clues that may indicate a nurse is chemically impaired by alcohol and/or other drugs while on duty.

10. Explain the difference between codependency and conscientious nursing.

11. Discuss the difference between recreation and relaxation.

12. Describe which source of relaxation is most effective for you.

Key terms

Burnout (p. 146)
Chemical dependency (dĭ-PĔN-děn-sē, p. 149)
Codependency (KO-ddĭ-PĔN-děn-sē, p. 151)
Empathy (ĔM-pă-thē, p. 146)
Subungual zone (sŭb-ŬNG-gwăl, p. 146)
Sympathy (SĬM-pă-thē, p. 147)

 Keep in Mind

Make time for yourself: build some pleasure into every day.

NEW LOOK AT NUTRITION AND HEALTH

As food, shelter, clothing, and the availability of each has improved, longevity has increased for past generations. Predictions are that longevity will not increase for the children of the current generation. The reasons given relate to lack of exercise and poor eating habits. Obesity and related health issues have become a serious issue not just for adults, but for children as well.

The U.S. Department of Health and Human Services (HHS) has expressed concern about the high rate of obesity in all age groups. The U.S. Centers for Disease Control and Prevention (CDC) underwrote an analysis that showed obesity to be a major factor in America's rising health care costs. Obesity is considered a major factor in having or dying from a heart attack, stroke or other cardiovascular disease; developing high blood pressure, high cholesterol, or diabetes; being diagnosed with postmenopausal breast cancer, cancer of the endometrium, colon, kidney; or being afflicted with some other chronic conditions (Willett, 2001). The CDC recommended that obesity be targeted as aggressively as smoking. Because government and ultimately the taxpayer are financing half the economic burden of obesity, it is no longer seen as just a personal or societal issue.

Low-fat snacks got the public's attention after the release of the 1992 USDA Food Guide Pyramid. The assumption was that if the label says "low-fat," it is healthy to eat the snack without further investigation. Although many people want to be healthy, the influx of contradictory information, powerful advertising, and availability of tempting low-fat, high–refined carbohydrate foods, has made choices confusing and overwhelming. Some people hook onto the low-fat label and often do not feel satisfied after they eat. They compensate by eating larger quantities. Meanwhile, serving sizes in restaurants and fast-food establishments have increased. Interestingly, food is the least expensive part of running most restaurants; they are not doing you a favor by giving you a larger serving of food. Studies show that the more food there is on our plate or on the table, the more we eat at the time. The rate of obesity has climbed and continues to do so, as do nutrition-related illnesses. As of 2004, HHS has moved to encourage weight loss, changes in school lunches, reduction of "junk" foods consumed by the general public, and exercise. As a result, many fast-food establishments are offering more wholesome choices and smaller portions of food and are deleting trans fat from their foods.

Research continues in the United States, Canada, and countries throughout the world on the effects of the food we eat.

 Learning Exercise

Making Good Food Choices

Make a list of current favorite foods you eat now while you are in nursing school. Next to each food listed identify if the food is a healthy choice. Look at the food labels for ingredients. Use your nutrition book as a resource.

2005 USDA MYPYRAMID FOOD GUIDE

The 2005 MyPyramid is distinctly different from the previous (1992) Food Guide Pyramid. The new guide is based on studies about nutrients and the way people eat in the United States. It takes into consideration the need for daily activity and makes recommendations in both areas (Fig. 10-1).

Learning Exercise

Make MyPyramid Work for You

Look carefully at Figure 10-1. In your own words, explain how you can make the MyPyramid work for you in each of the following areas, and include a target date for starting any changes you have identified.
- Activity—
- Moderation—
- Personalization—
- Proportionality—
- Variety—
- Gradual improvement—

MyPyramid emphasizes that nutrition be kept simple, be physically active, stay within calorie limits, and enjoy foods rich in essential nutrients from all five food groups (Fig. 10-2). No foods are off limits. Ten readily available foods that are high in phytonutrients and antioxidants such as vitamins A and E are apples, almonds, blueberries, broccoli, red beans, salmon, sweet potatoes, vegetable juice, wheat germ, and spinach.

Anatomy of MyPyramid

One size doesn't fit all

USDA's new MyPyramid symbolizes a personalized approach to healthy eating and physical activity. The symbol has been designed to be simple. It has been developed to remind consumers to make healthy food choices and to be active every day. The different parts of the symbol are described below.

Activity

Activity is represented by the steps and the person climbing them, as a reminder of the importance of daily physical activity.

Moderation

Moderation is represented by the narrowing of each food group from bottom to top. The wider base stands for foods with little or no solid fats or added sugars. These should be selected more often. The narrower top area stands for foods containing more added sugars and solid fats. The more active you are, the more of these foods can fit into your diet.

Personalization

Personalization is shown by the person on the steps, the slogan, and the URL. Find the kinds and amounts of food to eat each day at MyPyramid.gov.

Proportionality

Proportionality is shown by the different widths of the food group bands. The widths suggest how much food a person should choose from each group. The widths are just a general guide, not exact proportions. Check the Web site for how much is right for you.

Variety

Variety is symbolized by the 6 color bands representing the 5 food groups of the Pyramid and oils. This illustrates that foods from all groups are needed each day for good health.

Gradual Improvement

Gradual improvement is encouraged by the slogan. It suggests that individuals can benefit from taking small steps to improve their diet and lifestyle each day.

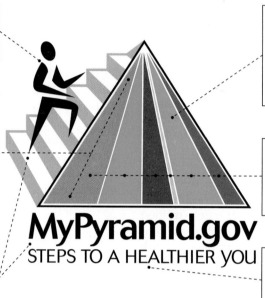

MyPyramid.gov
STEPS TO A HEALTHIER YOU

USDA U.S. Department of Agriculture
Center for Nutrition Policy
and Promotion
April 2005 CNPP-16

USDA is an equal opportunity provider and employer.

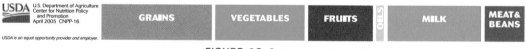

| GRAINS | VEGETABLES | FRUITS | OILS | MILK | MEAT & BEANS |

FIGURE **10-1** USDA MyPyramid.

MyPyramid can also be personalized by age, culture, and personal need. Check out *www. MyPyramid.gov.*

MAKING TIME FOR PHYSICAL ACTIVITY

It takes more than information on the importance of a healthy diet and daily exercise, and the increase in chronic disease and death, to improve health. We know from studies what works, but what will provide the personal motivation to make it happen in your life as a lifelong activity?

The motivating factor for individuals is something personal: "What is in it for me?"

Think about what is in it for you because that will be a part of the critical thinking exercise at the end of this section.

Learning Exercise

Making Room for Exercise

Make a list of the activities that you are involved with that count as exercise.

Rate the activities on a scale of 1-5 as light, moderate, or heavy, with 1 being light and 5 being heaviest.

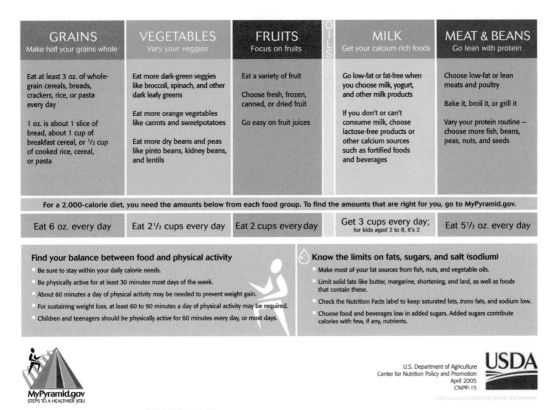

FIGURE **10-2** MyPyramid food groups and servings.

1. How often do you do each activity?
2. Does the activity increase flexibility?
3. Does the activity increase muscle strength?
4. Does the activity reduce stress?
5. Does the activity make you feel better about yourself?

MODERATE PHYSICAL ACTIVITY

A pleasant surprise is that any amount of exercise is helpful. As little as 30 minutes a day of moderate activity on most or all days of the week will make a noticeable difference in your health. The 30 minutes of activity can even be divided into 10-minute increments. Brisk walking, (meaning 3.5 miles per hour), is probably the easiest for most people to incorporate into a busy day. The important thing is to choose an activity that you like, and that fits in with your busy lifestyle. For example, maybe you are within walking distance from work, can park your car further than where you are going, use stairs rather than the elevator, can walk with a co-worker during your lunchtime, or are frequently the one who gets sent to another part of the building to pick up something. If you are fitting in a walk with a friend at lunchtime, a few minutes of slower walking at the beginning can be a useful preparation for more brisk walking. Slow your pace for a cool-down toward the end of the walk (Table 10-1).

If you have medical issues, check with your doctor before starting to exercise. Start slowly and listen to your body. Hurting all over your body is not a sign that you are doing the body a favor. Some activities that count as moderate activity include hiking; gardening and yard work; dancing; golf (walking and carrying clubs); bicycling (less than 10 miles/hour); and weight training (general light workout).

Table 10-1	*Examples of Moderate Activity*
ACTIVITY	**TIME**
Bicycling	5 miles in 30 minutes
Walking	2 miles in 30 minutes
Social dancing (fast)	30 minutes
Swimming laps	20 minutes
Walking stairs	15 minutes
Gardening	30-45 minutes
Playing volleyball	45 minutes
Pushing stroller	1.5 miles in 30 minutes
Shooting baskets	30 minutes
Running	1.5 miles in 15 minutes
Raking leaves	30 minutes

VIGOROUS PHYSICAL ACTIVITY

Being active for longer or doing more vigorous activity can provide greater health benefits. Vigorous physical activities include running/jogging (5 miles per hour); bicycling (more than 10 miles per hour); swimming (freestyle laps); aerobic exercise; walking very fast (more than 4.5 miles per hour); heavy yard work (such as chopping wood); weight lifting (vigorous effort); and basketball (competitive).

If an activity is too hard, conversation cannot be carried on during physical activity (the person is out of breath). Activities that do not increase your heart rate do not count toward the 30 or more minutes per day. The target heart rate during physical activity should be 60% to 90% of the maximum heart rate. To calculate the target heart rate, use the following formula:

1. 220 (beats per minute) minus age = maximum heart rate
2. Maximum heart rate multiplied by the intensity level = target heart rate

For example, a 50-year-old woman exercising at 60% maximum would use the following calculation:

1. 220 − 50 = 170 (maximum heart rate)
2. 170 × 60% = 102 (target heart rate)

This is her target heart rate regardless of the type of physical activity she elects to do (*www.nlm.nih. gov/medlineplus/ency/article/001941.htm*).

PARTS OF A WORKOUT

Ideally there are three important parts to a workout: a warm-up, main activity, and a cool-down.

The warm-up prepares the muscles, ligaments, and tendons for action before more vigorous use. The cool-down activity prevents the blood from pooling in the legs, which could limit the amount of blood returning to the heart. It also reduces muscle soreness, dizziness, and the amount of fatigue products, such as lactic acid, that build up in the blood. Adjust warm-up and cool-down according to what you have been doing (Mollard, 2003).

USING EXERCISE EQUIPMENT

If you are going to be using weight machines and other equipment, ask for instruction on how to warm up and cool down. It is also important to ask for specific directions on how to use the equipment so that you do not injure yourself. Be sure to state what your goal is for the exercise. Are you looking to improve muscle strength, increase flexibility, lose weight, relieve stress, generally "feel better," etc.? As always it will be important to listen to your body. Remember, exercise and fitness is personal: You do it for yourself and for your own reasons.

START THE DAY WITH STRETCH AND FLEX

Stretching and flexing cannot be overemphasized for the nurse.

- Before getting out of bed, start your day with *stretching*. Think of how a cat or dog stretches before they get busy with their activities. Follow their lead and prepare your sleepy muscles for the day by stretching while still in bed.
- If the back muscles are feeling uncomfortable, *lying on your back and drawing the knees to your chest* may be helpful. Stay that way until you sense some relief.
- The lower back may benefit from a *low-back stretch*. You are already lying flat with the previous exercise. Bend your knees slightly and keep your feet on the bed. Roll your knees to the side and back to the center. Reverse to the other side, keeping your back flat.

- *When ready to get up,* roll to the side with your knees bent. Use your elbow and arms to push yourself up gently. This is much easier on the back than bolting upright or jumping out of bed.

MAKING MINIMAL EFFORT PAY OFF AT WORK

Some of you will have to think small (i.e., items you can bring to work that will enable you to strengthen certain groups of muscles). For example, if you work at a desk for much of the day, a small, latex-free hand exerciser in the shape of a ball can be squeezed when one hand is free. It is useful in strengthening the muscles in the lower arm and hand. Even easier is to pick up something from the desk, such as a stapler, and flex your lower arm. Resistive, non-latex exercise tubing is color-coded according to the resistance desired. The tubing (or band) can be rolled up and takes limited space to transport. You can do any stretching exercise you do without it; the tubing just provides more resistance.

Once you are at work, stretching is essential for different reasons. Take a few minutes to stretch (warm up) the muscle groups before beginning patient care. Relax and breathe deeply while you stretch. It is worth finding stretching exercises that you can work in periodically throughout the day. They should become increasingly pleasant and soothing. For example:

- **Improve circulation and prevent muscle cramps** by doing a gentle, seated spinal twist. Sit up straight with your upper thighs at the edge of the seat. Cross your right leg over your left leg. Place your left hand on the inside of your left knee. Twist to the right as you exhale. Bring your right elbow or shoulder around toward the back of the chair. Hold the stretch for four to five breaths, twisting deeper when you exhale. Do this gently. Return to the starting position. Repeat in the opposite direction, crossing your left leg over your right leg, etc.
- **Correct poor posture.** Nurses often assume poor posture to do the work that they do. In fact, few of the tasks involved in direct

patient care permit you to maintain good posture. Poor posture is hard on the spine, interferes with breathing, and increases the risk of shoulder and back pain. Stand up straight. Clasp your hands behind you. Press your shoulder blades toward each other. Have your elbows bent slightly. Breathe deeply, and then exhale. Press your knuckles toward the floor, straightening your arms. Do not arch forward; keep the back straight. Breathe in. Lift your chest, lengthening your spine. Straighten your arms a little as you exhale. Hold the stretch for five breaths. Release. After some practice this stretching exercise will be easy to do and feel so good on the back.

- **Deep breathing** periodically throughout the shift helps to relieve tension in the lower back, neck, and shoulders. Place a hand on the abdomen and the other on the rib cage. Inhale deeply and feel the abdomen rise. As you exhale, feel the air move to the ribs and on up. Do this three to four times.
- A **head roll** helps to relieve tension in the neck, upper shoulders, and back. *Do not roll the head all the way around.* Instead, drop your head down, roll the neck to the right over the shoulder, and then back to the left shoulder. Repeat, reversing the direction.
- **Back stretches while sitting** stretch the back, neck, and arm muscles. Sit fully in a chair. Bring your torso over your knees and touch the floor with your hands. Sit up gently, raise your arms, and reach as high as you can with your fingers. Do this two to three times.
- **Relieve back pain** by sitting on the edge of a chair. Bend forward slightly. Lift a weight you are comfortable with: First with one arm and then with the other. Repeat several times.
- **Side stretches** may relieve tensed arm, hip, and lower back muscles. Stand with your feet apart. Hold a towel or tubing overhead and stretch your arms up and to the right side. Keep the hips still and facing front during the stretch. Switch sides and repeat.

Use exercises that you use to stretch muscles before working out. Obviously you will have to limit your exercises to those you can do while standing or sitting. Nursing is a form of working out and deserves the same thoughtful preparation you would use for an exercise activity.

Critical Thinking Exercise

Making Exercise a Daily Activity

1. What is in it for you to incorporate exercise, including stretching, into your daily routine? Think in terms of both home and work.
2. What are your reasons for exercising?
3. Make a plan that fits your need and works with your lifestyle.
4. Involve children as well if they are a part of your current life.

BACK INJURIES IN NURSING: WHAT WE DID NOT KNOW

Nurses have been taught body mechanics in the belief that if done properly during patient care, injury to the nurse can be avoided. If this is entirely true, why is the rate of back injuries in nurses double that among construction workers? "Manual lifting and other patient-handling tasks are high-risk activities for both nurses and patients. The prevalence of work-related back injuries in nursing is among the highest of any profession internationally; annual prevalence rates of nursing related back pain range from 35.9% in New Zealand to 47% in the United States to 66.8% in the Netherlands" (Nelson, Fragala, and Menzel, 2003). There are many related factors involved, including the rising rate of obesity in nurses and other staff who handle patients. "Duke University researchers found that the fattest workers had 13 times more lost work days due to work related injuries, and their medical claims for those injuries were seven times higher than their fit co-workers." The study was based on data from 11,728 people employed by Duke and its health system (Associated Press, 2007).

Body mechanics do help reduce the rate of nurse injury, but is not enough by itself. Interestingly, body mechanics were based on studies with men. Yet nursing remains primarily a female occupation. Women often have less upper-body strength than their male counterparts. Some of the early rationale was based on lifting boxes with handles, bending the knees, and keeping the back straight. Personally we do not recall seeing patients with handles, who can be lifted this way, close to our body! There are many other roadblocks involved, such as bedside clutter and small, awkward spaces. Many nursing tasks involve unnatural positions, such as bending forward with the torso twist. In the article, Nelson and colleagues offered the 16 most stressful handling tasks in order of rank (Box 10-1).

PREVENTING INJURIES

The ANA launched a "Handle with Care" campaign in 2003. The purpose is to re-educate nurses in principles of safe handling and movement of patients in a way that prevents injury to the patient and the nurse. In the fall of 2005, a safe patient handling and movement (SPHM)

Box 10-1 | *The 16 Most Stressful Handling Tasks for Nurses*

1. Transferring a patient from toilet to chair
2. Transferring a patient from chair to toilet
3. Transferring a patient from chair to bed
4. Transferring a patient from bed to chair
5. Transferring a patient from bathtub to chair
6. Transferring a patient from chair lift to chair
7. Weighing a patient
8. Lifting a patient in bed
9. Repositioning a patient from side to side in bed
10. Repositioning a patient in a chair
11. Changing an absorbent pad
12. Making a bed with a patient in it
13. Undressing a patient
14. Tying supports
15. Feeding a bedridden patient
16. Making a bed without a patient in it

Used with permission. From Nelson A, Fragala G, Menzel N. (2003). Myths and facts about back injuries in nursing. *AJN* 103:22–41.

pilot curriculum was funded in 26 nursing programs. Multiple pieces of ergonomically correct lifting devices were provided for the projects. The cost of equipment has been a factor in initiating similar programs across the country. In 2005, Texas, Ohio, and New York approved laws. In 2006, the state of Washington enacted legislation mandating the development of policies and the acquisition of lifting devices, and allowing tax credits for the cost of equipment (Crocker, 2006).

Back (gait) belts were initially thought to be a partial answer, but intensive study by the National Institute of Occupational Safety (NOSHA) has not been able to prove the claims. Lifting devices have proved to be of help when used properly, but not all lifting devices are created equal. An ergonomically correct device must be chosen for a particular lift, and the nurse must know how to operate it properly. Sometimes nurses avoid using a lift, even if that would be the best choice, because it is stored away from the area or improperly maintained. Sometimes nurses have forgotten how to use the device because of a time lapse. If properly used, mechanical devices can minimize injury. An interesting factor is that many nurses experience injury as a result of accumulative trauma—slowly over a period of time with repeated stress.

More attention on the part of administration is being given to cost savings. Having an ergonomic evaluation of their agency, buying the correct mechanical lift devices for their service, and training nurses to use the devices correctly have proved cost effective by decreasing the number of back and shoulder injuries. Compared with lost nursing days, insurance, medical costs, worker's compensation costs, etc., the benefits far outweigh the cost of the mechanical devices.

 Critical Thinking Exercise

Preventing Injury in the Clinical Area

Investigate what devices are available for you to use on the clinical area to minimize potential back, shoulder, and other injury. Where are they located? Do you know how to properly use all of the assists available? Who will train you to use the devices? Under what circumstances is each appropriate to use?

Do you currently have a back or other injury that will benefit from strengthening exercises? Who is available to teach you exercises and how to do them, so that the exercises do not cause additional injury?

HEALTH CARE-ASSOCIATED INFECTION: AN ISSUE OF SAFETY FOR THE PATIENT

Health care-associated infections (HAIs), formerly called nosocomial infections, (infections caught in the hospital), kill about 103,000 Americans per year. That number is about as many as are killed by AIDS, breast cancer, and auto accidents combined. One out of 20 patients picks up infection while in the hospital. Hospitals in Denmark, Finland, and the Netherlands once had similar rates of infection, but brought them down to below 1% through enforcing rules about hand washing, meticulous cleaning of equipment and hospital rooms, the use of gowns and disposable aprons to prevent doctors and nurses from spreading germs on clothing, and the testing of incoming patients to identify and isolate those carrying MRSA (methicillin-resistant *Staphylococcus aureus*) (McCaughey, 2005). According to Goldman (2006), "If every caregiver would reliably practice simple hand hygiene when leaving the bedside of every patient and before touching the next patient, there would be an immediate profound reduction in the spread of resistant bacteria." The recent widespread deployment of waterless, alcohol-based hand antiseptics has made this task even easier for harried caregivers. The CDC has recommended that health care workers use ethyl alcohol–based hand rubs for "routine" hand cleansing (referring to situations in which the hands are not visibly soiled or contaminated with blood or other body fluids). Yet compliance with hand hygiene remains poor in most institutions—often in the range of 40% to 50%. A study noted that "health care personnel were more likely to wash their hands if their peers or more highly ranked personnel did so, too (*AJN*, August 2004).

Clothes and uniforms worn while bending over a patient can pick up germs. *Clostridium difficile* is often caused by fecal material from one patient entering another patient's mouth (for example, the combination of emptying bedpans and delivering food trays). Using an alcohol-based hand antiseptic does not destroy this organism. Frequently, stethoscopes, blood pressure monitors, and other equipment are contaminated with live bacteria. If not cleaned between patient uses, the germs are passed on to the next patient and in the case of sharing equipment, to the caregiver. The British Medical Association has encouraged physicians to quit wearing neckties, a potential bug haven, and other functionless clothing to work. Ties are rarely washed and lab coats are often hung up at the end of the day and put on the next day.

Research has shown that another major culprit in the spread of health care-associated infection is artificial nails and exceptionally long natural nails (*http://www.nurseweek.com/news/features/03-06/nails.asp*). As early as 2002, the CDC recommended that health care workers not wear artificial nails or extenders when having contact with high-risk patients. Specific cases causing severe infection or deaths have been traced to nurses with artificial nails and long natural nails. Most hand-borne pathogens collect in the crook between the fingertip and the nail (i.e., subungual zone). Artificial, long natural, and nails with chipped nail polish are difficult to clean properly. Long natural nails can become a source of infection directly or through a glove that is punctured by a long nail. Even after careful hand washing or use of surgical scrubs or hand rubs, these personnel often harbor substantial numbers of pathogens in subungual spaces. Although the studies focus primarily on the serious hazard to the patient, artificial nails, long natural nails, and nails with chipped polish are also a way to take home pathogens to your friends and family. Some health facilities have banned long natural fingernails and artificial nails. There is additional concern about pierced fingernails.

DIFFERENTIATING BETWEEN BURNOUT AND STRESS

Burnout is different from stress. Although burnout can be the result of unrelenting stress, it is not the same as stress. In fact, your world can seem perfect: home, job, friends, and one day you realize that you feel empty and hopeless. Stress is related to too many physical and mental demands. The person cares too much and thinks if they can just do it right and do more, it will all be OK. The person who is stressed is aware of the stress, whereas the person with burnout may not be aware of being burned-out.

Some reasons for burnout include having unrealistic expectations imposed on you by yourself or someone else, being required to perform tasks that are against your personal values, working under severe rules, being bored by work that does not challenge you, or feeling trapped for economic reasons in a job or other life situation. Someone else may be pointing out that your attitude and behavior has changed. What is being identified is the cynicism, sense of hopelessness, detachment from others, and negative attitude toward patients and patient care. The major damage to the person with burnout is emotional. Check out *http://www.helpguide.org/mental/burnout_signs_symptoms.htm*. We are including a comparative table from that site (Table 10-2).

Learning Exercise

Your Life Choices and Burnout

When asked why you wanted to study nursing, what was your response? Is this statement related to burnout?

PREVENTING BURNOUT
Empathy vs. Sympathy

Differentiating between feelings of empathy and sympathy in regard to your patient is a major consideration in preventing burnout. Empathy is a respectful, detached concern. As a nurse you understand what your patient is experiencing,

Table 10-2 | *Stress vs. Burnout*

STRESS	BURNOUT
Characterized by over engagement	Characterized by disengagement
Emotions are overactive	Emotions are blunted
Produces urgency and hyperactivity	Produces helplessness and hopelessness
Exhausts physical energy	Exhausts motivation, drives, ideals, hope
Leads to anxiety disorders	Leads to paranoia, detachment, depression
Causes disintegration	Causes demoralization
Primary damage is physical	Primary damage is emotional
Stress may kill you prematurely; You won't have enough time to finish what you started	Burnout will never kill you, but life may not seem worth living

From *http://www.helpguide.org/mental/burnout_signs_symptoms.htm.*

but do not experience the emotion. Patients entering a medical facility are out of their own element. You can pick up the stress they experience as a sympathetic response, having lost perspective of the nurse-patient relationship.

The patient may be demanding a magical, dramatic change in his or her condition. Regression is almost always present in the patient. Needs are often expressed indirectly, perhaps through irritable comments or requests. The patient's emotional responses may elicit negative emotional responses in a sympathetic nurse.

Some patients do not respond to treatment no matter how hard they, and you, try. They may continue to go downhill to the point of death. Meanwhile other patients may not cooperate, and your sympathetic response of anger and frustration will get in the way of a therapeutic relationship with them. Some patients are negative in their responses to staff or constantly ask questions in a challenging way. Maybe you are beginning to think in terms of who does and does not deserve care. Nonassertive and aggressive, verbal and nonverbal communication styles can have other devastating effects.

Sympathy is a reaction that leaves you vulnerable to identifying with and experiencing the emotion along with the patient. This means that you are no longer in control of the situation, and your therapeutic value as a nurse is limited. A long-term sympathetic response is very stressful. What starts out as a caring relationship can become detrimental to you and your patient because of being over-involved.

Detached Way of Evaluating Self

Another significant step in preventing burnout is to develop a detached way of evaluating your daily performance. Waiting for a patient, doctor, or nurse manager to notice your performance is rarely helpful or rewarding. Perhaps they notice only what is missing. However, a detached, daily evaluation of your performance leaves you free to credit yourself for what you have done well. Furthermore, it alerts you to areas in which you need more study, assistance, or practice. Be your own most effective boss!

Time Management

Time management is another important factor in dealing with both personal and professional areas of your life. Because of its significance, Chapter 3 is devoted to this topic.

Humor

Humor—do not forget humor. No matter how seriously you take yourself, you are never going to get out of this life alive. So lighten up.

1. Humor shows you care.
2. Nurses are accepted better when they have a sense of humor.
3. Humor shows you your patient's personality with their defenses down.
4. Humor reduces tension and helps you get on with work.
5. Humor makes us equals, because we laugh at the same things (Balzer-Riley, 2000).

Remember that using humor with a patient is funny only if the patient thinks so, too. Many things happen in a nursing situation that can be lightened up through humor. Case in point: The nursing instructor walked into the room to see how the student nurse was doing with the patient. As the instructor approached the patient, she extended her hand and greeted the patient by name. As the patient opened his mouth to speak, he simultaneously expelled flatus—a thunderous clap! The patient's eyes opened wide, there was momentary silence, the student looked shocked, and then the instructor chuckled! "It happens," she said with a shrug. Soon all three were laughing; the embarrassment was gone. The real issue of the patient's condition and nursing care was again the priority.

Maintaining Nursing Skills

Maintaining nursing skills throughout your career is essential. Even if you are in a situation that requires less hands-on care, make time to perform nursing procedures. Learn how to perform new procedures as they are introduced to your facility. This helps feed your self-worth and makes you a more valuable employee. Both issues are closely related to burnout. Chances are that if you do not maintain nursing skills, you will develop a secret fear of being put on the spot and perhaps will lie your way out of requests to demonstrate or assist.

Some final tips for reducing stress and preventing burnout include the following:

1. Be clear about the reasons you want to be a nurse.
2. Set clear goals with realistic expectations.
3. Know your limits: learn when to say "no."
4. Work within your team structure.
5. Keep in mind that you cannot be all things to all people.
6. Maintain a clear understanding of what constitutes a professional, caring relationship: The patient needs a nurse, not a buddy.
7. To experience less guilt and anger, do not personalize the patient's response to you. Keep the patient in the patient role: See that the patient responds out of the patient's own needs.

8. Maintain a positive attitude (i.e., warm, caring, and hopeful), even if the patient is dying: The patient and the family will feel less hopeless.
9. Understand your own need, both personally and professionally. Maintain a balance and a clear distinction between your work and your personal role. It is necessary to tell the patient who wants to be involved in your personal life by calling and visiting that, "I will do my best as a nurse while I am at work, but my personal life is separate. You may *not* call my home or visit me in my home." Furthermore, developing personal relationships with patients is unprofessional and violates the Nurse Practice Act in many states.
10. Be alert to signs of burnout: lack of caring for your patient is a real danger signal.
11. Maintain perspective about your role as a nurse. Sometimes the whole world looks ill and grim! Remind yourself that you have a choice: *Nursing can be a limited part of your life or the dominant feature in your life.* You get to choose.

Critical Thinking Exercise

Where Am I Headed?

1. Inventory your feelings and physical health. Are friends making comments regarding your attitude and behavior?
2. Do you find yourself frequently focusing on home issues at work and work issues at home?
3. Are you often talking about work when you are with friends and family?
4. If your answers indicate that there are issues, do something about it now before you are overwhelmed physically and/or mentally.

SECONDARY TRAUMATIC STRESS

We want to briefly touch on this important issue of secondary traumatic stress. Nurses in burn units, emergency departments, neonatal intensive care units, or other high-stress environments are constantly exposed to traumatic horrors that may cause this type of stress. After a while some nurses will respond with hypertension, gastritis, peptic ulcers, and fatigue. There may be more sick days, problems with decision making, isolation, or withdrawal, or behavioral outbursts. The result will be a decrease in staff morale and errors in judgment, which will affect not only the patients, but the employer as well.

RECOGNIZING SIGNS OF SECONDARY TRAUMATIC STRESS

It is important to recognize signs of oncoming secondary traumatic stress and not attempt to hide it. Too often nurses think that they are not entitled to their feelings and that they must be kept to oneself. It is important that nurses are alert to their feelings, thoughts, and physical changes and how they are functioning with patients and other staff.

Sometimes journaling is a way to get the feelings out and identify the seriousness of what is happening for the nurse. When journaling, remember to include things you did that were right. Nurses tend to focus on the negative outcomes of traumatic situations. Remember that sometimes, no matter how many things we do that are correct, the patient still dies or is crippled in some way for life. That is just the way it is.

PREVENTION

It helps to get sufficient rest, which is not easy if you become focused on the negative outcomes. Proper diet and personal relaxation techniques such as meditation or yoga may be helpful. It is important to have positive relations with peers and to have those with whom you can share your feelings and concerns honestly.

If all these efforts do not work, then ask for a change in assignment to another nursing area. There is nothing wrong with requesting a change; it is not a sign of failure. Keep your options open for getting professional help. Sometimes what has happened now has ties to the past, which will need professional assistance to unravel, heal,

and make necessary changes. Participating in employer-sponsored or privately arranged support groups or counseling is helpful to many nurses.

CHEMICALLY DEPENDENT NURSES

Chemical dependency refers to abuse of alcohol and/or other drugs. Alcohol is listed separately to emphasize that it is the most commonly abused drug. Between 2% and 18% of nurses become chemically dependent on alcohol and/or other drugs (Weiss, 2005). These nurses tend to be perfectionists and often have a family history of chemical dependency. Nurses work taking care of others, and frequently ignore their own needs. The health care system uses medication to deal with symptoms and illness. Nurses diagnose themselves and begin to "treat" their symptoms. It often starts as an alcoholic drink and/or other drug to unwind at the end of a work shift. Gradually more of the alcohol or other drug is needed to attain the same effect. Finally the drug controls the user.

Eventually, the nurse may divert drugs from patients or ask physician friends for "hallway prescriptions." If the user is a nurse, the nurse is considered impaired when use of the drug(s) extends to the quality of work. When the impairment is discovered, there is so much humiliation for a nurse: The nurse is expected to know better. There is also the possibility of losing their nursing license and, as a result, their livelihood. According to the NCSBN, most state nursing board sanctions are drug related. If the nurse has been caught stealing drugs, he/she may face criminal proceedings.

Because of the prevalence of alcohol use, we will speak specifically about alcohol. The list of telltale signs that follows later, applies to all chemical dependency.

Alcohol is high in calories, but has no nutritional value. It provides 7% to 10% of total calories for the average American's diet. More than a moderate amount of alcohol can increase excretion of nutrients and decrease their use in the body. This in turn leads to decreased levels of nutrients in body tissues (e.g., folic acid, thiamine, vitamins B_6 and B_{12}, niacin). Alcohol is an irritant to all cells of the body. Consequently, all systems of the body are affected in some way. Possible negative health effects include esophageal varices; cardiomyopathy; chronic gastritis; cirrhosis; decreased resistance to infection; increased cancer (especially of the mouth, esophagus, pharynx, larynx, and pancreas); permanent brain damage; and polyneuropathy. Alcohol ranks as the third leading cause of death in the United States. According to the National Institute on Alcohol Abuse and Alcoholism, alcohol is implicated in 50% of all homicides, 50% of all fatal car accidents, 41% of all crimes, 33% of all suicides, and a large proportion of drowning, boating accidents, and aviation deaths (NIAAA, 2007). We do not have figures on the number of extended hospital stays or patient deaths related to impaired nurses.

Alcohol is a drug that acts like a depressant. Unlike food, alcohol does not have to be digested. It is absorbed directly into the bloodstream from the stomach and small intestine, reaching the brain within 5 minutes. At first alcohol stimulates you. If you continue to drink, it depresses you and may put you to sleep. However, the sleep may be short. Alcohol interferes with the necessary sleep cycle needed for a restful sleep.

When combined with other drugs (e.g., sedatives, anti-anxiety medication, and some over-the-counter [OTC] medications), alcohol will have a multiplying effect. *This means that the combined effect is more than 1 + 1.* Accidental overdoses can occur this way.

KNOW WHAT YOU ARE INGESTING

The body can metabolize *approximately* one drink per hour. Metabolism of alcohol is influenced by gender, presence of and type of food, body weight, muscle, and body fat content. A blood alcohol level of 0.4% to 0.7% can result in coma, respiratory failure, and death.

ALCOHOL ABUSE VERSUS ALCOHOLISM

What is the difference between alcohol abuse and alcoholism? Abuse is drinking so much that you get drunk. Alcoholism is an addiction. The body craves alcohol, and physical effects result from its withdrawal. For you as a nurse, either way impairs your judgment and places your patient in danger. Early intervention is essential. Not only are your health and life at stake, but also the lives and health of your patients. During work hours, consuming alcohol is absolutely forbidden by your employer and a violation of your state Nurse Practice Act.

Nurses would not drink while at work, you say? There are many examples through the years, but one that stands out is a nurse who always carried her coffee mug with her while supervising students. A student nurse who was being supervised discovered that the instructor had vodka and water in the mug.

The most telling sign of any chemical dependency in nurses is a gradual decline in performance, which usually becomes noticeable within 3 to 6 months (Box 10-2).

Box 10-2 *Telltale Signs of Chemical Dependency in Nurses*

Behaviors that need to be checked out include the following:
- Complaints by staff, students, and patients.
- Accidents, errors in documentation, a greater number of injuries caused while moving patients or equipment, errors in practice, and poor judgment.
- Increased visits to the employee health department or emergency room. Increased volunteering to take call for others (especially true for evening and night shifts if there is less staff; makes stealing patient drugs easier).
- Arriving early or staying late to assist in the narcotic count.
- Frequent absenteeism after days off and for personal emergencies, especially on a Monday.
- Irritability and mood swings.
- Performing only the minimum amount of work required.
- Inability to perform psychomotor skills owing to intoxication or tremors.

Two emotional characteristics of chemical dependency make it difficult to begin treatment: (1) The denial system is very strong, and (2) the person who drinks is usually a skilled manipulator. In approximately 40% of states, help is available from confidential diversion programs through the State Board of Nursing (called the Nursing Commission in some states). Nurses can be referred to treatment, and subsequent monitoring, including random drug tests, as an alternative to taking action against their license.

Contact the National Organization of Alternative Programs at *www.alternativeprograms.org* for additional information for yourself or a peer. For some nurses, Alcoholics Anonymous, Moderation Management, or Narcotics Anonymous provides assistance. Type in the name of the organization you desire using Google or another search engine to find confidential information on Alcoholics Anonymous, Moderation Management, Impaired Professional Programs Provided by State Boards on Nursing, or Narcotics Anonymous. The Yellow Pages list resource numbers under "alcohol abuse information and treatment" and "drug abuse information and treatment," and the White Pages, under "business and professional listings" (alcohol or drug abuse services and hotline numbers). It is worth the risk of making a telephone call to obtain information on your own or a friend's behalf. Most important, you have a duty to the patient and, in many states, a legal duty to report use of alcohol and/or other drugs.

Critical Thinking Exercise

How Am I Doing?

1. Do I turn to alcohol and/or other drugs for relief from pain or job stress on a regular basis?
2. If the answer to question No. 1 is yes, to whom will you go to seek intervention?
3. List the names of some facilities and persons in your area who assist with chemical dependency issues.
4. If you realize that a co-worker or someone else on the health care team is drinking and/or impaired by other drugs while on duty, consider the following questions.

5. What is your responsibility to the co-worker?
6. What is your responsibility to the patient?
7. What is your responsibility to your school or employer?
8. What is your responsibility to your State Board of Nursing (Nursing Commission)?

CODEPENDENCY: A PATHOLOGICAL NEED

Learning Exercise

Codependency: A Pathological Need

Before you read any further, answer the following questions:
1. What is your reason for making nursing your career choice?
2. Who supplies the most important critique of your day's work?
3. How do you feel if the patient and/or instructor do not tell you that you did a good job?

Codependency is when a person has a pathological need to be needed by others. The behavior of others affects them in a way that causes them to be obsessed about "fixing" the behavior (i.e., the need to control the behavior of others). Some writers have speculated that a large number of nurses may be codependent. Helping others is a way of meeting their own codependency needs. Codependent nurses become over involved in their patient's life and go to extremes to serve both their patients and coworkers. They react too quickly to feelings with a sense of intensity and urgency. Patients (and others) in their life are viewed disrespectfully (i.e., they are thought to be incapable of participating in their own care). This viewpoint takes away a sense of personal control.

The codependent nurse may think that no one else can give the patient care that is required. The codependent nurse readily accepts a patient's statement that "no one has ever given (me) such wonderful care (or understood me)." The nurse is equally devastated by any perceived criticism by the patient (e.g., "How can they say that after all

I did?"). Codependent nurses give the message that the patient, family, or staff member is more ill (or helpless) than initially perceived. For some codependent individuals, a painful childhood that included sexual abuse, violence, or chemical abuse may have paved the way to codependency (Table 10-3).

 Critical Thinking Exercise

Codependency: A Bothersome Behavior

Codependent behavior can be modified. As with any behavior that is bothersome, the sooner it is recognized, the easier it is to modify. Ask yourself:

1. Do any of the behaviors described in Table 10-3 apply?
2. Circle the behaviors that apply.
3. Choose one behavior that you think will cause the most difficulty as a nurse.
4. Make a plan for change that is attainable, measurable, and time-referenced.

The following true incident illustrates codependency in a future nurse. A man and his fiancée, both in their twenties, were involved in a car accident. The woman experienced serious injuries and was placed in traction. The man was admitted for observation. He was not placed on bed rest. The following morning a nursing student working as an aide during a summer break was assigned to him. Later in the day other aides were overheard talking about the male patient's description of his morning care. "He told me that it was the best care he had ever received. She insisted that he have a bed bath. She scrubbed him from top to bottom—and I do mean bottom! She even powdered his penis!" This nursing student interfered with his autonomy; the patient's activity order was up as desired.

A notable author on the subject of codependency has compared codependent behavior to the sides of Karpman's drama triangle (victim, rescuer, persecutor). Because codependent persons are caretakers or rescuers, they rescue, persecute, and ultimately end up feeling victimized. The author, Beattie (1992) has a self-help book, *Codependent No More*, with specific information on codependent characteristics and how to change the behaviors.

Table 10-3 | *Some Codependent Characteristics and Behaviors*

CHARACTERISTICS	BEHAVIORS
Says "yes"—really means "no."	Agrees to help another staff member and then complains to someone else about being taken advantage of.
Feels the fate of nursing care rests on their shoulders.	Takes on non-nursing duties that belong to other departments.
Feels responsible for solving other people's problems.	Sympathetic rather than empathetic response to patients and other staff.
Competes for attention rather than supporting coworkers.	Engages in one-upmanship and intershift rivalries over patient care.
Often feels angry, unappreciated, and used.	Comes in early and works late. Works extra shifts to "help" coworkers.
Does not support patient's need for autonomy and return to self-confidence.	Does for the patient what the patient needs to do to regain optimal health and self-sufficiency.
Makes excuses and conceals negative practices rather than working for change.	Feels powerless. Takes on extra duties because of chronic understaffing.
Shows feelings of anger indirectly.	Pouts, procrastinates, forgets, gets sick, or is late.
Perfectionist: gossips and judges.	Unrealistic expectations of others.
Avoids conflict.	Too nice, loving, and forgiving.
	Smiles when having negative feelings.

DEALING WITH NEGATIVE STRESS: SOME IDEAS

Learning Exercise

Avoid Negative Stress

List some things that cause excessive negative stress in your life.

It is interesting to note that it is *our reaction to a situation, rather than the situation itself, that causes stress.* Everything that happens to you—either pleasant or unpleasant—creates stress. Interpretation of stress as distress or negative stress is dependent on personal problem-solving skills and the intensity and duration of the situations involved. Ironically, a time of boredom and understimulation is accompanied by high adrenaline levels in the body, as is a time of high stress during over stimulation. In other words, individuals seem to do best with a moderate amount of stress in their lives. What is defined as moderate stress varies from person to person.

As a nurse you probably have better coping skills than most. You accept that acute stress is part of the vocation you are preparing for. During your clinical rotations, instructors assign you to increasingly more difficult tasks. They remain on the unit to assist you in dealing with the expected and unexpected situations as they occur. The clinical experience gives you an opportunity to experience the real world of nursing—an incredible plus in building your coping skills. However, you continue to be vulnerable to stress, and there are many factors that add to the vulnerability—a nursing shortage; patient acuity and rapid discharge; complexity of new medications, treatments, and equipment; personal issues not separated from work; and so on. The belief that good nurses are self-sacrificing has many nurses focusing on care for others (work and family) and ignoring their own needs.

Learning Exercise

Find a Good Role Model

Who will be a positive role model for you? Find someone who does a good job as a nurse and also finds time to focus on personal needs (good nutrition, exercise, recreation, relaxation, etc.).

RECREATION

Although work is necessarily commendable and personally satisfying, it is, of necessity, only one part of your life. Recreation is also important and must be part of your plan for living. Otherwise, it is too easy to brush it aside because "I have too much work to do." The ultimate choice in recreation may not be available to you consistently, but short-term recreation is available.

Learning Exercise

Make Time for Recreation

What kinds of recreation do you enjoy? List two activities that consume more time to accomplish and four recreational activities that can be accomplished in a short amount of time or on a continuing basis.

As you look at the answer to the previous learning exercise, remember that some forms of recreation may be high-stress activities for you. Recreation is not the same as relaxation. Rethink your list and choose one or two short-term recreational activities that you will be able to involve yourself with on an ongoing basis without causing distress in your life. There will be times to treat yourself to longer activities if you think it through—maybe play 9 holes of golf instead of 18; read your favorite author's work during breaks, while on appointments, on trains, or in the bathtub—use your imagination.

RELAXATION

Relaxation training is one way to manage stress. During a relaxed state the pulse and respiratory rates decrease, the metabolic rate and blood pressure are lowered, and muscular tension is decreased. Along with the positive physical changes experienced by all except 3% of the population, you also experience a sense of well-being. If you are part of the 3% that becomes more stressed during a relaxation exercise, there is nothing wrong with you. It just is, so think about what does bring about the physical changes for you, as previously described. For example, a student shared that relaxation exercises and soothing music made her "ready to climb the walls," whereas rock and roll had a calming effect on her. Knowing this, she insisted on listening to rock and roll during labor.

Many relaxation methods are available and need to be tailored to your lifestyle. Decide on a regular practice time. Some of you will want to start your day with a relaxation exercise. Some of you will want to end your day this way. Overall relaxation is accomplished most readily before meals or at least 2 hours after a meal because of the stimulant effect of food on the body. Caffeine-containing drinks, such as regular coffee and some soft drinks, are best avoided before a training session.

MEDITATION

For meditation, you need a quiet environment, a mental device, a passive attitude, and a comfortable position.

- A **quiet environment** helps eliminate distractions and permits you to concentrate on a mental device of your choosing.
- A **mental device** is any sound, word, or phrase that evokes a sense of calm in you as you repeat it.
- **Repeat the device silently or aloud** with your eyes closed. If you prefer to keep your eyes open, you can fix your gaze on an object. Either way, your mind is focusing on one thing. If you are feeling uncomfortable with your eyes closed, open them, look around, and close them again when satisfied, and return to the mental device.
- **Concentrate on your normal breathing pattern.** It enhances your repetition of the mental device. Breathe through your nose when you breathe out.

- A **passive attitude** is considered most significant for eliciting a successful relaxation response. Distracting thoughts may occur; simply let them pass and return to repetition of the mental device. Trying too hard usually creates tension.
- A **comfortable position** prevents added muscular tension. Sit with good posture, wear loose-fitting clothes, take off your shoes, and keep your feet on the floor. Lying down is not encouraged because you tend to fall asleep (unless that is your intent).
- To begin, breathe in and out (mental device), then repeat.
- To stop, sit for a while, note how you are feeling, open your eyes, look around, get up slowly, and continue your day.

IMAGERY

Imagery is an excellent way of learning to relax and, once learned, can be done in less structured settings, such as during break time. It is also a way of protecting yourself against situations you may face in the future, by visualizing the situation and how you will move through it successfully. It is also creative and fun. You already do it; you did so before embarking on your present career by imaging the steps to becoming a nurse and seeing yourself as a licensed practical/vocational nurse.

This kind of imagery is not the guided imagery that is used in psychotherapy, requiring a trained psychotherapist to deal with the symbolic material that may emerge. Some of you are better at imagining than others. Some may only see shadowy figures, whereas others see vivid, Technicolor images. Images need not be particularly vivid to be effective.

- Begin with a brief relaxation exercise, or a progressive relaxation, if very tense.
- Once relaxed, follow the imagery.
- Two or three deep breaths are helpful before the imagery. In practicing the imagery it is important to take sufficient time to include enough detail so that you can get into the imagery.

- When ready to conclude the imagery, count from 1 to 10, sit for a while with your eyes closed, open your eyes, and then stretch.

It is worthwhile to remember that if you experience anxiety any time during the imagery, you need only to open your eyes and continue with the imagery. Some of you will be comfortable with your eyes open during the entire process and do not seem to have any problems visualizing. Imagery, like other relaxation techniques, takes self-discipline; therefore, daily practice sessions are suggested. *It is often helpful to tape the steps of any of the relaxation exercises in advance so you do not interrupt yourself by trying to remember the next step.* Use your most comforting voice and pace the instructions. If you desire, tapes and videos are available in many libraries and bookstores.

Modify the instructions to meet personal needs. Instructions for using imagery to relieve anxiety are found in Box 10-3.

BRIEF RELAXATION

Brief relaxation techniques are useful as a method of preparing your body for other techniques like imagery. However, they are also useful throughout the day when you have limited time and can be practiced without any special effects (Box 10-4).

Box 10-3 | *Imagery: Relieving Anxiety*

- Design your own favorite place: Whatever is your idea of complete peace, harmony, and joy.
- See yourself appropriately dressed in the setting you have created.
- Take time to look around and visualize your surroundings with great detail.
- Use all of your senses to experience the sight, sound, smell, touch, and taste available in your special hideaway.
- See yourself staying there and feeling peaceful and calm. Remember that it is a safe place, and that you can return there to rest daily.
- When you are ready to leave, take one look back, knowing that you can return anytime.
- You will continue to feel relaxed and happy as you return to your daily activities.

Box 10-4 | *Brief Relaxation*

- **Brief relaxation.** This exercise prevents the rush of thought. It can be used to induce on-the-spot relaxation in a public place or to promote sleep. Directions: Part your lips slightly. Place the tip of the tongue behind the lower teeth. Keep it there without pressure for a while. Continue with normal breathing. Place: Walking down the hall, in the bathroom, in class, in a meeting (not in front of the boss or instructor), during break, while studying.
- **Yawning.** This is a 1-minute tension release exercise. The lungs expand; the back, jaw, mouth, and tongue relax. More oxygen comes into the system. Directions: Drop your jaw gently until it feels large enough to take in a whole fruit. As you begin to yawn, it feels as though it will never end. As you yawn, you are taking in a deep breath. When the yawn ends, you feel relaxed clear down to your stomach. Your lungs have expanded and your back begins to release its tension. Place: Nice to do near an open window.
- **Do Nothing.** Take 5 to 10 minutes to sit quietly and do nothing. Pay attention to the sounds around you, your emotions, and any tension in your body (Jaret, 2003).
- **Breathe Easy.** Take 5 minutes to slow down your breathing to approximately six deep abdominal breaths a minute; inhale for 5 seconds, then exhale for 5 seconds (Jaret, 2003).

PROGRESSIVE RELAXATION

Progressive relaxation is a method of tensing all of the muscle groups in order, resulting in deep relaxation.

- Taping the directions in advance with plenty of time to follow each direction can be helpful.
- Sometimes progressive relaxation is enhanced by taped (or natural) sound, such as the wind or seashore sounds, or by music that is close to body rhythm, such as certain Bach selections and Pachelbel's Canon in D.

- Some experimentation with sound will help you discover if it enhances or distracts.
- Both sides of the body can be relaxed at one time, or if especially tense, one side can be relaxed at a time. The order of relaxation can be reversed according to choice.

Directions are available in Box 10-5.

Critical Thinking Exercise

Personal Stress Management

Design a personal stress management plan for yourself. Include the date you will start and where you will seek instruction, if necessary.

SLEEP

All the methods of dealing with personal stress can be sabotaged unless you develop a regular pattern of sleep. Be aware that you can create your own insomnia by taking your worries to bed. Tell yourself firmly that you have done your best for the day and will not think about the issues until you awaken. Some hand their left-over worries to their God at the end of the day or put them on a bookshelf. Any of the relaxation techniques suggested in this chapter can be used for bedtime relaxation.

Research on sleep has shown that most people have 90- to 100-minute sleep cycles. Many individuals feel rested after 7.5 hours of sleep. To make use of this information, do the following:

- Go to bed at the same time; listen to what your body is telling you. Going to bed extra-early or later than your usual bedtime is not a favor for the body.
- Most important, when you naturally awaken, get out of bed. Better yet, do the stretching exercises and then get out of bed.
- Be alert to the number of hours you slept and if you feel rested. You will recognize a pattern if you track your sleep hours for several days.

No doubt you have at some point decided to treat yourself to a few extra minutes of sleep and

Box 10-5 | *Progressive Relaxation*

Sensations of warmth, tingling, and unusual heaviness or lightness are not unusual. If you become uncomfortable, open your eyes, look around, and resume relaxing. The exercise takes about 30 minutes. Take time to tape these directions in advance.

Directions: Lie down with eyes closed, arms at the side, legs uncrossed. Take two or three deep breaths. Breathe deeply enough so the abdomen rises while inhaling. Concentrate on your breathing for a while, and continue to breathe naturally throughout the exercise. During each step, do the following:

- Tense each of the muscle groups for about 30 seconds.
- Note the tension.
- Relax for about 60 seconds.
- Note the difference.
  - Point the feet and toes down.
  - Point the toes up.
  - Straighten the legs up and lock the knees.
  - Dig the heels into the floor.
  - Tense the groin and buttocks muscles at the same time.
  - Pull in the muscles of your stomach.
  - Push your shoulders down. Keep your buttocks down; bring your chin to your chest.
  - Press your arms against your body.
  - Shrug your shoulders.
  - Bend your wrists up.
  - Make a fist.
  - Turn your head to the left.
  - Turn your head to the right.
  - Bring your chin to your chest.
  - Smile. Make a tight "O" with your lips.
  - Close your jaw tightly.
  - Stick your tongue way out.
  - Frown and shut your eyes tightly.
  - Raise your eyebrows.

Continue to breathe normally. Stay with the feeling. When you are ready to return to an alert state, count slowly from 1 to 10. Open your eyes when you are ready.

ended up feeling tired much of the day. Research seems to indicate that the body is set on a 25-hour clock, and when you get up at a different time, the body tries to "reset" the clock throughout the day. No wonder the treat you offered yourself did not work. Nurses still work different shifts in some agencies. If there are many changes within a week, the body is struggling to reset its clock throughout the time that the change is taking place.

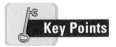

Get Enough Sleep

Evaluate your sleep habits. Do they work for you most of the time?

_____

_____

Key Points

- Poor eating habits and lack of exercise are major causes of increasing obesity and its health-related problems.
- The USDA MyPyramid can be personalized based on your need for nutrition and physical activity.
- As little as 30 minutes of moderate exercise, such as brisk walking on most days of the week, will affect personal health in a positive way. The 30 minutes of exercise can be broken down into three 10-minute periods, if necessary.
- Nurses are among the highest of any profession internationally to have work-related back injuries.
- Practicing good body mechanics alone cannot prevent all back injuries. Ergonomic evaluation of needs, taking time to use the right lifting device for the task, and keeping your body healthy, trim, strong, and flexible are all helpful in preventing back injuries.
- Artificial and long fingernails are linked to patient infection and deaths.
- Burnout and stress are not the same. With stress, the nurse cares too much, and is trying to work harder to solve the situation. Burnout leaves the nurse feeling hopeless, helpless, and cynical. Burnout is experienced emotionally and the sense of caring for patents is blunted.
- Nurses, who work in settings such as burn units, emergency departments, or neonatal units, are constantly exposed to traumatic horror. These nurses are especially susceptible to developing secondary traumatic stress.
- About 2% to 18% of nurses become dependent on alcohol and/or other drugs. The effort to self-medicate gets out of hand when additional amounts of the alcohol and/or other drug are needed to attain the same effect.
- Codependent persons have a pathological need to be needed by others. They become over involved in the patient's life and go to extremes to serve the patient.
- Our reaction to a situation, rather than the situation itself, causes stress in our lives.
- Limit work as one part of your life; enjoy a full personal life that includes friends, family, recreation, relaxation, other activities, etc.
- Recreation is not the same as relaxation. Some recreation activities increase distress in your life. Choose recreation based on need and time.
- Relaxation works to relieve both psychological and physical stress. Choose relaxation that fits into your lifestyle and meets your needs.
- Regular sleep habits help to avoid the fatigue caused by the body's attempt to reset the body clock when sleep patterns are disrupted.

REVIEW ITEMS

1. What symptom has become the most important factor in developing a chronic disease?

   1. Accidents
   2. Hypertension
   3. Obesity
   4. Alcohol

2. What is the most important way to protect patients from health care-associated infection?

   1. Use of masks during patient care.
   2. Consistent hand hygiene during patient care
   3. Reporting infractions in infection control
   4. Dispensing antibiotics 20 minutes before beginning care.

3. What explanation will you offer when a non-nurse friend asks you why so many nurses have back problems?

   1. Nurses are unable to consistently use good body mechanics because many nursing tasks cause unnatural positions.
   2. Lifting devices are stored too far from the central area of work and nurses do not have the time to dig them out.
   3. Nurses are expected to be strong and flexible, and many nurses perceive it as a sign of weakness to ask for help.
   4. Nursing shortage creates an atmosphere of urgency on the unit, so nurses have little time to care for themselves.

4. Select the priority strategy that would help the LPN/LVN stay alive and well in nursing.

   1. Ask for daily feedback from your immediate boss.
   2. Make patients and staff the focus of your daily life.
   3. Recall: nurses have better coping skills than most.
   4. Monitor yourself as you learn and make changes.

ALTERNATE FORMAT ITEM

You are the charge nurse on a unit in the nursing home. A staff nurse mentions that patients are not worth the time spent on them. "They just complain and finally die no matter what we do." Which of the following apply to this situation? *(Select all that apply.)*

_____1. We are all in the same situation.
_____2. Working here is your own choice.
_____3. Get over it. What did you expect?
_____4. When did this feeling start?
_____5. You are a poorly prepared nurse

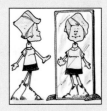

CHAPTER 11

The Health Care Team

evolve   http://evolve.elsevier.com/Hill/success/

Objectives

On completing this chapter, you will be able to do the following:

1. Explain in your own words the goal of the health care team.

2. List 10 members of the health care team. (All levels of nurses count for only one member on your list.)

3. Identify the nursing personnel who are part of the health care team, according to the following criteria:

   a. Education,

   b. Role and responsibilities,

   c. Licensing, and

   d. Sites of employment.

4. Define nursing.

5. Describe in your own words the following methods used to deliver nursing service:

   a. Case method,

   b. Functional method,

   c. Team method,

   d. Primary care,

   e. Case management method, and

   f. Patient-focused care.

6. Describe the practical/vocational nurse's role in the methods used to deliver the nursing services listed in objective No. 5.

7. Discuss solutions to the nursing shortage.

Key Terms

Advanced practice (p. 167)
Associate degree nursing (p. 165)

Baccalaureate nursing program (BĂK-ă-LŎR-ē-ĭt, p. 165)
Case management method (p. 174)
Case method (p. 172)
Certification (SŬR-tĭ-fĭ-KĀ-shŭn, p. 166)
Clerk receptionist (rĕ-SĔP-shŭ-nĭst, p. 171)
Clinical pathway (care maps) (p. 173)
Cross training (p. 176)
Decentralized (dĔ-SĕN-tră-LĪZD, p. 176)
Diploma program (dī-PLŌ-mă, p. 161)
Functional method (p. 172)
Independent (ĬN-dĕ-PĕN-dĕnt, p. 166)
Interdependent (ĬN-tĕr-dĕ-PĕN-dĕnt, p. 166)
Nursing assistant (p. 171)
Patient-focused care (p. 174)
Practical/vocational nurse (p. 162)
Primary care method (p. 173)
Registered nurse (RĔJ-ĭ-stĕrd, p. 165)
Skill mix (p. 176)
Standards of care (p. 166)
Student nurse (p. 170)
Team method (p. 173)
Unit manager (p. 172)
Unlicensed assistive personnel (UAP) (ŭn-LĪ-sĕnst, p. 171)

Keep in Mind

You can't tell the players without a program. Chapter 11 is your program to identify players on the Health Care Team.

WHO IS RESPONSIBLE FOR MRS. BROWN'S DISCHARGE?

Mrs. Amelia Brown, age 75, lives with her daughter on a 200-acre farm in rural Wisconsin. While working in the barn, Mrs. Brown fell and broke her right hip. She required surgery to repair the hip. Under general anesthesia during surgery, Mrs. Brown's blood pressure reached dangerously high levels, but it quickly stabilized under the anesthesiologist's interventions. Despite this setback, Mrs. Brown was discharged after 4 days in the hospital. She and her family agreed that she was not ready to return home at that point in her recovery, so she was discharged to an extended-care facility, where she was given physical therapy to learn how to function at home with her restrictions in ambulation. Two weeks later Mrs. Brown was discharged from the extended-care facility to her home.

Sounds like another success story for nursing, doesn't it? We will follow Mrs. Brown as she progresses through the health care system and then decide who should get credit for Mrs. Brown's discharge back to the farm.

MRS. BROWN'S EMERGENCY CARE

After Mrs. Brown falls, her daughter calls the emergency squad to transport her mother to the nearest hospital. The hospital is located 20 miles away in a city with a population of 98,000. The three people manning the emergency squad are **emergency medical technicians** (EMTs). Each EMT has taken an approximately 120-hour course in basic life support skills and has been certified as an EMT by means of a national test. The EMTs are currently taking a 5-month paramedic course, which is preparing them to provide more advanced life support skills. On the way to the hospital the EMTs monitor Mrs. Brown's blood pressure, pulse, respirations, and level of consciousness. They keep her right leg immobilized. The EMTs maintain contact with the hospital emergency room by means of a two-way radio.

On arriving at the **emergency room** (ER), the EMTs provide the **registered nurse** (RN) with verbal and written reports of Mrs. Brown's status. The emergency room doctor examines Mrs. Brown and orders an x-ray film of her right hip. The x-ray technician brings the x-ray equipment to the ER and takes an x-ray film of Mrs. Brown's right hip. The **x-ray technician** has taken a 2-year program conducted by a hospital or technical college to prepare herself to perform diagnostic measures involving radiant energy. The **radiologist** on duty reads the x-ray film of Mrs. Brown's right hip. On the basis of the physical examination and the results of the x-ray, the ER physician diagnoses a fracture of Mrs. Brown's right proximal femur. The ER physician notifies Mrs. Brown's **family physician** and contacts the **orthopedic surgeon** Mrs. Brown requests.

The RN receives Mrs. Brown in the ER, assesses her, and provides care until she is admitted to the hospital. The RN is a graduate of a diploma or 3-year program in nursing. This nurse has passed a national examination to become an RN. RNs who work in the ER participate regularly in continuing education courses at the hospital and at seminars given regionally and nationally for ER nurses. Mrs. Brown's RN prepares her for surgery.

To be qualified to be in charge of the medical care of Mrs. Brown, the family physician has attended 4 years of college, 4 years of medical school, 1 year of internship, and approximately a 3-year residency program. Medical school consists of a program that provides the basic knowledge and skills needed to be a medical doctor. Internship involves a program of clinical experiences designed to complete the requirements for licensure as a practicing physician. The residency program prepares physicians for practice in a specialty. The specialty in this situation is family practice. With some exceptions the ER physician, the radiologist, and the orthopedic surgeon have had the same education as the family physician, up to the residency experience. The ER physician has completed a residency program in emergency or trauma medicine. The radiologist has completed a residency program in the reading and interpretation of x-ray films. The orthopedic surgeon has completed a 3- to 5-year residency in performing surgery for problems of bones and joints. Each of these physicians has passed the board examinations, which licenses them as physicians and allows them to practice under the state medical practice act. Each physician in this scenario is board certified in his or her specialty area.

Laboratory studies are ordered preoperatively. **Lab personnel** draw blood for these studies. Lab personnel have varied educational backgrounds. Some have on-the-job training to obtain blood samples. A medical lab technician has 2 years of education. A medical technologist (MT) has more than 4 years of education and can be certified by a national examination. Lab personnel are responsible for collecting the specimens needed for lab tests, performing the tests, and reporting the results to physicians and staff.

The family members request that their parish priest be contacted to give Mrs. Brown the sacrament of the sick (see Chapter 13). Because surgery is imminent, the pastoral care department is notified. A Roman Catholic **priest**, a member of the pastoral care team, anoints Mrs. Brown with holy oils, prays with her, and gives her Holy Communion. To be able to meet Mrs. Brown's spiritual needs, the priest has had 4 years of college and 4 years of theological school before being ordained.

THE SURGICAL EXPERIENCE

In the ER the **anesthetist** prepares Mrs. Brown and her family for the anesthesia part of the surgical experience. This health care worker is an RN with a bachelor of science in nursing (BSN). This nurse has studied an additional 2 to 3 years in an approved school of anesthesiology after the 4-year BSN program. The anesthetist provides anesthesia to patients undergoing surgery. Mrs. Brown is transferred to the surgical suite, where she undergoes a right hip pinning procedure under general anesthesia. This type of anesthesia will put Mrs. Brown in a state of unconsciousness. During surgery, the anesthetist monitors Mrs. Brown's vital signs continuously while she is unconscious. The **surgical technician** assists the orthopedic surgeon. The surgical technician sets up the sterile environment in the operating room.

This health care worker makes sure the surgeon's instruments and supplies are available when he requests them for the pinning of Mrs. Brown's right hip. The surgical technician is a graduate of a 1-year **diploma program** at a local technical college. The professional nurse, who has a minimum qualification of a BSN, coordinates the overall functioning of the surgical team.

During surgery, the anesthetist notes that Mrs. Brown's blood pressure is rising to a dangerous level. She contacts the anesthesiologist STAT (i.e., immediately!). The **anesthesiologist**, a medical doctor with a residency in anesthesiology, orders antihypertensive drugs (i.e., drugs that lower the blood pressure). The situation is quickly brought under control. Surgery is completed, and Mrs. Brown is sent to the postanesthesia care unit (PACU).

POSTANESTHESIA CARE UNIT

The purpose of the PACU is to monitor the patient's vital signs, level of consciousness, movement, and any special equipment required by patients after surgery. When patients' conditions are stable, they are transferred to their hospital room. A PACU registered nurse, who is a graduate of a 3-year school of nursing program, assesses Mrs. Brown. After 1.5 hours, Mrs. Brown is assessed as being ready to leave the PACU. Because of the episode involving high blood pressure during surgery, Mrs. Brown's surgeon orders her to go to the intensive care unit (ICU) overnight for closer observation instead of to the postoperative surgical floor. A **transport aide**, who is trained on the job, and a **staff nurse** from the PACU take Mrs. Brown to the ICU.

INTENSIVE CARE: A TIME FOR CLOSE OBSERVATION

The ICU is staffed by RNs who went to school for 2 years (associate degree nurses), 3 years (diploma nurses), or 4 years (**baccalaureate** nurses). Each nurse has taken the same national examination to become an RN. None of these nurses are qualified to work in the ICU immediately on graduation from their nursing programs. Most institutions prepare a nurse for the responsibilities of this unit through in-service classes after a minimum amount of experience or through a postgraduate or continuing education course. Mrs. Brown's nurse, a **2-year graduate**, is responsible for the care and observation of two patients.

The family is unable to answer some additional questions about Mrs. Brown's medical history. The family physician asks the **clerk receptionist (ward clerk)** to obtain Mrs. Brown's medical records from the medical records department. The clerk receptionist assumes the responsibility for many of the clerical duties that are a necessary part of any patient care area. The clerk receptionist learns these skills by taking a course that varies in length, depending on the area of the country. The course averages approximately one semester of theory and clinical experience. The **medical records department** is staffed by personnel who have gone to school for 2 to 6 years to learn the skills required for indexing, recording, and storing patient records, which are legal documents. Thanks to Mrs. Brown's old records, which are sent to the ICU, the family physician receives answers to his medical questions.

The surgeon writes postoperative orders for Mrs. Brown, including an order for patient-controlled analgesia (PCA) to control postoperative pain. The hospital **pharmacist** has studied for a minimum of 4 to 6 years to become licensed to prepare, compound, and dispense drugs prescribed by a physician or dentist. The pharmacist fills the order for Mrs. Brown's drugs and intravenous solutions.

The **respiratory therapy department** is contacted to evaluate Mrs. Brown's respiratory status and suggest treatment to prevent respiratory problems. Certified respiratory therapists (CRTs) are graduates of 12- to 18-month programs in respiratory therapy and have passed a certifying examination. Registered respiratory therapists (RRTs) are graduates of associate degree or 4-year college programs in respiratory therapy and have taken three examinations to register. Within 24 hours of admission to the ICU, Mrs. Brown is judged to be in stable condition. A **transport aide** and an **ICU staff member** transfer her to the surgical floor.

SURGICAL FLOOR: AN EYE TO DISCHARGE

The **nurse manager** on the surgical floor at this hospital is an RN who has graduated from a 4-year nursing program. As manager of the unit, this nurse is responsible for all the care given to patients. Mrs. Brown's **team leader** is an RN from a 2-year nursing program. This nurse is responsible for formulating a plan of care for each of the assigned patients and modifying these plans as needed.

The team leader receives a verbal report and the current care plan for Mrs. Brown from the ICU personnel. The team leader begins assessment of her new admission. The practical/vocational nurse (LPN/LVN) helps put Mrs. Brown to bed and immediately takes her vital signs. The LPN/LVN is a graduate of a 1-year vocational program in nursing. The LPN/LVN has taken a national examination to become licensed as a practical/vocational nurse. The practical/vocational nurse is assigned to give Mrs. Brown bedside care.

A referral is sent to the physical therapy department. The **physical therapist** (PT) assesses the strength of Mrs. Brown's unaffected extremities. The PT sets up a program of exercises and ambulation with no weight-bearing on the right extremity. The goal of treatment is to restore function and prevent the development of complications. Physical therapy keeps up the strength of Mrs. Brown's unaffected extremity until she is able to bear weight fully on the right side. The PT has been educated in a 4- or 5-year college program. Some PTs have a master's degree in physical therapy. The **physical therapy assistant** (PTA) has been educated in a 2-year community college or technical school setting. The PTA carries out the plan of care developed by the PT.

Soon after the patient is transferred to the surgical floor, the **social worker** visits Mrs. Brown and her family to discuss discharge plans. The social worker suggests that Mrs. Brown stay in an extended-care facility for 2 weeks to participate in extensive physical therapy before returning to the farm. Social workers help patients and families solve problems with the financial concerns of hospitalization. They arrange for community agencies to provide appropriate care and services needed by patients after discharge from the hospital. Social workers also help the family communicate their health care needs more clearly. Social workers obtain a bachelor's degree in social work in 4 years and a master's degree in 1 additional year of college. Mrs. Brown's social worker talks to the PT and the family. All agree that with exercise and skills teaching, the family eventually will be able to care for Mrs. Brown at home.

As the time for discharge to the extended-care facility gets closer, a **patient care technologist** (PCT) is assigned to take Mrs. Brown's vital signs. PCTs perform treatments and skills assigned to them by the RN or the LPN/LVN. PCTs are trained by the hospital for the specific duties they are to perform. Training involves classes (sometimes autotutorial or self-study classes) and a clinical component. The training a PCT gets is short and varies among facilities. The job titles **"unlicensed assistive personnel" (UAP), "nurse's aide," "nursing assistant," and "patient care assistant"** are used in some facilities. The responsibilities of the LPN/LVN in relation to PCTs are discussed in Chapters 16, 18, and 20.

Because Mrs. Brown is 50 lbs overweight, her physician orders a weight-reduction diet. The **dietitian** teaches Mrs. Brown and her daughter the elements of weight reduction that will be carried out when Mrs. Brown returns to the farm. A hospital's dietitian is responsible for planning the meals and supplementary feedings for patients and the cafeteria meals for staff. The dietitian also supervises the preparation of food and counsels patients and their families about nutritional problems and therapeutic diets. This health professional is educated in a 4- to 5-year college program, followed by a year of internship in a health care agency.

The **housekeeper** cleans Mrs. Brown's room and bathroom during every day of her stay. Maintaining cleanliness is an effort to maintain medical asepsis (absence of germs) and to provide a pleasant environment. The housekeeper receives training in the needed skills by the employing institution or through a short course in a technical school.

Finally, Mrs. Brown is discharged from the hospital. She leaves by **Medi-Van** and is transported to the extended-care facility.

EXTENDED-CARE UNIT: ON THE ROAD TO REHABILITATION

Mrs. Brown's roommate in the extended-care facility is an 80-year-old woman who has had a stroke. The roommate is also preparing to go home after additional physical therapy. The **PT** conducts an initial assessment of Mrs. Brown and incorporates the hospital physical therapy plan of care with her findings. The **PTA** helps Mrs. Brown daily with exercises and ambulation, using a walker, and minimum weight-bearing on her right leg. A **nursing assistant** (NA) is assigned to assist Mrs. Brown with her personal care. NAs are educated to give bedside care through courses of a minimum of 75 hours. Successful completion of this course of study makes the NA eligible to be placed on the state registry as a certified nursing assistant (CNA).

A referral is sent to the occupational therapy department. The **occupational therapist** (OT) completes an assessment of Mrs. Brown. The **occupational therapy assistant** (OTA) carries out the plan of care. The goal for Mrs. Brown is to be as **independent** as possible when she returns to the farm, despite her physical limitations. Occupational therapy helps patients restore body function through specific tasks and skills. Educational requirements include a 4-year occupational therapy program. Some 4-year graduates pursue a master's degree in their field. A 2-year program prepares OTAs for their roles.

Mrs. Brown receives her newly prescribed blood pressure medication from the **practical/vocational nurse**, who also is functioning in her expanded role as charge nurse in this facility. The **day supervisor**, an RN with a BSN, checks Mrs. Brown daily to monitor her progress. Ten days later, Mrs. Brown excitedly waits for her family to take her back to the farm. She is pleased with her progress and is confident about going back to her home. She knows that at this time she is unable to gather the eggs each day, but she is anxious to get back in the kitchen.

Critical Thinking Exercise

Who Is Responsible for Mrs. Brown's Recovery?

Who is responsible for Mrs. Brown's return to the farm? After reading Mrs. Brown's story, you can see that it is impossible to give any one member of the health care team credit for sending Mrs. Brown home. Everyone needs to work together. It is a team effort.

HEALTH CARE TEAM

A primary goal of health care is to restore optimal physical, emotional, and spiritual health to patients. This goal is accomplished by promoting health, preventing further illness, and restoring health when illness or accident has occurred. Health care includes a large number of specialized services. It is necessary for groups of people to work together to provide patients with all the services they need to maintain comprehensive health care. These groups of health care workers are called the *health care team.*

For Mrs. Brown to be rehabilitated after her fall, it took a minimum of 123.5 years of education for all the health care workers in this scenario to learn how to perform their respective jobs. The x-ray technician's x-ray film confirmed the presence of a hip fracture. The pharmacist supplied the narcotic pain reliever that relieved pain after the surgical procedure, allowing Mrs. Brown to move more freely and avoid complications. The treatment by the RRT helped prevent pneumonia. The PTs, OTs, and nursing staff all helped restore Mrs. Brown's health and prevent further illness by avoiding complications. The dietitian's expertise allowed Mrs. Brown to receive the basic nutrients she needed to maintain her health, heal her fracture, and lose weight. Teaching about weight-reduction diets promoted health by pointing out the importance of keeping Mrs. Brown's weight within acceptable limits.

As you can see from Mrs. Brown's case, each member of the health care team, because of his or her specific preparation in a field of study, can increase the quality of health care for a patient. It is impossible for one person to provide the knowledge, expertise, and skills that the health care team as a whole can provide.

The members of the health care team are generally on duty in acute or residential health care organizations 24 hours a day, 7 days a week. Some members of the health care team may not be scheduled at night or on weekends or holidays, and some of these persons are available on an on-call basis. In the community, health care workers' hours vary depending on site of employment. Some sites are open Monday through Friday, during day hours only, whereas others also offer services in the evening. Other sites are open 7 days a week and sometimes 24 hours a day.

Each member of the health care team needs to have good communication skills. Good communication ensures that care is coordinated for the patient's benefit (see Chapter 9). Fragmentation of care can be avoided. Each health care team member has to be able to anticipate problems and avoid them when possible. This is accomplished by using critical thinking skills. When problems do occur, the health care team needs to use problem-solving skills to find solutions in the process of delivering care. In this way the quality of patient care is continuously improved. The team must strive continually to keep its care patient-oriented. The team needs to realize that a cooperative effort is needed to reach patient goals.

WHAT IS NURSING?

One definition of nursing is by Virginia Henderson, who stated that "the unique function of the nurse is to assist the individual, sick or well, in the performance of those activities contributing to health or its recovery (or to peaceful death) that he would perform if he had the necessary strength, will, or knowledge" (Henderson, 1966). Henderson refers to nursing's interest in illness and wellness. The direction of practical/vocational nursing has been channeled by this definition.

It is important for practical/vocational nurses to understand their role in Mrs. Brown's care. An understanding of the education, licensure, roles, and responsibilities of the varied members of the health care team is necessary.

NURSING'S PLACE ON THE HEALTH CARE TEAM

Nursing staff on the health care team includes **unit managers, RNs, LPN/LVNs, student nurses, NAs,** and **cross-trained staff.** UAPs assist the nursing staff. Clerk receptionists, although not nurses, are an important part of the unit staff. The public is unclear as to the different types of nurses on the health care team. Sadly, some RNs are unaware of the educational background of LPN/LVNs, and some LPN/LVNs are unaware of the education professional nursing entails. A common question from the public is, "What is the difference between a registered nurse and a licensed practical/vocational nurse?" Members of the health care team generally, and nursing specifically, need to know about each other. For this reason, general information about the education for and many roles of registered nursing is given in this section, which describes the members of the nursing team.

REGISTERED NURSES (PROFESSIONAL NURSES)
Education

Registered nurses (RNs) are the largest group of health care workers in the United States. There are 2.9 million RNs in the United States. Approximately 8.1% of RNs are male (Seago et al., 2007). The graduates of the three types of educational programs for professional nurses—2-, 3-, and 4-year programs—currently take the same licensing examination. On successful completion of this examination, all these graduates hold the title of registered nurse

Associate Degree Nursing (ADN) Program
- An associate degree nursing program is a 2-year educational program that can be found in community colleges, junior colleges, and technical schools.
- The ADN program includes general education courses (e.g., courses in the biological, behavioral, and social sciences), as well as nursing courses, and clinical practice.

- On graduation, the 2-year graduate receives an associate degree in nursing and is eligible to take the NCLEX-RN® examination to become a registered nurse.

Diploma Program
- A diploma program is a 3-year educational program conducted by a hospital-based school of nursing.
- The diploma program comprises the same general education courses as 2-year programs, with nursing courses and clinical practice. Diploma programs traditionally have emphasized clinical experience.
- On graduation, the 3-year nursing graduate receives a diploma in nursing and is eligible to take the NCLEX-RN® examination to become a registered nurse.

Baccalaureate Nursing Program
- A baccalaureate nursing program is a 4-year nursing program that can be found in public and private colleges and universities.
- The baccalaureate program emphasizes course work in the liberal arts, sciences, and nursing theory, including public health. Clinical practice is included.
- On graduation, the 4-year nurse receives a BSN and is eligible to take the NCLEX-RN® examination to become a registered nurse.

Role of Registered Nurses

Graduates of all three nursing programs are prepared for general duty staff nursing in a hospital or nursing home. Nursing education programs also prepare graduates of all three programs to function in a community-based, community-focused health care system. Although you may find 2- and 3-year RNs in supervisory and administrative positions, only baccalaureate graduates have been prepared in their nursing education programs for advancement to these positions. Baccalaureate graduates are also prepared for beginning positions in public health agencies.

Graduates of associate degree nursing programs outnumber BSN graduates. Since 2000, entry-level BSN enrollments have experienced a moderate upswing in numbers. The number of diploma programs and graduates continues to decline. This education mix is expected to continue.

All RNs function under the nurse practice act of the state in which they are working. RNs use the nursing process to identify patient problems, formulate nursing diagnoses, and plan and evaluate care. Standards of care are used instead of care plans in some acute care agencies. These standards include the priority nursing diagnosis for each patient, with appropriate assessments, nursing interventions, and expected outcomes (goals). Standards provide minimum guidelines for a consistent approach to delivering patient care. The RN uses standards as a reference when individualizing patient care.

Registered nurses assign routine care and the care of stable patients to assistive personnel. This allows RNs to do the following:

1. Plan care.
2. Coordinate all the activities of care.
3. Provide care that requires more specialized knowledge and judgment.
4. Teach patients, families, and other members of the health care team.
5. Act as patient advocate.

Independent Role of the RN. Registered nurses function **independently** in nursing, initiating and carrying out nursing activities. For example, to prevent complications in the respiratory and circulatory systems, RNs assess the patient on bed rest. They identify the need for a turning routine, deep breathing, leg exercises, and range-of-motion exercises. If not contraindicated by the patient's diagnosis and/or treatment, RNs add these nursing interventions to planned care. Because of their level of education, RNs can identify which patients can and cannot receive these nursing interventions. In the community, RNs will initiate dietitian and social worker orders. *It is the independent role in decision making that distinguishes RNs from LPN/LVNs.* Registered nurses have the ultimate responsibility for care given to patients.

Interdependent Role of the RN. When RNs carry out the legal orders of another health professional (e.g., the physician or physical therapist),

they are functioning in an interdependent role. Often, RNs function interdependently (collaboratively) when carrying out decisions about patient care that are made jointly by members of the health care team.

Education Beyond the Basic Nursing Programs for Registered Nurses

The postgraduate educational opportunities available to RNs are presented to explain the various RNs found on the health care team.

BSN Completion Program. After passing the NCLEX-RN® examination, associate degree and diploma graduates can enroll in a program that will grant a BSN. Programs vary in length, content, and mode of delivery.

Master of Nursing Programs. Master's of science in nursing programs prepare registered nurses for a specialty area in nursing, such as medical-surgical, pediatrics, nursing education, and geriatrics. The MSN is a requirement for teaching in associate degree programs. Generally, nurses with BSN degrees are the only nursing graduates who may elect to do graduate work in nursing at the master's and doctoral levels. However, MSN programs exist that offer an MSN degree to nurses with an undergraduate degree in an area other than nursing. The MSN then becomes the entry degree into nursing.

Certification. Passing the NCLEX-RN® examination provides initial licensure in nursing and ensures basic competence for entry into nursing practice. After gaining work experience, RNs can receive certification from numerous professional nursing groups. The certificate that is awarded after passing a comprehensive examination indicates that the nurse has demonstrated competence in a select area of practice. The American Nurses Credentialing Center (ANCC), a subsidiary of the American Nurses Association (ANA), makes certification available to all RNs. There is no longer a difference in credentials based on type of RN educational program from which one is a graduate for basic specialty certification. All basic specialty-certified nurses are board certified (American Nurses Credentialing Service, 2007). The requirement of a master's degree in nursing remains for certification as an advanced practice registered nurse. Because certification needs to be renewed periodically, certification through ANCC allows the registered nurse to demonstrate ongoing competence in a selected area of nursing.

Advanced Practice Registered Nurse. With an additional degree, RNs can pursue expanded roles, called **advanced practice**. These nurses acquire specialized nursing knowledge and skills and demonstrate a greater depth and breadth of nursing knowledge and an increased complexity of skills and interventions. The term advanced practice registered nurse (APRN) identifies the advanced practice roles of (1) a clinical nurse specialist, (2) a nurse practitioner, (3) a nurse anesthetist, and (4) a certified nurse-midwife. Each of these nurses has a minimum of a master's of science degree in nursing (MSN), obtained in a 1- to 2-year program of study.

- *Clinical nurse specialist (CNS).* This registered nurse has a minimum of an MSN in a specialty area (e.g., medical-surgical nursing). The CNS is a clinical expert in nursing practice based on the latest research and has certification as a clinical nurse specialist. When employed by acute care organizations, the CNS serves as a mentor, role model, and resource person for staff by setting standards for nursing care. The CNS provides direct care in challenging patient situations and shares knowledge, experiences, and resources with staff. The CNS also is employed by clinics, nursing homes, nursing schools as instructors, and in other community settings. In all sites of employment the CNS also serves as an educator, consultant, researcher, and administrator.
- *Nurse practitioner (NP).* This registered nurse has a minimum of an MSN and certification by a national body. There are many areas of specialization for nurse practitioners, such as family (FNP), geriatrics, pediatrics (PNP), primary, or acute care. Some NPs provide primary care in the community in physicians' clinics or in their own offices. Others provide acute care services in hospitals. NPs order and interpret lab and diagnostic tests, develop diagnoses, and prescribe treatments, including drugs, for acute and chronic diseases. Their care differs from medical care because of their interest in and awareness of psychosocial aspects of illness.
- *Certified Nurse-Midwife (CNM).* This registered nurse has a minimum of an MSN and certification as a nurse-midwife. The CNM manages women's health care in the area of prenatal low-risk pregnancy, childbirth, the postpartum period, care of the newborn, and family planning at home, in hospitals, and birthing centers and in the gynecological care of women. They diagnose and treat illness, including prescribing drugs.
- *Certified Registered Nurse Anesthetist (CRNA).* This registered nurse has a minimum of an MSN, is a graduate of an accredited nurse anesthesia educational program, and has certification as a nurse anesthetist. CRNAs work in every setting where anesthesia is given: operating rooms, clinics, and outpatient surgical centers. They prepare patients for anesthesia, induce and maintain local, regional, and general anesthesia, provide postanesthesia care, including pain management, and provide emergency resuscitation.

The American Association of Colleges of Nursing (AACN) has *proposed* a clinical nurse leader (CNL) role requiring a master's or post-master's CNL program of study that would make one eligible for the AACN CNL certification exam. This advanced generalist role was proposed to address the call for change in today's health care system.

Doctoral Degree Programs. Many nurses who have doctorates have a PhD, which is a *research-focused* degree. Although they hold a research degree, many doctoral graduates have *teaching* as their primary responsibility. A small percentage of doctoral programs offer a Doctor of Nursing Science degree (DNS, DSN, or DNSc). These programs focus heavily on science and research. All require an original research project and defense of a dissertation. Nursing leaders point out the need to prepare more expert clinicians (nurses working in health care agencies) and clinical faculty with clinical doctorates. Practice-focused doctoral programs prepare experts in specialized advanced nursing practice (AACN, *The Essentials of Doctoral Education for Advanced Nurse Practitioners*, 2006*). **AACN has proposed and voted** that by 2015, all new advanced practice nurses in the United States will be educated at the doctoral level and receive the Doctor of Nursing Practice (DNP) degree (ANCC, *Certification and Certification Renewal News and Announcements*, 2007).

Learning Exercise

Get to Know the Nursing Team

During an unhurried moment in the clinical area, ask the RN with whom you are working about the educational requirements to be employed for his/her position. If there are initials behind his or her name, ask for them to be explained.

PRACTICAL/VOCATIONAL NURSES
Background

Since little information about the exact number of **licensed practical/vocational** nurses can be found in the literature, information needs to be extracted from other information. Licensed practical/vocational nurses held about 726,000 jobs in 2004 (*Occupational Outlook Handbook*, 2006-07) and are the second-largest group of licensed health care workers in the United States. Males represent 4.4% of LPN/LVNs (Seago et al., 2007) but the numbers are increasing.

Education

There are more than 1200 practical/vocational nursing programs in the United States (*Occupational Outlook Handbook*, 2006-07). The educational program for practical/vocational nurses varies from 9 to 18 months. The practical/vocational nursing program is found in trade, technical, and vocational schools, as well as community colleges. These institutions are usually public, tax-supported institutions. Practical/vocational nursing programs are also found in private schools.

Practical/vocational nurse education concentrates on clinical care at the bedside, based on fundamentals of biological sciences. Courses in basic nursing care, the behavioral sciences, as well as the biological sciences, are included. Basic nursing care includes the administration of medications. Critical thinking is stressed, and the practical/vocational nurse's assisting role in nursing process is included in all phases of the nursing program, as determined by each state's Nurse Practice Act. Clinical experience in acute care facilities, extended care facilities, and the community is included. On graduation, the practical/vocational nurse receives a diploma in practical nursing and is eligible to take the NCLEX-PN® examination to become an LPN/LVN.

Role of Practical/Vocational Nurses

Practical/vocational nurses must be aware of the content of the Nurse Practice Act of the state in which they are employed (see Chapter 20). The LPN/LVN's role is found in this law, and the law differs from state to state. Regardless of the site of employment, LPN/LVNs provide care in basic and complex patient situations under the general supervision of an RN, physician, podiatrist, or dentist, as determined by the state nurse practice act.

Interdependent Role. Practical/vocational nurses function interdependently when they offer input to the RN about the effectiveness of patient care or offer suggestions to improve care. When practical/vocational nurses provide actual care at the bedside in acute care situations, their collection of data while engaged in giving care is valuable in determining whether progress is being made to meet patient outcomes. *A major criterion in differentiating* between the roles of the registered and practical/vocational nurse is that the practical/vocational nurse does not function independently. Practical/vocational nurses must function safely and are accountable for their actions. They should assume responsibility only for nursing actions that are within their legal role and that they feel competent in carrying out. Table 11-1 helps identify differences between the LPN/LVN and the RN role.

 Critical Thinking Exercise

The LPN/LVN Role in Assisting with Nursing Process

Identify the major difference between the RN's and LPN/LVN's role in the nursing process. How is the LPN/LVN's role in the nursing process determined?

Expanded Role of Practical/Vocational Nurses

In all settings practical/vocational nurses are being used in their expanded role. An example of the expanded role of the practical/vocational nurse is the charge nurse position in nursing homes/long-term care facilities. Because practical/vocational nurses work under another professional's direction, their role is called an interdependent one. While functioning in an interdependent role, employers expect practical/vocational nurses to think critically and solve problems in patient care situations. During implementation of care by the LPN/LVN, the RN is available to help in decision making when questions arise, either on-site (direct supervision) or by phone (general supervision). See Chapters 15 and 16 for further discussion of the expanded role of the LPN/LVN.

Table 11-1 *Differences Between the Roles of RN and the LPN/LVN*

FIVE NURSING ROLES	ROLES OF RN AND LPN/LVN
1. PROFESSIONAL	
RN	Belongs to and is actively involved in ANA at state and local levels.
LPN/LVN	Belongs to and is involved in NFLPN and/or NAPNES at state and local levels (see Chapter 23)
2. PROVIDER OF CARE	
RN	This is an independent role.
	Initiates all phases of nursing process; formulates nursing diagnoses.
LPN/LVN	This is a dependent and interdependent role.
	Assists with all phases of the nursing process.
	Works with established nursing diagnoses.
	Identifies possible new nursing problems and reports same to RN.
3. MANAGER OF CARE	
RN	Controls decisions regarding staff and care of patients.
LPN/LVN	First-line manager in nursing home/extended care.
	Responsible to RN nurse manager.
4. TEACHER	
RN	Initiates all health teaching.
LPN/LVN	Initiates health teaching for basic health habits (e.g., nutrition and cleanliness).
	Reinforces health teaching of RN in other areas.
5. RESEARCHER	
RN	Theory included in 4-year program.
	All levels interpret and implement research findings.
	Participates in the research process.
LPN/LVN	Theory not included in 1-year program.
	Assists in implementing research findings.

Critical Thinking Exercise

Expanded Role of the LPN/LVN

Refer to your state's Nurse Practice Act to determine the circumstances under which you may function with the direct or general supervision of an RN and in your expanded role.

Sites of Employment

Periodically, the National Council of State Boards of Nursing (NCSBN) performs a job analysis. The purpose of the job analysis is to determine the content areas for the NCLEX-PN® examination. The findings of the latest job analysis (2008) indicate that newly licensed practical/vocational nurses are continuing to provide care in all types of settings, with the majority continuing to be employed in long-term care settings (NCSBN: *NCLEX-PN® Examination Test Plan,* 2008). No statistically significant changes have occurred in work settings since the last job analysis.

The increasing number of patients requiring more complex care in acute care facilities reflects the practice of discharging patients from these facilities for continued recuperation in extended-care units and nursing homes. These sites are excellent places of employment for practical/vocational nurses. Generally, LPN/LVNs who work in nursing homes stay employed longer than other levels of nurses, and this ensures consistent care and availability of nurses to the patients and residents.

Although regionally LPN/LVNs are employed in acute care settings, their employment in hospitals declined 47% from 1985 to 2005 (Lafer and Moss, 2007). Nursing homes and long-term care units continue to be the major source of employment. The demand for practical/vocational nurses is expected to continue to increase. Practical/vocational nurses are also employed in the community, in such places as physicians' offices, weight-loss clinics, freestanding clinics, ambulatory care centers, home health care agencies, and industry. Sites of job placement for the practical/vocational nurse in the community

increase each year. These include clinics, dialysis centers, group homes, home health agencies, adult day care centers, Red Cross (as a phlebotomist), Alzheimer's disease units, companion centers, and various entrepreneurship opportunities (see Chapters 21 and 23).

Opportunities Beyond the Basic Program for Practical/Vocational Nurses

If you choose to stay in the practical/vocational nursing role, opportunities exist to take courses to increase skills and certify in various areas. If you choose to continue in nursing at a different level, various programs are available for the LPN/LVN to progress through the ADN and BSN programs and beyond. Chapter 23 explores the exciting options open to LPN/LVNs.

Critical Thinking Exercise

Difference Between Registered Nursing and Practical/Vocational Nursing

With a peer, role play the difference between an RN and an LPN/LVN in the areas of education, role, and sites of employment.

STUDENT NURSES

Student professional and practical/vocational nurses come to the clinical area under the supervision of clinical instructors. The clinical area is an extension of the classroom. It provides an opportunity to apply theory to practice. When assigned to patients, these student nurses have a responsibility to give safe care and function responsibly under the supervision of the instructor. Students are in the clinical area to learn, not to give service. It is possible that a clinical instructor can remove students from the assigned clinical site at any time for additional learning experiences.

Students are members of the health care team. They are expected to assist other team members in addition to performing their patient assignment. Examples of such assistance include passing trays, answering call lights in acute care and long-term care situations, and assisting patients and staff in the community. These activities help students learn how to get along in a team situation.

Student practical/vocational nurses are responsible for giving the same safe nursing care that licensed practical/vocational nurses provide. This is a legal matter. Therefore the student role demands preparation and supervision.

Critical Thinking Exercise

Your Assigned Patient Wants to Know

You are assigned to a patient in acute care who had a stroke and cannot move the left side of his body. While you assist him with bathing, the patient asks, "What is the difference between the registered nurse and the licensed practical/vocational nurse?" Answer his question.

NURSING ASSISTANTS

Nursing assistants are trained for their positions by combining federally mandated classroom instruction with close supervision by RNs while in the clinical area. Vocational schools offer programs that last a minimum of 75 hours and up to 12 weeks in length. These programs combine classroom or autotutorial instruction with clinical practice. During the course, testing for competence occurs to meet federal Omnibus Budget Reconciliation Act (OBRA) requirements. When test results are satisfactory, the names of NAs are placed in a registry. There are approximately 2.3 million nursing assistants in the United States.

NAs function under the direction of registered or practical/vocational nurses. NAs who work in hospitals, nursing homes, extended care units, or psychiatric hospitals assist in providing personal and comfort needs for stable patients. They are assigned routine tasks, sometimes involving housekeeping chores. A large number of NAs are employed by nursing homes. Currently the supply of NAs is not meeting the high demands of employers. People in some areas of the country refer to male NAs as orderlies.

Some states offer an advanced NA course that teaches more complex skills. These skills include many that are performed by the practical/vocational nurse. The demand for home health care workers continues to increase. NAs are allowed to perform a wider variety of skills in the home as home health care workers. Some states offer a postgraduate course for NAs to prepare them for the transition to home care. The comprehensive home care program may also be available to individuals without NA experience.

UNLICENSED ASSISTIVE PERSONNEL

In an effort to use health care workers more efficiently and effectively, health care organizations have added a new level of worker to the health care team. Unlicensed assistive personnel (UAP) are trained by health care organizations to function in an assistive role to RNs and LPN/LVNs. Some health care organizations require applicants for UAP positions to be registered as NAs. These workers learn selected skills, sometimes by the autotutorial method or module method, combined with some clinical teaching. Actual skills learned depend on which skills are needed in specific patient care units. UAPs are also known by the terms patient care technician, patient care associate, care pair, nurse extender, and multiskilled worker.

CLERK RECEPTIONISTS (WARD CLERKS, HEALTH UNIT CLERKS, HEALTH UNIT COORDINATORS)

The job of the clerk receptionist is mainly secretarial in nature, but the duties vary from site to site. With the clerk performing this job, nurses are freed from much of the paperwork involved in patient care. Clerk receptionists are trained on the job or in programs of several months' duration in technical schools. Clerks prepare, compile, and maintain patient records on a nursing unit. Duties include transcribing physician's orders; scheduling lab tests, x-ray procedures, and surgeries; scheduling other appointments for services; routing charts on patient transfers or discharges; compiling the patient census; answering the telephone; maintaining established inventories of supplies; distributing mail to patients; and generally ensuring that the unit functions smoothly.

UNIT MANAGERS

Some large health care organizations have unit managers to supervise and coordinate management functions for patient units. A college background and supervisory experience are desirable for this position. This job is combined with on-the-job training for specific duties. Responsibilities include budgeting, supervision of ward clerks, assignment and evaluation of clerical personnel, inventory of patient's valuables, coordination with housekeeping and maintenance, and clarification of hospital compliance with Medicare requirements. If a health care organization does not have unit managers, the clerk receptionist and the nurse manager assume these duties.

 Critical Thinking Exercise

Know Your Health Care Team

When on the clinical area, list the various members of the health care team with whom you have contact. Draw a concept map describing their role on the team and education required for their job.

DELIVERY OF NURSING CARE IN ACUTE CARE SETTINGS

With the goal of providing optimal care, the nursing team uses different methods to assign patients to staff. The methods evolved as a response to changing needs of the health care system, including staffing. Each of the methods is discussed in its general form, as it was intended to function. Health care organizations modify these methods to fit their individual needs.

CASE METHOD

At the turn of the twentieth century, families hired nurses to meet a patient's special needs in the home. By the 1920s private-duty nursing was popular. This case method of patient care continued in various degrees into the 1960s. Vestiges of

the case method, or a one-to-one relationship with a patient, are found today in acute care situations as total care nursing (comprehensive care). In the case method, one nurse is assigned to one or two patients and is responsible for planning, organizing, and carrying out the care for these patients. Today, total care nursing occurs in intensive care or special care units, as Mrs. Brown experienced in the ICU after she left the PACU. Nursing instructors frequently use the total patient care method when assigning beginning students to the acute care clinical area.

FUNCTIONAL NURSING

During WWII, the functional method was a popular method of patient assignment. Registered nurses were in scarce supply because of the war. Hospitals increased the number of LPN/LVNs and NAs to provide care for patients. The functional method of patient care is task oriented. The tasks that have to be done for patients are divided among the staff. For example, one person might measure all vital signs, another might do all treatments, and still another might make all the beds. This method's emphasis on efficiency and division of labor is based on the assembly line production concept found in industry.

The nursing home nearest Mrs. Brown's home schedules resident assignments by the functional method. An NA helped Mrs. Brown with her physical care. An LPN/LVN gave her medications and did her treatments. In addition to assuming responsibility for all care given to residents, the charge nurse, a practical/vocational nurse, would be kept busy with managerial (e.g., staff evaluations) and non-nursing duties (e.g., inventory of supplies).

Functional nursing can easily overlook holistic care, especially in the area of psychosocial needs. This results in fragmentation of care. Although this method is efficient and appears to be less costly to implement, it can discourage patient and staff satisfaction. The functional method, however, may work well in times of critical shortages or need of large numbers of personnel, such as disaster situations and emergencies.

TEAM NURSING

After World War II, the shortage of registered nurses continued. The team method of patient care was introduced, aided by the increasing number of LPN/LVNs and NAs. The team method is based on the belief that goals can be achieved through group action. The patients on a unit are divided into small groups. Small teams are assigned to care for the patients in each group. Assignments are based on the needs of each patient and the skills of the team members. The team leader, the RN, leads the team. The RN continues to have the final responsibility of planning, coordinating, and evaluating the implementation of care for each patient and supervising the personnel giving the care.

In team nursing the capabilities of each team member are used effectively. This increases the quality of care for the patient and the satisfaction of the team member. An integral part of the team method is the team conference. During this conference, which should be held daily, team members share information about specific patients. Patient problems are identified and solved, and plans of care are developed and revised. The team method is rarely carried out in this manner. When busy, the team leader may administer medications and perform treatments. Team conferences are often postponed. The team method then becomes a functional method of assigning care. Several years ago the nurses on the medical floor where Mrs. Brown was a patient used the team method, but often the team leader functioned as the medication nurse.

Modular nursing is a method to deliver nursing care that modifies team nursing by arranging the physical layout of units so that nurses can stay near the bedside of assigned patients for convenient patient access and record-keeping. For consistency, the same group of caregivers is assigned to a specific patient area.

PRIMARY NURSING

The hospital in which Mrs. Brown was a patient adopted the primary care method several years ago to replace the team method of assigning care. The intention was to increase the quality of care for patients. This method was instituted in the 1970s as a result of the dissatisfaction of professional nurses with their lack of direct patient contact and the fragmentation of care that resulted from functional and team nursing. In primary nursing, RNs individualize patient care and accept responsibility and accountability for total patient care, generally eliminating the need to delegate to other licensed staff persons (Lafer and Ross, 2007). Ideally, staffing for this method requires a nursing staff composed entirely of RNs. Each nurse is assigned a maximum of six patients. There are no team leaders in this method. Each primary nurse is a bedside nurse, who has received the assignment from and in turn reports to the nurse manager.

The major characteristic of this method is the responsibility and accountability of the primary nurse. The primary nurse is assigned to a patient on admission, develops the nursing diagnoses after the admission interview, develops a plan of care, and is responsible for the care of that patient 24 hours a day until he or she is discharged. When the primary nurse is off duty, an associate RN continues care as planned by the primary nurse. If any changes are contemplated in patient care, the primary nurse must be contacted.

Primary nursing facilitates continuity of care. Positive aspects of the primary method include shorter hospital stays for patients, improved communication among staff, and a more holistic focus of care. Negative aspects include the difficulty of recruiting a sufficient number of RNs. But the greatest negative aspect of this method is the cost of a staff composed entirely of RNs. Practical/vocational nurses are used as assistive nurses in primary care situations and have performed safely and effectively.

NURSING CASE MANAGEMENT

In acute care, **nursing case management** focuses on achieving patient outcomes within a specified time frame. Clinical pathways (care maps) or **critical paths** are used as a tool by all health care workers involved with the patients care to identify incidents that must occur at specific times to achieve patient outcomes within an appropriate length of stay. These pathways provide a blueprint for care that includes a time frame of significant events that are expected to occur each day a patient with a specific diagnosis is in the hospital. Figure 11-1 is an example of a clinical pathway.

Nursing case management became popular in the 1980s in response to the increasing complexity of patient care, the need to use scarce nursing resources, and meeting patient needs in a *cost-effective* manner in acute care. Depending on patient needs, this method uses baccalaureate registered nurses, diploma and associate degree registered nurses, licensed practical/vocational nurses, nursing assistants, and unlicensed assistive personnel in varying ratios to deliver nursing service.

Some institutions use care maps, which are a combination of care plans and critical paths. The case manager keeps an eye on timely discharge and continuity of care in the community by planning, directing, and evaluating care throughout the patient's stay in acute care. The strength of the case management method of delivering nursing services is its focus of delivering cost-effective, quality care to patients with complex needs. **Quality, service,** and **cost** are timely considerations for health care in the twenty-first century.

 Critical Thinking Exercise

Just a Routine Morning on the Medical/Surgical Floor

Have you ever experienced the following situation in an acute care setting?

Rhonda, an LPN/LVN, tried to find out when her nauseated, elderly patient was scheduled to have his chest x-ray, physical therapy session, and special lab studies. When Rhonda called to find out, staff in these departments were unable to give even a ballpark time frame for the procedures. Instead they answered, "We'll come when we can." So Rhonda started the bath. After Rhonda finished washing the patient's face, a transport aide appeared at the door to take the patient to the radiology department. Rhonda cautioned the transport aide that the patient was nauseated, but the aide said she was not trained to take care of things like that.

After 40 minutes, the patient returned to his room. Fortunately, he did not have to vomit while he was in the x-ray department. After Rhonda started the bath again, lab personnel came to take the patient to the laboratory for the special blood test that had to be done in that department. The lab personnel looked shocked when Rhonda included the emesis basin with the patient, with instructions that they might need to assist him. Forty-five minutes later, the patient returned to his room.

Rhonda continued the patient's bath from where she thought she left off. Then the physical therapy transport aide came to take the patient to his physical therapy session. Thirty-five minutes later the patient was back, but he had not had his physical therapy session. The patient was waiting for his turn for therapy when he had to go to the bathroom, but nobody was available to help him get to the bathroom. The patient could not have his physical therapy because he had been incontinent.

Identify two ways of doing things differently in this acute care situation that could help make the situation more patient-focused, efficient, and effective, and that would make more sense.

The patient would benefit if the following things were done differently:

1. _____

2. _____

The following are innovations created by management people to apply to acute care situations similar to the one just described:

1. Relocate small departmental units to the nursing area instead of making the patient go to them.
2. Cross-train health care workers so that each has the skills and can perform the tasks of other health care workers

PATIENT-FOCUSED CARE: ANOTHER METHOD FOR DELIVERING PATIENT CARE

Patient-focused care is an attempt to be more competitive and effective in today's health care system and improve the quality of care by organizing hospital resources and personnel around the needs of patients. It combines and changes inpatient services that affect all departments

1 - 7-3
2 - 3-11
3 - 11-7

LAST □ Chemotherapy Date ___
     □ Radiation Date ___

CARE NEED	DAY 1 ADMIT DAY date ___	DAY 2 date ___	DAY 3 date ___	DAY 4 date ___
ASSESSMENTS/ TREATMENTS	Postural BP on admission & prn / Weight documented / I&O / Baseline vital signs documented / Vital signs q shift and prn / Review old chart / Previous admit for n/v/d date:___ / Safety/fall assessment	AM weight / I&O / Vital signs q shift — stable / Evaluate lab results	AM weight / I&O / Vital signs ONLY 7-3 and 3-11 if stable	
FLUIDS/ NUTRITIONS	Start IV hydration @ admit / 1000cc D_5 ½ NS 20 KCL @ 100 / IV antiemetics / Adjust IV fluids based on lab results within 8 of admit / Clear liquids as tolerated	IV fluids continue / Start PO or PR antiemetics q 6 around-the-clock / Cont. IV antiemetics for BREAKTHROUGH / Clear liquids-Intake: / 7-3 500; 3-11 400; 11-7 100 / Advance to full liquid dinner or as tolerated	DC or HL IV by noon / Antiemetics AC and HS PO only / Advance to regular diet for lunch / Fluid Intake: / 7-3 600; 3-11 500; 11-7 100	
LAB/ DIAGNOSTICS	CBC—if not available from MD office / SMA 20-SMA 7 stat	SMA-7		
ACTIVITY	Up to BR / Ambulate in room 1x day/evenings	Up to BF / Ambulate ½ length of hallway TID	Ambulate full length of hallway TID	
SELF-CARE	Mouth care / Face/hand washing / Feeding	Mouth care / Self bath @ bedside / Feeding	Mouth care / Shower	
DISCHARGE PLANNING	Evaluate home care support / Refer to Social Services if: / Social Work intervention needed	Document discharge plan: / Social Services or Nursing	Finalize home care needs	Discharge by 11:00 AM
TEACHING	___ Assess current knowledge of antiemetics; document on kardex	___ Medication instruction / ___ Dietary consult evaluate need for diet counseling	___ Review/reinforce med instruction / ___ Review/reinforce diet instruction	___ Verbalizes understanding of meds for home care and diet
	RN ___ D E N / Initial / Signature	RN ___ D E N / Initial / Signature	RN ___ D E N / Initial / Signature	RN ___ D E N / Initial / Signature

Good Samaritan Hospital
A division of Good Samaritan Community Healthcare
407-14th Ave SE, PO Box 1247, Puyallup, WA 98371-0192 (206) 848-6661

Oncology
Clinical Pathway
Nausea/Vomiting/Dehydration

FIGURE 11-1 Oncology clinical pathway; nausea, vomiting, and dehydration in patients with cancer.

found in hospitals. The major change in patient-focused care is "decentralizing" centralized service departments within hospitals and locating them in each patient unit. For example, in this system of delivering care the radiology department would cease to be a department of its own. Each patient care area might have its own radiology suite, and an x-ray technician would be assigned to this area. Each unit might also have its own pharmacy and lab areas and even an admitting desk.

These health care workers would also undergo cross-training, learning to perform specific skills on the unit when needed by patients. Examples of cross-trained skills would be drawing blood, feeding patients, assisting patients with basic needs, providing health teaching about medications, and so on. As coordinator of the team, the RN would assign care duties to this team of health care workers. Patient-focused care can build a stronger team delivering higher quality care because the resources of the health care organization are focused on the patient.

SKILL MIX

Skill mix refers to the different levels of educational preparation of members used to staff the nursing team. The skill mix on the nursing team can be varied. Some hospitals are converting to all RN staffs. Some hospitals utilize LPN/LVNs, nursing assistants, and unlicensed assistive personnel to deliver patient care.

Research and data are needed to evaluate the quality of care provided by variously composed teams of RNs, LPN/LVNs, and nursing assistants in a variety of health care settings.

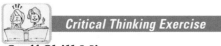
Critical Thinking Exercise

Staff Skill Mix

Investigate the skill mix of nursing staff in health care agencies at which you have clinical experiences.

NURSING SHORTAGE

The literature contains little current information about the supply and demand of licensed practical/vocational nurses. Articles about the nursing shortage generally refer to the shortage of registered nurses. The shortage of RNs continues to be a national and worldwide problem. Buerhaus estimates the shortage of RNs at 340,000 in the U.S. and serious enough to significantly damage the health care delivery system (Nursing Shortage Update: A Conversation with Peter Buerhaus: 2007). There is an increased demand for RNs in all areas of employment and health care facilities. The aging of 80 million U.S. baby boomers alone will increase the need for health care in the future.

Can LPN/LVNs fill in "the gap" in a nursing shortage? A study by Needleman and Buerhaus in 2005 simulated the effect of several options that would increase staffing to a feasible level for most hospitals. (An article about this study can be purchased by typing Needleman and Buerhaus +2005+staffing+LPN in Google search box and selecting Nurse Staffing in Hospitals: Is There a Business Case for Quality?) The key findings were:

- Greater use of RNs translates into fewer patient deaths, reduced hospital stays, and decreased rate of hospital-linked complications.
- Increasing the number of hours of nursing care by both RNs and LPNs would result in fewer deaths, avoidable complications, and days of care.
- Expanding both the proportion of RNs and the number of hours provided by LPNs to reach the top quarter of hospitals (a combination of the other two options) saves the most lives and greatest number of patient days (*The Business Case for Nurse Staffing*, 2006).

In addition to lack of information about the supply and demand of LPN/LVNs, there is little information in the literature about their education and scope of practice (scope of practice is discussed in Chapter 20). A study entitled *Supply, Demand,*

and Use of Licensed Practical Nurses (Seago, et al., 2004) explored the question of whether the LPN/LVN could help alleviate the nursing shortage. (The study can be retrieved at *http://bhpr.hrsa.gov/healthworkforce/reports/lpn/LPN1_5.htm.*) Based on their findings of demographics, education, scope of practice, and demand for LPNs and RNs, the authors believe LPNs can help address the current nursing shortage. Even though the scope of practice of LPN/LVNs is more limited and they cannot replace or substitute for RNs, they do contribute to the severe need for nursing manpower. Nursing leaders and focus group members who participated in the study acknowledged that much of the work that RNs perform could be performed by LPN/LVNs.

A report by Lafer and Moss (2007) stated that "the combination of LPN's education, skills, commitment and diversity enable them to make a vital contribution to hospital care. LPNs who are utilized to their full scope of practice are highly qualified, cost-effective members of the nursing team." The report can be accessed by typing into Google, Lafer and Moss and *The LPN: A Practical Way to Alleviate the Nursing Shortage.*

Box 11-1 lists some additional causes of the nursing shortage, and Box 11-2 lists some additional solutions to the nursing shortage.

 Critical Thinking Exercise

Promote Practical Nursing

Starting as a student, what can you do as a practical/vocational nurse to help promote practical nursing?

Box 11-1 | *Some Causes of the Nursing Shortage*

There is need for nurses in all sites of employment and this will increase in the future.
- In 2006 there were 118, 000 RN vacancies in hospitals.
- Predictions of actual numbers for the shortage differ. By 2020, Auerback states 340,000 RNs will be needed and HRSA estimates 1 million RNs will be needed. *Occupational Outlook Handbook* estimates that 1.2 million RNs will be needed by 2014. The nursing workforce is aging.
- The average age of RNS and LPN/LVNs in 2003 was 43 years.
- Thirty percent of nurses are younger than age 30.
- Sixty percent of nurses are older than age 40.

Nurses are leaving nursing for retirement and personal reasons.
- Younger nurses in the nursing workforce do not equal the number retiring and leaving.

- Fifty-five percent of nurse managers plan to retire between 2011 and 2020.
- We can expect a large number of LPN/LVNs to retire in the next 20 years.

Nursing schools cannot admit all qualified applicants because of a shortage of faculty, classrooms, and clinical facilities.
- The average age of faculty members is 55. They face retirement in about ten years or less.
- Nurses tend to postpone pursuing nursing doctorates until their mid-forties.
- In 2006-07 U.S. nursing schools turned away almost 43,000 qualified applicants.
- The modest increase in enrollment of students in BSN programs, after years of declining enrollments, is not enough to meet the demand for nurses.

Box 11-2 | *Some Solutions for the Nursing Shortage*

Attract more nursing students.
- Starting in grade school, promote nursing careers.
- Continue television advertisements promoting nursing; for example, the television advertisements sponsored by Johnson & Johnson.
- Nurses for a Healthy Tomorrow (NHT) is a coalition of 43 nursing and health care organizations that wage a campaign to attract people to the nursing profession.
- Create more accessible nursing programs for LPN/LVNs who elect to become RNs.

Change the culture of health care agencies to make nurses feel more "welcome."
- Recognize that people have decreased energy when getting older and make adjustments in schedules, routines, etc., to accommodate decreasing energy levels and improve efficiency on clinical units by providing devices that decrease physical strain, for example, mechanical lifting devices.
- Educate RNs about the role and the scope of practice of the LPN/LVN in the hospital and other health care settings.
- Improve staff morale.
- Identify staffing and workload problems.

- Develop a wellness program.
- Offer benefits, including retirement benefits.

Encourage more RNs to pursue graduate degrees earlier in their careers so the number of eligible faculty increases.
- Offer scholarships that support the preparation of nurse educators.
- Encourage Congress to appropriate funds for Title VIII—Nursing Workforce Development Programs— the largest source of federal funding for nursing education programs, including students.

Enlist the support of philanthropic (charitable) organizations.
Examples:
- The Robert Wood Johnson Foundation (RWJF), the largest charitable organization devoted to nursing has focused on retaining nurses in medical-surgical nursing.
- Partners Investing in Nursing's Future-RWJF and the Northwest Health Foundation encourage investment in nursing workforce solutions.
- The Betty Irene Moore Nursing Initiative funds projects to increase and retain the number of qualified nurses in the San Francisco area.

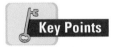

Key Points

- Health care organizations include a large number of specialized services and health care workers to provide these services. As a result, patients in the United States have some of the best and most expensive health care services in the world.
- Each member of the health care team provides a valuable service to the patient. All members of the health care team are equal in importance to each other.
- Members of the nursing team are registered nurses, practical/vocational nurses, student nurses, and cross-trained staff. Unlicensed assistive personnel, clerk receptionists, and managerial personnel round out the nursing team.

- To understand where the practical/vocational nurse fits into the picture, it is important to be aware of the educational background, role, responsibilities, and possible licensing requirements of all levels of personnel on the health care team.
- To understand your position on the health care team, it is necessary to keep up-to-date about new levels of health care workers and the method of delivering nursing care in your health care agency.
- The nursing shortage is expected to extend into the future.
- In the twenty-first century, practical/vocational nurses are recognized as important members of the health care team in acute care facilities and the community.

REVIEW ITEMS

1. Which of the following nurses on the health care team, with the following initials after their name, has the most education?

   1. RN
   2. BSN
   3. ADN
   4. MSN

2. Select the statement that indicates understanding of a major difference between the RN and LPN/LVN.

   1. The LPN/LVN initiates all health teaching for patients.
   2. The registered nurse formulates nursing diagnoses.
   3. By law, the LPN/LVN functions in an independent role.
   4. The LPN/LVN interprets the results of research studies.

3. Which of the following statements best describes nursing case management as a method of delivering nursing care?

   1. The method based on the level of staff skill and patient need.
   2. Task-oriented efficiency is divided among staff of all shifts.
   3. The RN plans and is accountable for total patient care 24 hours a day.
   4. This method utilizes scarce nursing resources in a cost-effective way.

4. Which of the following practical/vocational nurses is working in a typical LPN/LVN position?

   1. A visiting nurse on the day shift of a public health agency in the community.
   2. A charge nurse on the evening shift of an acute care agency in her community.
   3. A staff nurse assuming nurse manager responsibilities on a surgical unit.
   4. An office nurse preparing a child for a physical examination in a pediatrician's office.

ALTERNATE FORMAT ITEM

Which of the following statements differentiates the role of the practical/vocational nurse from the professional nurse? *(Select all that apply.)*

1. The LPN/LVN is responsible for formulating all nursing diagnoses.

2. The LPN/LVN has a more limited role in health teaching for patients.

3. The LPN/LVN is not employed in any management positions.

4. The LPN/LVN joins and is actively involved in NFLPN and NAPNES.

5. The LPN/LVN interprets many research findings in the clinical area.

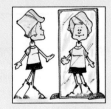

evolve http://evolve.elsevier.com/Hill/success/

Objectives

On completing this chapter, you will be able to do the following:

1. Define in your own words the following terms:
   a. Culture
   b. Cultural competence
   c. Cultural diversity
   d. Cultural uniqueness
   e. Ethnocentrism
   f. Cultural bias
   g. Cultural sensitivity
   h. Stereotype
2. Explain in your own words nine basic daily needs of all persons.
3. Describe your culture in the areas of:
   a. Family
   b. Religion
   c. Communication
   d. Educational background
   e. Economic level
   f. Wellness, illness, birth, and death beliefs and practices
4. Identify how all persons are unique and similar.
5. Explain in your own words the philosophy of individual worth as it applies to health care.
6. Describe general differences among cultural groups frequently served in your geographical area that may have importance in patient care situations.
7. Explain the importance of the following in developing an ability to provide culturally competent care:
   a. Increasing awareness of your own cultural self,
   b. Obtaining general knowledge about culturally diverse groups,
   c. Gathering data about specific beliefs and health practices of individual patients to be used in care plan development, and
   d. Negotiating plans of care for culturally diverse patients.

Key Terms

Assimilation (ă-SĬM-ă-LĀ-shŭn, p. 183)
Biomedicine (BĪ-ō-MĔD-ĭ-sĭn, p. 193)
Complementary and alternative medicine (CAM) (KŎM-plĕ-MĔN-tĕ-rē ăl-TŬR-nă-tĭv, p. 193)
Cultural bias (BĪ-ăs, p. 182)
Cultural competence (KŎM-pĭ-tĕns, p. 181)
Cultural diversity (dĭ-VŬR-sĭ-tē, p. 187)
Cultural sensitivity (SĔN-sĭ-TĬV-ĭ-tē, p. 181)
Culture (p. 181)
Customs (p. 181)
Discrimination (dĭ-SKRĬM-ĭ-NĀ-shŭn, p. 182)
Enculturation (ĕn-KŬL-chŭr-Ā-shŭn, p. 181)
Ethnic groups (ĔTH-nĭk, p. 187)
Ethnocentrism (ĔTH-nō-SĔN-TRĬZ-ĕm, p. 182)
Melting pot (p. 187)
Naturalistic system (NĂCH-ŭr-ăl-LĬS-tĭk, p. 195)
Nonjudgmental (NŎN-jŭj-MĔN-tăl, p. 188)
Personalistic system (PŬR-sŏ-năl-LĬS-tĭk, p. 195)
Prejudice (PRĔJ-ŭ-dĭs, p. 182)
Repatterning (p. 202)
Stereotype (STĔR-ē-ō-TĪP, p. 182)
Wellness and illness (p. 193)
Worldview (p. 182)

Keep in Mind

With knowledge comes responsibility. With knowledge of cultures, that responsibility entails respect for differences.

You have chosen a career that will give you an opportunity to meet people who are different than you. Some of these people will be your patients. Some will be your peers at school. Some will be your co-workers. Some will be a different age than you. Some will belong to a different social class. Some will have disabilities. Some will have different health care beliefs about what causes them to get sick. Some will have different values. In addition to all these differences, some of your patients and coworkers will have different cultural backgrounds, owing to ethnic group status. Regardless of cultural background, some differences will be the result of a growing diversity in individual and family lifestyles. You will discover that people think, feel, believe, act, and see the world differently from you and your family and friends. Log on to *www.minoritynurse. com/about/index.html*, sign up for the free quarterly email newsletter, check out featured articles about issues facing minority nurses, and find out if your school subscribes to *Minority Nurse Magazine.*

Review the standards of the National Association for Practical Nurse Education and Service, Inc. (see Appendix B: NAPNES Standards of Practice and Educational Competencies of Graduates of Practical/Vocational Nursing Programs) and the National Federation of Licensed Practical Nurses (Appendix C: NFLPN Nursing Practice Standards for the Licensed Practical/Vocational Nurse). You will note that both organizations have embraced statements that describe the need of the practical/vocational nurse to provide health care to all patients regardless of race, creed, cultural background, disease, or lifestyle. This is an ethical expectation. Review your state's Nurse Practice Act. You might find that failing or refusing to render nursing services to a patient because of the patient's race, color, sex, age, beliefs, national origin, or handicap is listed as unprofessional conduct. The ethical expectation now becomes a legal mandate. Nurses could risk legal suits because of their ignorance of the culture of the patient and resulting poor nursing judgment.

Not only do practical/vocational nurses need to provide care for all persons, but they also need to provide *culturally competent* care. Cultural competence is the *continuous* attempt of practical/vocational nurses to gain the knowledge and skills that will allow them to effectively provide care for patients of different cultures. Cultural competence is not gained by reading a chapter in a textbook, nor is it gained by looking up a culture in a reference book. It is developing an awareness of different cultures (cultural sensitivity) and continually learning about people who are different than you.

When differences are identified in a health care situation, the practical/vocational nurse needs to suggest adaptations to the plan of care so that the plan recognizes these differences. In doing so the patient will be encouraged to follow suggestions, avoid treatment failures, and return to health as quickly as possible. Practical/vocational nurses will then be able to say that they have truly met the patient's needs.

DEFINITION OF CULTURE

Culture is a way of life. It is the total of the *ever-changing* knowledge, ideas, thoughts, beliefs, values, communication, actions, attitudes, traditions, customs, and objects that a group of people possess and the ways they have of doing things. Culture also includes standards of behavior and sets of rules to live by. Customs are the generally accepted ways of doing things common to people who share the same culture. Basic concepts about culture can be accessed at *http://www. culturediversity.org*.

CHARACTERISTICS OF CULTURE

An important point about culture is that it is *learned behavior*. The culture of a group is passed on from generation to generation. From the moment you were born you began to learn about the culture of the group into which you were born. The process of learning your culture (the way your group does things) is called enculturation. A result of enculturation is a worldview that is generally shared by persons with the same cultural background. The worldview, or similar ways of seeing and understanding the world, becomes the reality of the group. This reality fills every aspect of life. It is a cultural bias (a mental leaning) that is never proved or questioned by the individual. The worth of everything, either within or outside of the group, depends on whether it fits the worldview of the cultural group. One's worldview can lead to ethnocentrism, prejudice, and discrimination, unless modified by knowledge and experience.

Socialization is the process by which a person of one culture learns how to function within a larger culture. Right now you are being socialized into the career of practical/vocational nursing. You are learning how to think and act like a practical/vocational nurse.

DANGER: ETHNOCENTRISM, PREJUDICE, AND DISCRIMINATION

People who belong to the same cultural group may develop the attitude, through their worldview, that their way of doing things is superior, right, or better than that of groups with different cultures (ethnocentrism). The group uses its culture as the norm against which to measure and evaluate the customs and ways of others. The group is uncomfortable with people who display customs and behaviors that differ from their cultural group. Ethnocentrism is common to all cultural groups. When intolerance of another cultural group occurs, prejudice results. When rights and privileges are withheld from those of another cultural group, discrimination is the result.

AVOIDING FALSE ASSUMPTIONS (STEREOTYPES)

Nursing students sometimes think that somewhere there is a manual that will tell them how to care for people who are different from themselves. This type of approach can lead to false assumptions, which are called stereotypes. A stereotype is an assumption used to describe all members of a specific group without exception. It is an expectation that all individuals in a group will act exactly the same in a situation just because they are members of that group. Stereotypes ignore the individual differences that occur within every cultural group. Members of any culture may have modified the degree to which they observe the values and practices of the culture.

Critical Thinking Exercise

Example of a False Assumption (Stereotype)

During a seminar on business practices, the presenter, while talking about a specific business practice, singled out an engineer in the group who was of Japanese descent. He used the engineer as an example of someone who thinks differently from "Americans" because he is Asian. The engineer was a third-generation American and had no clue what the presenter was talking about.

How did the presenter in this situation go wrong in his assumption?

THINK LIKE AN ANTHROPOLOGIST!

Anthropologists are scientists who study physical, social, and cultural characteristics of human groups. It is helpful to understand how these scientists conduct their studies.

- Anthropologists start the study of cultural groups by identifying common trends in a cultural group.
- These common trends found in the group are called "generalizations."
- Then anthropologists gather data to determine if the common trends (generalizations) apply to all individuals within that cultural group.

To automatically generalize cultural information about health practices that were obtained for a group to an individual in that group might be drawing a wrong conclusion. Does the individual follow the traditional practice of the group? Has the individual rejected the practice? Does the individual use the practice only in certain situations?

If so, what situations? Is the person an immigrant? How recently? When people immigrate to a new country, culturally different groups do adopt some of the culture of the new country. The process of giving up parts of their own culture and adopting parts of the culture of the dominant group is called assimilation. Complete assimilation rarely occurs. *Members of the generations that follow the original immigrants may retain some elements of their original culture in addition to assimilating parts of the new culture.* For these reasons, generalizations help explain observed behavior. They do not *predict* behavior.

KNOWING YOURSELF

WHAT MAKES YOU UNIQUE?

To become aware of different cultures, you need to be aware of yourself as a person. Several activities are included in this chapter to help you with cultural self-awareness. The exercises also help you develop an awareness of cultural differences with peers.

 Learning Exercise

What Makes You Unique?

Let your uniqueness show! Divide the class into small but equal sized groups. Find one item that makes you unique from other members of the group. Share with your class the item that makes you unique.

HOW MANY HATS DO YOU WEAR? WHAT ROLES DO YOU PLAY?

Each of you fills many roles in your daily life. Sometimes you refer to this situation as wearing many hats or your plate is full. Some of these roles are played out individually, one at a time. Sometimes you play many roles at the same time. The following learning exercise, "Identifying the Roles You Play in Your Life," will give you the opportunity to identify your roles.

Learning Exercise

Identifying the Roles You Play in Your Life

The following categories describe the roles you play in several areas in your everyday life.

Category 1: Economic Status Role

Although standards are available to assign persons to each of the following economic classes, people generally place themselves in one of the following categories by how they perceive their economic status.

Place a check mark next to the economic class that best describes you.

I am in the

_____ Lower economic class
_____ Middle economic class
_____ Upper economic class

Category 2: Political Role

Put a check mark next to the word(s) that best describes the political role you play in society.

I am

_____ Republican
_____ Democrat
_____ Independent
_____ Liberal
_____ Conservative
_____ Moderate
_____ Indifferent
_____ To the left of liberal
_____ To the right of conservative
Other _____

Category 3: Racial or Ethnic Role

Place a check mark beside the racial or ethnic terms that best describe you.

I am a (an)

_____ African American
_____ American
_____ American Indian
_____ Amerindian
_____ Anglo
_____ Anglo-Saxon
_____ Arab American
_____ Asian American
_____ Asian
_____ Black
_____ Chicano
_____ Ethnic
_____ Gypsy

Continued

_____ Hispanic
_____ Indian
_____ Latin American
_____ Latvian American
_____ Native American
_____ Spanish-speaking
_____ White
Other _____
Category 4: Social Role
Circle the social roles that describe you.
I am (a)
female, male
married, single
separated, divorced
blended family
wife, husband
significant other
mother, father
daughter, son
sister, brother
stepmother, stepfather
stepdaughter, stepson
stepsister, stepbrother
half-sister, half-brother
godmother, godfather
godchild
grandmother, grandfather
granddaughter, grandson
aunt, uncle
niece, nephew
cousin
Other _____
Category 5: Work Role
Place a check mark beside each work role you play in your life.
I am (a)
_____ Blue-collar worker
_____ Business person
_____ Laborer
_____ Professional
_____ Service provider
_____ Skilled worker
_____ Student
_____ Technician
_____ Unemployed
_____ White-collar worker
Other _____
Summarize the hats you wear by listing the items you have checked and circled in the five categories.
Category 1: Economic status role _____
Category 2: Political role _____

Category 3: Racial or Ethnic role _____
Category 4: Social role _____
Category 5: Work role _____
_____
_____

 Learning Exercise

Who Am I Based on My Roles?
Make up a sentence using all the words you listed in the five role categories. This sentence describes you by the roles you play in your life. Have each student write the sentence on a piece of paper (no name of writer!) and put it in a paper bag. Have someone pick one of the papers out of the bag, read the sentence, then give the class the opportunity to guess whom the sentence describes (adapted from Randall-David, 1992).
_____
_____

WHAT WE SHARE IN COMMON

Because of our genes, each individual the world over is different from every other person. The only exception is identical twins. Before you start to think about the differences among people, it is a good idea to think about what people share in common.

 Learning Exercise

What We Have in Common
When you are among a group of your peers (e.g., eating lunch in the cafeteria or walking to the parking lot), take a few minutes to play the "What We Have in Common" culture game. Excluding sex, age, marital status, and culture group, try to find five items you share in common with each member of the group. This activity is especially helpful when the group includes classmates you perceive as "different" from you.
1. _____
2. _____
3. _____
4. _____
5. _____

1. In a class situation, discuss the items you have in common. Did any items you share in common with other members of the group surprise you?
2. Did you discover any stereotyping in *your* thinking regarding your peers?

BASIC DAILY NEEDS: ANOTHER COMMONALITY

All people share the same basic daily needs regardless of age, sex, economic status, lifestyle, religion, country of origin, or culture. Chapter 15 discusses human needs as understood by the psychologist Abraham Maslow. In 1974 registered nurse Vivian Culver listed nine essential daily needs of all persons (Culver, 1974). This list has stood the test of time. These essential needs are a simple, yet good place to start in learning to understand that all people, regardless of background, share the following things in common:

1. Personal care and hygiene
2. Sleep and rest
3. Nutrition and fluids
4. Elimination
5. Body alignment and activity
6. Environment
7. Emotional and spiritual support
8. Diversion and recreation
9. Mental hygiene

These nine basic daily needs can form the basis for planning patient care. However, you need to understand the meaning of these basic needs for well persons, including yourself, before you can apply them to individuals in the clinical area. Once you gain understanding of these needs and the varieties of ways persons meet them, applying these needs to patients will be easier. As you read about the nine basic needs of all people, think about how you specifically meet each need in your own daily life. Do some of your peers meet their daily basic needs in different ways than you meet your needs? So too will it be with patients in the clinical area.

Personal Care and Hygiene

Clean hair, skin, nails, teeth, and clothing serve two general purposes: protection from illness and promotion of well-being. Skin constantly secretes sebum, the cold cream–like substance of the body, to keep the skin supple. Daily, epidermal skin cells (the outer layer of the skin) are shed as new cells push toward the outer layer. Skin eliminates fluid in the form of perspiration to help keep body temperature stable. Sebum and perspiration are odorless substances. Ever-present bacteria on the skin are responsible for the body odor we associate with the body's oils and perspiration. We meet personal care and hygiene needs by bathing, shampooing, hand washing, maintaining oral hygiene, and grooming.

- Do you prefer a shower, a bath, or another method of cleansing your body?
- How often do you cleanse your body?
- During what part of the day do you cleanse your body?
- How often do you shampoo?
- What products do you use to style your hair?
- How often do you visit the dentist?

Sleep and Rest

Sleep is needed to refresh ourselves. The actual number of hours of sleep required varies with the individual. Rest and periodic relaxation are just as important because they also help the body restore itself.

- How many hours of sleep do you get each night or day?
- Where do you rest or relax?
- What do you do to rest or relax?
- Do you take naps during the day?

Nutrition and Fluids

Preparing meals from the suggested food selections, as you studied in nutrition, is needed to stay healthy. We all need a variety of food daily. Fluids help our body complete its many chemical reactions, transport nutrients, regulate temperature, and lubricate body parts. Fluids include the water content in food, as well as the beverages we drink.

- How many calories do you consume each day?
- How many meals do you eat each day?
- When do you eat your meals?

- How many glasses of fluid do you drink each day?
- What fluids do you prefer to drink?

Elimination

Elimination of wastes from the body is primarily accomplished by the kidneys (in the form of urine) and the large intestine (in the form of feces). The skin is not as good at elimination as these organs, but it does eliminate some body wastes through perspiration.

- What do you consider to be "normal" time intervals for urinary and intestinal elimination?

Body Alignment and Activity

Body alignment, or the relationship of the body parts to one another, is better known as posture. When posture is "good," the body can be used in a comfortable manner without danger of injury. Good posture also enhances the functioning of the respiratory, gastrointestinal, and circulatory systems. You will not tire as quickly if good posture is maintained. Daily exercise may also enhance the function of these body systems. Exercise also helps maintain muscle tone.

- Have a peer evaluate your posture while you are sitting and walking
- How much exercise do you get each day?
- How do you get your exercise?

Environment

Environment refers to the space that surrounds us. Our environment changes many times during a day. Regardless of our specific environment, the most essential component of our surroundings is oxygen. After that environmental need has been met, the next most important need is safety. When oxygen and safety needs have been met, the individual can focus on changing his or her environment to accommodate comfort and personal taste.

- Describe your home environment.
- Do you feel safe in your environment?

Emotional and Spiritual Support

Our emotions greatly influence our health because the body and the mind are linked. This link enables the body to influence the mind and the mind to influence the body. All emotions, including excitement, fear, anger, worry, grief, joy, surprise, and love, can influence our bodies positively or negatively. Spiritual and emotional needs are closely related, yet different. People meet their spiritual needs in a variety of ways that are unique to their personal beliefs (see Chapter 13). Do you acknowledge spiritual needs? If so, how do you meet them?

- How do you express anger, worry, joy, grief?

Diversion and Recreation

We all need to turn aside (diversion) from our usual activities and refresh our bodies and minds with activities other than work (recreation). What is work to one person can be play to another.

- How much time do you spend studying each week?
- How many hours do you work outside school?
- What type of recreation do you engage in each week?
- How many hours do you devote to recreation each week?

Mental Hygiene

Mental hygiene involves the care and hygiene of the brain. Just as there are good health habits for the body, there are also good daily health habits for the mind. You need to strive to understand and accept yourself, be optimistic, work well with others, accept criticism, know your abilities and limitations, trust and respect others, and accept responsibility for yourself.

- Who is responsible for your success in the practical/vocational nursing program?
- What is your attitude toward constructive evaluation?
- What kind of a team member are you in the clinical area?
- How do you control your stress level?

Learning Exercise

Basic Daily Needs

Choose one basic daily need and discuss with class-mates how you meet that need.

KNOWING OTHERS: CULTURAL DIVERSITY

In the nineteenth century, waves of immigrants from throughout the world entered the United States. The United States was referred to as a melting pot. This term indicated that the immigrants had given up their native cultures and adopted the culture of the people already in the United States.

The 2000 U.S. Census included the following categories for respondents to select: Spanish/Hispanic/Latino (if so, indicate if Mexican, Mexican American, Chicano, Puerto Rican, Cuban, or other group), white, black, African American or Negro, American Indian or Alaska native, Chinese, Filipino, Japanese, Korean, Vietnamese, other Asian, Hawaiian, Guamanian or Chamorro, Samoan, other Pacific Islander, or other race. The melting pot is now more like a "casserole," with each ingredient (i.e., different culture) adding to the quality of the whole. The concept of the melting pot has been replaced by the concept of cultural diversity. The many differences in the elements of culture in groups of people in American and Canadian society are called "cultural diversity." Traditionally, examples of groups that have been identified as culturally diverse in the United States are Hispanics, African Americans, Asians, American Indians, and whites.

Cultural diversity goes beyond racial and ethnic groups. As a practical/vocational nurse, you need to define this concept more broadly. Defined more broadly, examples of culturally diverse groups include single parents, people who live in poverty, homosexuals, bisexuals, the wealthy, the poor, the homeless, the elderly, and people with disabilities.

The concept of race as a means of categorizing people by biological traits has come under attack by social scientists. These scientists suggest using ethnicity as a more accurate means of capturing the great diversity found in over 6.5 billion people in the world (*http://www.census.gov/main/www/popclock.html*). Members of ethnic groups are a special type of cultural group, composed of people who are members of the same race, religion, or nation, or who speak the same language. They derive part of their identity through membership in the ethnic group. Examples of ethnic groups in the United States include Irish Americans, African Americans, American Indians, Asian Americans, German Americans, Mexican Americans, Jews, Arab Americans, Greek Americans, and many more.

IMPORTANCE OF CULTURAL DIVERSITY

Health care today and into the future needs to be able to accommodate patients of many differing cultural backgrounds. Failure to develop sensitivity to and competence in handling this diversity could lead to misunderstanding between the patient and you, resulting in stress for care-giver and patient. The plan of treatment for the patient could fail. You could make false assumptions based on generalizations. You might label patients as difficult or uncooperative when their lack of cooperation with the plan of care could be related to a conflict with their personal health belief system. Patients may experience less-than-adequate care when cultural diversity and the differences it represents are overlooked or misinterpreted.

Philosophy of Individual Worth and Celebrating Our Uniqueness

The philosophy of individual worth is a belief shared by all members of the health care team. The philosophy includes the uniqueness and value of each human being who comes for care, regardless of differences that may be observed or perceived in that individual. Practical/vocational nurses need to realize that each individual has the right to live according to their personal beliefs and values, *as long as they do not interfere with the rights of others*. Each individual deserves respect as a human being.

Many factors are responsible for differences in patients. They may think and behave differently because of social class, personal income, religion, ethnic background, or personal choice. Regardless of these differences, all patients have the right to receive high-quality nursing care. As a practical/vocational nurse you cannot decrease the quality of the care you give because of differences you observe or perceive.

Practical/vocational nurses need to guard against making judgments about people who are culturally different. This does not mean you must adopt differences as part of your behavior. It means being open-minded and nonjudgmental. It means taking the difference at face value, accepting people as they are, and giving high-quality care. Be aware of your own attitudes, beliefs, and values as they affect your ability to give care. If you do identify biases, see them for what they are. Become sensitive to cultural differences, and acknowledge that they exist. Gather knowledge about them so that you can work on trying to modify your biases and provide more culturally competent care.

LEARNING ABOUT CULTURAL DIVERSITY
How to Begin

You have been given exercises that help you to discover your own uniqueness and that of others, as well as similarities. Unless you understand your own culture, it will be difficult to understand the culture of others. You need to look inside yourself to learn about your own cultural beliefs, values, and worldview, and how they influence how you think and act. Some elements of your culture are obvious; for example, your language, celebrated holidays, and how and what you eat. However, other aspects of your culture are hidden. Elements such as aspects of communication, beliefs, attitudes, values, sex roles, use of space, concept of time, structure of the family, and family dynamics may be more difficult to recognize and discuss. There are areas of cultural diversity that might ordinarily be taken for granted in patient situations. Examples include food preferences, religion, educational background,

economic level, wellness and illness beliefs and practices, the birth experience, and terminal illness and death beliefs and practices.

The first step to developing knowledge about patient differences in these areas is to become aware of and explore *your* cultural patterns in these areas. Read the general information about each area. Develop an awareness of your own cultural patterns in these areas by answering the group of statements or questions included with each area. Sharing this information with peers will highlight the cultural diversity that exists in your nursing class, regardless of cultural background. **The questions also provide examples of areas to be discussed with patients when collecting data about their personal beliefs and health practices.**

AREAS OF CULTURAL DIVERSITY
Family Structure

No matter what culture is being discussed, the family is the basic unit of society. The role of the family is to have children, if desired or as they come, and to raise them to be contributing members of the group. Actual child-rearing practices vary from culture to culture. Families generally socialize the young to the culture of the group. They meet the physical and psychological needs of the young in culturally specific ways. Some cultures expect only the nuclear family (mother, father, and children) to live in the same house. Others may expect the extended family (the nuclear family plus the grandparents and other kinsmen) to do so. Some Vietnamese families are examples of extended families, with three or more generations living in the same house. In many of these families, ties are strong. Behaviors that enhance the family name are encouraged, such as obedience to parents and those in authority.

The single-parent family continues to challenge the traditional nuclear family as the typical family structure. A parent may become a single parent on the death of a spouse, by electing not to marry at the time of pregnancy, or by divorce. Health care workers who have not been in the same situation may be unaware of, and insensitive to, the special way of life of this type of family.

Learning Exercise

Cultural Patterns: Family

Respond to the following statements. Your responses will help you discover your own cultural patterns in regard to the family.

1. Describe your family structure (nuclear, extended, or alternative lifestyle).
2. Describe the role of children, if any, in your family.
3. Discuss who gives permission for hospitalization in your family.
4. List factors that influence the decision of your family members to visit or not visit the hospital when a member is ill. If visiting is acceptable, how long does your family think it is appropriate to visit?
5. Describe the effect that your hospitalization today at 4 PM for emergency surgery would have on you and your family.

Food Preferences

All cultures use food to provide needed nutrients. However, what they eat, when they eat, and how they eat differ vastly by cultural group. Knowledge of nutrition as a science differs by culture. It is interesting that the soil of some cultures (e.g., Mexico) encouraged the growth of two complementary foods that together make up a complete protein source (corn and beans) and became a staple of that culture's diet. Specific foods in different cultures have different meanings. All cultures use food during celebrations. Through generations of experience, different cultures have learned to use different foods to promote health and cure disease.

Learning Exercise

Cultural Patterns: Food

To assist you in identifying your own cultural patterns in regard to food preferences, respond to the following statements or questions.

1. State your favorite food.
2. Identify one special occasion in which your cultural group participates. What foods, if any, are part of this celebration?
3. Describe your favorite recipe/meal from your mother and from your grandmother. What special ingredients or techniques are used to make the recipe? Is there a written recipe?

Religious Beliefs

Religious beliefs are personal to the individual. Religion is an important aspect of culture. Religion can have different meanings in people's lives. For some, religion is a brief, momentary, and sporadic part of daily life. For another person, it may influence every aspect of life and have a profound effect on personal outlook and on how one lives his or her life. For others, religion may not play a part in their lives. Chapter 13 deals with spirituality and religious differences. This aspect of life cannot be excluded from this chapter. There is a close relationship between religious beliefs and the concept of wellness and illness in some groups. Practical/vocational nurses need to be aware of their own religious beliefs, obligations, and attitudes. They need to know whether these beliefs and attitudes influence the care that is given to patients.

Learning Exercise

Cultural Patterns: Religion

The questions that follow give you the opportunity to discover your own cultural patterns in regard to religion.

1. Do you have a religious affiliation? If so, indicate your affiliation.
2. What role does religion play in your life?
3. Is prayer helpful to you?
4. What is the source of strength and hope?
5. What rituals or religious practices are important to you?
6. What symbols or religious books are helpful to you?
7. What dietary inclusions or restrictions are part of your religious beliefs?
8. How does your religion view the source and meaning of pain and suffering?
9. When ill, does your religion prohibit people from the opposite sex from giving care?
10. Does your religion have special days when certain behaviors/activities are mandatory or prohibited?

Concept of Time

Some persons follow clock time. An hour has a beginning and an end (after 60 minutes). People who follow clock time eat, sleep, work, and engage in recreational activities at definite times each day. Some persons live on linear time. For them, time is a straight line with no beginning and no end. People who follow linear time eat when they are hungry and sleep when they are tired.

 Learning Exercise

Cultural Patterns: Time

The questions that follow give you an opportunity to discover your own cultural patterns in regard to time.
1. What determines when it is time for you to eat or sleep?
2. Do you wear a watch if you are not in the clinical area?
3. Are you on time for appointments?

Communication

Chapter 9 introduced you to types of communication and barriers to the communication process. A major barrier to communication in health care is a different language spoken by the patient or nurse. A person's language gives a view of reality that may differ from yours. For example, in English the clock runs, but in Spanish it walks. This illustrates the different concept of time between the two cultures. For a person who speaks English as a first language, time could move quickly, and there may be a rush to get things done. For some who speak Spanish as a first language, time may move more slowly. The following is a list of areas of communication that may vary for people who are culturally different.

Forms of Greetings and Goodbyes
- You may greet your patient and want to get right down to business.
- The patient might expect some light conversation before getting to the matter at hand.
- In some cultural groups people take an hour to say good-bye, whereas people from other cultures may get up and leave without saying anything.

Appropriateness of the Situation
- Some groups prefer people to sit, not stand, while they converse.
- In some groups the sharing of food is a good way to relate to others and get them to verbalize.

Confidentiality
- All information the patient gives the nurse is considered confidential.
- Some patients do not want their spouse questioned or informed about their problems of the reproductive organs. They fear the spouse may think they are less desirable sexually.

Emotions and Feelings and Their Expression
- Emotions are universal, but the cues to those emotions vary considerably. A lack of awareness of this fact can cause unnecessary stress between the patient and the nurse.
- In some cultural groups people cannot display affection in public, show disapproval or frustration, or vent anger.
- Some members of cultural groups cannot take criticism.
- You may show dissatisfaction with other members of the health care team by approaching them directly, whereas some team members may show dissatisfaction with you by being polite to your face but then complaining about you to the rest of the staff. The same applies to your classmates.

Pain Expression
- Pain has two parts: sensation and response. All individuals experience the same sensation of pain.
- One's culture influences the definition of pain and the response to the sensation.
- Pain is whatever the person says it is. It exists whenever the person says it does.
- One's culture provides guidelines for approved ways of expressing one's response to the pain sensation and ways to relieve the pain.
- Some cultures teach individuals that it is acceptable to cry, moan, and exhibit other behavior that calls attention to the pain. These behaviors may be considered a cure for pain in their culture.

- Other cultures encourage uncomplaining acceptance of pain and passive behavior when pain is experienced (stoic behavior).

Tempo of Conversation

- You may tend to speak quickly and expect a quick response.
- The patient may be accustomed to pausing and reflecting before giving a response.

Meaning of Silence

- Silence can mean anything from disapproval to warmth, but generally it does not indicate tension or lack of rapport.
- Silence can be difficult for some nurses to tolerate. Resist the temptation to jump in at a pause in the conversation by forcing yourself to concentrate on listening.

 Critical Thinking Exercise

Stoic Behavior in Patients

Discuss some nursing situations in which a stoic reaction to pain could have negative consequences, if a practical/vocational nurse lacked knowledge of cultural differences in pain expression (e.g., a woman in labor or a patient having a heart attack).

 Learning Exercise

Cultural Patterns: Communication

Develop an awareness of your own cultural patterns in communication by answering the following questions:

1. What is your first (native) language?
2. Do you speak additional languages?
3. What facial or body habits are you aware of in yourself while you are talking?
4. How do you greet people, and how do you say good-bye?
5. How do you express the following emotions:
   a. Love?
   b. Hate?
   c. Fear?
   d. Excitement?
   e. Disappointment?
   f. Dissatisfaction?
   g. Humor?
   h. Anger?

   i. Sadness?
   j. Happiness?
6. Do you make eye contact when talking to people?
7. Do you touch people while talking?
   a. If so, how do they react?
   b. How do you react when people touch you while they are talking to you?
8. How do you express pain? How do you react to pain?

Additionally, you should keep the following hints in mind when using interpreters or other language resources (Box 12-1).

Educational Background

The 2003 National Assessment of Adult Literacy assessed the English health literacy of adults in the United States and found that 14% have below basic health literacy skills (able to understand a simple health pamphlet). Twenty-two percent have basic health literacy (able to understand a more complex health pamphlet). Both groups got most of their information about health issues from radio and television (Kutner, 2006). Differences in educational background and literacy need to be taken into consideration when teaching patients. When in the clinical area, adapt your explanations to the patient's level of understanding.

 Learning Exercise

Cultural Patterns: Education

Responding to the following statements will help you identify your own beliefs and practices in regard to education.

1. Calculate the number of years of education you have had.
2. State your ultimate educational goal.
3. Discuss the role education plays in your life.
4. Describe your feelings toward a person who has less education than you.
5. Describe your feelings toward a person who has more education than you.
6. Describe your feelings if you were referred to your school's skills center.
7. Discuss the effect of your cultural background on your values and practices with regard to education.
8. Who in your family has graduated from high school, technical school, junior college, or college or university?

Box 12-1 | *Hints for Using Interpreters and Other Language Resources*

Interpreters provide an invaluable service when patients do not speak English or do not have sufficient experience with the English language to understand complex medical information. Another communication skill for the nurse is learning to work with an interpreter. To decrease the possibility of difficulties in an interpreter situation, follow these suggestions:

- The ideal interpreter should be trained in the health care field, proficient in the language of the patient and the nurse, and understand and respect the culture of the patient.
- If the ideal interpreter is not available, make sure that the individual chosen has training in medical terminology, understands the health matter that needs to be translated, and understands the requirements for confidentiality, neutrality, and accuracy.
- Use family members as interpreters cautiously. Patients of specific cultures may be embarrassed to discuss intimate matters with family members who are younger or older or of the opposite sex. Family members may censor information to protect the patient or the family.
- Make sure the interpreter is acceptable to the patient.

- Look and speak directly to the patient.
- Speak clearly and slowly in a normal voice. Use short units of speech.
- Avoid slang and professional jargon.
- Observe the nonverbal communication of the patient.
- Be patient. Remember that interpretation is difficult work.

Other resources to assist with patients with language other than English include foreign language classes offered to staff in the language of patients commonly served. Language Line is a telephone-based interpreting service. Information about Language Line is available at *http://www.languageline.com*. You can sign up for their Healthcare enewsletter at *http://www.languageline.com/page/newsletter*.

Say It in Spanish, by Joyce and Villanueva de Gonzalez (2004), is a reference book for health care workers that contains commonly used Spanish phrases.

Hablamos Juntos is a program whose mission is to improve communication between health care providers and their patients with limited proficiency. Information about this program can be accessed at *http://www.hablamosjuntos.org/mission/default.mission.asp*.

Adapted from Reinhardt E: *Through the Eyes of Others—Intercultural Resource Directory for Health Care Professionals.* Minneapolis: University of Minnesota School of Public Health, 1995.

Economic Level

Economic level is often related to educational background. Sociologists use these two factors to determine the social class of individuals. You will meet patients who are very wealthy and patients who are at or near the poverty level. Others have midlevel incomes. Patients' annual income determines the type of house they live in, the neighborhood where they live, the availability of food, and the ability to participate in certain types of preventive health care. Practical/vocational nurses need to take economic level into consideration while reinforcing patient teaching and should adapt their approach accordingly.

Learning Exercise

Cultural Patterns: Economic Level

Identify your personal patterns in regard to economic level by responding to the following statements or questions.

1. Describe how your economic background affects your daily life in the following areas:
   a. Availability of food,
   b. Availability of shelter,
   c. vailability of clothing, and
   d. Amount and type of recreation
2. Discuss your feelings toward a person who has less money than you.
3. Discuss your feelings toward a person who has more money than you.

4. Describe how these feelings fit with those of your cultural group.
5. Discuss your ability to afford to go to a physician when you get sick.
6. If you work, do you have health insurance benefits?

Wellness and Illness Beliefs and Practices

Wellness and illness can have different meanings for persons who are culturally different. *Wellness* and *illness* are relative terms. What is good health to one person can be sickness to another. Wellness may not be a high-priority matter to some patients.

Preventing Illness. Some patients believe that illness can be prevented; they practice elaborate rituals and engage special persons to carry out those rituals in an attempt to prevent disease. Other patients look at prevention as an attempt to control the future. They may consider this an impossible feat in the way they view their lives. They may wonder about the necessity of making a trip to a health care provider for preventive care, such as immunizations. Others may think prevention is tempting fate or the gods; to follow through with prevention would be risky.

Curing Illness. When disease does strike, some people blame pathogens (germs), some blame spirits, and others blame an imbalance in the body. Some cultural groups have folk medicine practices, such as rituals, special procedures (e.g., rubbing the skin with the edge of a coin to release the toxins causing illness), and special persons in the group to cure disease (e.g., physician, herbalist, shaman). Some groups believe that special foods or food combinations (e.g., "cold" foods for "hot" illness) and herbs (e.g., echinacea and feverfew) can prevent or cure illnesses. Others see no relationship between diet and health.

Complementary and Alternative Medicine. The dominant health system of the United States is biomedicine (Western medicine). Biomedicine focuses on symptoms. The goal of biomedicine is to find the cause of disease and then eliminate or correct the problem. Nearly 50% of Americans are seeking methods that avoid side effects from medications and treatments and/or that focus on the whole body and not just symptoms when treating disease. They are spending billions of dollars a year, mostly out of pocket, on complementary (used in conjunction with biomedical treatments) and alternative (substitute for conventional medicine) medicine. Complementary and alternative medicine (CAM) focuses on assisting the body's own healing powers and restoring body balance. The diversity of non-Western health care practices among the many cultural groups in the U.S. has helped increase the interest and use of CAM. The National Center for Complementary and Alternative Medicine (NCCAM) of the National Institutes of Health conducts research and evaluates the effectiveness and safety of CAM. NCCAM's website (*http://www.nccam.nih. gov*) provides information about CAM.

Modesty. Individuals in some cultures are embarrassed when they have to discuss bodily functions or allow certain body parts to be examined. This does not bother others. Hygiene practices vary according to beliefs, living conditions, personal resources, and physical characteristics.

Mental Illness. Some cultural groups attach a stigma to mental illness and psychiatrists. They may not attach the same stigma to impairments of physical health. Some groups may feel that the mental symptoms manifested are a healthy reaction to an emotional crisis. Some cultural groups believe that the mind and body are united and are not separate entities. These cultures may have traditional healers who are expert at healing both the mind and the body. Some people may seek out traditional healers to heal the mind, while at the same time consult Western medicine to heal the body.

Learning Exercise

Cultural Patterns: Wellness Beliefs and Practices

To assist you in identifying your own cultural patterns in regard to wellness beliefs and practices, respond to the following statements and questions.
1. Describe what it means to you to have good health.
2. What are some of your own practices or beliefs about staying well?

Continued

3. Describe what it means to you to be sick.
4. List some foods in your diet that you believe help prevent illness.
   a. How does eating these foods prevent illness?
   b. What are some foods you must avoid to prevent illness?
5. List some foods in your diet that help you recover when you are sick.
   a. What illnesses do they cure?
   b. How do they cure illness?
6. Discuss complementary and alternative medicine (CAM) used by your family.
7. If you use CAM and biomedicine, do you inform the physician of CAM use, including herbs, during a clinic visit?
8. Describe your attitude toward mental illness.
   a. Describe what you think causes mental illness.
   b. Who do you think should treat mental illness?
   c. How do you believe mental illness is best treated?

Pregnancy and Birth Beliefs and Practices

There is a variety of ways different cultures welcome a new member into the world.

Learning Exercise

Cultural Patterns: Pregnancy and Birth Beliefs and Practices

To assist you in identifying your own cultural patterns in regard to birth beliefs and practices, respond to the following statements and questions about your family's customs regarding pregnancy and birth.

1. Do the females in your family receive prenatal care?
2. How is pain expressed during labor?
3. Who attends the birth?
4. Where does birth take place?
5. Who delivers the baby?
6. Is bonding encouraged?
7. What special practices take place after birth and during the postpartum period?
8. Are there special practices regarding the placenta and umbilical cord?
9. Is breast-feeding encouraged?
10. Are there precautions regarding breast-feeding?
11. Is birth control encouraged? Allowed?

Terminal Illness and Death Beliefs and Practices

Generally, death and dying bring out strong emotions in most people. Be aware that some cultures have special taboos and prohibitions when death occurs. Roles that family and friends carry out at the time of death may vary. There are many differences in the way different cultures handle terminal illness for a member. When death does occur, the rituals practiced are numerous and varied.

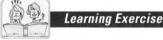

Learning Exercise

Cultural Patterns: Terminal Illness and Death Beliefs and Practices

To assist you in identifying your own cultural patterns in regard to terminal illness and death beliefs and practices, respond to the following statements and questions pertaining to a death in your family.

1. Is it acceptable to tell a terminally ill family member the diagnosis? If yes, who tells the family member?
2. Where does an anticipated death occur?
3. Who should be present when the death occurs?
4. Does your family require specific treatment of the body after death?
5. Does your family permit/encourage autopsy or organ donation?
6. Who makes the burial arrangements?
7. Describe what you believe happens to the spirit after death.
8. Does your family permit cremation?
9. Does your family have a funeral or memorial service?
10. Do you have a get-together after the burial? If so, for whom? What occurs during the get-together?
11. How does your family remember the dead?
12. Is autopsy, organ donation allowed?

Learning Exercise

Areas of Cultural Diversity

With your classmates, discuss your answers to statements and questions about various areas of cultural diversity, especially wellness and illness, birth, and death practices.

Regardless of which cultural group you belong, these exercises about cultural diversity have given you the opportunity to think about the many ways you and your peers differ. You will observe some of these differences in patients in the clinical area. Along with that awareness of and sensitivity to differences, a tolerance may develop for ways of doing things that may be different from yours.

INCREASING YOUR KNOWLEDGE OF CULTURALLY DIVERSE GROUPS

No one can be an expert on every culture in the world. Even "experts" of one culture are cautious about being labeled an expert. These people are aware of the ever-changing nature of cultures and of the important individual variations that occur within any cultural group. Experts are always cautious about stereotyping persons in any particular cultural group.

CATEGORIES OF MAJOR HEALTH BELIEF SYSTEMS

Anthropologists have developed a helpful framework for generally discovering and understanding health belief systems of groups. They divide health beliefs into three major systems: biomedicine, personalistic, and naturalistic.

- Biomedicine is the primary belief system of the United States and is also called "Western medicine." There is an effort to transform nursing curriculums so that they reflect multicultural concepts in nursing. However, it is possible that the curriculum of your school of practical/vocational nursing is set up to reflect biomedicine (Box 12-2).
- The personalistic system is found among groups native to the Americas, as well as those south of the Sahara (e.g., Chad and Niger) and among the tribal peoples of Asia (Jackson, 1993) (Box 12-3).
- The naturalistic system of beliefs developed from the traditional medical practices of the ancient civilizations of China, India, and Greece. Variants of this belief system are found today in the Philippines and among low-income African Americans and indigent white southerners (Jackson, 1993) (Box 12-4).

Box 12-2 Biomedical Health Belief

Cause of disease
- Abnormalities in structure and function of body organs, bacteria, viruses, biochemical alterations, immune system disturbance, environmental factors

How disease is diagnosed
- Physical exam, x-ray, CT scan, MRI, identification of pathogens by lab studies

How disease is treated
- Drugs, surgery, diet

Who cures the disease
- Physician

How disease is prevented
- Handwashing, covering mouth when sneezing, lifestyle (diet, exercise, etc.), immunizations, etc.

Adapted with permission from Jackson L. Understanding, eliciting, and negotiating patients' multicultural health beliefs. *Nurse Practitioner* 18(4):30-32, 37-38.

Box 12-3 Personalistic Health Belief

Cause of disease
- Punishment by a ghost, god, evil spirit, sorcerer, ancestor spirit, witch
- Breach of taboo, sin, evil eye, curse
- Above results in soul loss or theft, possession of spirit, poisoning, curse

How disease is diagnosed
- By a person with magic or supernatural powers

Who cures the disease
- Shaman, diviner, herbalist, magic/religious specialist

How disease is treated
- Counteract cause with herbs, prayer, rituals, laying on of hands

How disease is prevented
- Faithful observance of rituals (for example, honor ceremonies for ancestors), protective spells, wearing objects that have magic properties against evil eye, or injury (amulets)

Adapted with permission from Jackson L. Understanding, eliciting, and negotiating patients' multicultural health beliefs. *Nurse Practitioner* 18(4):30-32, 37-38.

Rarely does a group ascribe to all the beliefs in one system. You might see elements of each of the three systems at work in one individual. For example, a Hispanic patient with a strep throat

Box 12-4 | *Naturalistic Health Belief*

Cause of disease
- Imbalance of body elements
  Yin (cold)/yang (heat)
  Wet/dry
  Emotions
  Bad luck

How disease is diagnosed
- Cause of excess heat or cold identified

How disease is treated
- Regain body balance, foods, acupuncture, coining, cupping

Who cures the disease
- Physician or herbalist—no supernatural or magical powers

How disease is prevented
- Maintain balance of hot and cold in body, mind, spirit, and environment

Adapted with permission from Jackson L. Understanding, eliciting, and negotiating patients' multicultural health beliefs. *Nurse Practitioner* 18(4):30-32, 37-38.

might take an antibiotic as prescribed by the medical doctor, drink herbal teas as suggested by the curandero, and say prayers as suggested by the religious authority.

DIVERSITY PROFILES OF PREDOMINANT CULTURAL GROUPS IN THE UNITED STATES

At the beginning of the twentieth century the majority of immigrants to the United States were of European ancestry. If current immigration and birth trends continue, it is projected that by the year 2050 nearly 50% of Americans may be members of an ethnic minority (U.S. Census Bureau, 2004; *http://www. census.gov/ipc/www/usinterimproj/*). The Hispanic population will be 24.4%, Asian 8%, African American 14.6%, American Indian/Alaskan Native 1.4%, and the white population 50.1%, of the total population (U.S. Census Bureau, 2004). Box 12-5 profiles these culturally diverse groups.

Box 12-5 | *Diversity Profiles of Predominant Cultural Groups in the United States*

These profiles are intended to be a general sketch of the culture of the group.

African Americans
- **Origin:** from Africa as slaves
- **Family structure:** matriarchal, nuclear and extended family, fictive kin (not really relation, for example, "Aunt" Bessie)
- **Religion:** Protestant denominations, Catholicism, and Islam
- **Food preferences:** chicken, fish, leafy greens, yams, grits, and cornbread
- **Illness beliefs:** illness results from bad spirits, a hex, a spell, as punishment from God. May treat illnesses with home remedies, teas, herbs, compresses. May wait until illness becomes serious before seeking medical care. May visit a spiritualist or folk healer.

Hmong
- **Origin:** Vietnam, Laos, Thailand, Burma
- **Family structure:** patriarchal. Nuclear family plus extended family (father, mother, brothers, sisters, uncles, aunts, nieces, and nephews) considered one family.

- **Religion:** animism (worship of deceased ancestors). This may be replaced by or combined with Catholicism and Buddhism.
- **Food:** rice the main food and served at each meal. Noodles, rarely eat fruit, adults rarely consume dairy products.
- **Illness beliefs:** imbalance between spirit and the body. Natural and supernatural causes of illness. Natural plants, roots, and herbs used to cure a sick person. Shaman may be called to visit sick person in hospital. Healing rituals performed at home. May use cupping, coining, and pinching of skin as cure.

Hispanics
- **Origin:** Mexico, Puerto Rico, Cuba, Spain, Central America (El Salvador, Guatemala, Honduras, Nicaragua, Panama, Costa Rica, Belize), South America (Colombia, Ecuador, Peru, Argentina, Venezuela, Chile, Bolivia, Uruguay, Paraguay).

The following information may vary by country.
- **Family structure:** nuclear, extended, patriarchal. Family not always defined by blood or marriage.

Box 12-5 | *Diversity Profiles of Predominant Cultural Groups in the United States—cont'd*

- **Religion:** Catholic but changing to various Protestant Evangelical religions, Pentecostal and other sects/groups, African spirit religion, voodoo or a combination of these.
- **Food:** rice, beans, spices, food choices vary due to socioeconomic status, country of origin and location within country. Many have "hot" and "cold" foods. Some think American food is bland.
- **Illness beliefs:** a punishment from God for bad behavior or God's will, evil eye (*mal de ojo*), evil spells, fright (*susto*) magic, "hot" and "cold" imbalance, lack of cleanliness, humoral (body fluids) imbalance.

American Indians/Alaskan Natives

- **Origin:** North America. The federal government of the U.S. recognizes 550 tribes, bands, and nations with additional 200 tribes not federally recognized. This population is very diverse and retention of traditional customs and the level of acculturation is vastly different. Tribes within geographic areas differ as do people within tribes (Lipson and Dibble, 2006).
- **Family structure:** matriarchal, patriarchal, kinship roles extensive and fictive at times.
- **Religion:** traditional beliefs, Christian, combine different religious practices.
- **Food:** diet high in fat, salty, and sugary.
- **Illness beliefs:** violation of taboos, body, mind, spirit out of harmony with God, nature. May use native healers and ceremonies to restore harmony

in conjunction with Western medicine. Sacred objects should not be touched or moved by staff.

Arab Americans

- **Origin:** There are 21 Arab nations and, as with other cultural groups, there is great variation based on country of origin, social class, education, urban or rural origin, and time in the United States. Most are Muslim (Lipson and Dibble, 2006). Approximately 128 countries have people of the Muslim religion. Not all of these people are Arab but the culture of the Islam religion links people from these various countries. Islam and how it affects your patient care is presented in Chapter 13.

Notes:

Information about "yin" and "yang" can be accessed at *http://www.feng-shui-institute. org/yinyang.htm.*

Information about cupping, coining, and pinching can be accessed at *http://ethnomed.org/ ethnomed/clin_topics/cambodian/ethno_ wind.html#traditional.*

Information about "evil eye" can be accessed at *http://skepdic.com/evileye.html.*

Information about humoral pathology can be accessed at *http://anthro.palomar.edu/medical/ humoral_pathology.htm.*

Information about curanderos can be accessed at *http://www.tsha.utexas.edu/handbook/ online/articles/CC/sdc1.html.*

Adapted from Reinhardt E: *Through the Eyes of Others—Intercultural Resource Directory for Health Care Professionals.* Minneapolis: University of Minnesota School of Public Health, 1995, pp. 5–6, 8–14; Lipson J, Dibble S: *Culture and Clinical Care.* The Regents, Univ. of CA, School of Nursing, 2006, UCSF Nursing Press.

DEVELOPING CULTURAL COMPETENCE IN HEALTH CARE SITUATIONS

You have started the long road to becoming a practical/vocational nurse who gives culturally competent care. Up to this point, participating in this chapter has given you the opportunity to do the following:

- Identify your culture and its strengths and limitations.
- Recognize how your culture affects your thinking and behavior.

- Discover how persons are similar despite their cultural group.
- Discover how persons are unique despite their cultural group.
- Gain knowledge of the three major health belief systems to increase your awareness of different worldviews about the cause, treatment, and prevention of disease.
- Gain awareness of ethnocentrism that can help you respect health beliefs and practices of others when they are different from your health beliefs and practices.

• Learn to respond flexibly when your values and assumptions differ from those of your patients.

Your next step to cultural competence is to develop a knowledge base for a few cultures different than your culture.

IDENTIFY YOUR AGENCY'S CULTURAL GROUPS

Identify the cultural groups in your community that are served by local health care agencies. Use the following blank lines to list the groups. It is necessary to be knowledgeable about the cultural groups that you frequently come across in your community.

_____

_____

_____

_____

Learning Exercise

Your Area's Cultural Groups

1. A helpful learning activity is to hear reports from peers about various cultural groups.
2. Remember to think beyond the more traditional cultural groups, based on ethnicity. Include the disabled, elderly, single parents, alternative lifestyles, etc.
3. Read about the different cultures that are served in your area. Use the References and Suggested Readings listed at the back of this book for this chapter, internet sources in the text, and the resources of your learning resource center (LRC), as suggested in Chapter 5, to find texts and articles about specific cultural groups. Google a specific group to obtain information (*http://www.google.com*).
4. View documentaries on television about cultural groups.
5. Attend community events sponsored by cultural groups.
6. Attend graduations, weddings, birth celebrations, and funerals of different cultures when the opportunities present themselves.
7. Attend a religious service of a cultural group.
8. Read novels involving different cultures.
9. Attend seminars about cultural groups.

10. Invite a member of a cultural group to class to talk about the health/illness beliefs of the group of whom he/she is a member.

MODIFY YOUR WORK SETTING

The health care environment can be made more "welcoming" to culturally diverse patients. Many of these changes require little cost or time to implement, but the results can promote better health and compliance among culturally diverse patients. Box 12-6 includes suggestions for modifying the workplace environment for the practical/vocational nurse working in health care agencies with culturally diverse patients.

Box 12-6 | ***Modifying the Environment to Accommodate Culturally Diverse Patients***

• Identify the various cultural groups that use the health care facility.
• Post welcome signs in the languages of the groups you serve.
• Arrange for messages on answering machines to include the languages of the patients you serve. Place magazines in waiting rooms that reflect the diversity of the patients you serve.
• Include background music that reflects the diversity of the patients you serve.
• Provide handouts, appointment cards, and patient education materials in the languages of the patients you serve.
• Decorate the environment (pictures, posters, objects, etc.) to reflect the diversity of the patients you serve.
• Stock adhesive bandages that do not match any specific skin tone-for example, Walt Disney characters for children and fluorescent or varied colors for adults.
• In waiting areas, provide books, toys, and multicultural videos for children that promote acceptance of diversity. Barney, Sesame Street, Blues Clues, and Spongebob Squarepants themes are especially effective and accepted.

Adapted from Reinhardt E: *Through the Eyes of Others—Intercultural Resource Directory for Health Care Professionals*. Minneapolis: University of Minnesota School of Public Health, 1995, pp. 19-20.

CARE PLANNING FOR CULTURALLY DIVERSE PATIENTS IN YOUR SERVICE AREA

Because of short staffing and heavy workloads, your 55-year-old Hmong patient's cultural assessment on admission was not done. This patient speaks limited English. For the past 2 days while in the hospital, this patient has not eaten his breakfast, which comes to the floor at 7:30 AM. You refer to the topic Hmong *in* Culture and Nursing Care: A Pocket Guide *(Lipson and Dibble, 2006). The guide states that Hmong usually eat two to three meals a day. But if only two meals are eaten a day, the first meal is usually eaten at 9 AM or 10 AM. The licensed practical/vocational nurse sends a note to the Dietary Department to schedule two meals a day for this patient (breakfast at 9:30 AM and the evening meal at the regular time that trays are delivered).*

Each patient of a different culture needs to have data gathered regarding activities of daily living (ADLs) and personal health beliefs and practices. Develop a fact sheet for collecting data for each patient (Box 12-7). Use your culture resources and select topics and questions from the exercises found in this chapter. Clarify ADLs and health beliefs and practices for your patient.

Use reference guides that present general information about different cultural groups. These guides are helpful because they offer general information about, for example, wellness and illness beliefs and practices, nutritional preferences, and communication issues, when you come across a patient of a culture with which you are unfamiliar. These quick sources of **generalities of various cultural groups** are a starting point that make you aware of the topics to

---

Box 12-7 | *Sample Data Gathering Sheet using a Traditional Hmong Patient as an Example*

The following twelve questions are assessment items for all patients. *In italics in parentheses are generalizations from the text about traditional Hmong culture that explain the data collected for this patient. The explanations are applicable to the culture of the traditional Hmong group only.*

   Patient: Culture: **Traditional** Hmong

1. What language do you use to speak/read? *(The Hmong written language developed in the 1950s. Most elderly Hmongs are illiterate in their own language.)*
2. Observe eye contact during questions. *(Consider prolonged, direct eye contact rude.)*
3. Observe reaction to handshake when introducing self. *(Handshakes are appropriate.)*
4. How long have you lived in the United States? *(Assimilation may occur the longer a person is in the dominant culture.)*
5. What is your religion? What is its importance in your daily life? *(May have animistic beliefs in which spirits inhabit objects and natural settings. Worship ancestors with ceremonies so that ancestors will bring good fortune and protect the family from harm. Buddhism.)*

6. What caused your present illness? *(Traditional causes of illness might be soul loss or illness caused by an ancestral spirit.)*
7. How can your illness be best treated? *(In traditional religious/spiritual beliefs, a shaman is necessary to communicate with the spirit world to learn why the person is ill and what sacrifice is required to make the person well.)*
8. Do you use home remedies to cure illness? *(Cupping, coining, and pinching are used to release evil spirits or illness-causing toxins from the body.)*
9. What is your usual meal pattern at home? *(Hmong usually eat two to three meals a day. If two meals are eaten, the first meal is usually eaten at 9 AM or 10 AM.)*
10. What foods are in your usual diet? *(Rice with small amounts of meat, fish, and green vegetables. Fruit is rarely eaten.)*
11. Will you accept visitors while in the hospital? *(Visitors are welcomed and helpful in recovery.)*
12. Who in your family has decision-making authority? *(Women allowed opinions; father/husband makes final decisions.)*

Topics and explanations for data gathering sheet were taken from Lipson and Dibble: *Culture and Nursing Care: A Pocket Guide.* San Francisco: UCSF Nursing Press, 2006, pp. 250–263.

include when collecting data (assessing) that need to be clarified and validated with the individual patient. Examples of reference guides include the following:

- **Lipson:** *Culture and Nursing Care: A Pocket Guide.* **San Francisco: UCSF Nursing Press, 2006.** This reference lists information for the same topics used for learning activities, plus more topics for 24 ethnic groups found in the United States.
- **D'Avanzo:** *Pocket Guide to Cultural Assessment.* **St. Louis: Mosby, 2008.** This *truly* pocket-sized reference book contains information for many of the topics you have been using for learning activities, plus more general information for 180 different cultures throughout the world, listed by country.
- **The Transcultural Nursing website** (*http://www.culturediversity.org*) provides information pertaining to people from diverse cultural backgrounds with a range of cultural behaviors in health and illness.

The references explain the limitations of their use in introductory chapters. *Be sure to read the preface and introductory material!* The website presents generalizations about cultural groups. When using this information, it is important to avoid stereotyping your patient. Use Box 12-8 as a guide to help you avoid falling into the stereotype trap.

Suspect cultural differences when a patient is not following the plan of care, refuses treatment, is a "problem" patient, etc. Question the patient about his or her ADLs and wellness and illness beliefs. When cultural differences are identified, follow Jackson's (1993) suggestions for negotiating patient care with culturally diverse patients. These examples follow. Doing so will result in fewer dissatisfied patients and more compliance with the plan of care.

If the Hmong patient in the situation at the beginning of this section did have a cultural assessment on admission, or if his nurse had questioned him as to the reason for refusing to eat breakfast, it would have been discovered that he did not like oatmeal and bacon and eggs. The items were foods selected by the staff because

---

Box 12-8 | *How to Avoid Stereotyping Culturally Diverse Patients*

- Avoid automatically applying the information you gain to all individuals in a cultural group. To do so is called the "cookbook method" of learning about different cultures.
- To apply information by the cookbook method makes you guilty of stereotyping individuals; that is, assuming that everyone in that cultural group is the same.
- You have learned that classifying people as being the same, just because they share the same religion, lifestyle, or ethnic background, is stereotyping.
- Expect personal variations within each cultural group about which you gather information.
- Behaviors found in articles, reference books, and on the Internet containing culture and nursing care for various cultural groups can be applied generally to cultural groups as a whole but cannot automatically be applied to every individual in that group.
- Variable, individual differences exist because of the changing nature of the culture, the patient's personal life experiences (including hospitalization), age, religion, and adaptation to a new culture.
- No individual is a stereotype of one's culture of origin. Individuals are a unique blend of the diversity found within each culture.
- Gather cultural data for each patient. Discover the behaviors in your culture guide that apply to your patient.
- Look at information about cultural groups as explaining behavior in patients, not predicting behavior.

Adapted from D'Avanzo C: *Pocket Guide to Cultural Assessment.* St. Louis: Mosby, 2008.

---

they were uncertain if he could read the hospital menus. Because "Hmong people are very polite and reticent" (Lipson, 2006), he did not bring this matter to the attention of staff. He merely did not eat. When questioned about his continued refusal of breakfast, he admitted that he likes Rice Krispies and frequently eats this cold cereal for breakfast at home. The principle governing this situation is that general group behavior *sometimes explains* observed behavior (he did not complain out of respect), but it is *not predictive* of individual behavior (he did not eat because the meals were served at inappropriate times; he did not eat breakfast because he did not like the foods that were served).

SPECIFIC EXAMPLES OF ADAPTING PLANS OF CARE FOR CULTURALLY DIVERSE PATIENTS

Jackson (1993) offers suggestions for discovering the health beliefs of patients, along with guidelines to develop plans of care that incorporate those beliefs through a process of negotiation with the patient. Jackson points out that discovering specific health beliefs is easier if the nurse is familiar with a specific culture, but this is not absolutely necessary. She suggests ways of negotiating a treatment plan with culturally diverse patients. The practical/vocational nurse can collaborate with the professional nurse to incorporate these beliefs into the patient's plan of care:

1. *Discover the health beliefs of the individual.* Be respectful and open-minded when you question the patient about the cause of the health problem, when it started, its severity, its course, the problems it has caused in the patient's life, and the treatment the patient thinks will cure the disease. *Avoid assuming anything.* When you are unsure of anything, ask! In situations of cultural diversity our patients are the teachers and we are the students.

2. *Negotiate treatment plans with the patient.* Avoid trying to change patients' beliefs. This is an impossible feat. Cultural health practices are deeply ingrained. Tradition means more than your word does, even though you are a person representing a health profession. Instead, involve the patient in making decisions about his or her own care. Do so in a way that does not threaten the patient's beliefs and practices or conflict with them. Explain from the biomedical point of view the cause of the disease, how the body is altered by the disease, the role of treatment, and the expected outcome. Then

compare the patient's belief system with that of biomedicine. All patients need to have this information to help ensure their cooperation with the plan of care. See Box 12-9 for an example of **negotiating** treatment plans with the patient.

| Box 12-9 | *Negotiating Treatment Plans with the Patient*

SITUATION
Nancy Thai, a Cambodian refugee, resides in Chicago with her husband and three children. She delivered an 8-pound boy early this morning at St. Mary's Hospital. The practical/vocational nurse who was assigned to Mrs. Thai on the day shift reported to the evening staff that the patient was "uncooperative." Specifically, Mrs. Thai refused to eat and take her pills. In frustration the nurse said, "I just don't know what to do with her."

CULTURAL HEALTH BELIEFS IN THIS SITUATION
Mrs. Thai's health beliefs include the belief that pregnancy and birth weaken the body. Also, blood loss during delivery is considered a yin (cold) condition. Mrs. Thai believes that for 1 month after delivery a mother must have a yang (hot) diet to restore strength, keep the stomach warm, counteract heat loss, prevent incontinence, and prevent itching at the site of the episiotomy. Among preferred foods are rice, pork, and chicken. Cold foods (e.g., beef, salad, sour foods), as well as cold water, are viewed as bad for the stomach and the teeth.

NEGOTIATING TREATMENT PLANS
The nurse assigned to Mrs. Thai on the evening shift informed her that the doctor had ordered pills to help prevent bleeding after delivery. After discussing this, Mrs. Thai agreed to take her pills with warm water. In a respectful manner the evening nurse asked if Mrs. Thai did not like the hospital food. Mrs. Thai smiled and explained her need for a yang diet. The evening nurse said that she could arrange to have the dietary department send rice, chicken, or any other food Mrs. Thai would find helpful after childbirth. Mrs. Thai said her husband would bring rice and chicken from home. The nurse canceled Mrs. Thai's food order but requested a pot of hot water, silverware, and napkins for her use.

3. *Preserve the beliefs and practices that are helpful to the patient.* Starting in 1993 the Office of Alternative Medicine of the National Institutes of Health began to identify, study, and bring together the best healing practices of other cultures with those of Western medicine. Many of the beliefs and practices of non-Western systems of health beliefs have proved beneficial. Examples are acupuncture and acupressure. More are about to be approved. Other practices of your patient may not yet have been researched or found effective. Collaborate with your professional nurse about these practices. If they seem to help the patient and do no harm, include them in the plan of care, regardless of your ability to see the benefit of the practice. These practices have special significance and meaning to some individuals, despite the fact that you may be unable to see how or whether they help. See Box 12-10 for an example of **preserving** the beliefs and practices that are helpful to the patient.

4. Repattern harmful practices. Harmful practices prevalent in Western society include smoking, diets high in fat, refined grains and refined sugar, and lack of exercise. In Burma, when a woman is pregnant, extreme dietary restrictions are imposed. In Cambodia, mud is placed on the umbilicus of newborns. These practices are dangerous. If followed, these practices could lead to high blood pressure, heart disease, maternal toxemia, poor fetal development, and tetanus in the newborn. Explain your reason for opposing a harmful practice and offer alternatives. See Box 12-11 for an example of repatterning harmful practices.

When practical/vocational nurses demonstrate (1) awareness of and respect for the many cultural groups in their service area, (2) knowledge about these cultural groups, and (3) skill in applying their knowledge in a caring manner, they are on the road to delivering culturally competent care.

Box 12-10 | *Preserving the Beliefs and Practices That Are Helpful to the Patient*

SITUATION

Ted Washington, a 72-year-old African American, lives in a rural area of South Carolina. He was admitted to Brent Hospital with pneumonia and advanced osteoarthritis. An LPN, John, is his nurse. John cannot understand how anyone can get to such a state of ill health without seeing a doctor. John is especially upset because Mr. Washington could have prevented much of his disability from arthritis if he had followed a preventive program when he first developed symptoms of this disease.

CULTURAL HEALTH BELIEFS IN THIS SITUATION

Mr. Washington has been poor during his entire life. As with any person experiencing poverty, his main concern in life has been the present and getting through his problems on a day-to-day basis. Mr. Washington's time orientation is the moment (present), not the future; therefore, preventive regimens have not been central to his way of thinking. Persons with similar backgrounds and situations delay care until the disease interferes with their ability to work or results in a disability.

It cannot be said that Mr. Washington ignored his condition. He participated in self-treatment by using cultural health practices in the form of topical application of oils and ointments to his aching joints. These self-treatments helped Mr. Washington deal physically and psychologically with his condition. Mr. Washington looks at his disability as a punishment from God, who let something get into his joints. His belief stems from the wellness and illness beliefs brought to this country from Africa. These beliefs center on wellness as a state experienced when one is in harmony with nature. Illness is experienced as a state of disharmony with nature.

PRESERVING THE BELIEFS AND PRACTICES THAT ARE HELPFUL TO THE PATIENT

John supported Mr. Washington's application of oils and ointments. He applied massage lotion to Mr. Washington's joints at bedtime. John made arrangements for a friend of Mr. Washington's to bring his ointment from home. After clarifying self-treatment with the patient, John realized that such applications could give psychological comfort to the patient, as well as relieve pain. In the future John will make it a point to ask all newly admitted patients about self-treatment for their diseases.

Box 12-11 | *Repatterning Harmful Practices*

SITUATION
Over a 2-month period during the summer, a Chinese infant was seen in a New York clinic for diarrhea that did not respond to treatment. Stool cultures showed no unusual organisms. A change in formula did nothing to stop the diarrhea. During a home visit, the visiting nurse found a hot apartment with several bottles of home-prepared formula on the windowsill. Several other full bottles were in the refrigerator.

CULTURAL HEALTH BELIEFS IN THIS SITUATION
The child's mother explained that she had recently given birth. Because of this, she had to avoid cold. To avoid her exposure to the cold of the refrigerator, her husband would remove the bottles from the refrigerator that she needed during the day before he left for work, and line them up on the windowsill.

REPATTERNING THE PATIENT'S HARMFUL PRACTICES
The visiting nurse explained that by being exposed to the heat of the day, the formula would grow germs that could cause diarrhea. She asked if there was a way that the bottles could be kept cold until needed. After some thought, the mother said she could put on a hat, coat, and gloves before removing bottles from the refrigerator. The nurse agreed with this plan. The baby had no further episodes of diarrhea.

Reproduced with permission from Jackson L: Understanding, eliciting and negotiating patients' multicultural health beliefs. *Nurse Practitioner* 18:30-32, 37-38, 42, 1993.

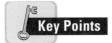 **Key Points**

- A good place to start learning about how people are different is to remind yourself that all persons are unique but also have similarities.
- Everyone shares the nine basic daily needs. How individuals meet these needs varies with their culture, the learned ways they have of doing things.
- One guideline in health care is the philosophy of individual worth, the confidence that all persons are unique and have value regardless of the way they view their world, and they deserve the best nursing care you can give.
- Awareness of cultural diversity is important for practical/vocational nurses so that they can avoid false assumptions and misunderstandings about the patients in their care.
- The first step in understanding other people's culture is to understand your own culture. It is important to be aware of your personal beliefs and practices in the areas of family, religion, communication, educational background, economic level, pregnancy, wellness and illness beliefs and practices, and death and dying.
- Some ways to learn about cultural diversity include reading about different cultures, especially those found in your geographical area, and actively listening to reports from your peers who are culturally different.
- Cultural characteristics of groups are not predictive of behavior of individuals in a group. They are generalizations. *Always allow for individual variations within specific groups.*
- Understanding your own culture, attaining sensitivity to cultural diversity, gaining knowledge about other peoples' culture, and adapting the plan of care to reflect the patient's health and illness beliefs puts you well on the road to providing culturally competent nursing care.

REVIEW ITEMS

1. Select the term practical/vocational nurses need to avoid when studying different cultures.

   1. Stereotyping
   2. Socialization
   3. Enculturation
   4. Assimilation

2. Select the statement that best illustrates the philosophy of individual worth.

   1. All individuals are unique and have value regardless of their differences in how they meet daily needs.
   2. People belonging to ethnic groups and minority groups have different daily needs in most needs categories.
   3. People of different cultures need to be approached as if their culture is the best of all culture groups in the area.
   4. People of color are sensitive about their differences and need to have them downplayed in patient situations.

3. An Asian-American resident in a nursing home does not want to follow the nursing care plan regarding diet. The best course of action for the nursing staff would be to:

   1. Insist the resident accept the diet as ordered.
   2. Document the stubbornness of this resident.
   3. Avoid making an issue of his noncompliance.
   4. Consider the possibility of cultural differences.

4. Mr. Metoxen, a member of the Oneida Tribe of Indians, was admitted to the medical floor, diagnosed with angina. He is to receive nitroglycerin PRN for chest pain. Select the priority cultural concern of the practical/vocational nurse for administering pain medication to a patient whose culture values stoic behavior.

   1. That the drug be kept in a dark container to protect it from light.
   2. That the drug is always kept with the patient when he is walking.
   3. That nonverbal signs of pain not be overlooked in this situation.
   4. That the patient's pain level be assessed at the beginning of the shift.

ALTERNATE FORMAT ITEM

Practical/vocational nurses use culture and nursing care guides to gather information about different cultures. Which of the following suggestions apply to the use of culture reference guides? *(Select all that apply.)*

1. Avoid applying information automatically to all members of a culture.

2. Variation in any member of the same cultural group does not occur.

3. Assume that all members of a cultural group are the same in all aspects.

4. Information obtained explains behavior but does not predict behavior.

5. Once you gather data for one patient, this info can be applied to others.

Spiritual Needs, Spiritual Caring, and Religious Differences

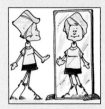

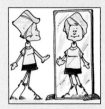 **evolve** http://evolve.elsevier.com/Hill/success/

evolve http://evolve.elsevier.com/Hill/success/

Objectives

On completing this chapter, you will be able to do the following:

1. Differentiate between spirituality and religion.
2. Identify the difference between the spiritual and emotional dimensions of individuals.
3. Discuss the practical/vocational nurse's role in providing spiritual care to the patient and the family.
4. Discuss nursing interventions that can be used to meet the spiritual needs of patients.
5. List members of the health care team who can help provide spiritual care for patients.
6. Discuss personal religious and/or spiritual beliefs, or the absence of them, and how these beliefs will influence nursing practice.
7. Discuss the general beliefs and practices that account for the differences among various Western, Middle Eastern, and Eastern religions, philosophies, and groups in the United States and Canada.
8. Describe nursing interventions/considerations of patients of various religions, philosophies, and groups.

Key Terms

Agnostic (ăg-NŎS-tĭk, p. 209)
Allah (ĂL-ă, p. 217)
Atheist (Ā-thē-ĭst, p. 209)
Buddha (BŪ-dă, p. 221)
Christ (p. 212)
Emotional needs (p. 206)
Parish nurse (p. 207)
Pastoral care team (PĂS-tĕ-RĂL, p. 208)
Reincarnation (RĒ-ĭn-kăr-NĀ-shŭn, p. 221)

Religion (p. 206)
Religious denomination (dĕ-NŎM-ĭ-NĀ-shŭn, p. 209)
Rituals (p. 209)
Spirit (p. 206)
Spiritual caring (p. 206)
Spiritual dimension (dĬ-MĔN-shŭn, p. 206)
Spiritual distress (p. 209)
Spiritual needs (p. 206)
Spirituality (SPĬR-ĭ-chū-ĂL-ĭ-tē, p. 206)

 Keep in Mind

How important would it be to you to have your spiritual practices known by staff if hospitalized?

Jan, the evening nurse, found Thomas Bernes, age 32, sitting up in bed crying and moaning with what she interpreted as pain after a testicular biopsy that was positive for cancer. After assessment, she volunteered to get Thomas some pain medication, but he refused. Thomas shouts, "Why did I have to get cancer? Why me?" Then he says, "Oh, I'll be fine. Just let me meditate and pray and I will get rid of the pain myself." Jan quickly and quietly leaves the room so Thomas can be alone.

The North American Nursing Diagnosis Association (NANDA-I) includes spiritual distress as one nursing diagnosis in its listing. In the foregoing patient situation Thomas was in spiritual distress. A minister or priest might have been able to address Thomas' problem, but Thomas needed immediate spiritual care. It would have been helpful to Thomas if his nurse had offered to spend time with him and encouraged him to talk about what he was thinking and feeling at that time. Nursing has always embraced a holistic approach to patient care—care of the body, mind, and spirit. Despite the NANDA-I diagnosis, some nurses are uncomfortable with matters of the spirit. Some have not had adequate education in how to deal with patients in this aspect of care. This chapter will help you to do the following:

- Differentiate spiritual matters from religious matters.
- Provide interventions for the patient in spiritual distress.
- Develop awareness of various religious beliefs and practices of patients and peers.

SPIRITUALITY AND RELIGION

Spirituality is an essential part of being human. The word comes from the Latin word *spiritus*, which means "breath" or "air". The spirit is the very essence of a person, the innermost part of a person that provides animation. The spirit is a life force that penetrates a person's entire being. It includes the beliefs and value system that provide strength and hope to persons. The spirit gives meaning to life. It is hoped that the spiritual self grows and matures throughout one's life. In the past, on her daytime television show, Oprah Winfrey provided a good look at the meaning of one's spirit with a segment called "Remembering Your Spirit." Segments included examples of individuals simplifying everyday life, spending time in nature, and using relaxation techniques.

Spirituality and religion are related terms but with different meanings. Religion may be a spiritual experience that contains specific beliefs and rituals. Religion may include spirituality. Spirituality, one's life force, does not necessarily include religion. Participation in a religion may include spirituality, but spirituality does not necessarily include participation in a religion. LeGere (Carson, 1989) differentiates between religion and spirituality as follows: Spirituality is not a religion. Spirituality has to do with experience; religion has to do with giving form to that experience. Spirituality focuses on what happens in the heart. Religion tries to make rules and capture that experience in a system.

SPIRITUAL VERSUS EMOTIONAL DIMENSION OF THE INDIVIDUAL

Meeting the spiritual needs of patients through spiritual caring differs from providing emotional support. The spiritual dimension of a person gives insight into the meaning of life, suffering, and death. This dimension refers to the relationship of an individual to a higher power. Emotional needs include how people respond and deal with feelings of joy, anger, sorrow, guilt, remorse, and love, among others. The spiritual dimension of a patient's life requires the same emphasis that other daily needs receive. When spiritual needs of patients exist and are met, practical/vocational nurses can say they have directed care to the total person.

IMPORTANCE OF SPIRITUAL CARE

Spiritual care involves helping patients develop awareness of and maintain the following:

- Inner strength,
- Self-awareness,
- Life's meaning and purpose,
- Relationship to others, and
- Relationship to a higher power.

Florence Nightingale encouraged nurses to be instruments of spiritual caring in all situations. Avoid waiting for crisis situations to occur to be concerned about spiritual care. The Joint Commission requires spiritual assessments and interventions to support the spiritual needs of patients and families. As a practical/vocational nurse, you have the responsibility to provide spiritual care to patients and families.

WHO NEEDS SPIRITUAL CARE?

An individual's spiritual dimension is a very private and personal area. Although all people have a spiritual dimension, needs that arise in this area depend on a variety of situations and the individual's ability to cope with them. An example of nurses who routinely recognize spiritual needs are nurses working with patients in various church settings in a health ministry. The goal of these parish nurses is to keep their groups happy and healthy by treating the whole person—body, mind, and spirit. **Parish nurses** recognize the relationship between spirituality and health and encourage spiritual growth in their patients.

Crisis situations occur in all health care situations. They frequently surface in acute health care situations. Patients' beliefs and values can profoundly affect their response to these crises, their attitude toward treatment, and their rate of recovery. Be alert for the following patient situations that may intensify the need for spiritual care for patients and families:

- Hospitalization,
- Patients who are in pain,
- Patients who have a chronic or incurable disease,
- Patients who are dying,
- Families who have experienced the death of a loved one,
- Patients who are facing an undesirable outcome of illness, such as an amputation, and
- Patients who have lost control of themselves.

"When the body and mind are battered by time and use, the spirit, the very essence of the patient remains". (Schoenbeck, 1994)

GATHERING DATA FOR SPIRITUAL ISSUES

The first step to providing spiritual care for patients is to strive to be personally comfortable with spiritual matters. The second step is to become aware of your own spirituality and the spirit that is the essence of you. Gather data about your spiritual self. The following learning exercise can help you increase awareness of your personal spirituality.

 Learning Exercise

Your Personal Spirituality

1. How do you cope?
2. Who is your source of support?
3. Who are the significant people in your life?
4. With whom do you laugh?
5. Do you feel loved?
6. Do you have someone with whom to cry?
7. What gives your life meaning?
8. What brings joy to your life?
9. Do you believe in the power of prayer?
10. What are your beliefs about a higher power?
11. Do you have a relationship to a higher power?
12. Do you have a religious affiliation? If so, how do your religious beliefs affect your spirit?
13. What is your philosophy of life and death?

Critical Thinking Exercise

My Spiritual Sensitivity

Have you ever said or heard others say, "My spirit is broken"? What does this remark mean to you?

HOW DO I MEET THE SPIRITUAL NEEDS OF MY PATIENTS AND THEIR FAMILIES?

Once you know your spiritual self, you will be better able to help others meet their spiritual needs. When you acknowledge that your beliefs are effective for you but not necessarily for others, you will be able to set your beliefs aside when helping patients and families meet their spiritual needs. The questions in the previous learning exercise, "Your Personal Spirituality," can also be used to gather data for patients' spiritual condition. Respect for the belief system of patients and families can give strength, hope, and meaning to their lives. When working with patients and families, try to do the following steps:

- Ask questions to help patients and families verbalize beliefs, fears, and concerns, such as, "What do you think is going to happen to you (your father/mother?)" and "Who is your source of support?"
- Show interest through supportive statements (see Chapter 9).
- Listen with an understanding attitude. Be sure your body language and affective response reflect what you are saying.
- Respond as naturally to spiritual concerns as you do to physical needs.
- Help patients face the reality of a terminal illness without abandoning hope.
- Encourage the patient's active involvement in self-care, which can help uphold hope.
- Allow families to participate in care giving (e.g., offering fluids/ice chips, when allowed; wiping the patient's brow).
- Avoid false assurances; for example, "Everything will be okay."
- When a patient faces death, you can help to make the remaining days meaningful by attending to needs, respecting their beliefs and death practices, and approaching the patient in a supportive and empathetic manner. Feeling loved helps bring peace to the dying.

Box 13-1 lists spiritual care interventions that can be used by practical/vocational nurses.

| Box 13-1 | *Spiritual Care Interventions* |

- Ask open-ended questions.
- Actively listen to the patient. Sit beside the patient. Make eye contact.
- Be nonjudgmental of patients and their responses.
- Avoid giving advice or a lecture to the patient.
- Avoid being a proselytizer (i.e., a person who tries to convert another person to one's religion).
- Be aware of nonverbal messages from the patient.
- Understand the feelings of the patient, but avoid adopting those feelings for yourself. (See Chapter 9 for a discussion of sympathy versus empathy.)
- Expect to learn from patients.
- Stay with the patient after the person has received an unfavorable diagnosis.
- When patients request help with prayer, offer to pray with them.
- When a patient requests help with specific readings, offer to read to him or her.
- Assist the patient to participate in desired religious/spiritual rituals.
- Protect the patient's religious/spiritual articles.

PASTORAL CARE TEAM

The **pastoral care team** is made up of ministers, priests, rabbis, consecrated religious women (i.e., nuns/sisters), representatives of other religious organizations, and laypersons. All are educated to meet spiritual needs, in addition to religious needs, in a health care setting. The members of this team are allies with nurses in providing spiritual care. You can notify this team with a patient request to be visited. When members of the pastoral care team come to the unit to fill the request, inform them of the patient's background and condition. Describe the interventions you have incorporated into the patient's care to provide spiritual care. Remember that the pastoral care team does not relieve you of your responsibility to provide spiritual care.

By visiting, talking, and listening, the pastoral care team explores the patients' fears, hopes, and sources of strength. Because of federal privacy standards (see the Health Insurance Portability and Accountability Act [HIPAA] in Chapter 20), the health care facility may not make a patient's name available to church representatives without the patient's permission. Before being hospitalized/admitted, patients can personally notify their clergy regarding the planned hospitalization and desire for a visit. If an admitted patient requests a visit of personal clergy, follow the facility directive for arranging this request. Agency policies vary and are being tested nationwide.

HOW THE PATIENT MEETS SPIRITUAL NEEDS

PATIENT'S SPIRITUAL PRACTICES

Regardless of religious beliefs, or lack of them, *all* patients have a spiritual self. They also have spiritual needs and personal spiritual practices to meet those needs. Spiritual practices help individuals develop awareness of self, understanding of the meaning and purpose of life, and their relationship to a higher power. Examples of personal spiritual practices may include gardening, reading inspirational books, listening to music, meditating, watching select TV shows and movies, communing with nature, walking a labyrinth, practicing breathing techniques, enjoying art, enjoying fresh flowers, volunteering, expressing gratitude, counting blessings, walking, talking with friends and relatives, and participating in crafts and hobbies.

 Learning Exercise

My Spiritual Practices

Identify the spiritual practices that you use to meet spiritual needs.

_____

_____

RELIGION AND THE PATIENT

The religious self refers to the specific beliefs held by an individual in regard to a higher power. Some patients help to meet their spiritual needs by belonging to a specific religious denomination. A religious denomination is an organized group of people who share a philosophy that supports their particular concept of God or a higher power, as well as worship experiences.

Agnostics hold the belief that the existence of God can be neither proved nor disproved. Atheists do not believe that the supernatural exists, so they do not believe in God. Christians may find comfort and solace in their refuge in God, including passing into another life after death. The atheist does not have this belief. It may be difficult for the nurse who believes in the supernatural to relate to a person with atheistic beliefs. The nurse may feel unsuccessful in meeting the total needs of the patient who is an atheist because atheists do not believe in the supernatural. The spiritual aspect, however, is present in all individuals. Spiritual assessment and interventions are appropriate for agnostic and atheist patients. Encourage these patients to express personal feelings about life, death, separation, and loss. Avoid imposing personal beliefs and values on the patient.

VALUE OF RITUALS AND PRACTICES

The different rituals and practices of a religion are stabilizing forces for the patient. Rituals are series of actions that have religious meaning. They can bring the security of the past into a crisis situation. Concrete symbols such as pictures, icons, herb packets, rosaries, statues, jewelry, and other objects can affirm the patient's connection with a higher power.

The value of patients' rituals and religious practices is determined by their faith. Value is not determined by scientific proof of their benefit. There have been studies that have shown that people who have faith can recover more quickly from illness, surgery, and addiction and are less likely to die prematurely from any cause. When patients are not allowed to practice their religious rituals, practices, and responsibilities, they may feel guilty and uneasy. This can also affect their recovery. As a practical/vocational nurse, you need to develop an awareness of the general religious philosophy of the patient's belief system. If membership is claimed in a specific denomination, question the patient about the rituals and exercises that the patient believes in and practices. Spiritual distress can be observed in patients who are unable to practice their religious rituals. It also can be observed in patients who experience a conflict between their religious and spiritual beliefs and the prescribed health regimen (e.g., a Catholic patient with continuous, severe psychiatric problems who is advised to avoid pregnancy).

PATIENT AND PRAYER

Prayer is a spiritual practice of some individuals whether or not they are members of an organized religion. Prayer can put a patient in touch with a personal higher power. Sometimes prayer can decrease anxiety as effectively as a drug. Prayer helps some patients cope with their illness or situation. Honor the request of the patient who wants to pray privately. If the patient requests prayer, the nurse needs to assist the patient or seek assistance in this matter. When patients express an interest in praying, ask what prayer they would like to say. Try to accommodate the request.

Carson (1989) comments on conversational prayer, one of the many forms prayer can take. In this type of prayer the specific concerns and needs of the patient are included in the prayer. Carson provides the following interaction between a patient awaiting a cesarean section and a nurse who noticed the patient had been crying. It is an excellent example of the simplicity and effectiveness of conversational prayer.

Nurse: You have been crying. What's wrong?
Patient: I wanted to see my minister this morning, but he will not be able to get here before my surgery. I wanted him to pray for me and my baby.
Nurse: Well, I'd be happy to pray for you and the baby. Would that be okay?
Patient: Oh yes, would you please? This surgery really scares me.
Nurse: Dear God, please comfort this mother as she enters surgery.
Lift her fear and in its place give her peace and strength.
Let her know that you are with her and the baby.
Patient: Thanks so much, that really means a lot to me.

WHO IS THE RELIGIOUS AMERICAN?

Examples of the religious American include Hindu, Jew, Buddhist, Muslim, Lutheran (Evangelical Lutheran Church in America, Wisconsin Synod, Missouri Synod, and English Synod), Catholic (Roman Rite, Eastern Rite as Ukrainian Catholic, and Greek Catholic), Eastern Orthodox (Russian Orthodox and Greek Orthodox), Quaker, Presbyterian, Methodist, Church of Christ, Mennonite, Seventh-Day Adventist, Assembly of God, Mormon, Baptist (Independent and Southern Baptist Convention), Wiccan, Jehovah's Witness, Episcopalian, African Methodist Episcopalian, Christian Science, United Church of Christ, Moravian, Evangelical, Salvation Army, and nondenominational.

The First Amendment of the U.S. Constitution allows the free exercise of religious choice. Starting with the pilgrims, America has a long history of religious freedom and tolerance. *The United States is religiously diverse, as the aforementioned listings from the "Churches" section of the Yellow Pages of a telephone book indicate.*

RELIGION IN THE UNITED STATES

The U.S. Census Bureau does not ask about religion on the census questionnaire. The number of persons belonging to specific religious denominations and groups in the U.S. can be found at *http://www.adherents.com*. The approximate size of Protestant, Catholic, Jewish, and Islamic denominations in the U.S. follows:

- The 2000 Religious Congregations & Membership Study conducted by the Glenmary Research Council identified that all Protestant denominations accounted for 66 million members. Since the 2000 study, the number of mainline Protestants has decreased, and it is predicted that in the future Protestantism will not be a majority religion.
- The *2005 Yearbook of American and Canadian Churches* identified the Catholic Church as the largest single denomination in the United States with over 67 million members (Lindner, 2005).
- According to *The World Christian Encyclopedia*, 5.6 million Jews comprise the largest non-Christian, organized religion (Barrett, 2001).

- *The World Christian Encyclopedia* identified 4.1 million Muslims (Barrett, 2001). However, Muslim groups estimate that there are almost 8 million Muslims in the United States (Aita, 2006).

AVOIDING FALSE ASSUMPTIONS AND STEREOTYPES

The suggestions presented in Chapter 12, regarding the avoidance of false assumptions and stereotyping when caring for culturally diverse patients, also apply when caring for patients of different religions. Some nursing students may think that there is also a guidebook that will list nursing interventions when caring for patients who belong to different religions. As with different cultures, this type of approach can lead to false assumptions and stereotyping. Not only is there diversity among religious groups, but there is also diversity among members of a specific religion or group. It is a false assumption to expect that all individuals of a specific religion or belief system will believe exactly the same just because they are members of that religion or belief system. Avoid assuming that all Protestants, Catholics, Jews, Muslims, Buddhists, and Hindus, for example, believe in all the aspects of their formal religion/belief system. *Individual differences occur within every religious or belief systems group.* Members may have modified the degree to which they observe the practices of their religion or belief system based on age, experience, education, social group, etc. Avoid judging patients if there are variations in their beliefs. Each patient needs to have data gathered about their specific beliefs and religious practices (Box 13-2).

The nursing interventions provided in Boxes 13-3 to 13-8 and Tables 13-1 and 13-2 will serve as a reference to be used in meeting the religious needs of specific patients during your time as a student practical/vocational nurse. This information can also be used in your nursing career after you graduate. Each religion has specific beliefs and practices. Sometimes an individual will adapt them to fit his or her own circumstances. Clarify with the patient the specific beliefs and practices that offer comfort to them,

---

Box 13-2 | *Gathering Data for Religious Beliefs and Practices of Patients*

- Do you have a religious affiliation? If so, state it.
- What role does religion play in your life?
- Is prayer helpful to you?
- What is your source of strength and hope?
- What brings you comfort and joy?
- What religious rituals or practices are important to you?
- What symbols or religious books are helpful to you?
- What dietary inclusions or restrictions are a part of your religious beliefs?
- How does your religion view the source and meaning of pain and suffering?
- When ill, does your religion prohibit people of the opposite sex from giving care?
- Does your religion have special days when certain behaviors are mandatory or prohibited?
- (If death is imminent) Does your family have any special practices at the time of death?

---

and are preferred by them. Develop awareness of health issues and decisions that may involve religious or philosophical beliefs. The references at the end of this book can be used to learn more about a specific religion when such information is needed. Also, check *http://www.beliefnet.com*.

WESTERN AND MIDDLE-EASTERN RELIGIONS IN THE UNITED STATES AND CANADA

Judaism, Christianity, and Islam will be discussed as examples of monotheistic (belief in one God) Western and Middle Eastern religions found in the United States.

JUDAISM

Judaism is the oldest of faiths that have a belief in one God. In 1990 there were almost 18 million Jews worldwide. The prophet Abraham founded Judaism in approximately the twentieth century BC. The Holy Books of the Jews are the *Torah* and the *Talmud*. The *Torah* contains the written teachings, laws, and stories of Judaism. The

Talmud contains the oral teachings and explanations. Followers of Judaism are called Jews. Jewish clergy are called rabbis. Jews worship in buildings called temples or synagogues. The following are the major divisions of Judaism:

- **Orthodox Judaism:** Orthodox Jews follow the traditional faith and strictly adhere to rituals, including a kosher diet and keeping of the Sabbath. They consider the *Torah* and the *Talmud* as revealed by God and do not believe in completely integrating into modern society. Hasidism is an ultraorthodox form of Judaism.
- **Conservative Judaism:** Conservative Jews follow most traditional practices but adapt traditions to the modern world.
- **Reform Judaism:** Reform Jews stress the ethical and moral teachings of the prophets and autonomy of the individual. Rituals are performed that will promote a Jewish, God-filled life. Reformed Jews regard Judaism as evolving and subject to change. Reform Judaism does not accept the binding nature of Jewish law and believes that the *Torah* was written by human sources, rather than by God. Traditionally, Jewish identity is considered to be passed on through the mother. Reform Jews accept Jewish identity passed on through the father. Reform Judaism is the largest, fastest growing division of Judaism.

Box 13-3 lists beliefs and practices that need to be clarified for each patient and nursing interventions that have importance for health care workers in contact with patients who are Jewish.

CHRISTIANITY

Christianity is a 2000-year-old religion based on a belief in Jesus Christ as the Son of God. Followers of Christianity are called Christians.

General Beliefs of Christians

The Bible. The *Bible* is the sacred book of Christians. It contains writings divided into two sections: (1) the Old Testament, written before the birth of Christ; and (2) the New Testament,

---

Box 13-3 | *Beliefs, Practices, and Nursing Interventions for Jewish Patients*

GENERAL
Beliefs and Practices
- Jews believe in God but do not have a belief in Christ.

Nursing Interventions
- Avoid references to heaven or Jesus.

OBSERVATION OF SABBATH
Nursing Interventions
- If observed, provide time for rest, prayer, and/or study from sunset on Friday until after sunset on Saturday.
- If observed, provide yarmulke (skullcap) or prayer shawl. Ask family to provide these items.

OBSERVANCE OF DIETARY RULES (KOSHER DIET)
Beliefs and Practices
- If following a kosher diet, meat may be consumed a few minutes after drinking milk, but 6 hours must pass after eating meat before drinking milk.
- Some Jews do not eat pork, ham, Canadian bacon, eel, oysters, crab, lobster, shrimp, or eggs with blood spots.

Nursing Interventions
- Clarify if patient follows these dietary rules.
- If desired by patient, make arrangements for separate utensils for preparing and serving meat and milk dishes. If separate dishes are not available, these foods can be served in the original containers or on paper plates.

DYING JEWISH PATIENT
Beliefs and Practices
- Family and friends may want to be with the patient at all times.
- Some Jews do not believe in autopsies, embalming, or cremation.
- Some Jews may not want the nurse to touch the body of a deceased Jew.

Nursing Interventions
Some Jews may request that the nurse notify the Burial Society for preparation of the body for burial.

written after the birth of Christ. Different Christian groups use different versions of these writings. The number and names of books in the Bible differ between Catholics and Protestants.

Many Christian patients will find comfort in reading or having someone read to them selected passages from the *Bible*. Treat the patient's *Bible* with respect. In addition to believing it contains the inspired word of God, some people have received their *Bibles* as gifts commemorating special occasions, such as a wedding, graduation, confirmation, anniversary, or jubilee. Some *Bibles* list passages that can be used in specific patient situations, such as pain, sorrow, sleeplessness, etc.

Baptism. Baptism is the rite of admission to the Christian community. Christian groups give different meanings to Baptism. Some consider this rite a means of salvation, a way of washing away sin, a means of receiving the Holy Spirit (the third person of the Trinity, the belief of some Christians of the three persons in one God), an imprinting of character on the soul, and/or a promise of divine grace. Christian groups differ as to the age (infant, adult) at which a person may receive baptism. Although water is used for baptizing, the method differs among groups (pouring, sprinkling, immersion).

If an infant is in danger of death, baptism may be given if the religious beliefs of the parents include infant baptism. If the patient is Protestant and baptism is desired, it is preferable to have a witness. If death is imminent and the patient is Catholic, a witness is not necessary and anyone with the right intention may baptize. The procedure for baptism can be found in Box 13-4. Baptism beliefs and practices of Catholics and some Protestant denominations are included in Boxes 13-5 and 13-6.

Communion. Communion is partaking of consecrated (blessed) elements of bread and wine. Depending on the group, the bread is leavened (with yeast) or unleavened. Some groups use grape juice instead of wine. Communion has different meanings for different denominations. Examples of these differences include a remembrance of the Last Supper and a remembrance of Christ's death. Some groups look at the bread and wine as a symbol of Christ. Other groups believe

---

Box 13-4 | *Procedure for Baptism*

If baptism is desired/allowed:

Nursing Interventions
- Allow water to flow over and contact the patient's skin while saying the words, "Name (if known), I baptize you in the name of the Father, and of the Son, and of the Holy Spirit."
- If the patient is Catholic, death is imminent, and it is uncertain whether baptism was received in the past, baptism is administered conditionally. In this situation the following words are used: "If you are not baptized, I baptize you in the name of the Father, and of the Son, and of the Holy Spirit."
- Report the baptism to the chaplain or pastoral care team and the family.
- Document the baptism in the patient's record.

---

in the real presence of Christ. When caring for a patient of a specific affiliation, question the patient and family regarding specific beliefs and practices regarding communion. Boxes 13-5 and 13-6 include communion beliefs and practices of Catholics and some Protestant denominations.

Major Divisions of Christianity

The major divisions of Christianity are Catholicism, Protestantism, and Eastern Orthodoxy.

Catholicism. *Catholicism* consists of the Western or Roman Catholic Church, including Catholics of the Eastern Rite. Sometimes there is confusion between the Eastern Churches and Roman Catholicism. The Eastern Churches are either Catholics of the Eastern Rite or Eastern Orthodox

Catholics of the Roman Rite. The Catholic religion is the largest religious organization in the world. Catholics trace their faith from Christ through an unbroken line to the Pope. The Pope is considered to be the representative of Christ on earth. He is considered to be infallible, that is, incapable of being in error when speaking of matters of faith and morals. Beliefs are found in the *Bible* and tradition. Catholic clergy are called priests. Roman Catholic priests cannot marry. Women cannot be ordained. The administrative hierarchy of the Catholic Church consists of

Box 13-5 *Beliefs, Practices, and Nursing Interventions for Catholic Patients*

ROMAN CATHOLIC (WESTERN)
Baptism Beliefs
- Necessary for salvation and initiation into the community. This sacrament removes all sin. Person receives the Holy Spirit. Infant or adult may be baptized, usually by pouring or immersion.

Nursing Interventions
- If the patient is a gravely ill infant, a stillbirth, or a fetus, the nurse may baptize without a witness.
- If a patient or family member requests baptism and death is imminent, the nurse may baptize before the priest arrives.

Communion Beliefs
- Believe the bread and wine are the body and blood of Christ.

Nursing Interventions
- If sacrament is desired, follow agency privacy policy, developed to carry out HIPAA guidelines, to receive communion.
- Medicine and water may be taken before communion.
- If the patient's mouth is dry, water may be given after communion.

Sacraments
Nursing Interventions
- If requested, follow agency privacy policy to arrange for the sacrament of reconciliation and provide privacy when the priest hears the patient's confession.
- If desired by patient, follow agency privacy policy for arranging the sacrament of the anointing of the sick. (Some Roman Catholics may refer to this as the Sacrament of the Sick. Older Catholics may refer to this as the Last Rites.) This sacrament is for anyone seriously ill or weakened by old age. This sacrament is believed to offer hope, consolation, and peace; assist in physical, mental, and spiritual healing; and provide strength to endure suffering.
- If requested, follow agency's privacy policy to make arrangements for the priest to administer this sacrament.

Dietary Restrictions
If there are no health restrictions, Roman Catholics 14 years of age and older are to abstain from meat on Ash Wednesday and all Fridays during Lent. Catholics ages 14 to 59 are to fast (eat one full meal and two lighter meals) on Ash Wednesday and Good Friday. Fasting and abstaining is excused during hospitalization. Eastern Rite Catholics may be stricter about fasting.

Nursing Interventions
- Clarify practices with patient.

Sexuality
Abortion is not allowed. Natural methods of family planning are allowed.

Dying Catholic Patient
Catholic patients facing death may want to receive the last sacrament of the Christian. In addition to the anointing of the sick, the sacraments of reconciliation and Viaticum (the last communion that provides food for the journey from this life to the next) are administered.

Nursing Interventions
- Follow agency privacy rules to make arrangements for the priest to administer this sacrament. Cremation and organ donation are allowed.

EASTERN ORTHODOX CHURCHES
Baptism Beliefs
- Necessary for salvation. Infants are baptized by sprinkling or immersion.

Communion Beliefs
- Believe the bread and wine are the body and blood of Christ.
- Follow procedure for communion as with Catholic patient.

Sacraments
- Celebrate seven sacraments.

Nursing Interventions
- Follow procedure for anointing of the sick as with Catholic patient.

Dietary Restrictions
Abstain from meat and dairy products on Wednesdays and Friday during Lent.
- Ill patients are excused from this requirement.

Sexuality
Birth control and abortion are not allowed.

Box 13-5 | *Beliefs, Practices, and Nursing Interventions for Catholic Patients—cont'd*

Dying Eastern Orthodox Patient
The Last Rites are obligatory.

Beliefs and Practices
- Autopsy and organ donation are not encouraged. Euthanasia and cremation are discouraged.

Nursing Interventions
Follow agency privacy policy to arrange for priest to administer the Last Rites, preferably while the patient is conscious.

Box 13-6 | *Beliefs, Practices, and Nursing Interventions for Protestant Patients of 10 Denominations*

NURSING CONSIDERATIONS THAT PERTAIN TO ALL PROTESTANT PATIENTS
Nursing Interventions
- Because of federal privacy laws, inform patient that if a visit by personal minister or pastor is desired for communion, anointing, etc., patient needs to follow agency policy.
- Provide privacy if patient reads Bible.
- **Include on data-gathering list:**
- If patient is an infant and condition is serious, do parents desire baptism if child is not baptized?
- If patient is dying, what are family's beliefs about death and dying?

OLD ORDER AMISH (HOUSE AMISH)
Amish are a conservative division of the Mennonites. Old Order Amish worship in private homes. The Amish do not believe in health insurance and social security and rely on mutual aid in time of need. Patients may believe that sudden fright or blood loss may cause loss of the soul. Female patients may object to cutting their hair because of their belief that Holy Scripture forbids it.
- ***Baptism***: Adult baptism.

ASSEMBLY OF GOD
One of several American Pentecostal denominations. May believe in the power of prayer for healing.
- ***Baptism***: Receive Jesus Christ as Lord and Savior. Administered by immersion when person understands the meaning of baptism.
- ***Communion***: Yes.

BAPTIST
Started in the seventeenth century in the United States. Baptists regard the Bible as a complete, sufficient, and final authority in matters of faith. Interpret the Bible literally. Stress personal relationship with Jesus Christ. Discourage alcohol consumption.

- ***Baptism***: No infant baptism. Person needs to understand the meaning of Baptism. Adults are baptized by immersion. Baptism not considered a means of salvation.
- ***Communion:*** Considered a symbol and a remembrance of Christ's death.

EPISCOPALIAN
Began in the sixteenth century in England. Also called the Anglican Church in England. Service book is Book of Common Prayer. Clergy include bishops, priests, and deacons. Priests may marry. Women may be ordained.
- ***Baptism:*** Believe baptism is necessary for salvation. Infant baptism is performed by sprinkling.
- ***Communion:*** Believe that Christ is present in the bread and wine.

LUTHERAN
There are several Lutheran bodies in the United States. Ministers may marry. Believe in anointing and blessing when ill.
- ***Baptism:*** Conveys grace. Infants are baptized at 6 to 8 weeks of age by pouring, sprinkling, or immersion. In case of illness, invasive procedures, and emergent situations, infants may be baptized by their pastor, if possible. Baptism by a layperson is acceptable.
- ***Communion***: Believe the presence of Christ is real. Conveys grace.

METHODIST
Methodism started in the eighteenth century. There are several branches of the Methodist Church.
- ***Baptism:*** An outward and visible sign of an inward and spiritual grace. Infant and adult by sprinkling or immersion.
- ***Communion:*** Conveys grace. Open to everyone.

Continued

Box 13-6 | *Beliefs, Practices, and Nursing Interventions for Protestant Patients of 10 Denominations—cont'd*

PRESBYTERIAN

Began in Scotland and evolved from John Calvin in the sixteenth century. May avoid alcohol.

Baptism: Infant, usually by sprinkling. Signifies the beginning of life in Christ and not its completion.

Communion: Believe Christ is present in spirit.

QUAKERS (RELIGIOUS SOCIETY OF FRIENDS)
Beliefs and Practices

- Believe they receive Divine Truth from "inner" light supplied by the Holy Spirit. Services called meetings. Generally regard sacraments as nonessential to Christian life.

Nursing Interventions

- Clarify Baptism beliefs with patient. At birth, infant's name recorded in official church book.

SEVENTH-DAY ADVENTIST

Adventists observe the Sabbath from sunset on Friday to sunset on Saturday. Do not pursue their jobs or worldly pleasures during this time. Many Adventists are vegetarians and use soybean products as a protein source. These dietary practices are not mandatory. Adventists generally do not smoke or drink alcoholic beverages. Some Adventist patients may avoid beverages with caffeine. They believe that at death the body rests in the grave until the second coming of Christ.

Nursing Interventions

- Clarify diet restrictions.

Baptism: Makes one a church member. Adult by immersion. Opposed to infant baptism.

Communion: May practice washing of the feet in preparation.

UNITED CHURCH OF CHRIST

Formed in 1957 by merger of Congregational and Evangelical and Reformed Churches.

Baptism: Infant by pouring, sprinkling or immersion. When baptized, become church members.

Communion: Celebrated and open to all.

---

cardinals, archbishops, bishops, priests, and deacons. Buildings of worship for Catholics are called churches and cathedrals. A cathedral is the headquarters of a bishop, archbishop, or cardinal. Celebration of the Mass is the center of worship. The Eucharist (communion) is a commemoration of Christ's death and resurrection. There are seven sacraments: baptism, confirmation, Eucharist, penance, anointing of the sick, holy orders, and matrimony. The Society of Pius X is an example of an ultraconservative branch of the Roman Catholic Church that is in schism (separated from Rome).

Catholics of Eastern Rites. Catholics of Eastern Rites have the same beliefs as the Western or Roman Catholic Church. They recognize the Vatican and the Pope. They keep their own canon law, customs, and liturgy. Clergy are priests and bishops. Priests of this Eastern Rite, but not monks, may marry. Bishops are selected from among monks. Examples of Catholics of Eastern Rites include Armenian Catholic, Chaldean Catholic, Maronites, and the Catholics of the Byzantine Rite (e.g., Greek Catholics, Bulgarian Catholics, and Russian Catholics).

Orthodox Eastern Churches. There are approximately 250 million members of Orthodox Eastern churches worldwide. The Orthodox Eastern Church considers itself catholic (that is, universal) but does not recognize the Pope. The Roman Catholic Church considers these churches to be in schism because they refuse to submit to the authority of the Pope. Beliefs come from the Bible and tradition. Clergy are bishops, priests, and deacons. Priests may marry before ordination. *Matuska*, meaning Little Mother, is a title given to wives of Orthodox priests. Monks may not marry. Bishops are selected from among monks. There is no central authority in these Eastern churches. They are self-governed by a board consisting of a bishop and laymen. Some of these churches are headed by a patriarch. Seven sacraments are celebrated. The Virgin Mary is respected. Liturgies differ among nationalities but have similarities to the Roman Catholic Church; but services are more elaborate than Roman Catholic liturgies. Examples of Orthodox Eastern Churches are Orthodox of the Byzantine Rite (e.g., Greek Orthodox and Russian Orthodox), Armenian

Orthodox, and Jacobite churches. Box 13-5 lists beliefs and practices that need to be clarified for each patient and nursing implications for patients who are Catholic (Roman and Eastern). Eastern Orthodox beliefs and practices are also listed.

Protestantism. In the sixteenth century, Germany was part of the Holy Roman Empire and nearly all Roman Catholic. Protestantism began in 1517, when Martin Luther separated from the Catholic Church because of scandals in the church. Thus started the Reformation and the beginning of Lutheranism. As Lutheranism spread throughout Germany, Catholic clergy tried to limit changes affecting the Catholic Church and retain its authority in all church matters. John of Saxony led a group to a Catholic Church assembly. The group objected to the Catholic Church's plans to limit innovations in doctrine and practices in the Catholic Church. However, the group was never heard by the Catholic Church at the assembly. The group signed a *protestation* and became known as *Protestants* from then on (Gritsch, 2002). Protestants believe that their convictions are closer to New Testament Christianity. The chief characteristic of Protestantism is the acceptance of the Bible as the sole authority in matters of faith. It is believed that Christians are justified in their relationship to God *by faith alone* and *not by good works.* Examples of denominations and sects that came from the Reformation include Lutheran, Reformed, and Presbyterian. Depending on denomination, Protestant clergy are called ministers, pastors, etc. Protestant places of worship are called churches, temples, etc. During the second half of the nineteenth century, opposition to changes in Protestantism resulted in a conservative type of Protestantism called Fundamentalism. Southern Baptists are an ultraconservative form of Protestants. Box 13-6 lists beliefs and practices that need to be clarified for each patient and nursing interventions for patients of 10 Protestant denominations.

ISLAM

The word *Islam* implies peace. In the sixth century AD the prophet Muhammad founded Islam in Arabia. Followers of Islam are called Muslims. Muslims comprise approximately 20% of the world's population. Muslims believe in one God, Allah. Salvation depends on one's commitment to Allah and his teachings in the *Qur'an (Koran)*. This holy book contains the words of Allah as he spoke to Muhammad. Muslims pray in Arabic and worship in mosques. The imam is the leader of the Muslim congregation.

Muslims have many beliefs that are similar to Judeo-Christian doctrine. Examples include the belief in angels and God's prophets, such as Abraham, Moses, and Jesus. Muslims believe in paradise, hell, final judgment, prayer, fasting, and giving to the poor.

Islam is not one entity but has many interpretations resulting in diversity in its practice. There are two main divisions in Islam: the Sunni and Shi'ite sects. The majority of Muslims worldwide are Sunnis. Since Muhammad did not designate a successor when he died, the Sunni sect chose a successor who became the political leader of the community. Sunnis believe they must follow the Sunnah, the ethical and religious code from the sayings of Muhammad and vest religious and political authority with the community as guided by Islamic law and consensus of the *Qur'an* and the leaders. The Shi'ite sect believes that Muhammad designated his cousin and son-in-law, Ali, to be the leader of Islam after his death and vest all authority with the imam (the leader of a Muslim congregation) and ultimately the ayatollah (a high-ranking religious and political leader) and these leaders guide the teachings of Islam (Gellman and Hartman, 2002). Wahhabism is an ultraconservative form of Islam. Information about this reform movement can be obtained at *http://www.infoplease.com/ce6/society/A0851259.html.*

Despite different sects and divisions, the Five Pillars are the essential and obligatory practices all Muslims accept and follow. The Five Pillars are the following:

1. **The Profession of Faith:** This is a verbal pledge that there is only one God, Allah, and that Muhammad is the messenger of God. (Muslim mothers may whisper this pledge into a newborn's ear.)
2. **Prayer:** Muslims are called to prayer five times a day.

3. **Almsgiving:** This involves an annual payment of a certain percentage of a Muslim's wealth and assets. This money is distributed among the poor.

4. **Fasting:** During Ramadan, the ninth month of the Islamic calendar, adult Muslims abstain from dawn to sunset from food, drink, and sexual activity.

5. **Pilgrimage:** Adult Muslims who are physically and financially able are expected to perform the pilgrimage to Mecca (Islam's holiest shrine) at least once in their lifetime.

Jihad, meaning "to strive or struggle" in the way of God, is sometimes referred to as the sixth pillar of Islam, although it has no such official status. "In its most general meaning, it refers to the obligation incumbent on all Muslims, as individuals and as a community, to exert themselves to realize God's will, to lead virtuous lives, and to extend the Islamic community through preaching, education, and so on. A related meaning is the struggle for or defense of Islam, a holy war. Despite the fact that jihad is not supposed to include aggressive warfare, this has occurred, as exemplified by early extremists like the Kharijites and contemporary groups like ... Jihad organizations in Lebanon, the Gulf States, and Indonesia" (Esposito, 1998).

Male infants are circumcised. Islamic law does not prohibit contraception for married couples. No permanent damage to reproductive organs is allowed. Abortion is permitted if the mother's life is at stake and the fetus is not older than 4 months' gestation. Saving a life is one of the greatest merits and imperatives in Islam. Box 13-7 lists beliefs and practices that need to be clarified and nursing considerations for Muslim patients.

Box 13-7 *Beliefs, Practices, and Nursing Interventions for Muslim Patients*

GENERAL BELIEFS

Members of Islam may desire to pray to Allah five times a day (after dawn, at noon, in mid afternoon, after sunset, and at night).

Beliefs and Practices
- Rules of cleanliness may include eating with the right hand and cleansing self with the left hand after urinating and defecating.

Nursing Interventions
- If patient requests to face Mecca, the holy city of Islam, a bed or chair may be positioned in a southeast direction from the United States.
- If a Muslim brings the Koran, the holy book of Islam, to the health care facility, do not touch it or place anything on top of it.
- If a Muslim wears writings from the Koran on a black string around the neck, arm, or waist, these writings need to be kept dry and remain on the patient, because they are passages from the Koran.

OBSERVATION OF DIETARY RULES
Beliefs and Practices
- Some Muslims might not eat pork and pork products, eel, oysters, crab, lobster, shrimp, and meats from animals that have not been bled to death by a Muslim.
- Some Muslims might not drink alcoholic beverages.

Nursing Interventions
- Clarify dietary restrictions.

OBSERVATION OF FEMALE MODESTY
Beliefs and Practices
- Some Muslim women prefer to be clothed from head to ankle.

Nursing Interventions
- During a physical examination, female Muslims may prefer to undress one body part at a time.

DEATH PRACTICES
Beliefs and Practices
- Women may be barred from the room of a dying family member.
- The family may pray for the dying family member. The Imam usually reads from the Koran for the patient after death.
- After death, the body is turned toward Mecca.
- After death, the family washes the body, including all orifices, and seals them with cotton.

| Box 13-7 | *Beliefs, Practices, and Nursing Interventions for Muslim Patients—cont'd* |

- The body is wrapped in a white cloth for burial.
- The family may not permit organ donation, autopsies, or cremation in order to keep the body intact so that the person may meet God with integrity. These decisions may vary by country of origin.

- No embalming of bodies after death.
- Muslims try to bury the dead within 24 hours.

Nursing Interventions
The nurse may touch the body only after donning gloves.

Critical Thinking Exercise

Avoid Stereotyping Your Patients

Draw a concept map (see Chapter 4, Clustering) to show how to avoid stereotyping and avoiding false assumptions for a Muslim patient who is dying. Do the same for a patient of an ethnic group that is frequently seen in your community.

ADDITIONAL CHRISTIAN AND NON-CHRISTIAN RELIGIOUS/ SPIRITUAL GROUPS

Box 13-8 lists beliefs and practices that need to be clarified for each patient and nursing interventions for patients of various religious groups.

EASTERN RELIGIONS AND PHILOSOPHIES IN THE UNITED STATES AND CANADA

Because the Western and the Eastern worlds contain different value systems, the two worlds represent different ways of thinking that have molded the culture, including the worldview, of two different parts of the world. In the twenty-first century, cultures and religious practices of other countries have become more known to us because of travel, the mass media, and immigration of people from all over the world to the United States and Canada.

The Eastern world (e.g., India, China, Japan, and Korea) emphasizes the following virtues:
- Self-discipline and control,
- The inner nature of self,
- Moderation in all things,
- Nonattachment to worldly things,

- Awareness that selfish desire is the cause of much suffering,
- Tolerance to other religions and points of view,
- Respect for family, elders, and authority, and
- The principle of not harming any living creature.

The Western world (e.g., Europe, Canada, and the United States) emphasizes the following virtues:
- The value of individual worth,
- The need to be responsible for each other, which gives rise to many social programs, and
- A personal relationship with one God that translates into love of neighbor and environment.

Because of immigration and acculturation of Eastern peoples and interest in and adoption of Eastern philosophies by Western society, both traditions can be seen in the other. For example, there are a large number of Christians among Eastern peoples. Westerners have adopted meditation, yoga, complementary therapies (including use of herbs), and a focus on inner development.

HINDUISM

Hinduism dates back to prehistoric times. This oldest religion is the third largest religion in the world and is comprised of a diverse system of thoughts and beliefs. The essence of Hinduism is based on a vast body of scriptures, including the *Vedas* and the *Bhagavad-Gita*. These texts teach the path to the proper way of living through *dharma* (ethics, duties), *karma* (action, deeds), and *bhakti* (devotion and knowledge that God is the ultimate power, and exists in many forms).

Box 13-8 *Beliefs, Practices, and Nursing Interventions for Additional Christian and Non Christian Religious/Spiritual Groups*

CHRISTIAN SCIENTIST (CHURCH OF CHRIST, SCIENTIST)

Founded in nineteenth century by Mary Baker Eddy, who wrote *Science and Health with a Key to the Scriptures*.

Beliefs and Practices

- Believe sin causes sickness and studying Eddy's book and the Bible will heal them.
- Patient may believe that sickness can be overcome through prayer and spiritual understanding that God is good and the only reality.
- Healing considered an awakening to this belief.
- There are no clergy, but patient may want a Christian Science practitioner to give treatment through prayer.
- No Baptism.
- Consider the Lord's Supper a spiritual communion with God and may sit quietly during this time.
- No smoking or drinking alcohol. They do not accept blood transfusions or surgery.

Nursing Interventions

- Clarify Baptism beliefs with patient.

JEHOVAH'S WITNESSES

Originated at the end of the nineteenth century in the United States. Witnesses base their beliefs on the Bible.

Beliefs and Practices

- Believe the Second Coming has begun, Armageddon is imminent, and will be followed by the millennium. At that time, repentant sinners will have a second chance for salvation.
- They do not believe in the Trinity. Consider Jesus inferior to God, the Father, Jehovah.
- No ordained ministers.
- No churches but worship in Kingdom Halls. Publications include *Awake* and *Watch Tower*.
- Witnesses will refuse to receive whole blood products, including plasma. To receive such products is viewed as a violation of the law of Jehovah (Genesis 9:3,4, Leviticus 17:14, Acts 15:28,29). They will accept blood transfusion alternatives.
- Alcohol and tobacco are discouraged.

- Believe the soul dies at death. Autopsy decided by family.
- Cremation is acceptable.
- Organ transplants are a private decision. Before transplant, organs must be cleansed with a nonblood solution.
  Baptism: Necessary for salvation. Considered a symbol of dedication to Jehovah. Adult by immersion. No infant baptism.
  Communion: Occurs one time a year.

MORMONS (CHURCH OF JESUS CHRIST OF LATTER DAY SAINTS)

In the nineteenth century, Joseph Smith founded the Mormon Church. The headquarters are in Salt Lake City.

Beliefs and Practices

- Revelation is emphasized to establish doctrine and rituals.
- The Book of Mormon contains accounts of ancient peoples in America. This book is considered complementary scripture to the Bible.
- Mormons emphasize tithing and community welfare.
- Mormons worship in temples and tabernacles.
- There is no ordained clergy. High priests are members of the Church and form the Council of Twelve and exert spiritual leadership. Three high priests vested with supreme authority form the first presidency of the church.
- A Mormon may be anointed and blessed before going to the hospital.
- Abortion is not allowed unless the mother's life is in danger.
- Natural methods of birth control are allowed. Artificial means may be used when the physical or emotional health of the woman is in question.
- May avoid tobacco, alcohol, coffee, and tea.
  Baptism: Considered necessary for salvation. Causes remission of sins. Allows the person to receive the gifts of the Holy Spirit. Baptism is given at age 8 or older by immersion. Baptism may be given after death by proxy.
  Communion: The Lord's Supper with bread and water. Considered a symbol and renewing of covenant with Christ.

Box 13-8 *Beliefs, Practices, and Nursing Interventions for Additional Christian and Non Christian Religious/Spiritual Groups—cont'd*

BAHA'I Founded in the nineteenth century in Persia (now southern Iran). **Beliefs and Practices** • Believe in world peace, the unity of all religions and humanity, and the equality of men and women. • There is no clergy. • Members meet in homes. The house of worship in the United States is in Wilmette, IL.	• There is an annual 19-day fast from sunrise to sundown during the last month of the Baha'i calendar. • May avoid alcohol. • At death the soul, the real self, journeys through the spiritual world, which is the timeless, placeless extension of the universe. • No embalming, unless required by state law. • Burial to take place within 1 hour's travel time of death. • There is no baptism or communion. • Their special book is *The Book of Certitude*.

With these in mind, Hinduism is more a way of life than a religion. Hindus believe in reincarnation: One is reborn to a higher or lower level of existence based on one's moral behavior in the prior phase of existence. The cycle of birth and death continues until the soul achieves *moksha* (or Nirvana), the self-realization and unification of the soul with the ultimate being.

There is no common creed or doctrine in Hinduism; it is based on the accumulated treasury of spiritual laws discovered by different people in different times. Most Hindus venerate many gods and goddesses, including the Trinity—*Vishnu*, the Protector; *Shiva*, the destroyer; and *Brahma*, the Creator. These gods, along with their equally powerful consorts, are worshipped in their various incarnations and forms. Information about Hinduism can be accessed at *http://en.wikipedia.org/wiki/Hinduism*.

Tables 13-1 and 13-2 present general beliefs and practices of Buddhist and Hindu patients, nursing interventions, and items that need to be clarified.

BUDDHISM

Siddhartha Gautama (Buddha) founded Buddhism in the sixth century BC in India. Buddhism can be considered a religion, a philosophy, and a way of life. Much of Eastern beliefs have evolved from Buddhism. Well before Christianity, Buddhism originated in India, as did Hinduism. It shares much with Hindu philosophy, but also radically departs from it (Table 13-1). Buddhism spread to China, Japan, Korea, Tibet, Burma, Sri Lanka, Laos, Cambodia, and Vietnam. As Buddhism spread, the core beliefs were adapted to the culture of the host country. The beliefs were shaped and influenced by rituals and the belief system of each country. Two core beliefs of Buddhism remained constant, however. They are the Four Noble Truths and the Noble Eightfold Path leading to Nirvana, as follows:

1. Life is suffering.
2. Suffering is caused by desire. Desire is described as the craving or longing for the pleasures of the senses and life itself. Suffering is also caused by ignorance, which is interpreted as not being able to see things as they are.
3. Suffering can be eliminated by eliminating desire (craving or longing for the pleasures of the senses and life itself).
4. To eliminate desire, follow the **Noble Eightfold Path:**
   a. **Right views**
   b. **Right intention**
   c. **Right speech**
   d. **Right action**

Table 13-1 | *General Religious Beliefs/Practices and Nursing Interventions for Buddhist and Hindu Patients*

BELIEFS/PRACTICES	NURSING INTERVENTIONS
Not having a central authority or dictated doctrine, the approximately 550,000 **Buddhists** *and 1.3 million* **Hindus** *in North America exhibit a variety of traditions, beliefs, and practices.*	Clarify with the patient his or her preference of practices to be observed.
Buddhists *believe pain and suffering result from actions in this or a past life.*	Accept the patient's right to this belief; neither agree nor disagree.
Buddhist *and* **Hindu** *patients accept traditional medical treatment. However, to maintain a clear state of mind,* **Buddhists** *may refuse drugs that alter the state of the mind.*	Inform physician of patient's concern. Explain to patient/family the action of all medications before administering them. Report to physician and chart any medications refused and reason for refusal.
Generally, **Buddhists** *do not believe in healing through faith. Healing for* **Buddhist** *patients may be promoted by awakening to the laws of Buddha. After many years of searching, Siddhartha Gautama, the founder of Buddhism, finally found the truth of existence and became the Buddha—the Enlightened One. Many persons since then have become Buddhas by becoming enlightened.*	Avoid references to "God" (e.g., "God will help you get through this.").
Hindu *patients may prefer a light diet in the morning and evening and a heavy meal at noon. Some* **Hindu** *patients may fast on a specific day of the week or month.*	Allow patient/family to select diet for each meal. Encourage patient/family to write in food preferences when not listed. Arrange for visit by dietitian.
Hindus *may practice Ayurveda, the traditional Indian science of health that uses herbs to treat disease. Some* **Hindus** *also practice folk medicine.*	As with patients of all cultures and in all settings: Question use of herbs in daily life, so possible drug interactions can be avoided. Question use of folk medicine. If practice is not harmful, include practice in plan of care. If practice is harmful, repattern practice. (See examples of adapting care plans for culturally diverse patients, p. 203).
Buddhist *patients may use incense, images of Buddha, and/or prayer beads in worship.*	Respect these objects if used by patient. Provide these personal objects if patient asks for them.
Hindu *patients may have a thread on their torso or around their wrist to signify a blessing.*	Avoid removing the thread.
Buddhist *patients may have a visit from a Buddhist priest, monk, or nun to conduct a religious ceremony.* **Hindu** *priests generally are not involved with illness care.*	Provide privacy for visit of priest, monk, or nun.
Buddhist *families may perform traditions with patient.*	Arrange the environment to accommodate the family.
Significant others of **Hindu** *patients may do the same.*	Provide quiet and privacy.
Buddhist *patients may chant or meditate to help calm and clear their minds.*	Avoid interrupting the patient during meditation or chanting.
Puja, the worship of **Hindu** *deities, is preceded by outer purification.* **Hindu** *patients may request a daily bath.*	Provide necessary equipment for bathing for ambulatory patients. If patient requires assistance, assist with bath before meal. If bathing required in bed, add hot water to cold water (Lipson, 1996).

Table 13-2 *Death Beliefs, Practices, and Nursing Interventions for Buddhist and Hindu Patients*

Buddhists *believe in many reincarnations until they achieve Enlightenment and are freed from worldly illusion, passions, and suffering. Until this is achieved, death provides the opportunity to improve in the next life. Understanding of the Four Noble Truths and the Noble Eightfold Path will allow one to achieve Enlightenment and enter Nirvana (a state, the absence of self, extinguishing desire and suffering), at which time the cycle of rebirths and deaths ends. Resources within the person to achieve Enlightenment are stressed rather than reliance on ancient gods*

Hindus *believe in the wheel of birth, life, and death (reincarnations) until they break through the illusions of the world and participate in the manifestation of the true self (Atman, the deathless self, the soul). Meditation and grace will help the Hindu believer to realize the Supreme self, which is hidden in the heart. When this occurs, eternal peace or Brahman (the universal soul and source, the Absolute Truth) is the reward.*

BELIEFS/PRACTICES	NURSING INTERVENTIONS
Buddhists and **Hindus** *believe in re-birth and death (reincarnation). They do not believe in the concept of an immortal soul.*	Accept the patient's right to this belief; avoid agreeing or disagreeing.
Buddhists and **Hindus** *believe in karma, the law of cause and effect by which thoughts, words, and deeds of each person create his or her own destiny. One reaps what one sows. Karma is carried over to the next life and determines the form of each new existence.* **Buddhists** *believe it is the state of one's consciousness at the time of death that usually determines one's rebirth.*	For dying patients, make provision for rites and ceremonies by the family and/or spiritual leaders. Avoid interfering with praying, singing, and chanting. **Buddhist Patients** Provide an environment for the dying patient that will allow a clear, calm state of mind and a peaceful death. **Hindu Patients** Allow the family/spiritual leader to place water in the mouth of Hindu patients.
Buddhists and **Hindus** *treat the body with respect. Cremation is common for* **Buddhists** *and* **Hindus.** *The* **Hindu** *patient's ashes are saved, to be disposed of in a holy river (e.g., the Ganges). Family may want to wash the body in preparation for cremation.*	Inform funeral director of patient's religion. **Hindu Patient** When requested, provide family with equipment to wash the body. Present possibility of organ donation to family in a private environment.
ORGAN DONATIONS **Buddhists** *may allow organ donation if it will help someone pursue enlightenment.* **Hindus** *allow organ donation.*	Follow agency policy for obtaining permission for organ donation.
AUTOPSIES **Buddhists** and **Hindus** *permit autopsies.*	Follow agency policy for obtaining permission for autopsy.

e. **Right livelihood**
f. **Right effort**
g. **Right concentration**
h. **Right ecstasy**

Because of the variation in beliefs and history of Eastern groups, the time interval since immigration, and the degree of enculturation, it is difficult to provide clear cut examples of what a Japanese American or East Indian Hindu American believes and practices. As much diversity exists among Eastern religions and philosophies as exists among Christians.

NURSING INTERVENTIONS FOR EASTERN RELIGIONS/PHILOSOPHIES

In patient care the practical/vocational nurse can come in contact with a Japanese Buddhist,

Korean Buddhist, and Tibetan Buddhist, among others, as well as American/Canadian patients who have blended Buddhism with their chosen religion. Apply principles from Chapter 12. Develop awareness that not everyone sees the world as you do. Avoid stereotyping individuals and considering them all the same, because they are Buddhist or Hindu. Table 13-1 presents a comparison of general religious beliefs and practices that *may* be found in Buddhist and Hindu patients, and appropriate nursing interventions. Table 13-2 presents general death beliefs and practices of Buddhist and Hindu patients and appropriate nursing interventions.

 Learning Exercise

Learning About Different Belief Systems

Gather information about a religion, philosophy, or group not discussed in this chapter, that interests you but for which you are not a member. Focus on nursing interventions appropriate for the topic you chose to research. Use Chapter 5 as a resource to gather information.

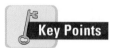 **Key Points**

- The practical/vocational nurse has a responsibility to care for the total person, including physical, emotional, and spiritual needs.
- Spiritual needs of patients arise from their desire to find meaning in life, suffering, and death.
- Gathering data about spiritual needs and providing spiritual care is a routine part of all patients' care, not only in times of crisis.

- To meet the spiritual needs of patients, you need to be aware of the patient's personal spiritual beliefs or the absence of them.
- Members of the health care team who assist the practical/vocational nurse in providing spiritual care to patients are the minister, priest, rabbi, chaplain, and other representatives of religions, groups, and philosophies and the pastoral care team.
- Many patients help to meet their personal spiritual needs by their participation in an organized religion.
- Spirituality can be part of religion, but religion is not necessarily part of spirituality.
- Spiritual distress can occur when patients cannot fulfill the rituals and practices of their religion or when they experience conflict between their spiritual beliefs and their health regimen.
- For these reasons, you need to develop an awareness of religious differences and an understanding of the basic beliefs, rituals, and practices of the many religious denominations, groups, and philosophies that exist today.
- Avoid assuming that patients who belong to a specific religion or belief system adopt all beliefs and practices of that religion or belief system.
- Clarify personal religious beliefs and practices for all patients.
- Although many patients in the United States are Protestant, Catholic, and Jewish, you will encounter other denominations and groups, such as Muslims and members of Eastern religions and philosophies, as well as persons who have no religious affiliation. By learning more about these groups, you will be able to accommodate their beliefs and practices and will be able to say you have met the needs of the total person.

REVIEW ITEMS

1. The God a Muslim patient prays to is:

   1. Christ

   2. Zeus

   3. Allah

   4. Yahweh

2. Select the statement that **best** describes the role of the pastoral care team.

   1. The pastoral care team is the social services department in acute care facilities and extended care.

   2. The pastoral care team works with the nursing staff to help meet the spiritual and religious needs of patients.

   3. Religious care and spiritual support is offered to seriously ill and dying patients by the pastoral care department.

   4. Because of pastoral care, the nursing staff does not have to worry about meeting the spiritual needs of patients.

3. If a Catholic patient requests Last Rites before surgery, the practical/vocational nurse responds by:

   1. Reassuring the patient that he is not going to die during surgery.

   2. Notifying the patient's family that his condition has changed.

   3. Calling the patient's physician to report patient's mental state.

   4. Notifying the pastoral care team of the patient's preoperative request.

4. If a patient with a bleeding peptic ulcer is a Jehovah's Witness and refuses to receive an ordered blood transfusion preoperatively, select the **priority** action of the licensed practical/vocational nurse.

   1. Notify the nursing supervisor STAT and report the patient's refusal.

   2. Encourage the patient to accept the transfusion as a life-saving measure.

   3. Explain that the transfusion is needed because of severe blood loss.

   4. Alert family members of the crucial need to notify church authorities.

ALTERNATE FORMAT ITEM

A Jewish patient is admitted to the extended care unit on your shift. Which of the following nursing interventions apply to this situation? *(Select all that apply.)*

1. Provide quiet time for prayer on the Sabbath.

2. Ask the family to bring in patient's yarmulke.

3. Order all meals to be served using kosher preparation.

4. Arrange for milk to be delivered at least a half hour before meals.

5. Clarify personal beliefs and practices with patient.

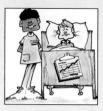

CHAPTER 14

Assertiveness: Your Responsibility

evolve http://evolve.elsevier.com/Hill/success/

Objectives

On completing this chapter, you will be able to do the following:

1. Explain why assertiveness is a nursing responsibility.
2. Differentiate among assertive, aggressive, and nonassertive (passive) behavior.
3. Describe three negative interactions in which nurses can get involved.
4. Maintain a daily journal that reflects your personal interactions and responses.
5. Explain the use of the problem-solving process to make a personal plan for change toward assertive behavior.
6. Discuss positive manipulation as a cultural choice.
7. Discuss codependency as an attempt to find relief from unresolved feelings.
8. Discuss the prevalence of physical assault against nurses in the workplace.
9. Discuss dealing with sexual harassment in nursing.
10. List two to three behavioral changes in an individual that may clue you in to possible employee violence.
11. Identify steps you can personally take to make the place you work a happier and safer environment.

Key Terms

Aggressive (ă-GRĔS-ĭv, p. 228)
Assault (ă-SŎLT, p. 239)
Assertiveness (ă-SŬR-tĭv-nĕs, p. 229)
Automatic responses (ĂW-tō-MĂT-ĭk, p. 227)
Choice (p. 227)

Compensation (KŎM-pĕn-SĀ-shŭn, p. 233)
Denial (dē-NĪ-ăl, p. 232)
Manipulation (mă-NĬP-ū-LĀ-shŭn, p. 238)
Nonassertive (passive) (nŏn-ă-SŬR-tĭv, p. 227)
Problem solving (p. 233)
Projection (prŏ-JĔK-shŭn, p. 231)
Rationalization (RĂSH-ăn-ă-lĭ-ZĀ-shŭn, p. 231)
Sexual harassment (HĂR-ăs-mĕnt, p. 243)

 Keep in Mind

Assertiveness is an expectation in nursing—a responsibility for you as a patient advocate.

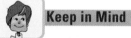 *Critical Thinking Exercise*

Personal Expectations

Imagine for the next few minutes that the nurse-patient roles are reversed and that you are the patient. What are your expectations of the nurse assigned to you? List the rationale for each expectation you identify.

Expectations   Rationale
_____   _____
_____   _____
_____   _____
_____   _____

Completing the previous exercise has already begun to give you insight into the need for assertiveness in the nurse. At the end of this chapter you are encouraged to do this exercise again. Evaluate any changes in expectations.

Verbal, nonverbal, and affective communication translates into three major behavior patterns. You will *hear, see,* and *feel* the message acted out. The most effective communication style is open and honest. It promotes positive relationships and a healthy sense of self. Ineffective communication or behavior is hurtful. It blames, attacks, or denies and is harmful to the self as well.

An *assertive* style separates the person from the issue. Most important, you speak out of choice. An emotional hook catches you when you use either an *aggressive or a nonassertive (passive) style of communication.* Both types of responses are automatic responses. You no longer respond from choice.

The three major behavior styles are **nonassertive** (passive), **aggressive**, and **assertive**.

NONASSERTIVE (PASSIVE) BEHAVIOR

Nonassertive (passive), fear-based behavior is an emotionally dishonest, self-defeating type of behavior. Nonassertive nurses attempt to look the other way, avoid conflict, and take what seems to be the easiest way out; they are never full participants on the nursing team. *Nonassertive individuals do not express feelings, needs, and ideas when their rights are infringed on, deliberately or accidentally. There may be a lack of eye contact, swaying and shifting from one foot to another, and whining and hesitancy when speaking.* The overall message is, *"I do not count. You count."* This personal pattern of behavior is reflected in their nursing as well. Consequently, they are unable to recognize and meet patient needs. A number of examples of nonassertive behavior observed in one nurse follow. With each example, the type of behavior is given in parentheses.

- Tells another nurse how "stupid" the doctor is for ordering a certain type of treatment (indirect, nonassertive behavior).
- Limits contact with a patient he or she is uncomfortable with to required care only (indirect nonassertive behavior).
- Routinely tells patients who ask questions about their illness, test, medications, or treatment to "ask the doctor" or "ask the RN." Although this answer is advisable some of the time, it certainly is a form of brush-off. Part of nursing responsibility is to seek answers for the patient (takes the easy way out).
- Experiences inability to continue with a necessary, uncomfortable treatment ordered for the patient (interprets patient's expression of discomfort personally ("The patient will not like me if I do this").
- May assume, without checking, that the patient wants to skip daily personal care when a visitor drops in (avoids conflict).
- Experiences a feeling of being "devastated" when a patient, doctor, nurse, or other staff person criticizes his or her work (interprets criticism of work as criticism of self).
- Responds to patient's questions about own personal life and that of other staff (afraid of not being liked).
- Patient asks nurse to pick up some personal items on the way home. Nurse frowns but agrees to do so (communicates real message nonverbally).
- Becomes angry with the team leader and drops hints to others about own feeling (communicates real message indirectly).
- When asked by another nurse to take on the care of assigned patients, responds by saying, "Well, uh, I guess I could," although already too busy (hesitance, repressing own wishes).
- Needs help with assignment but says nothing (refrains from expressing own needs).
- After making an error, overexplains and overapologizes (is unaware of the right to make a mistake; should take responsibility for it, learn from the error, and go on).
- Plans on finding a new job because of fear of approaching supervisor to tell own side of what has happened (avoids conflict).
- When "chewed out" by the doctor in front of patient, nurse is angry but says nothing (refrains from expressing own opinion—internalizes anger).

Nonassertive Behavior

Identify nonassertive behaviors in which you have been involved. Describe how each behavior worked or did not work for you.

By not taking risks and not being honest, nonassertive nurses typically feel hurt, misunderstood, anxious, and disappointed and often feel angry and resentful later. Because they do not allow their needs to be known, they are the losers.

Nonassertive Behavior

Develop a plan for change for each one of the nonassertive behaviors that you identified as having unsatisfactory outcomes.

AGGRESSIVE BEHAVIOR

Outspoken people are often automatically considered assertive; when in reality their lack of consideration for others may be a sign of aggressive **behavior**. *Aggressive (anger-based) behavior violates the rights of others.* It is an attack on the person rather than on the person's behavior. The purpose of aggressive behavior is to dominate or put the other person down. This behavior, while expressive, is self-defeating because it quickly distances the aggressor from other staff and patients. Examples of aggressive body language include leaning forward with glaring eyes; pointing a finger at a person to whom you are speaking; shouting; clenching fists; putting hands on hips and wagging the head. The overall message is, *"You do not count. I count."* The following examples are some of the ways by which aggressive behavior can be recognized. An explanation of the rationale is included in parentheses.

- You have asked to go to a workshop, and the supervisor says, "Why should you go? Everyone else has worked here longer than you have" (attempts to make you feel guilty for making a request).
- Another nurse points out your error in front of other staff and adds, "Where did you say you graduated from?" (attempt to humiliate as a way of controlling).
- A peer approaches you with a problem. You don't want to listen and say, "If it isn't one thing, it's another for you. Why don't you get your act together?" (disregards others' feelings).
- A new rule is instituted without requesting input from or informing those it will involve. You protest but are told, "That's tough; this is the way it's going to be from now on" (disregards others' feelings and rights).
- The patient has had his call light on frequently throughout the morning. You walk in and say, "I have had it. You have had your light on continuously for nothing all morning. Do not put your light on again unless you are dying or I will take it away" (hostile overreaction out of proportion to the issue at hand).
- You attempted to express your feelings to a peer about his or her behavior toward you. Today the peer greets you with an icy stare when you say hello (hostile overreaction).
- The patient tells you, "I thought this was a pretty good hospital, but none of you seem to know what you are doing" (sarcastic, hostile).
- You push yourself in front of others in the cafeteria line (rudeness).
- You ask the nurse manager a question. Instead of answering, he just stares at you with lips curled slightly upward (attempt to make you uncomfortable, a put-down).

Learning Exercise

Aggressive Behavior

Circle the aggressive behaviors in the previous example that are similar to behaviors you have experienced.

Critical Thinking Exercise

Aggressive Behavior

Develop a plan for dealing with the aggressive behaviors you identified in the previous learning exercise.

Aggressive behavior certainly is a way of saying what you mean at the moment. It often does produce temporary relief from anxiety. However, the feeling does not last. Very often the aggressive person is left with residual angry feelings that simmer until the next stressful situation or person comes along. It is interesting to note that sometimes an aggressive person was once passive and made a decision that "no one will step on me again." However, instead of practicing assertiveness, such a person practiced and became involved in another form of destructive, self-defeating behavior. Aggressive nurses, like nonaggressive nurses, are unable to function as true advocates for the patient because they are too busy taking care of what they perceive to be their personal needs.

ASSERTIVE BEHAVIOR

Assertiveness is a current name for honesty—that is, it is a way to live the truth from your innermost being and to express this truth in thought, word, and deed. The concept seems simple enough, but to actually practice being truthful all the time is difficult. According to *Webster's Dictionary*, taking a positive stand, being confident in your statement, or being positive in a persistent way characterizes assertiveness. You, the nurse, work in a setting that requires speaking frankly and openly to others in such a way that their rights are not violated. *Assertiveness is a tool, not a weapon.* As with any new behavior (or skill), becoming truly assertive will take practice and time. Avoid being harsh with yourself or giving up just because old behavior emerges initially when you are under pressure. Resolve to try again until assertive behavior is integrated as a part of your being. Although it is not the nurse's right to hurt others deliberately, it is unrealistic to be inhibited to the point of never hurting anyone. Some people are hurt because they are unreasonably sensitive, and some people use their sensitivity to manipulate others. Assertiveness is not only what you say, but also how you say it. Examples of assertive body language include: standing straight, steady and directly facing the people to whom you are saying it while maintaining eye contact; speaking in a clear voice, loud enough so the people to whom you are speaking can hear you; and speaking fluently without hesitation and with assurance and confidence.

Nurses have a right to express their own thoughts and feelings. To do otherwise would be insincere. It would also deny patients and other staff the opportunity to learn to deal with their feelings. Assertiveness, then, is a way of expressing oneself without insulting others. It communicates respect for the other person, although not necessarily for the other person's behavior. The overall message is, *"I count, you count."* Being assertive does not guarantee that you will get your way. What it does guarantee is that you will experience a sense of being in control of your emotions and your responses. Win or lose, you gave it your best shot. The real bonus is freedom from residual feelings of fear and anger. Later in this chapter, we will deal with exceptions, when you are faced with a potentially violent situation.

The following examples, with the rationale in parentheses, are expressions of assertive behavior. As an assertive nurse, you claim responsibility for your own feelings, thoughts, and actions. Use of "I" in the statements shows acceptance of responsibility for your thinking, feeling, and doing.

- The doctor orders a medication or treatment that seems inappropriate. You request to talk to the doctor privately and ask about expected outcomes. You present any new information you have that may potentially affect the decision to continue with the order (direct statement of information).

- The patient has been giving you a bad time. Pulling up a chair and sitting down, you say, "Mr. Smith, I would be interested in knowing what is going on with you. I have noticed that whatever I do, you are critical of my work." Then you listen attentively and with understanding (comprehension) and respond nondefensively (direct statement of feelings; does not interpret patient's criticism as a personal attack).

- When the patient requests information you are unfamiliar with regarding the illness and treatment, you say, "I do not know, but I will find out for you." You follow through by checking with appropriate staff. You determine who is to inform the patient (respects the patient's right to know).

- The doctor has ordered the patient to be walked for 10 minutes out of each hour. The patient complains that it hurts and asks to not walk. You respond by saying, "I know it is uncomfortable, but I will walk along beside you. We can stop briefly any time you like. I will also teach you how to do a brief relaxation technique (see Chapter 10) that you can use while you are walking." If pain medication is available, you will also make sure that this is given before walking and in enough time for the medication to take effect (respects patient's feelings but supports the need to carry out doctor's orders).

- Unexpected visitors arrive when it is time for you to help the patient with personal care. You ask the patient directly if care should be done now or postponed briefly. You state the time that you will be available to assist with care (respects the patient's right to choose, as long as it does not compromise the care).

- You have just been criticized for your work. You respond by saying, "Please clarify. I want to be sure I understand." If the error is yours, ask for suggestions to correct it or offer alternatives of your own (separates criticism of performance from criticism of self).

- The patient asks for personal information about you (or another staff member). You respond by saying, "That information is personal, and I do not choose to discuss it" (stands up for rights without violating rights of others).

- Your patient asks you to pick up some personal items from the store. This would mean doing it on your own time, which is already very full. You respond by saying, "I will not be able to do the errand for you" (direct statement without excuses).

- The team leader has been "on your case" constantly and, you think, unfairly. You approach the team leader and say, "I want to speak with you privately today before 3 PM. What time is convenient for you?" (direct statement of wishes).

- You are being pressed by other staff members to help with their assignments but are too busy to do so. You say, "No, I do not have the time to help today, but try me again on some other day" (direct refusal without feeling guilty; leaves the door open to help at a future date).

- Your day is overwhelming. You approach your team leader and say, "I know you would like all of this done today. There is no way I can get it all done. What are your priorities?" (direct statement of information and request for clarification).

- The doctor has criticized your work in front of the patient. You feel embarrassed and angry. You approach the doctor and ask to speak privately. Using "I-centered" statements, you begin by saying, "I feel both embarrassed and angry because you criticized me in front of the patient. Next time, ask to talk to me privately. I will listen to what you have to say" (stands up for your rights without violating the rights of others).

- You are ready to leave work when a peer approaches you about a personal problem. You respond by saying, "I have to leave now, but I'll be glad to listen to you during our lunch break tomorrow" (compromise).
- Another staff person moves into the cafeteria line ahead of you with a nod and a smile. You are in a hurry too, and feel this is an imposition. You say firmly, "I do not like it when you get in line ahead of me. Please go back to the end of the line" (stand up for your rights).

Complete the following learning exercise.

 Learning Exercise

Identify Assertiveness

List examples of assertiveness you can identify in your own behavior or in people around you.

_____

_____

The following three rules are helpful overall in being assertive:

1. Own your feelings. Do not blame others for the way you feel.
2. Make your feelings known by being direct. Begin your statements with "I."
3. Be sure that your nonverbal communication matches your verbal message.

NEGATIVE INTERACTIONS: USING COPING MECHANISMS

With the availability of so many types of preparation for nurses, and the lack of differentiation in roles based on preparation, nurses sometimes experience insecurity in their role and the worth of the role as they understand it. Projection is a coping mechanism during which individuals attribute their own weaknesses to others. The interaction can be characterized as "my education is better than yours," or "I'm more competent than you are," or "you're only a practical nurse," and so on. Unfortunately, this negative, aggressive interaction wastes energy that could be used to provide the patient with the care that is being alluded to. Nurses who are confident and assertive enhance each other's knowledge base and legal responsibility. The patient benefits from the assertiveness.

Another negative interaction is based on a previous unresolved incident between the patient and the nurse. The nurse uses the coping or mental mechanism of rationalization, in which a logical but untrue reason is offered as an excuse for the behavior. The nurse quickly informs others that this patient is a "troublemaker" or a "manipulator" or "uncooperative." This is a nonassertive, indirect type of behavior on the part of the nurse. Obviously, if other nurses incorporate this information into their transactions with patients, patients will never be seen as their true selves. Anything the patient does can be interpreted within the context of the label given by the nurses. A vicious circle can ensue. If the patient's needs are not met because of this labeling, this increases their frustration. This in turn is a threat to self, resulting in anxiety. Depending on the patient's personal strength at this time, the situation can lead to **problem solving**, use of coping/mental mechanisms, or symptom formation (Fig. 14-1).

An honest, assertive response on the part of the original nurse involved would consist of dealing with the patient directly in regard to the previous situation. It would not involve other nurses as allies in "getting this patient." An example of an extreme situation resulting from just such a seemingly innocent rationalization occurred at a nursing home. A young man who was paralyzed from the waist down as a result of a car accident was being transferred from one nursing home to another. A transfer form arrived before he did. The information on the form created immediate anxiety for the nurses involved before they had even met the man. The form labeled the man as

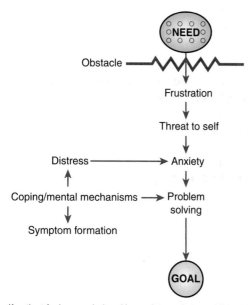

If patient feels overwhelmed by anxiety and stress (distress), coping/mental mechanisms may be resorted to in order to deal with the distress. If coping/mental mechanisms fail, the result will be mental or physical symptom formation. Unmet needs are a threat to self, resulting in stress and anxiety. If the patient has the personal strength to problem-solve, needs can be met.

FIGURE **14-1** A vicious circle showing a negative interaction from an unresolved incident between the patient and the nurse.

"manipulative." It explained "he will be pleasant and polite at first, but watch out because it is a trick. When he has won you over, you will see his 'true colors.'" The nurses discussed the prospective admission. They expressed gratitude that their colleagues in the other nursing home had warned them. After all, that is what colleagues are for. They felt, "forewarned is forearmed."

When the patient arrived and attempted to get acquainted, he was dealt with coldly and abruptly and made to wait. The nurses intended to show him that he could not manipulate them. As his frustration and discomfort increased, he began to demand that his treatments be done on time. He shouted angry comments at the nurses when they finally arrived to assume his care. The nurses called him "demanding" and "hostile." The original title of manipulative was supported when the patient asked his roommate to put on the call light to get help to take him to the bathroom. Each day seemed worse than the day before. The showdown finally came when a long-time nurse employee left, saying that she would not come back until the patient was transferred to another facility. She would even volunteer to do the transfer note. Other nursing staff threatened to follow suit. Finally, the administrator gave in. The patient was transferred, and the nurses congratulated each other for having worked together! Complete the following critical thinking exercise on negative interactions.

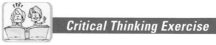

Critical Thinking Exercise

Negative Interactions

1. What factors contributed to the patient's behavior?
2. What factors contributed to the nurses' response to the patient?
3. How could this situation have been handled differently?
4. Was the behavior of the nurses passive, aggressive, or assertive? Explain your answer.

Another negative transaction involves the patient's right to know (for example, a patient being transferred from a skilled nursing home facility to an intermediate nursing home facility). This transaction can be known by many titles, depending on the issue. It can be called: "I've got a secret," "it is not my responsibility," "she will be upset," or "she is too weak to know." The responsibility of informing the patient about his or her condition or transfer plans is not carried out so that the present staff does not have to deal with the full impact of the patient's reaction to the information. The coping or mental mechanism used by the nurses is denial. The nurse refuses to recognize the existence and significance of the patient's personal concerns. The nurse further uses denial as a way of excusing personal responsibility: "The doctor should tell him" or "It's the team leader's responsibility." Although the decision may not be entirely yours, it is clearly your responsibility to check out what portion of the information is yours to give. You also have the responsibility to check out who is going to present the information and when. Complete the following learning exercise.

Learning Exercise

Identify if Behavior is Passive, Aggressive, or Assertive

Is the nurse's refusal to take responsibility to seek out the information the patient needs to know a passive, aggressive, or assertive transaction? Explain your answer.

GOSSIP HURTS

Although it has many possible negative interactions, certainly the passive or aggressive game of gossip—for example, "Did I tell you?" or "I just found out"—is a destructive interaction that has the potential to ruin the reputations of both patients and personnel. The coping or mental mechanism is compensation. The nurse is covering for real or imagined inadequacies in his or her work by developing what he or she considers desirable traits of observation, listening, and reporting. The energy is misguided because reputations are at stake, and time spent socializing while at work is time away from providing quality patient care. A listener can squelch this game by saying assertively, "I will work on a relationship with you and me, but I do not wish to have you talk to me about others." Instead, if the listener, while calling the other nurse a gossip, listens with interest, continuation of this behavior is supported. Complete the following critical thinking exercise.

Critical Thinking Exercise

More Damaging Interactions

1. What other damaging interactions between staff or between patients and staff are you familiar?
2. Provide examples of how continuation of this type of interaction is supported by others.
3. What can you do or say to avoid being drawn into these interactions?

GUIDELINES FOR MOVING TOWARD ASSERTIVENESS

Read the poem, "Myself," in Box 14-1. It captures the reason for working toward assertiveness-being able to feel good about yourself as you continue to grow as a person.

Changing behavior is difficult. After all, the behaviors have been practiced and perfected for years. It is so much easier to tell others what *they* should do to change. The decision to change must come from inside you so that it becomes yours alone.

PROBLEM-SOLVING PROCESS

The problem-solving process is a series of steps used to solve problems long before the nursing process was developed. You will note similarities between problem-solving and nursing processes. The nursing process is a more advanced method of using the problem-solving steps. We reintroduce you to problem solving in this chapter because of its continued usefulness in dealing with self.

It is easier to begin the problem-solving process before feelings and behaviors about a troublesome problem are deeply rooted. A common response to unresolved problems is the cycle

| Box 14-1 | *Myself* |

I have to live with myself and so,
I want to be fit for myself to know.
I don't want to stand with the setting sun
And hate myself for the things I've done.
I want to go out with head erect.
I want to deserve all men's respect.
But here in this struggle for fame and self,
I want to be able to like myself.
I don't want to look at myself and know
That I'm bluster and bluff and empty show.
I never can fool myself, and so
Whatever happens, I want to grow
More able to be more proud of me,
Self-respecting and conscience free.

Author: Unknown.

of worry→fear→anger→rage. This cycle can be interrupted and resolved at any stage, but requires different levels of nursing skill. When dealing with the underlying problem, ask the person, "What do you want?" Putting the problem-solving steps into action is work! Without resolution the cycle continues and intensifies with time. This behavior, for example, can be seen in the nursing home patient who strikes out, seems calm for a period, gets irritable, and eventually strikes out again. If the underlying problem is not resolved, the cycle continues. The person gets labeled as one who strikes out without warning, so, "Watch out." Ask a more skilled staff to do the behavioral intervention if you are uncomfortable. You must not set yourself up for injury (Fig. 14-2).

The self tries to find relief of unresolved feelings through behavior such as codependency, self-medicating with alcohol and/or other drugs (or food), and projecting the anger toward patients (burnout). Prolonged, unresolved negative emotions such as worry, fear, and anger create changes in the body at a cellular level and can result in physical illness. We first get clues in our thoughts of how we will

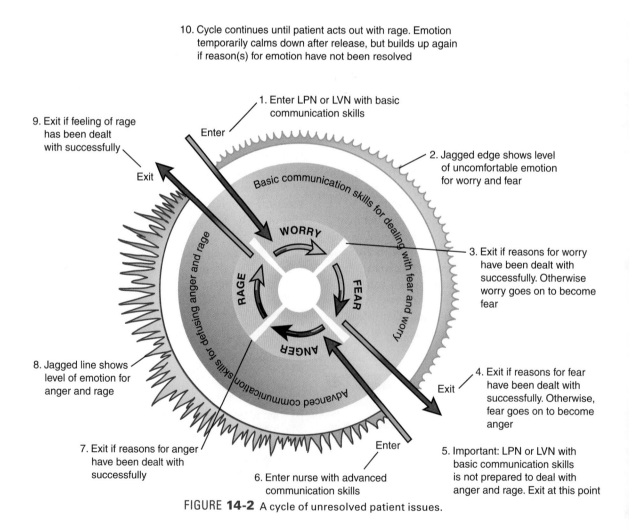

10. Cycle continues until patient acts out with rage. Emotion temporarily calms down after release, but builds up again if reason(s) for emotion have not been resolved

9. Exit if feeling of rage has been dealt with successfully

1. Enter LPN or LVN with basic communication skills

2. Jagged edge shows level of uncomfortable emotion for worry and fear

3. Exit if reasons for worry have been dealt with successfully. Otherwise worry goes on to become fear

4. Exit if reasons for fear have been dealt with successfully. Otherwise, fear goes on to become anger

5. Important: LPN or LVN with basic communication skills is not prepared to deal with anger and rage. Exit at this point

6. Enter nurse with advanced communication skills

7. Exit if reasons for anger have been dealt with successfully

8. Jagged line shows level of emotion for anger and rage

Basic communication skills for dealing with fear and worry

Advanced communication skills for defusing anger and rage

WORRY FEAR ANGER RAGE

FIGURE **14-2** A cycle of unresolved patient issues.

become ill. Listen to your self-talk: "I'm sick of—I'm heartsick—I feel like I have the weight of the world on my shoulders—He's a pain in the neck (or butt)—Oh, my aching back—I'm so upset I can't speak—I can't stomach this much longer"—and so on. If your self-talk is negative, pay attention. These statements give clues to potential areas of physical involvement. We also read or hear news almost daily of mild-mannered, nice people who suddenly acted out because of rage. No one wants to get there. Rage can be turned against others (including homicide), or it can be turned against oneself. Passive means of rage turned against oneself include adopting personal habits damaging to one's health. Active rage against self includes the extreme act of suicide. The risk of suicide for nurses is real and ranks "among the top five causes of death in nurses, and all nurses—from students to retirees—have higher rates of suicide than the general population" (Belanger, *RN*, Oct 2000).

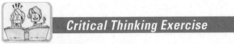

Critical Thinking Exercise

Plan for Living

Begin a plan for living in a personal, confidential journal. Include specific examples of positive health habits that you currently practice.

The problem-solving process is a conscious growth-producing method of dealing with challenges in your life. It is important to note that problem solving is an active process and is more than simply developing an intellectual awareness of the challenge at hand.

PROBLEM-SOLVING STEPS
Step 1: Define the Problem

Sometimes what is perceived as the problem is not the problem. For example, you may have been blaming another individual for talking you into behaviors of which you do not approve. Before making a commitment to change, it is important to look objectively at the gains and losses associated with the present behavior. For example, blaming someone else for your behavior may be gaining you sympathy and care taking by friends. However, you lose by not taking responsibility for your own behavior and dealing with it in a growth-producing way. Your present way of responding to others developed as a response to anxiety-producing situations in life. The behavior usually has its roots in childhood. Complete the following critical thinking exercise about gains and losses.

Critical Thinking Exercise

Gains and Losses

Answer the following questions in your confidential journal: What are you gaining from staying nonassertive/aggressive? What are you losing from staying nonassertive/aggressive?

Another consideration is that when you change the way you act toward others, you change the way they act toward you. What has been a predictable reaction will no longer be predictable. Initially the "others" will test you. They will increase their old way of behaving as a way of getting you to give up the new behavior. If you persist with your new way of dealing with and responding to situations, their behavior toward you will gradually change. *This is the only way to influence change in anyone's behavior.* No amount of "telling" or "scolding" makes a difference as long as others can count on you to continue behaving in the old, predictable way.

Defining the problem depends on collecting data for 2 or 3 days and writing your problem statement based on this information. Collecting data needs to be done in an objective manner, as though you were observing someone else.

Learning Exercise

Keep a Daily Journal

Maintain a daily confidential journal to help pinpoint specific situations that create worry, fear, anger, and rage in you. Track:

1. What happened,
2. When it happened,
3. How you felt physically,
4. The emotion you felt,
5. What you would have liked to have done instead, and
6. What kept you from doing it.

Critical Thinking Exercise

Defining the Problem

Review the data you have collected for 2 or 3 days in your daily journal. It will give you insight into the pros and cons of your current behavior. Develop a problem statement that is personal and specific for you. Before writing the problem statement, read the sample that follows.

Sample

I am afraid to say what I mean for fear that others will get angry with me.

This behavior is characterized by the following situations:

* Saying "yes" to requests to babysit when I need the time for homework.
* Not asking for help with household chores, even though I am a full-time student plus homemaker.
* Saying "yes" to added requests not related to responsibilities for school that I must complete on my own time.
* Feeling tired and resentful much of the time and eventually blowing up over something insignificant.

Step 2: Decide on a Goal

Review the problem statement and write it out, applying the nursing process. Ask yourself what you want to do differently. This can be stated as

a single goal. Often it is more useful to break the goal down into a long-term goal (what change or outcome you want) and several short-term goals (steps needed to attain the desired long-term goal). All goals must be realistic (attainable), measurable (tells how you will know the goal has been attained), and time-referenced (an educated guess on when you will see results). Complete the following critical thinking exercise on deciding on a goal.

Critical Thinking Exercise

Deciding on a Goal

At this time, write a goal about assertiveness for yourself. Before you write the goal, read the sample that follows.

Sample

Long-Term Goal	**Short-Term Goal**
Within 6 months I will say what I mean without fear that others will be angry with me (give actual date—this is your best "guesstimate").	Within 2 weeks I will say "no" to babysitting requests when I need the time for homework (give actual date—this is your best "guesstimate").

As you read each of the goals you have written, ask yourself whether they are realistic. Are they reasonable to attain? Next, review each goal and ask whether it is measurable. Are they so specific that you can use the senses to detect the change? Note that each goal begins with the phrase "I will." This phrase signals a personal commitment to work on the goal. Note that the goals are to be attained within a designated period—that is, they are time-referenced. This is also the only way to give yourself a personal push to get started.

All the changes are not going to occur exactly by the projected date. You will have to revise the goal dates from time to time. Most important, they provide target dates to strive for. As you accomplish each short-term goal, cross it out and go to the next one. Do not be alarmed if you find yourself working on more than one goal at a time. This is possible and even desirable when the opportunity presents itself. It is important to continue recording your progress in the confidential journal that you began initially to obtain data. Its value now lies in keeping a record of the process you are going through and seeing the changes taking place. Unless you do this, you may not fully appreciate your work and its progress. Many changes will be subtle and will not be accompanied by bells and claps of thunder.

Step 3: Choose Alternatives

Alternatives are the approaches that you will be using to attain each of the established goals. When you make a list of alternatives in your journal, let your imagination run wild. Consider all the possible solutions, from serious to humorous. This may even provide some comic relief from the serious challenge with which you are dealing. Remember to include "do nothing" in the list of alternatives. Doing nothing is a *choice* and therefore an alternative. Look at each of the goals and think of specific things you can do or say to help support the goal. Complete the following critical thinking exercise about personal alternatives.

Critical Thinking Exercise

Personal Alternatives

Write alternatives to support the short-term goal(s) you chose in the previous critical thinking exercise. Before you write in your journal, read the sample that follows.

Sample

Approach: Practice in front of a mirror. In an even tone of voice say, *"No, I will not be able to babysit tonight, but try again another time."* If the person persists, say, *"No, I do not have the time tonight."* Repeat as needed until heard. Compliment yourself for not giving in.

How does the approach (alternative) correspond specifically to the short-term goal from the assertiveness exercise?

Step 4: Try Out the Alternatives

The initial plan has been made. It is time to put the plan into action. For many of you, the paperwork is far easier than taking the first step to make the "paper trip" a reality. You may also have discovered that it is far easier to offer ideas to peers than to take the first step into action with your own plan.

It is a good idea to build in an incentive to continue using the new assertive approaches. Promise yourself something that is worthy of you (a worthy goal). As you go along, you will sometimes slip back into old familiar ways of behaving. Do not be dismayed. This is normal. Simply reinstitute the newly planned approaches immediately and continue. The more you practice the new approaches, the more they will become part of you. Ultimately, new assertive behaviors will replace old nonassertive or aggressive behaviors.

Learning Exercise

Celebrate Attaining Your Goals

Identify a worthy incentive to celebrate attaining your goal. To make it work, the goal must be within your budget and not create a new problem for you to solve!

Step 5: Evaluate the Effectiveness of Your Approach

The evaluation mechanism is built into the overall plan for change by making the goals time-limited. This tells you that each goal, along with the alternatives you have chosen, will be evaluated at the time indicated. Do not change a goal or approach too quickly. Give it at least 2 to 3 weeks. There are two reasons for this: (1) The negative behaviors of other individuals toward you will increase initially as they attempt to resist the change created by the change in you; and (2) It takes a minimum of 3 weeks for the new behavior to catch on. (It takes approximately a year for a new behavior to become part of you.)

Learning Exercise

Review Your Journal

As a part of the evaluation process, review your entire confidential journal. This is an excellent source of information for what happened, how you dealt with it, and whether the present course is effective.

Step 6: Repeat the Process if the Solution Is Not Effective

Step 5 gave you information about whether to pursue the established course of action. If changes are needed, go back to step 3, identify additional alternatives, or perhaps choose alternatives that you originally identified but did not use. Then go through the rest of the steps as before.

As you pursue an assertive way of behaving, monitor your nonverbal messages. The nonverbal communication you provide is even more powerful than your words. It is possible to have the words just right but to sabotage the words by hesitation, a sarcastic tone of voice, or emphasis on certain words. Practice in front of a mirror. Busy schedule? Try bath time. Listen to the way you sound. A tape is helpful, as is speaking into an empty corner and hearing your words bounce back. Try lowering your tone of voice. Be sure that the last word of a sentence is no higher than the one before it. Listen for this in others. It makes a statement sound like a question.

Posture plays an important role. Sit up straight; walk with the shoulders back and a confident stride. Make eye contact when speaking. If this is new and difficult for you, look at the area between the eyes of the person you are addressing. This provides an illusion of eye contact. Periodically look away so that it does not look as though you are staring. Avoid annoying characteristics such as staring, nail biting, finger or foot tapping or jiggling, playing with your hair, chewing on a pencil or glasses, artificial laughter, putting hands in and out of pockets, etc.

When someone asks you what you think of an issue or what you would like to do, answer the person. Instead of saying, "I really do not know," or "Whatever you like," or "It does not matter," risk expressing your opinion. Life is an adventure. Your ideas count, and the more you express your opinion, the easier it becomes.

CULTURAL DIFFERENCES: MANIPULATION

With feedback from valued teachers, students, and reviewers we have learned that it is not safe to assume that all cultures are focused on moving toward assertive behavior. In some cultures, manipulation is an accepted norm. Although the term *manipulation* has a negative connotation in our society, manipulation in itself is not a maladaptive behavior. In some cultures it is taught and accepted as a purposeful way of meeting one's needs. Skillful manipulation is especially applauded in some cultures. Persons are taught to be indirect in their comments, polite, and avoid confrontation or direct expression of disagreement, so as not to give offense, and cause loss of face (Lipson and Dibble, 2006).

It is easy to jump to the conclusion that a manipulative person is trying to "trick" you when you do not share the same cultural background. Make time to talk. The differences will be interesting and revealing for both of you.

NEGATIVE MANIPULATIVE INTERACTIONS

Manipulation is considered maladaptive if: (1) the feelings and needs of others are disregarded, or (2) other people are treated as objects to fulfill the needs of the manipulator. The following examples of negative manipulative interactions show a lack of consideration for others' feelings and needs.

- The *seducer* initiates a relationship with someone (e.g., a nurse with a supervisor). They share what seem to be common goals and insights. Ultimately, the seducer asks for special favors or privileges. If denied, the seducer pushes the guilt button, saying, "I thought you liked me," or

"I thought we understood each other." The other person is left feeling guilty, angry, or both.

- The *passive-aggressive* manipulator focuses on the other person's weaknesses. He or she uses this knowledge to exploit or create anxiety for the victim. For example, a physician might point out a nurse's errors or personal or professional problems in front of a patient or other staff. The nurse is left feeling guilty, angry, embarrassed, or all of these emotions.

- The *divide-and-conquer* manipulator "confides" half-truths, rumors, gossip, and innuendo. A skilled manipulator can sever work relationships by sowing seeds of distrust. As the staff squabbles, there is less energy to unite and focus on common patient issues. For example, a divide-and-conquer manipulator who is an established member of the community might "confide" to another department head that a newer employee cannot be trusted. By the time this information proves to be untrue, valuable time has been lost in patient planning and care. Meanwhile, the divide-and-conquer manipulator has continued to tell the same story to other listeners. Because the feelings and needs of others are not considered, they are left with anger and seeds of distrust.

Dealing with a negative manipulator is difficult. An assertive approach is the best recourse. This will, however, be met with resistance and resentment. You may end up backing off if the problem cannot be worked out. Set limits on any inappropriate manipulative behavior toward you. Refuse to play the game any more.

As a nurse, you must learn to take care of yourself. In turn, you will be more effective in meeting patients' nursing needs. In taking care of yourself assertively, you serve as a positive role model for your coworkers, those you lead and manage, and your patients. How you view and deal with an event determines the outcome for you.

AGGRESSIVENESS AND WORK-RELATED ISSUES

ASSAULT

Workplace violence has always existed in nursing facilities. It is the increase in violence, however, that is making nurses take notice. "Whether it is violence, hostility, **sexual harassment** or discrimination, nurses are near the top of the victims list. Statistics show that health care workers, especially nurses, are physically assaulted more often in the workplace than any other group, including prison guards and police" (Taken from *www.nurseweek.com/news/features/*). OSHA (U.S. Department of Labor's Occupational Safety and Health Administration) guidelines for security in health care facilities reports that in general hospitals, 41% of assaults occur in psychiatric units; 18% in medical units: 13% in surgical units; and 7% in pediatric units. Patients do most of the assaults, and almost three fourths of those assaulted are staff nurses. Some of the worst attacks on nurses are from within their own medical community. The attacks range from nasty words and vicious threats to physical assaults from physicians with whom they work. Many nurses accept the violence as the norm and do not report an attack to their supervisor. A lack of action on the part of the nurse gives approval and permission for the perpetrator to continue the behavior. As a nurse, you have the responsibility to act assertively together with other nurses to advocate for a safe workplace.

In March 1996, OSHA released its first Act of Violence Prevention Guidelines (1996) geared toward protecting health care and social service workers on the job. The national guidelines are designed to protect employers and employees with a framework for deterring violence and increasing safety. Box 14-2 lists OSHA guidelines.

Not all agencies have complied with the OSHA guidelines, but some state nurses' associations are working toward increased penalties against people guilty of assaulting a health care worker, or to establish task forces to study workplace violence.

Box 14-2 *OSHA National Guidelines for Deterring Violence*

- Safer nurses' stations: bullet-resistant glass
- Unit arrangement with staff safety in mind
- No toleration of violence policy
- At least two exits in rooms to prevent entrapment of staff
- Adequate, qualified staff coverage at all times
- Policies and procedures for protecting home care providers
- Prompt medical evaluation and treatment regardless of severity of incident
- Victims' right to prosecute perpetrators
- Investigation of all incidents and installation of corrective action
- Alarm systems: security devices such as panic buttons and cell phones
- Metal detectors
- Closed-circuit televisions
- Curved mirrors in hallway intersections
- Time-out rooms for upset patients
- Bright lights

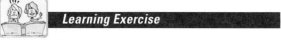

Learning Exercise

ANA Bill of Rights

The ANA *Bill of Rights for Registered Nurses* states, "Nurses have the right to a work environment that is safe for themselves and their patients (*ANA Bill of Rights arms Registered Nurses with critical information*, 2002). Research what your state practical/vocational nurses' association is doing to minimize risks of violence in the workplace.

CONTRIBUTING FACTORS

Many of the findings regarding factors contributing to violence apply to all of nursing.

Personal Factors

These factors relate to verbal, nonverbal, and affective communication, including nurses' attitudes and behaviors. Attitude and body language are considered more significant than the sex and age of the nurse. The manner of approaching a

patient, such as with respect and confidence, emerged as important.

Workplace Practices

Shortage of staff and reduction of trained, regular staff contribute to incidences of assault on staff. Assaults are often associated with meal times, visiting times, and times of increased staff responsibilities at night when staffing is reduced (OSHA, 2004).

The quality, performance, and availability of security personnel are important. Nurses believe they are safer when security officers wear police-type uniforms. Officers convey authority in uniform more so than when they wear a customer-friendly jacket and tie—a nonverbal form of communication. Incidents are also more common when nurses and security personnel lack aggression management skills. Finally, not all administrators back nurses on reporting incidents of physical and verbal abuse, including those involving supervisors and physicians.

Environmental Factors

The type of patient seen and the location of the care facility (for example, high crime risk area), determine the type of patient admitted to a hospital. An important risk factor at hospitals and psychiatric facilities is the carrying of guns by patients, family, or friends of the patient. Other issues include early release of acute or chronic mentally ill, the right to refuse psychotropic medication, inability to voluntarily hospitalize mentally ill persons unless of immediate danger to self or others, and use of hospitals for criminals instead of incarceration.

Risk Diagnosis

Majority of assaults are by a minority of persons. A history of previous violence is the best indicator but sometimes this information is not available to staff. Mentally ill persons commit a small percentage of assaults. More common are gang members, drug users, social deviants, distraught relatives, and those who feel threatened.

Nurses need to learn how to read cues for potential risk of violence in the patients (and others) with whom they are dealing. Some diagnoses that can cue you to possible risk include affective disorders, paranoid delusions, chemical abuse/dependency, dementia, impulse control disorders, and personality disorders.

If you find yourself in **potential** danger, take the following immediate steps:

- Have an escape route in mind.
- Stand at the side of the door; do not block a door.
- Maintain an open position: hands out of pockets, uncrossed arms and legs, hands visible.
- Call the person by name.
- If their voice is raised, speak softly and maintain a quiet, controlled voice.
- Remain calm: sit or stand still; do not fidget.
- Keep 5 to 7 feet of distance between you and the person.
- Do not touch, point, order, challenge, argue, plead, belittle, threaten, or intimidate the person.
- Never turn your back on the person.
- Match eye contact.
- If overtly threatening, some people will respond to being told firmly, "You may not harm me" or "You do not want to harm me" or "It's against the rules."
- If the behavior continues to escalate, throw anything (e.g., a blanket or coat) over the patient's head and run to get help.

Many other practical suggestions are available from experienced nurses like your instructor. This is a time to keep a cool, calculating head (function now, and shake later). Complete the following learning exercise.

Learning Exercise

Evaluate Protection Against Potential Dangers

Do the health care agencies where you receive your clinical experience train their employees in management of assault behavior and/or gentle self-defense? Are assaults at this facility reported to the police? Under what circumstances are charges pressed against the perpetrator?

Investigate where in your nursing program you learn about identifying signs of possible danger to you, and techniques of gentle self-defense to protect yourself.

Critical Thinking Exercise

Preventing Possible Assault

Depending on what you discovered in the previous learning exercise, make a plan for learning what you need to know to better protect yourself from possible assault.

EMPLOYEE VIOLENCE

Workplace violence is classified according to the following four categories:

1. Employee: Violence is directed toward supervisors or management.
2. Domestic: The issue is personal, but the violent act takes place in the workplace.
3. Property: Violence is directed against the employee or employer's property.
4. Commercial: The employee engages in activities such as stealing from employers. Violence may ensue as a result of the activity.

Signs of Workplace Violence

Be alert to signs of violence. Early signs of workplace violence might include the following:

- Unusual behavioral change,
- Lack of cooperation with nursing supervisors,
- Cursing and other hostile forms of communication,
- Short fuse and frequent arguments,
- Spreading gossip or rumors to harm others deliberately,
- Uninvited sexual remarks,
- Hostile responses to other nurses, patients, or family members,
- Sleep disturbances mentioned at work, and
- Increased irritability and anxiety.

The next stage of violence might include the following signs:

- Conversation focused on "poor me, the victim,"
- Notes with threats or violent or sexual content,
- Verbalization that includes plans or a desire to harm someone,
- Stealing workplace property,
- Less interested in work and workplace assignments,
- Increased arguments, and
- Increased physical accidents or injuries.

As the anger intensifies, and if conflicts remain unresolved, the result can be violence against oneself or others.

- Behaviors directed toward oneself might include depression or suicidal threats.
- Behaviors directed toward others might include physical fighting, property destruction, or use of a weapon to harm others.

Prevention of Workplace Violence

Prevention entails management commitment and employee involvement.

- Prevention begins when each nurse makes a personal commitment to practice prevention guidelines.
- Participate in the training and refresher courses offered by the health care agency.
- Take advantage of programs offered by your police department or other agency.
- Remember that your focus is on *gentle self-defense*, not offense.
- Be prepared before workplace violence becomes an issue.
- There are policies in every workplace that cover forms of violence, as well as harassment. Check them out.
- Be alert to warning signs. Think through what you can do.
- **Take all threats seriously.** Report them to management and advocate assertively for implementing prevention guidelines (Box 14-3).

Box 14-3 | *Some General Safeguards for Preventing Workplace Violence*

- Do your part to promote a supportive, congenial, yet professional work environment.
- Whenever possible, resolve conflicts as they arise. Know that there are times when you have to back off. However, most of the time people want to have their point of view heard. A technique called *creative communication* encourages you to do the following:
  - Listen carefully to the other person's point of view.
  - Ask questions to clarify what you do not understand. (Remember that this step is not a sneaky way to argue or interject your own opinion!)
  - Tell the person what you think he or she said and what you think he or she is feeling. If your version is inaccurate, have the person repeat the explanation. When you can repeat back accurately what the person thinks and feels, then it is your turn to present your view. Use these steps as well when you present your point of view.
- Deal directly with unwanted or unwelcome behavior, including uninvited sexual advances. Review your own behavior to determine whether:
  - A clarification of the person's signals is in order.
  - Limits must be stated clearly and firmly on what you consider unacceptable behavior.
  - Supervisor or management intervention may be needed.
- Get to know your fellow workers and look out for each other.

Box 14-3   *Some General Safeguards for Preventing Workplace Violence—cont'd*

- Promote workplace integrity. Treat each other, your patients, and their families with respect, courtesy, and professionalism. Negative comments by patients and relatives usually are a response to their fear of the unknown. Rarely are the comments meant to be personal. Check out the fear. What are the questions? What can you do to help find answers?

- Be alert to changes in behavior that may signal violence.
- Avoid putting yourself in obvious danger. Make use of security guards for escort to parking lots and out-of-the-way areas. Listen to your intuition. This is making conscious use of affective communication.

 Critical Thinking Exercise

Personal Violence Prevention Plan

What additional ideas do you have to put into action to defuse or prevent violence of any kind in the workplace? Create an assertive approach.

SEXUAL HARASSMENT

Sexual harassment is about abuse of power. It is not about sex or passion. More than 50% of female nurses report that they have been sexually harassed. However, it is not limited to female nurses. Nearly a third of male nurses and nursing administrators believe that they too have been sexually harassed (Kurz, *RN*, July 2000). Most nurses do not report the incidents. The nurse puts up with harassment in order to remain employed, is embarrassed, or perhaps fears that he or she will not be believed. According to the Equal Employment Opportunity Commission (EEOC), sexual harassment includes unwanted sexual advances or other verbal or physical conduct of a sexual nature, such as: (1) a condition of employment or advancement, or (2) a hostile environment, where the advances intimidate, offend, or interfere with the nurses' ability to do their work. The key word is "unwanted." A distinct difference is made between consent and unwanted.

If you are the target, confront the person harassing you. Your assertive response is to tell the person clearly what they are doing—that this behavior is offensive to you and is unwanted. Be sure that your response is firmly assertive. Your message must be congruent so that the verbalization, body language (nonverbal), and affective communication all say the same thing. Mere words do not justify a physical response on your part. Document for yourself what happened, as well as what you said and did. Employers have the responsibility to correct unwanted (unwelcome) behavior that they know about or should know about in the workplace. If the unwanted behavior does not cease, report it to the supervisor, union representative, department head, etc., as needed, until you are heard. Take along your documentation. If the employer is convinced that someone is responsible for harassing, they can reprimand, require counseling, demote, transfer, deny a promotion or raise, or dismiss the harasser. The seriousness of sexual harassment can no longer be ignored. The nurse's work is usually affected; some leave their jobs to get away. For others, their emotional and/or physical health is affected, sometimes with long-term consequences. Complete the following learning and critical thinking exercises.

 Learning Exercise

Sexual Harassment Policy

Locate your school policy regarding sexual harassment.

Critical Thinking Exercise

Personal Plans for Safety

Make a plan for yourself on how you will deal with any harassment attempts during future employment.

COUNSELING AND FILING CHARGES

Levine et al. (1998) concluded that assault-related injuries are preventable. Only physical injuries are treated; all employees who have been verbally or physically assaulted should be referred for postincident debriefing. Hospital managers should implement violence prevention programs. If you are harmed or threatened by a patient or a patient's family member, you have the option to file charges. Some agencies will do this for you after a review board hearing, or they will support your filing charges yourself. Legal redress becomes an assertive stance for you and your fellow nurses (Carrol, 1997).

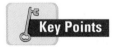

Key Points

- Communication translates into behavior.
- Assertiveness is honest and open behavior. It considers others' feelings and needs. It is based on choice.

- Nonassertive (passive) and aggressive behaviors are based on emotional hooks. These styles are ultimately damaging to both parties involved. Be alert to unresolved feelings leading to a cycle of worry→fear→anger →rage.
- Using the steps of the problem-solving process can change undesirable behaviors and interactions. Verbal, nonverbal, and affective interactions must be dealt with during this change.
- Some cultures value skillful positive manipulation. Positive manipulation involves consideration of others' needs and feelings. Furthermore, other individuals are treated with respect rather than as objects to be used for personal gain.
- Violence in the workplace has always been there, but it is on the increase in some areas.
- OSHA has established national guidelines to deter violence toward health care workers.
- Nurses are physically assaulted more often than are police and prison guards.
- Violent incidents are more common when nurses and security lack assertive management skills.
- Some patient diagnoses provide clues to potential violence.
- Legal redress is available to nurses injured during physical violence.
- Both female and male nurses report sexual harassment as a condition for employment or advancement.
- Focusing on learning to be assertive in nursing benefits both you and the patient.

REVIEW ITEMS

1. What is assertiveness?

   1. A level of communication that few nurses attain.
   2. Outspoken, anger-based, honest communication.
   3. Indirect method of getting others to do what you wish.
   4. Taking a positive stand without violating others' rights.

2. Which of the following best describes sexual harassment?

   1. You and a co-worker have been sharing sexual jokes since you started working.
   2. The immediate supervisor has asked you to spend a weekend together.
   3. A patient asks you if you are willing to go out on a date after he is discharged.
   4. Your co-worker calls you at home after you have firmly refused to date him.

3. What is an assertive response to a boss who is beginning to talk to you about problems with another nurse on the unit?

   1. I am honored that you trust me to problem-solve this issue with you.
   2. Maybe you and I can meet over coffee after the shift, so it's private.
   3. I'll talk to you about problems we have, but I won't discuss others.
   4. If you don't tell anyone of our conversation, I'll tell you what I know.

4. Which of the following recommendations will you offer the committee to promote unit safety?

   1. We need to look at staff attitude and body language in dealing with patients and visitors.
   2. Safety is an issue that must be placed in the hands of nonuniformed, outside security staff.
   3. It is necessary to go back to the strict visiting rules and limit hours and visitors to family.
   4. Violence is a part of our current culture, and there is very little you can do to effect change.

ALTERNATE FORMAT ITEM

Which of the following is not an example of an "I"-centered statement? *(Select all that apply.)*

1. I feel you are not quite working up to your potential.

2. I think that you could do your work a lot more carefully.

3. I saw that you had a problem getting the patient in the chair.

4. I will watch you demonstrate putting in a catheter today.

15 Leadership Skills

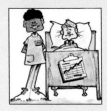

evolve http://evolve.elsevier.com/Hill/success/

Objectives

On completing this chapter, you will be able to do the following:

1. Describe the expanded role of the practical/vocational nurse (LPN/LVN), as described in your state's Nurse Practice Act.
2. Identify the location of the practical/vocational charge nurse on the organizational chart of a long-term care facility.
3. Explain the difference between leadership and management.
4. Identify your personal leadership style.
5. Explain the following leadership styles in your own words:
   a. Autocratic,
   b. Democratic, and
   c. Laissez-faire.
6. Identify ways to attain competency in the following five core areas, in which knowledge and skills are needed to be an effective first-line leader:
   a. Motivate team members to accomplish goals.
   b. Communicate assertively.
   c. Problem solve effectively.
   d. Build a team of cooperative workers.
   e. Manage stress effectively.
7. Identify ways to obtain competency in the following three specific areas, in which knowledge and skills are needed to be an effective first-line leader:
   a. Occupational skills
      1) Nursing (clinical) skills, including the nursing process
      2) Documentation

3) Legal aspects
4) Federal, state, and private organization regulations
   b. Organizational skills
      1) Time management
      2) Continuous quality improvement
   c. Human relationship skills
      1) Anger management
      2) Performance evaluations for nursing assistants
      3) Empowering team members
8. Describe how the Howlett Hierarchy of work motivators can help the practical/vocational nurse leader influence nursing assistants to motivate themselves.
9. Identify the importance of documenting objective, not subjective, charting entries in long-term care.
10. Use the problem-solving approach to set up a plan to solve a clinical problem.
11. Read the mission statement for your current area of clinical assignment.
12. Using suggestions in this chapter, write a plan that could be used to build a team to work on a unit in long-term care.
13. Develop a plan to decrease stress in the clinical area.
14. Using the ABCD method of Ellis, identify an irrational thought you have had on the clinical area, and convert it to a rational thought.
15. In your own words, explain specific skills required of the practical/vocational charge nurse in long-term care because of Omnibus Reconciliation Act of 1987 (OBRA) regulations.

16. Prioritize tasks that need to be completed for your next clinical assignment.

17. Identify areas to improve efficiency in your current area of clinical assignment.

18. Practice giving positive and negative feedback, in measurable terms, to peers in a mock clinical situation.

19. Develop a plan for personal growth as a practical/vocational charge nurse.

Key Terms

Autocratic style (p. 252)
Centers for Medicare and Medicaid Services (CMS) (p. 263)
Conflict resolution (p. 266)
Continuous quality improvement (CQI) (kŏn-TĬN-ū-ŭs, p. 265)
Continuum (kŏn-TĬN-ū-ŭm, p. 252)
Empower (p. 271)
Howlett hierarchy (HĪ-ē-RĂR-kē, p. 254)
Irrational thinking (p. 261)
Leadership (p. 251)
Management (MĂN-ĭj-měnt, p. 250)
Mission statement (p. 259)
Omnibus Budget Reconciliation Act of 1987 (OBRA) (RĒ-kŏn-SĬL-Ē-Ā-shŭn, p. 263)
Patient outcomes (p. 265)
Performance evaluation (p. 269)
Quality Improvement Organizations (QIOs) (p. 266)
Stress management (p. 261)
Subjective versus objective (p. 262)
Team building (p. 259)
The Joint Commission (p. 264)
The Nursing Home Reform Act of 1987 (p. 263)
Time management (p. 264)

Keep in Mind

"The manager does things right. The leader does the right things." Warren Bennis: On Becoming a Leader (1989)

Grace and Emily, nursing assistants at Quality Care Home, collapsed in their chairs in the lunchroom. "I had forgotten how hectic mornings can be," said Grace. "I am exhausted." This was the first day back on the day shift on the Evergreen Wing for both nursing assistants.

Both women had substituted for a week for vacationing nursing assistants—Grace on nights and Emily on the evening shift.

"I don't care how tired I am, I sure am glad to be back with our charge nurse," said Grace. "I missed Sal Sytchuashun's way of running things," she continued. "On nights, being with that LVN, Gina Ivanapleze, was like working with mass confusion. Anything you wanted to do was fine with her. It seemed the most important thing to her was the happiness of the nursing assistants, not the resident's care. Anything we wanted to do was hunky-dory. Sal listens to my suggestions but also offers input when I need it."

"That sure is different from my experience," said Emily. "Being with RN Priscilla Pittbul taught me the real meaning of her initials—real nasty. She commanded us to do everything; she never suggested. Never a 'thank you' or 'good job.' We had a task list and a time sequence to follow and, despite what cropped up, heaven help us if we didn't stick to it precisely. We couldn't even ask questions about her assignment sheet. The only time I appreciated Priscilla barking her orders was the evening we had a code. I was shaking in my boots but she knew exactly what to do. And the resident pulled through."

"I'm glad we didn't have a code with Gina in charge," said Grace. "We have so few codes around here. That is a situation in which I would appreciate having some direction.

"I liked the way Sal handled the situation this morning in the lounge, when a resident complained of chest pain," Grace added. "Sal gave us each something to do STAT. After the situation was over, we all discussed the emergency as a team. Sal listened to our suggestions on how to make things go more smoothly in the next emergency situation. Sal makes me feel like a real team member and not a slave!"

Grace and Emily finished their lunches. As they went back to Evergreen Wing, they both agreed that LVN Sal has a way about him that gets the job done, makes you feel comfortable about going to him with a concern or question, and makes you want to come back to work for the next shift. Both agreed he is a good role model for the vocational nurses and nursing assistants.

PRACTICAL/VOCATIONAL NURSE AS FIRST-LINE LEADER

Have you ever experienced employment situations similar to the ones just described with Gina and Priscilla? Perhaps you received directions as a nursing assistant or in another job capacity and did not like the way you were approached by your supervisor.

Nurses at all levels need to manage patient care. Some nurses will also be leaders. Licensed practical/vocational nurses have proved themselves effective as first-line leaders. First-line leaders are responsible for supervising nursing assistants who deliver care in long-term care situations. Such positions are referred to as charge nurse positions. If you are a manager of patient care and a leader, you will be more effective in this expanded role in practical/vocational nursing.

Practical/vocational nurses need to develop **leadership** and **management** skills so they can direct and supervise others in a manner that will effectively meet the goals of the employing agency. In your practical/vocational nursing program you started to build a strong, solid base in these skills. The purpose of Chapters 15 and 16 is to help you continue to develop skills to lead and manage. This chapter will focus on the leadership role and provide 21 Leadership Hints, 5 Leadership Activities, and 1 Critical Thinking Exercise to get you started thinking in a leadership mode.

Chapter 16 provides 10 Management Hints, 14 Management Tools, and 3 Critical Thinking Exercises to help you apply the knowledge and skills needed to be a charge nurse. The interactive format of both chapters, especially Chapter 16, will have you thinking as a new charge nurse and solving some of the problems new charge nurses face. Chapters 15 and 16 can be used as reference tools of skills while orienting to a practical/vocational charge nurse position. They can also be used in a future job when you function in your expanded role as a licensed practical/vocational charge nurse.

ORGANIZATIONAL CHART

The organizational chart is a picture of responsibility in an employment situation. In the traditional organizational chart, individuals who are lower on the organizational chart report to the person directly above them on the chart. Figure 15-1 shows where the practical/vocational nurse fits into the traditional organizational chart as a first-line leader. In Figure 15-1 the practical/vocational nurse reports to the nurse manager, who is a registered nurse. Nursing assistants report to the practical/vocational nurse. To whom does the nurse manager report?

Because of changes in the structure of organizations, organizational charts have become more horizontal than vertical in appearance. Figure 15-2 provides an example of a contemporary

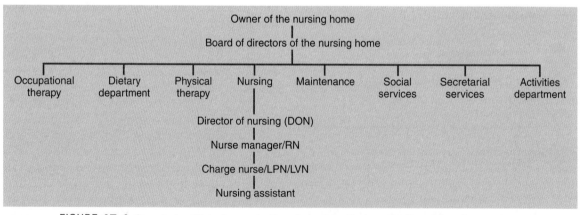

FIGURE **15-1** Sample traditional organizational chart for the practical/vocational nurse in the Charge Nurse role.

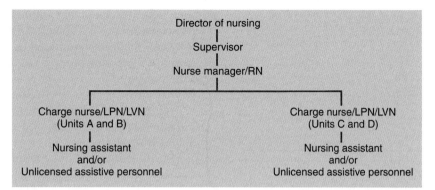

FIGURE **15-2** Sample contemporary organizational chart for the practical/vocational nurse in the Charge Nurse role.

organizational chart. This "flattening out" has eliminated some of the middle manager positions in organizations. As a result, remaining middle managers have taken on more responsibilities and are spread thin. Middle managers in this system have more persons reporting to them than in the past. Middle managers depend on the people who report to them, such as the practical/vocational charge nurse, to think critically and problem solve. Middle managers expect to be contacted when you have tried and are unable to solve your own problems. See Leadership Activity: Examining Organizational Charts.

Leadership Activity

Examining Organizational Charts

Resources Needed:
- Organizational charts from clinical sites used by students in your practical/vocational nursing program

Organizational charts may differ by region of the United States. Obtain organizational charts of long-term care facilities in your area. Clarify specific levels of responsibility as they apply to the practical/vocational nurse. Identify whether these charts reflect a traditional or contemporary style of organization.

EXPANDED ROLE OF PRACTICAL/VOCATIONAL NURSING

It is important for you to review the current Nurse Practice Act of your state. This law legally defines the exact role and boundaries for practical/vocational nurses. Also review the following for more guidelines related to the expanded role of the practical/vocational nurse:

1. Appendix B: NAPNES Standards of Practice and Educational Competencies of Graduates of Practical/Vocational Nursing Programs
2. Appendix C: NFLPN Nursing Practice Standards for the Licensed Practical/Vocational Nurse

See Leadership Activity: Determining Your State's Requirements to Assume the Position of Practical/Vocational Charge Nurse.

Leadership Activity

Determining Your State's Requirements to Assume the Position of Practical/Vocational Charge Nurse

Resources Needed:
a. Your state's Nurse Practice Act

1. Obtain a current copy of your state's Nurse Practice Act. Nurse Practice Acts can be purchased from your state's Board of Nursing for a nominal fee, which covers printing costs. Identify the part of the act that addresses your state's position on the

practical/vocational nurse assuming the charge nurse position in the following areas:

a. Requirements before assuming the practical/ vocational charge nurse position

b. Site of employment

c. Scope of practice

2. If your state's Nurse Practice Act does not address the issue of charge nurse, how can this information be obtained?

An example of the expanded role of the practical/ vocational nurse is the first-line manager position, also called charge nurse, in a nursing home or long-term care facility. In these situations the practical/vocational nurse has the responsibility of supervising the care given by nursing assistants and other personnel. The practical/vocational nurse will direct, guide, and supervise these health care workers as they attempt to meet the goals of the resident's plan of care.

The most recent practice analysis of entry-level practical/vocational nurses by the National Council of State Boards of Nursing (NCSBN), for which data is available, occurred in 2006. This survey identified that 48.2% of practical/vocational nurses responding to the survey reported they had one or more administrative roles with 72.4% of these respondents working in long-term care. Fifty-eight percent of respondents in long-term care reported the charge nurse position as their administrative responsibility (Wendt, 2007). To carry out the first-line manager/charge nurse role effectively, you will need the abilities found in a leader **and** a manager. The 2006 practice analysis can be obtained at *http://www.ncsbn.org/359.html*.

HOW YOU ARE ALREADY PREPARING FOR A LEADERSHIP AND MANAGEMENT ROLE

The topic of leadership and management for the practical/vocational nurse is a vast one. All practical/vocational nurses are managers in the sense that they consistently need to direct, handle, and organize care for assigned patients. It is worthwhile for you to review the ways in which your practical/vocational nursing program helps

prepare you for a management position. The practical/vocational nursing program encourages development of the following skills, which are necessary for functioning successfully as a first-line manager:

1. Basic nursing skills, including the nursing process,
2. Time-management techniques for home and clinical time,
3. How to learn new information, including use of resources for learning,
4. The power of positive self-talk and thinking,
5. Rules for assertiveness,
6. Communication skills,
7. Ethical aspects of health care,
8. Legal aspects of health care,
9. Problem solving and critical thinking,
10. Stress management, and
11. Participation in clinical evaluation.

Learning leadership and management involves much more than taking one course or reading one chapter about becoming a leader. Learning leadership is a process (continual development) that includes many skills and is something that evolves over time. This chapter will encourage you to think specifically of a leadership role, and it will provide leadership hints needed by practical/vocational nurses.

DIFFERENCE BETWEEN MANAGEMENT AND LEADERSHIP

Management is the organization of all care required of patients in a health care setting for a specific period.

- The focus of management is planning and directing to meet patient goals.
- Management is a formal role given to a person by the employer.
- Managers are appointed by their employers.
- The tools needed for management could be written in a step-by-step manner and given to you to follow.
- Following the directions for using the management skills would possibly get the job done in an efficient manner.

Leadership is the manner in which the leader gets along with coworkers and accomplishes the job.

- The focus of leadership is to produce changes in the workplace that will meet the goals of the employing agency.
- Leadership is an informal role that is given to a person by a group of workers. You become a leader when your team members decide to follow you.
- Leaders cannot be appointed.
- The leader needs to influence others in the work setting to want to implement desired change.
- Directions for leadership skills can also be written, but it is through experience that leadership skills are truly developed.

The practical/vocational nurse who has the skills of management **and** leadership will get the job done in the most efficient and effective manner, and the practical/vocational nurse manager and coworkers will enjoy the experience that much more! A manager is not automatically an effective leader. A leader is not automatically an effective manager. Your goal will be to develop skills of leadership *and* management.

WHAT KIND OF LEADER ARE YOU?

There are several different ways to lead. What is your predominant leadership style? Each of the statements given in Leadership Activity: Discovering Your Personal Leadership Style is an extreme. The responses are not positive or negative. One answer does not have value over another answer. They just are.

 Leadership Activity

Discovering Your Personal Leadership Style

Put a check mark next to the statement that *best* describes the way you *might* be at work, not how you want to be.

A Short Test of Leadership Style:

1. My primary goal at work is to:
   a. Get the job done.
   b. Get along with the people with whom I work.
   c. Do the job correctly.
   d. Hope the work I do is noticed.
2. My clinical co-workers would say I am:
   a. Domineering in my relationships.
   b. Friendly and personable in my relationships.
   c. Likely to attend to details of the resident care plan.
   d. Creative and energetic in giving care.
3. At work, I feel like I have to be:
   a. In control of the resident situation.
   b. Liked by my co-workers.
   c. Correct in giving care.
   d. Recognized and praised for my care.
4. When I communicate on the nursing unit:
   a. I am usually direct and to the point.
   b. I am more considerate of the person to whom I am talking rather than strongly getting my point across.
   c. I usually give detailed information.
   d. I usually elaborate on the point at hand.
5. My co-workers would say I am a person who:
   a. Gets the job done regardless of what shift I work.
   b. Is very likable and patient.
   c. Is precise and accurate in giving nursing care.
   d. Is optimistic and has good verbal skills.
6. My charge nurse might describe my behavior while on my shift by saying that:
   a. Sometimes I alienate people.
   b. Sometimes I waste time and fall for excuses others may give.
   c. Sometimes I can be stubborn with co-workers.
   d. Sometimes I appear flaky to my co-workers.
7. I react to a stressful incident on the nursing unit:
   a. By being rude, blaming other departments, and yelling at co-workers.
   b. By being accommodating to the person in charge, and by passive behavior.
   c. By becoming silent and withdrawing from the situation.
   d. By talking faster and louder.
8. When I deal with my co-workers on the nursing unit regarding patient matters, I like them to:
   a. Get to the point and be business-like in their behavior.
   b. Be casual and sincere in their behavior.
   c. Use the facts of the matter and go step-by-step when explaining a resident-care situation.
   d. Be enthusiastic about the situation and use demonstrations to explain their points.

Continued

Add up your "a" and "c" answers. These answers are more characteristic of a task-oriented person. In leadership terms this person is called an *autocratic* leader. Add up your "b" and "d" responses. These are more characteristic of a people-oriented person. In leadership terms this person is called a *laissez-faire** leader. Your score can give you a rough estimate of the tendency of your leadership style.

---

*French: Noninterference in the affairs of others.

LEADERSHIP STYLES

The literature abounds with examples of leadership styles. Figure 15-3 illustrates a continuum (a line with extreme opposites at each end) of leadership styles. Box 15-1 compares and contrasts the leadership styles found on this continuum.

BENEFITS AND DISADVANTAGES OF LEADERSHIP STYLES

A purely task-centered leadership style (autocratic style) thrives on power. It involves telling someone what to do, with little regard for the employee as a person who may have ideas about how to improve resident care or reach the goals of the employer. Adopting the autocratic or laissez-faire style in Box 15-1 to use consistently as a leadership style is unrealistic. Its consistent use could be disastrous. However, there is room for an autocratic leadership style; for example, in times of emergency. On the following lines, list two additional examples of situations that might require the autocratic style of leadership.

1. _____

2. _____

A purely people-oriented style (laissez-faire) focuses on people's feelings but ignores the task at hand. It allows employees to act without any direction. The goals of the employer will be compromised when the laissez-faire leadership style is used. At times, persons in leadership roles may feel the need to be liked by all team members and use this leadership style, but the task of accomplishing goals will be seriously compromised.

Focusing on both the task and the employee is characteristic of the democratic style of leadership. In this style the practical/vocational charge nurse displays concern for the work that needs to be done, as well as for the team performing the work. When using this leadership style, the practical/vocational charge nurse encourages supervised nursing assistants to discuss resident care, make decisions, and problem solve improvements in care. It may take longer than the autocratic style for work to be accomplished, but patient goals (outcomes) will be achieved, with staff having positive feelings about their supervisor and the experience. Examples of situations in which the democratic style of leadership is useful include daily nursing care situations, unit meetings, and reviews of patient care plans.

Situational Leadership

A popular system of leadership for the twenty-first century is called *situational leadership*. Situational leadership involves varying your leadership style to meet the demands of the situation in the work environment. According to this system, the practical/vocational nurse needs to pick a leadership style that fits the work situation at hand.

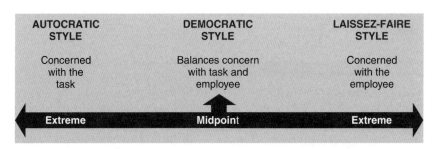

AUTOCRATIC STYLE	DEMOCRATIC STYLE	LAISSEZ-FAIRE STYLE
Concerned with the task	Balances concern with task and employee	Concerned with the employee
Extreme	**Midpoint**	**Extreme**

FIGURE **15-3** Extremes of leadership styles on a continuum.

Box 15-1 | *Comparing Autocratic, Democratic, and Laissez-Faire Styles of Leadership*

GENERAL DESCRIPTION
Autocratic: Does not share responsibility and authority with employees
Democratic: Shares responsibility and authority with employees
Laissez-faire: Gives away responsibility and authority to employees

IMPORTANCE OF AGENCY'S POLICIES
Autocratic: Emphasis is on policies
Democratic: Enforces policies but with concern for employees
Laissez-faire: Puts employees before policies

HOW LEADER GETS THE JOB DONE
Autocratic: Tells employees what tasks to do; does not seek input from employees
Democratic: Seeks input from employees and encourages problem solving
Laissez-faire: Tries to please everyone

WHAT GETS DONE
Autocratic: May reach goals
Democratic: Because of involvement of employees, goals may be achieved with positive staff feelings
Laissez-faire: Maybe nothing, but staff feels good.

WHEN STYLE CAN BE USED
Autocratic: Crisis situations, code situations, emergencies
Democratic: Daily nursing care situations, meetings, committees, review of care plans
Laissez-faire: When agency goals/policies are not a consideration

USING THE LEADERSHIP CONTINUUM AS A GUIDE

The value of a continuum, as shown in Figure 15-3, is that as you move along the continuum from each extreme toward the center or midpoint, the two extremes begin to blend together. You have some of each style, depending on where you are on the continuum. A blend, to some degree, of the two extremes in the appropriate work situation would be the leadership style needed at the moment.

Leadership Activity

Plotting My Leadership Style Score

Using your leadership style score from Leadership Activity: Discovering Your Personal Leadership Style, place an "X" on the continuum in Figure 15-3 to indicate where you are at this point in general leadership style tendencies.

Remember, this score is your tendency. If your "X" is far to the left or right, it will benefit you to be aware of this tendency and to avoid using this style consistently. Remember the continuum and the need to be flexible in your style. Balance task and people orientation as needed. Knowing what your predominant style of leadership is will be helpful in your evaluation of work situations and the style needed at that time. Some situations require a supportive style, whereas others require a more directive approach.

CORE KNOWLEDGE AND SKILLS NEEDED FOR LEADERSHIP

To function well in your expanded role as practical/vocational charge nurse, you will strive to be a good leader. The scenario at the beginning of this chapter provides examples of what not to do as a nurse leader. Much research in learning about the business of leading others and the theories that go with leading is available in the literature. *Core knowledge and skills lay the foundation for leadership.* They will help you develop other necessary knowledge and skills for your leadership role. We identify five **core areas** of knowledge and skills that are necessary for the practical/vocational charge nurse to be an effective leader. These core areas include the ability to do the following:

1. Motivate team members to accomplish team goals,
2. Communicate assertively,
3. Problem solve effectively,
4. Build a team of cooperative workers, and
5. Manage stress effectively.

UNDERSTANDING MOTIVATION AND HUMAN NEEDS

As a leader, you will have the task of getting your team members to meet goals set by your employer. Getting people to do what needs to be done is a complex task. What motivates one person does not necessarily motivate another. However, generally understanding motivation and human needs will help you get started.

Motivation

Motivation is a drive that causes individuals to set personal goals and behave in a way that will allow them to reach those goals. The motivation drive comes from within an individual and thus is said to be *intrinsic*. Because motivation is intrinsic, an LPN/LVN manager, or anyone else for that matter, cannot motivate another person to do something.

Human Needs

All individuals have needs that must be filled to meet goals. Individuals are internally motivated to engage in various activities to meet these needs. The activity they engage in is called behavior and can be observed. Abraham Maslow, a psychologist, presented a pyramid of human needs that can assist the learner in understanding self and ranking human needs. You have studied Maslow's Hierarchy of Needs in your nursing courses.

The human needs theory developed by Maslow in 1962 outlines our basic needs in a hierarchy (Fig. 15-4). Meeting needs on one level of the pyramid acts as a motivator for meeting needs on the next highest level. However, progression through these levels is not clear-cut. In reality, as most of your needs are met on one level, you are already beginning to check out the next level. When faced with overwhelming difficulties, physical or emotional, some regression takes place. For example:

1. Physiological needs become a priority if you have lost your job or housing.
2. Safety and security needs become a major issue if you are facing a serious illness, move into an unsafe neighborhood, or are facing a divorce.

Once these issues have been dealt with or resolved, higher needs will reemerge.

Adapting Maslow's Hierarchy

Maslow's Hierarchy of Needs can be adapted to help the first-line LPN/LVN leader understand motivation of team members in a health care setting, based on needs. Refer to Figure 15-5, the Howlett hierarchy of work motivators. Remember, all behavior is internally motivated.

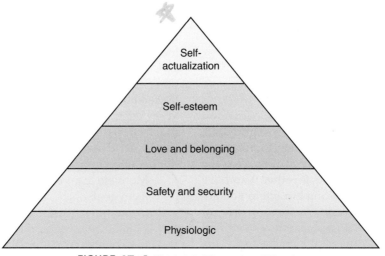

FIGURE **15-4** Maslow's Hierarchy of Needs.

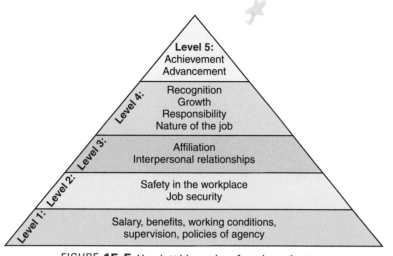

FIGURE **15-5** Howlett hierarchy of work motivators.

All levels of the pyramid in Figure 15-5 are considered to be needs of employees in an employment situation. With some exceptions, the opportunity to meet these needs can be encouraged or discouraged by the employer and the work environment, including the charge nurse (extrinsic motivators). If these needs are met, the person can proceed to the next highest level of the pyramid. If these needs are not met, a person may become dissatisfied with the work situation.

At a time when it is difficult to find and keep quality nursing assistants to work in a long-term care facility, retaining staff is very important. As an LPN/LVN manager, you can influence what nursing assistants might be motivated to do. You can encourage the motivation your nursing assistants already possess. If nursing assistants can see that doing a good job is in their best interest and helps them meet personal needs, they will work hard to meet the goals of their employing agency.

Using the Howlett hierarchy to meet needs of employees can help LPN/LVN managers influence and direct employees to act in certain ways to benefit the employer, as well as meet personal needs. It is a challenge for the leader to channel the motives of team members to meet the goals of the employer. As you go up the Howlett hierarchy (see Figure 15-5), begin identifying strategies that could be carried out to encourage meeting needs of nursing assistants

at each level. Also, identify whether the employer needs to initiate the strategy or whether the strategy could be initiated by the first-line practical/vocational nursing leader. As needs are met on one level, movement can then be encouraged to the next level of the hierarchy. Strategies for levels 3 and 4 can play an important role in motivation for team members at any level of the Howlett hierarchy. Praise, recognition, and rewards are extremely important tools for leaders. Research has shown that rewarding desired behavior of employees is instrumental in having that behavior repeated. Research also indicates that employees find personal recognition more motivating than money (Herzberg, 1993). See the following Critical Thinking Exercise: Using the Howlett Hierarchy in Leadership Situations.

Critical Thinking Exercise

Using the Howlett Hierarchy in Leadership Situations

Resources Needed:
* Readings on motivation, the Howlett hierarchy, and your creativity to find ways to meet needs of nursing assistants.*

This critical thinking exercise encourages the nurse to be creative in finding ways to encourage motivation in nursing assistants. The exercise gives you an opportunity to assume responsibility as an LPN/LVN leader.

- Examples of behaviors that encourage meeting needs at each level of the hierarchy are given.
- The person responsible for the behavior is listed in parentheses.
- Space is provided for you to fill in additional suggested behaviors at each level, which shows how you can meet needs of nursing assistants and therefore encourage their motivation.

Level 1: Salary, Benefits, Working Conditions, Supervision, and Policies of Agency

Examples
- Explanation of policies that affect employees (first-line LPN/LVN leader)
- Cafeteria-style benefits—pick and choose benefits (employer)

Level 2: Safety in the Workplace and Job Security

Examples
- Provision of adequate equipment to carry out standard precautions (employer and first-line LPN/LVN leader)
- Establish policy for hostile patients (employer and first-line LPN/LVN leader)

Level 3: Affiliation and Interpersonal Relationships

Examples
- Plan monthly potluck dinners, pizza lunches, get-togethers (first-line LPN/LVN leader)

_____

_____

Level 4: Recognition, Growth, Responsibility, and Nature of the Job

Examples
- Encourage attendance at continuing education seminars, in-service training, etc. (employer and first-line LPN/LVN leader)
- Recognize employees when working short-staffed (employer and first-line LPN/LVN leader)

Level 5: Achievement and Advancement

Examples

Recognition of successful completion of class or seminar (employer and first-line LPN/LVN leader)

Provide objective examples of how you can implement each of your suggested behaviors. For example, level 5 could be implemented by the following examples:

- A written account in the facility's newsletter,
- Posting an announcement on a special section of the bulletin board, and/or
- A personal note of congratulations from the charge nurse.

_____

*Appendix F, The Howlett Style of Nursing Leadership, contains additional suggestions.

APPLYING COMMUNICATION SKILLS AS AN LPN/LVN LEADER

One of the LPN/LVN leader's most productive tools is the effective use of verbal and nonverbal communication. The principles of communication in Chapters 9 and 14 are building blocks for the communication skills you will need as a practical/vocational charge nurse. See Leadership Hint: Communication of the Practical/Vocational Charge Nurse and Leadership Hint: Encouraging Verbal Communication from Nursing Assistants.

Leadership Hint

Communication of the Practical/ Vocational Charge Nurse

Verbal

1. In talking to nursing assistants, deliver your message with clear, specific language. Spell out objectively what has to be done for residents. If you work with nursing assistants who do not speak English as a first language, determine their proficiency with English. Verify that intended messages were received.
2. As a practical/vocational charge nurse, you are a role model for nursing assistants. Discourage profanity, personal criticisms, gossip, and rumors.
3. Use "I" instead of "you" messages. "I" messages indicate you take the responsibility for the message. For example, "I saw you tie the patient's wrist restraint to the side rail. This could cause injury to the patient when the side rail is lowered. I suggest you review the videotape on application of restraints. Also review the policy this home has about the danger of restraint application." "You" messages imply you blame the person to whom you are speaking. For example, "You did a poor job applying that wrist restraint." Take responsibility for your messages.

4. In talking with your supervisor, be valued for your input. Avoid being known as someone who just brings up problems. After objectively stating the problem, offer solutions.

Nonverbal

1. Be sure your body language and message are consistent and professional. For example, avoid smiling when you are delivering a needed reprimand. Face the person to whom you are speaking.
2. When delivering your message, appear sure of yourself. Have an attentive posture.

Written

1. Use language that all staff will understand.
2. Review your written messages before posting them to be sure the intent of the message is clear.
3. Provide written work assignments that do not require the nursing assistant to make judgments.
4. Provide written reports of all meetings. If information is not restricted, a report from a meeting with management can dispel/prevent rumors about what "they" are planning now. The reports can be placed in a loose-leaf binder in an area that is accessible for nursing assistants.

Telephone

1. Gather your thoughts before you make a call. This includes the purpose for the call.
2. With a smile in your voice, greet the person by name, identify yourself, and offer a brief inquiry as to their well-being, if you know the person you called. For example, "Hello, Mrs. Kylie, this is Tricia Zak from The Home. How are things going?"
3. State the reason for the call: "I need to order a video and wanted to know if you had any specific needs."
4. You initiated the conversation. Terminate it when your business is completed. The exception is when the person you called brings up a work-related question.
5. Avoid long conversations about non-work-related topics. This is what is considered allowing the telephone to extend into your time.
6. Arrange to have incoming calls answered quickly, by the second or third ring.
7. When you answer, identify the facility and give your name and title: "The Home, Tricia Zak, charge nurse."
8. Speak clearly in a moderate tone of voice. Most people talk too loudly on the phone.
9. Callers are "customers." Treat the caller respectfully and cordially.

10. If it is necessary to put the person on hold, ask permission to do so.
11. If it is necessary to put the person on hold, try to get back to her or him within 30 seconds. If you are still delayed, ask for a number so you can call back.
12. Provide the information requested.

Leadership Hint

Encouraging Verbal Communication from Nursing Assistants

1. Actively listen to nursing assistants. Avoid distraction and inattention.
2. Stay focused on what the nursing assistant is saying.
3. Avoid forming a response while the nursing assistant is speaking.
4. Avoid judging the message or the nursing assistant.
5. Rephrase the message when the nursing assistant is done to verify that you understand the message.
6. Encourage comments. Your goal is to have the nursing assistant go back to the team and say, "That charge nurse really listened to me!"
7. Encourage constructive evaluation. Create an environment in which nursing assistants are encouraged to give their input, whether positive or negative.
8. Respect all opinions. Nursing assistants need to feel safe to speak up, ask questions, identify problems, and suggest solutions to those problems.

APPLYING PROBLEM SOLVING AS AN LPN/LVN LEADER

The basic hint for successful problem solving is: **identify the real issue and solve it**. What is the problem? Avoid spending precious time on finding solutions for what is not really the problem. Chapter 6 introduced you to the nursing process, an excellent problem-solving process. You have been using this problem-solving method throughout your student practical/vocational nursing program. For problem solving, the nursing process can be used to solve resident problems as well as staff problems. The nursing process also works at home, as well as in the clinical area. See Leadership Hint: Decision Tree for Problem Solving (Fig. 15-6).

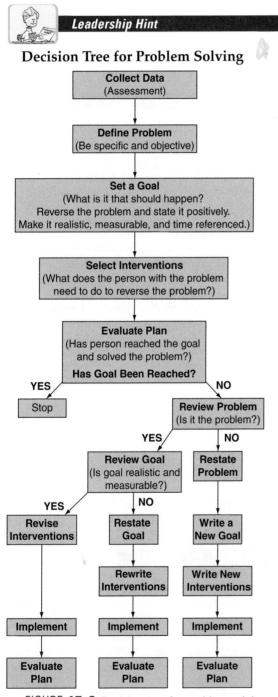

Leadership Hint

Decision Tree for Problem Solving

FIGURE **15-6** Decision tree for problem solving.

Scenario: Late for Assigned Shift

Penny, a nursing assistant, is assigned to the day shift in a long-term care facility. Her shift begins at 6:45 AM with a verbal report from the day practical/vocational charge nurse for her wing. All nursing assistants are expected to attend this report and receive their assignments at this time.

Data Collection. On May 8, 10, 15, 16, 23, and 24, Penny came to work either during the charge nurse report or after the charge nurse had finished. When questioned about this behavior, she states she has problems getting her teenagers up and ready for school.

Problem. A record of Penny's tardiness indicates this is a recurring problem and not an isolated incident. A pattern has been established in being late for report.

Goal. Starting immediately, Penny will be on time for the day charge nurse's report, and will hear the entire report.

Intervention. As the charge nurse, it is your responsibility to talk to Penny about this tardiness. This includes the times and days of her tardiness. Select a private location for your discussion. Encourage Penny to think through why this behavior is inconvenient for the staff and residents. Review the long-term care unit's policy on punctuality. Encourage Penny to come up with ideas that will allow her to be on time. Set limits with Penny. Identify that she needs to be on time for her assigned shifts. Plan to meet with her in 1 week to discuss her performance. At that time, if she has not improved her performance, a written reprimand will be given and included in her personal file. At the end of the meeting compliment Penny on an area of her work that has been going well.

Evaluation. During the next week, continue to document Penny's arrival for her assigned shifts. If she complies, note and praise her change in performance.* If she continues to be

---

*In the next week Penny actually arrived a few minutes before the other nursing assistants. The practical/vocational charge nurse allowed her to choose her break and lunch time. Penny had never experienced this before and was pleased.

late for her shift, issue a written reprimand. Place a copy in her file, give a copy to your supervisor, and keep a copy in your file. Be sure the warning contains objective information, such as the following:

1. Days and times late for shift,
2. Date of oral warning,
3. Seriousness of situation, and
4. Consequences.

TEAM BUILDING
Mission Statements

Mission Statement of The Home

- The Home is a private, nonprofit, long-term care facility. The Home provides 24-hour nursing care in a manner and setting that maintain or improve each resident's quality of life, health, and safety.

The practical/vocational charge nurse needs to be aware of the mission statement of the long-term care facility. A mission statement defines the purpose and goals of the organization. The foregoing mission statement contains what staff must do to meet the goals of The Home.

Each unit in the long-term care facility can write a specific statement of goals that spins off the facility mission statement. This will get the nursing assistants on your team thinking about what they believe and value in regard to resident care. One example of a unit mission statement that is a spin-off of The Home's mission statement follows.

The Home—Team A Goals

- Nursing assistants of Team A of The Home are committed to providing competent, caring, safe, and personalized service to residents and their families.

The team you supervise has the goal to carry out the mission statement of the long-term care facility. As charge nurse, you are in charge of creating the climate of the work environment that will motivate staff to meet this goal. In this situation the goal is maintaining or improving quality of life, health, and safety of residents at The Home. You are a role model for attitudes and behavior.

Your team will model the attitudes and behavior you expect of them. Suggested practical/vocational charge nurse attitudes to convey while attempting team building include the following beliefs:

1. Most employees want to do a good job at work.
2. Most employees want to reach their full potential.

See Leadership Hint: Using Unit Mission Statements and Leadership Hint: Practical/Vocational Charge Nurse Behaviors That Encourage Team Building.

Leadership Hint

Using Unit Mission Statements

1. Using input from nursing assistants, develop a unit mission statement for your unit.
2. Unit mission statements can be printed on small cards and carried in the pockets of nursing assistants.
3. Unit mission statements can be handed to residents and families on admission. Nursing assistant's first name and title can be included on the card.
4. Unit mission statements need to be reviewed on a regular basis to refresh nursing assistants about their goals. These cards are a written reminder of common values in resident care.

Leadership Hint

Practical/Vocational Charge Nurse Behaviors That Encourage Team Building

1. Review the mission statement of the facility with nursing assistants.
2. Review the unit mission statement with nursing assistants.
3. Use teamwork language, such as "we" and "us." Convey the attitude, "We have common goals, and together we will meet them."
4. Encourage politeness, cooperation, trust, and respect among nursing assistants.

5. Encourage honest feedback among nursing assistants.
6. Provide an opportunity for sharing of ideas among nursing assistants.
7. Ask nursing assistants for ideas on how to do unit tasks more effectively.
8. Provide occasions for nursing assistants to spend time together.
9. Create a positive environment in the clinical area that nursing assistants will want to be a part of.
10. Use rewards to provide positive reinforcement of behaviors that contribute to team goals.
11. Reward group accomplishments.
12. Treat nursing assistants on your team as you would like to be treated.

STRESS MANAGEMENT

Stress is a part of all work environments. The long-term care area has its fair share because of increased workloads (especially when a nursing assistant calls in sick) and conflicts with nursing assistants, physicians, families, and residents. Stress and anxiety in the clinical area can result in dysfunctional behavior on the job. Examples of dysfunctional job behaviors include the following:

1. Decreased performance of nursing assistants,
2. Negative interactions with nursing assistants,
3. Ineffective communication,
4. Inappropriate body cues, such as sharp tone of voice,
5. High staff turnover, and
6. Unhappy residents, families, physicians, and nursing assistants.

As a practical/vocational charge nurse, you have the responsibility to be a stress manager and role model for the team. Your goal will be to do the following:

1. Display the ability to cope with stress as it affects you.
2. Create a work environment with decreased stress levels.
3. Guide and support nursing assistants when they experience stress.

The practical/vocational charge nurse needs to learn how to detect stress in the clinical environment. A good place to start is to be aware of your own stress level. See Leadership Hint: Life Skills That Help Control Stress and Leadership Hint: Creating a Less Stressful Work Environment.

Leadership Hint

Life Skills That Help Control Stress

1. The actual stress reduction/relaxation technique you choose is personal. Whatever works for you is the skill to choose.
2. Review Chapter 10 regarding meditation, relaxation techniques, imagery, etc.
3. Massage.
4. Daily exercise: Walking is the easiest and least expensive form of exercise. No special equipment is required, except good walking shoes.
5. Apply the principles you learned in nutrition and let the food pyramid be your guide for getting the fuel your body needs. Review Chapter 10 for nutrition updates.
6. Get the amount of rest you need to function at your best.
7. Take your breaks when at work. You will be reenergized and increase your productivity.
8. Develop leisure activities you enjoy (or rediscover activities you put on the back burner during nursing school).

Leadership Hint

Creating a Less Stressful Work Environment

1. Your ability to organize your shift will help prevent some stressful situations.
2. Have available the equipment that nursing assistants need to get their job done.
3. Encourage nursing assistants to take breaks.
4. Create a calm environment.
5. Treat nursing assistants with respect. Remember your communication skills, especially "please," "thank you," and "I sure appreciate _____."

Leadership Activity

Identifying Signs of Stress

Resources Needed:
- Any text identifying physical and emotional signs of stress

The next time you feel yourself getting stressed, identify how you are feeling and what you are thinking. List the physical and emotional symptoms you experience.

Stress Control Skills for the Practical/ Vocational Charge Nurse

Controlling Stress by Altering How You Think. Stress is the body's reaction to the mind's analysis of a situation. It is not the situation, but your reaction to the situation, that creates stress. You have the only stress management tool you will ever need right inside your head. If you learn to manage how you think about the many interactions you have daily with nursing assistants, residents, and family members, you can control your reaction and therefore your stress level. See Chapter 10 for additional stress-reduction techniques.

Thinking Before "Irrational Thinking" Class
Nursing Assistant (on telephone): "I cannot come in today. I have a headache."
Practical/Vocational Charge Nurse *(thinking):*
I bet she has a headache. She probably spent half the night partying.

The LPN/LVN becomes abrupt with the nursing assistant and hangs up. She feels angry and allows the incident to ruin her entire day. Nursing assistants can sense that the charge nurse is upset and will try to avoid any contact with her.

Ellis (1994) discusses rational versus irrational thinking. When we are in a situation, we engage in self-talk about what is happening. This self-talk is often irrational because it is based on judgments we make about the situation. Judgments are subjective and have no bearing on facts. The irrational thinking then causes negative emotions, and stress often results. Ellis offers the ABCD way of increasing awareness of irrational thinking and changing how we think to a more rational way. In learning to do so, we control our emotions, and therefore the stress that results. The following are examples of how Ellis's ABCD method of controlling irrational thinking applies to the practical/vocational charge nurse.

A—Activating Event
The nursing assistant called in sick with a headache.
B—Belief (Self-Talk) About the Situation
The charge nurse thinks the nursing assistant must have been out partying.
C—Consequences
The LPN/LVN manager was abrupt with the nursing assistant on the telephone. She allowed herself to feel angry about the absence. She allowed it to ruin her whole day. Nursing assistants avoided her like the plague.
D—Dispute Irrational Thoughts
Choose a more rational, assertive response to the situation. Focus on the objective facts (nursing assistant has a headache). Avoid the subjective judgments that your beliefs (self-talk) call up (the nursing assistant was partying). You will avoid the anger over this incident and its effect on nursing assistants. Stress is avoided for all.

Thinking After "Irrational Thinking" Class
Nursing Assistant (on telephone): "I cannot come in today. I have a headache."
Practical/Vocational Charge Nurse (tempted to use irrational thinking but remembers Ellis's ABCD instead): "I'm sorry to hear that. I hope you will feel better with rest."
See Leadership Hint: Avoiding Irrational Thinking.

Leadership Hint

Avoiding Irrational Thinking

1. Be aware that beliefs about the situation are self-talk. Self-talk sometimes makes judgments. These judgments, if negative, can cause an emotional reaction. The emotional reaction leads to stress.
2. See situations objectively. Rational thinking is based on facts. Objective facts do not cause emotion. The situation "just is."

3. Avoid thinking that nursing assistants should, must, or always do something. This is another example of irrational thinking and can lead to anger. When you use these words for yourself, they can lead to anxiety and guilt.
4. We do not have the power to make nursing assistants do anything. We can encourage or prefer that nursing assistants do something.
5. For yourself and team members, use the words want, choose, and prefer in your thinking.

SPECIFIC KNOWLEDGE AND SKILLS NEEDED FOR LEADERSHIP

To be a leader in long-term care, it is necessary to use the aforementioned core areas of knowledge as a base and to develop the following skills in three specific areas:

1. **Occupational (clinical) skills:** The knowledge and skills of nursing.
2. **Organizational skills:** Skills necessary to function in the organization that delivers health care.
3. **Human relationship skills:** The ability to get along with and relate to people.

OCCUPATIONAL SKILLS FOR FIRST-LINE LPN/LVN LEADERS
Nursing (Clinical) Skills, Including the Nursing Process

Solid clinical skills are a must to be a good nursing leader. Visible expertise in clinical skills is a plus with the nursing assistants and also gives you an informal power base. See the resident situation for yourself, assist in providing care, and demonstrate nursing skills to nursing assistants as needed. This conveys the attitude that resident care comes first. This action demonstrates that the facility mission statement and unit goals are not just a written exercise. It communicates that practical/vocational charge nurses are there to support their staff.

Knowledge of your role in nursing process is an important part of organizational skills. Your practical/vocational nursing program has started your skill development in this area. You will

need to keep this area current and fresh. Refer to Chapter 8 for more about your role in the nursing process.

Documentation

Use the guidelines in Chapter 20 for your charting. Practical/vocational charge nurses need to be aware of the documentation requirements of federal and state laws and accrediting agencies. Specific, objective documentation demonstrates whether or not the standard of care has been met. Effective nursing documentation is the basis for payment of resident fees or denial of payment by Medicare, insurance, and/or the state. This is especially important when these agencies mandate **patient outcomes**. Incomplete or questionable documentation could also result in a citation for the facility. It cannot be emphasized often enough that you must make sure all your charting is specific, objective, and complete. Avoid subjective comments and personal judgments in your charting. Students sometimes find this area of charting difficult, especially if they see examples of general and subjective entries on charts by licensed staff in the clinical area. The following four situations are examples of subjective versus objective charting.

Subjective Versus Objective Charting

Subjective: Resident is drunk, confused, and uncooperative.
Objective: Odor of alcohol on breath, off balance, mistook nurse for a county sheriff, and refuses to stay in assigned room.
Subjective: Resident is noncompliant.
Objective: Found in room eating a large fast-food hamburger. Reminded of the need for restricted diet because of diabetes and receiving an intermediate-acting insulin.
Subjective: The family is nasty, abrasive, and difficult.
Objective: Resident's daughter yelled out when charge nurse entered room. Yelled that staff was out to get her father. Daughter refused to participate in health teaching regarding her father's diabetes.
Subjective: The pressure ulcer area is healing.

Objective: Border of pressure ulcer area on right trochanter is flat and pink. Area is 1 cm wide, 1.5 cm long, and 1.5 cm deep. Inner open area is reddish-pink. Small amount of clear, pink drainage on dressing.

Legal Aspects

The nursing assistants and you, the practical/vocational charge nurse, are the people who have direct contact with residents and their families on a daily basis. You have the ability to ensure resident and family satisfaction with care. You are also a vehicle to voice concerns. This in turn will decrease the need for legal action to resolve disputes. Chapter 20 provides you with information for being legally sound in your nursing career.

Be aware of your state's Nurse Practice Act, health care facility policies and procedures, state and federal regulations, and published standards of your nursing organizations and codes of conduct (NAPNES and NFLPN in Appendices B and C). The standards and codes are guidelines to evaluate safe practice. Keep current and informed.

Federal Regulations. Your facility must be in compliance with federal, state, and local laws. The impact of federal regulations in your facility is most strongly felt in the Omnibus Budget Reconciliation Act of 1987 (OBRA) and the Centers for Medicare and Medicaid Services (CMS).

The Omnibus Budget Reconciliation Act (OBRA) of 1987. OBRA contains The Nursing Home Reform Act. The basic objective of the Nursing Home Reform Act is to ensure that residents of nursing homes receive quality care that will result in their achieving or maintaining their "highest practicable" (reasonable) physical, mental, and psychosocial well-being. The act also established a Resident's Bill of Rights (The 1987 Nursing Home Reform Act: Fact Sheet: 2001). OBRA regulations will be reviewed with you at the time of your orientation. The Resident's Bill of Rights can be found at *http://www.aarp.org/research/legis-polit/legislation/aresearch-import-687-FS84.html.* See Leadership

Hint: OBRA Provisions That Deal Specifically with Nursing Assistants.

Leadership Hint

OBRA Provisions That Deal Specifically with Nursing Assistants

1. Nursing assistants require 75 hours of instruction before taking a state-approved written and skills competency evaluation. This establishes a baseline proficiency and competence of nursing assistants.
2. Each state must have a nursing assistant registry. This registry is an official listing of persons who have successfully completed nursing assistant training and competency evaluation. To be listed in a state directory, the history of the nursing assistant must be free of incidents of abuse, neglect, or dishonest use of property.
3. Your state's registry must be notified by the employer before employment of nursing assistants. The registry of some states is online.
4. Nursing assistants' work must be evaluated "regularly."
5. Nursing assistants must have 12 hours of in-service training per year.
6. If two consecutive years have passed without a person being employed as a nursing assistant, training and competency evaluation must be repeated.

Centers for Medicare and Medicaid Services. This agency was formerly called the Health Care Financing Administration (HCFA). CMS, a federal agency of the Department of Health and Human Services (HHS), certifies nursing homes for Medicare and Medicaid reimbursement. To receive payment, facilities are required to meet conditions of participation. The long-term care unit will have the conditions of participation in its policies. Current CMS regulations will be presented during your orientation.

Your State's Regulations. Long-term care units and nursing homes are licensed by the state in which they are located. Each state sets regulations that must be met to be licensed. Periodically, inspectors will visit the facility to determine whether the facility has any deficiencies. Being cited for deficiencies can affect licensing. Your state's regulations will be reviewed at orientation.

The Joint Commission is an independent, not-for-profit organization. The purpose of this organization is to improve quality of care by creating a safe environment for patients through the accreditation process. The Joint Commission reviews organizations such as hospitals, long-term care facilities, and home health agencies. Accreditation is a voluntary activity. If your facility participates in The Joint Commission accreditation, their requirements will be explained to you at your orientation. Detailed information about The Joint Commission and long-term care can be obtained at *http://www.jointcommission.org/AboutUs/joint_commission_facts.html*.

ORGANIZATIONAL SKILLS FOR FIRST-LINE LPN/LVN LEADERS

Organizational skills are an essential ingredient for leaders as well as team members. The emphasis on the personal and vocational issues/concepts course in your student practical/vocational nursing program has given you the opportunity to learn and apply principles of **time management** (see Chapter 3). **Continuous quality improvement** and conflict management are also necessary skills for the development of any nursing leader in today's health care organizations, including long-term care.

Time Management

Whether your dominance is on the left or right side of the brain, you have been given the opportunity this year to develop time management skills by applying the content of Chapter 3. Your school year has certainly provided the need to use your time effectively (doing the right thing) and efficiently (doing it right the first time, and in the appropriate amount of time) for class, clinical, and home. The step-by-step procedures learned in the nursing skills lab helped you prioritize your care for efficiency and the safety and comfort of the patient. You have experience organizing work for one or two patients in the clinical area. As a practical/vocational charge nurse, you will direct the care of approximately 30 residents and supervise a team of four to five nursing assistants.

Time management is more about management and less about time. Your ability to manage time will help you organize tasks and allow you to be successful as a charge nurse. Once again, the nursing process will be the tool to help you get organized. See Leadership Hint: Applying the Nursing Process to Organize Your Shift.

Leadership Hint

Applying the Nursing Process to Organize Your Shift

Assessment (Data Collection) of Tasks

1. Make a "to do" list that reflects unit routines and schedules. When new to the job, listing unit routines and schedules is helpful until you experience the actual routine. This list includes break times, staff meal times, resident meals and nourishments, scheduled physician rounds, and routine times for vital signs, capillary blood testing, medicine administration, treatments, and so on.

2. Develop a *worksheet* to use during report. Develop a form with which you are comfortable. Some charge nurses develop a list according to a sequence of room numbers. Others list residents that need special assessments. Others list treatments, vital signs, and so on by time.

3. *Prioritize* the list. Use Maslow's Hierarchy of Needs to set priorities for residents. Remember, physiological needs must be met before other needs are considered. As are most important needs and must be done. They could be life-threatening or urgent resident needs. Bs must be done, but there is more leeway in the exact time they are accomplished. Some Cs are necessary but not of urgent status. Some of the Bs and Cs can be assigned to unlicensed assistive personnel (UAPs) or postponed. Some Cs might not need to be listed at all. Examples follow:

Tasks	Examples	Comments
"A" tasks	STAT med, PRN med, q2h neuro check after resident's fall on prior shift.	New "A" tasks always surface during the shift, requiring modification of the "To Do" list. These needs are unpredictable and cannot be planned in advance.
"B" tasks	Routine medicine administration, dressing changes, routine resident personal care, ambulation, activities, routine treatments, nourishments, meals	These needs are recurring and predictable.
"C" tasks	Mail and flower delivery, chit-chat with family	Important but can be delayed.

Planning Use of Time (Goal Setting)

1. Plan tasks within a time frame of 2 to 3 hours. Arrange blocks of time according to unit routine. Planning allows you to have the feeling you are in control of the situation. Take resident preferences into consideration when you are planning. For example, one resident prefers to eat breakfast at 6 AM; however, breakfast is at 8 AM. Arrangements could be made for coffee and crackers at 6 AM, if diet allows.
2. Use the same guidelines for setting goals for planning time as with care plans or personal goals. Focus on goals as outcomes (the results expected after a given period). Using action verbs, make sure goals are realistic and measurable. A measurable goal states specifically and objectively what results are expected after a specified period. Set minigoals for timed tasks to keep you on task.
3. Planning involves having the equipment and supplies that the team needs for the shift and the shift that follows. As you collect data about residents when first starting your shift, check rooms and treatment closets for needed supplies. This includes linen, a well-stocked floor refrigerator, supplies for treatments, supplies for medicine administration kept on med cart, and so on.

4. Make sure you have your personal tools for the shift: your watch (working), a pen that writes, bandage scissors, a stethoscope, and a small notebook. Use the notebook to quickly jot down the equipment that is needed and results of data collection.

Implementing Your Plan

1. Remember, your plan is written in soft, non–trans fat margarine, not marble. Be flexible.
2. As you carry out your plan for the shift, expect interruptions of your planned activities. You know they will occur but not when. These include telephone calls, changes in residents' conditions, transfer of a resident, and staff injury.
3. When unexpected events occur, planning assists you to rearrange tasks. If you have a plan, you can return to the plan after interruptions. You can continue or revise the plan as needed.

Evaluating Your Use of Time

1. As nursing assistants give you reports for their assigned residents, seek input from them about the effectiveness and efficiency of the shift.
2. Ask for suggestions to improve staff and your use of time the next shift you work.
3. Keep a log of your shift activities. Look for a pattern of inefficient use of time. Examples of time wasters are putting things off, allowing unnecessary interruptions, socializing with staff, inability to say "no," allowing telephone calls to exceed needed time for business.
4. At the end of your shift, take a few minutes to plan for the next day. This will allow you to leave work-related activities at work, and it will allow you to enjoy your much-needed leisure time.

Continuous Quality Improvement

Continuous quality improvement (CQI) is a program found in all health care facilities. The principles of CQI found in health care are borrowed from those of the business world. The focus of CQI is quality of care. Quality is indicated by patient outcomes. Patient outcomes are observable, measurable results of nursing activities. The CQI program involves all **departments** of health care facilities, including long-term care. You will receive information about the CQI program during orientation at your facility. See Leadership Hint: CQI Components That the Practical/Vocational Charge Nurse Needs to Incorporate into the Leadership Role. Total quality management (TQM) involves all **employees** in improving the quality of their services to ensure customer satisfaction (Huber, 2006).

The Centers for Medicare and Medicaid Services (CMS) is involved with quality improvement in nursing homes and long-term care facilities. The Quality Improvement Organization (QIO) Program consists of a national network of 53 QIOs that are under the direction of CMS. The requirements of QIO include:

- Improve quality of care for beneficiaries
- Ensure that Medicare pays only for services that are reasonable and medically necessary and that are provided in the most appropriate setting.
- Protect beneficiaries by expeditiously addressing individual complaints, notices, and appeals, such as non-coverage (Quality Improvement Organizations, 2006).

Leadership Hint

CQI Components That the Practical/Vocational Charge Nurse Needs to Incorporate Into the Leadership Role

1. Review job descriptions with your nursing assistants. Emphasize the role they have in achieving quality care and resident service for a reasonable price (do it right the first time).
2. Remember that CQI is a continuous, daily part of your unit.
3. Encourage nursing assistants to report inefficiencies in resident care and the work environment.
4. Encourage nursing assistants to offer suggestions to solve the problems in Number 3 of this list.
5. When inefficiencies are noted, initiate a plan for improvement.
6. Consider volunteering for a CQI committee. Policies and nursing procedures are revised based on the input you and your nursing assistants provide regarding resident care and the functioning of the unit. It is personally rewarding to be included in policy and procedure revision because revisions improve resident care.
7. Document resident information in an objective and specific manner. Your documentation will be used to measure the effectiveness of CQI efforts.

Example of CQI in Action. A nursing home in northeastern Wisconsin experienced a 100% incontinence rate on one resident unit. Nursing assistants were concerned about the team time that it took to wash residents and change linens, the risk for skin breakdown, and the cost of laundry to wash the mountains of bed linens, protective pads, and resident personal items. With the help of their practical/vocational charge nurse and the director of nursing, the nursing assistants developed a plan to cut down on incontinence. They set a goal to decrease the amount of incontinence on the unit by 25%. Several months later they were quite surprised and pleased to see the results of their planning. The rate of incontinence decreased to 0%. The residents were pretty pleased about it, too (Mary Ann Kehoe, RN, Good Shepherd Nursing Home, Seymour, WI).

Conflict Resolution

Conflict can occur whenever two or more persons interact. In long-term care, conflicts can arise with nursing assistants, staff, residents, families, and physicians. Conflict is not always a bad thing; sometimes it is an opportunity for growth and learning. Other times the presence of conflict can point out the need for change in an organization. When conflicts are out in the open, the opportunity exists to settle issues. This is preferable to leaving conflicts unsettled. Unsettled conflicts can act like cancer, slowly growing into something much larger that may be more difficult or impossible to resolve. Tools to reduce conflicts include clear communication and the ability to work well as a team. Conflict resolution involves people settling their differences. Resolution of the conflict is an exercise in problem solving. See Leadership Hint: Applying the Nursing Process for Conflict Resolution.

Leadership Hint

Applying the Nursing Process for Conflict Resolution

Data Collection—Obtain All the Facts

1. When a conflict arises, avoid pursuing it on the spot. Arrange for the involved parties to meet in an area that will provide privacy.

2. Separate the person from the problem. Attack the problem, not each other.
3. Each party has its own perception and strong emotions about what happened. Unclear communication may result. Clarify subjective statements and generalizations. You need to obtain objective and specific facts. For example, clarify what is meant by "she always does that" and "they."
4. Actively listen to the person presenting "the facts."
5. Avoid formulating your response while the other party is giving "the facts."

State the Problem—Identify the Specific Issue
1. After hearing all sides, state in your own words what you understand is the conflict. Use "I" messages when presenting your perspective. For example, "Emma, I heard you say that Hannah always leaves the utility room in disarray and does not offer to help the other nursing assistants when she has completed her work and they are swamped."
2. Ask parties for feedback as to the accuracy of your understanding of the conflict: "Emma, am I clear about the nature of your complaint? Is there anything you would like to add or correct?" and "Hannah, is there anything you would like to add or correct about the situation?"

Interventions (Planning)
1. Convey the attitude of working side by side to settle the conflict. For example, sit side by side to work on the problem.
2. Involve all parties in identifying and discussing possible solutions to the conflict. The more alternatives the better. The goal is a solution that will be agreeable to everyone's interests.
3. *Avoid* bargaining over *positions (what you want)*. Egos are identified with positions. The parties involved will focus on defending their positions. In the end, all parties need to save face.
4. *Focus* on *interests (why something is wanted)*. Behind a *position* is a *motivating interest*. Behind opposite *positions* lie shared and compatible *interests. Compromise* involves giving up aspects of an issue that are important to one of the parties involved. This is not a good intervention. *Collaborate* for a win-win solution that focuses on shared or compatible interests.

Implementation—Implement the Selected Solution
On a sunny, cool day in the fall, two residents are sitting in the sun porch of a long-term care facility.

Resident A's *position* is that he wants a window open, and Resident B's *position* is that he wants the window shut. The practical/vocational charge nurse asks Resident A why he wants a window open. He replies, "So I can get some fresh air." The charge nurse asks Resident B why he wants the window closed. He replies, "So it won't be drafty."

A solution built on *collaboration* would involve the charge nurse wrapping Resident B in a blanket and moving his wheelchair to the north end of the sun porch. She would move Resident A to the south end of the sun porch and open a window near him. This is a "win-win" solution. A solution built on *compromise* would involve the practical/vocational charge nurse returning one of the residents to his room and accommodating the other in the sunroom. This is an "I win-you lose" solution.

Evaluation—Evaluate the Effectiveness of Interventions in Meeting the Goal
In the preceding situation, the practical/vocational charge nurse returns 30 minutes later and finds both residents peacefully asleep in their wheelchairs.

HUMAN RELATIONSHIP SKILLS FOR FIRST-LINE LPN/LVN LEADERS

Practical/vocational charge nurses can have excellent clinical skills, use the nursing process expertly, and document to the letter of the law. The practical/vocational charge nurse can have a good understanding of federal and state laws and requirements of accrediting agencies. Charge nurses can get the job done efficiently, but perhaps human relationship skills are the most important skills for an LPN/LVN leader to have. Gina Ivanapleze and Priscilla Pittbul *might* get the job done. Leaders with human relationship skills will get the job done with style and tact, without sacrificing quality. Nursing assistants will value their leader's style a whole lot more and be more effective in reaching the goals of the unit. Because success depends on what is accomplished through others, the ability to relate well to others is crucial.

Practical/vocational nurses are well versed in clinical skills. They risk bringing **clinical** problem-solving skills to the practical/vocational charge nurse role when leadership/management skills, in the area of human relationship skills, are needed in this position.

Anger Management

Besides providing money on which to live, work provides people with the opportunity to be recognized for what they do, to belong to a group, and to display their competence. (Review the Howlett hierarchy of work motivators.) When any of these needs is threatened in the course of the workday, or when you feel like a victim in a workplace with lack of control, you may get angry. Anger is not automatically bad. Anger gives you a cue that something is wrong. If your anger is justified, it can help you get your needs met by stimulating you to action. Harassment and discrimination are examples of situations in which anger is justified. If your anger is unjustified, or displayed inappropriately, it can get you and others in trouble. See Leadership Hint: Preventing Anger in Nursing Assistants, Leadership Hint: Personal Anger Management Techniques for the Practical/Vocational Charge Nurse, and Leadership Hint: Prevention of Workplace Violence.

Leadership Hint

Preventing Anger in Nursing Assistants

1. Meet the needs above level 2 (e.g., belonging, affiliation, and recognition) on the Maslow and Howlett hierarchies.
2. Use assertive communication, especially "I" messages. This will decrease the practical/ vocational charge nurse's being perceived as a threat. In your "I" messages, remember to include what you observed, the possible result of that observation, and your recommendations.
3. Actively listen, using direct eye contact and alert body posture to convey to nursing assistants that you are interested in understanding their point of view.
4. Successful team building helps nursing assistants feel like part of the group.
5. Seek input of nursing assistants to find solutions for unit problems. This provides a sense of control over one's work environment.

6. Use win-win strategies in conflict resolution to provide a feeling of having control over situations and being treated with respect.
7. Encourage nursing assistants to participate in objective evaluation of their clinical performance to maintain self-esteem, and give nursing assistants some control over what happens to them.
8. Encouraging self-evaluation also helps tone down an important but potentially volatile area, especially when areas for improvement are noted.
9. Attempt to help nursing assistants become self-confident, reach their full potential, and achieve the higher levels of the Maslow and Howlett hierarchies. When needs are met at these higher levels, nursing assistants are more satisfied in their work environment.

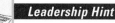
Leadership Hint

Personal Anger Management Techniques for the Practical/Vocational Charge Nurse

1. Learn your personal signs that communicate you are becoming angry. Pay attention to what you are thinking and feeling.
2. How you appraise events causes the anger response. Change irrational thoughts to rational thoughts.
3. If your heart is pounding, take deep breaths.
4. If you feel tension in a body area, rub the area for a few seconds.
5. When angry, speak slowly and in a lower tone of voice, acknowledge how you feel, and take a time-out.
6. View a stimulus to anger as a problem. Use the problem-solving process to arrive at a solution.

Leadership Hint

Prevention of Workplace Violence

1. Suggest in-service education in anger management for all employees.
2. Create a work environment that is respectful and fun.
3. As practical/vocational charge nurse, be a positive role model for anger management.
4. Take conflicts in the work environment seriously.

5. Refer to/use your facility's employee assistance program (EAP).
6. If your facility does not have an EAP program, suggest that such a program be developed.

Performance Evaluation of Nursing Assistants

The thought of performance evaluation can send shivers up the spine of the person doing the evaluating, as well as of the person being evaluated. Perhaps this goes back to bad evaluation experiences in prior situations. Perhaps it even goes as far back as grade school. Perhaps you and the nursing assistants have learned to associate evaluation with constructive criticism and weaknesses. Keep sight of the main purpose of evaluation, which is to encourage personal and career growth. Constructive evaluation gives you and your team members a profile of strong behaviors and behaviors for improvement, along with a plan to improve. Evaluation encourages the development of employees who will meet the facility's objectives and fulfill the mission statement. See Leadership Hint: Providing Feedback to Nursing Assistants.

 Leadership Hint

Providing Feedback to Nursing Assistants

Positive Feedback Identifies Strong Behaviors to Be Encouraged
1. Most nursing assistants know what it is like to be caught doing something "wrong." Catch them doing something "right." This encourages them to repeat the behavior.
2. Let nursing assistants know you notice their efforts, believe in them, and feel good about their contributions to the long-term care facility.
3. Praise people in measurable terms (specific and objective) so that the behavior can be repeated. For example, "When you disinfected the shower, I noticed that you paid special attention to the corners and the shower chair. Great job!"

Negative Feedback Identifies Behaviors That Need Improvement

1. Provide verbal feedback as close to the event as possible. The purpose of negative feedback is to point out behaviors that need to be modified. Focus on the behavior as one needing improvement. Avoid addressing the behavior as a criticism.
2. Without emotion, objectively point out what is wrong with the behavior and its consequences. You want the nursing assistant to remember the message, not the manner in which it was delivered. You also want the team member to know it is performance that is being evaluated.
3. Negative feedback needs to be accompanied by suggestions to correct the behavior. These suggestions need to be so specific that the nursing assistant will be able to correct behavior by following them. For example, "I noticed that the ties of your isolation gown were untied while you were in the room with the patient who has TB. Once you removed the gown, it risked spreading the bacteria to other patients, staff, and your family because the back of your uniform was not protected. When getting into an isolation gown, be sure to cover the back of your uniform and tie the gown at the waist."
4. Mention behaviors that need improvement first. Offer praise at the end of a reprimand. The message will be heard more clearly. The impact of the praising will not be ruined.

Ideas for feedback from Blanchard K, Lorber R (1992) *Putting the one-minute manager to work.* Berkeley Publishing, New York.

As a practical/vocational charge nurse, your responsibilities in evaluating nursing assistants include the following:
1. Observing skill performance and attitudes of nursing assistants.
2. Providing daily oral/written feedback, including suggestions for improvement.
3. Documenting observations.
4. Presenting a final evaluation form.

Review the evaluation process and form for your facility. What you are evaluating is not subject to your personal judgment. You will be objectively evaluating skills and attitudes of nursing assistants. These work-related activities are expected of nursing assistants and are found in their job description and the facility's policy manual. If a checklist format is used for daily observations, be sure you understand the scale used by the long-term care facility. In observing nursing skills, you will be evaluating the application of nursing assistant knowledge of a skill to actual skill performance. Attitudes are more difficult to evaluate. They are stated as observable behaviors and usually involve areas such as dress and grooming, attendance, functioning as a team member, and interpersonal skills.

The performance evaluation is written documentation of what you have been discussing and documenting throughout the period before the formal process of evaluation. Documentation is a time-consuming task. When you are used to the system for the long-term care facility, you will find it can be completed more quickly.

OBRA mandates regular evaluations for nursing assistants. In addition to scheduled performance evaluations, you will be giving spontaneous feedback to nursing assistants. Evaluation is the responsibility of the practical/vocational charge nurse and the nursing assistant. No one needs ever to "give" another person an evaluation. Evaluation needs to be a joint process. Evaluation is not a secret that you surprise team members with at the end of the evaluation period. It is a tool for personal and career growth. A team member has the right to be able to correct areas for improvement as time goes by. It is unfair to have your discrepancies unloaded on you (i.e., dumped) during the final evaluation interview. See Leadership Hint: Encouraging Nursing Assistants to Participate in the Evaluation Process and Leadership Hint: Meeting for the Final Evaluation Interview.

Leadership Hint

Encouraging Nursing Assistants to Participate in the Evaluation Process

1. Provide nursing assistants with a copy of the evaluation form at the beginning of the evaluation experience. Tell them it contains the elements you will be evaluating. Encourage them to read it.
2. Encourage nursing assistants to evaluate themselves daily and record their evaluation on the form. This also gives them the opportunity to become familiar with the form.

3. Remind them to include their strong areas. People are good at identifying areas for improvement but sometimes need reminders to acknowledge their strong points. Dispel the myth that to do so is egotistical or boastful. It is merely a statement of what is.
4. Encourage nursing assistants to include a plan on the evaluation form for improving areas that need improvement.

Leadership Hint

Meeting for the Final Evaluation Interview

1. Remember that the goal of evaluation is to encourage personal and professional growth. In preparation for the evaluation, summarize strong behaviors of the nursing assistant and behaviors that need improvement on your copy of the evaluation form. Develop a suggested plan for improvement. Attach this summary to the front of the evaluation. Remind nursing assistants to do the same and to bring their copy of the completed evaluation form to the meeting.
2. Schedule the interview for a private location.
3. Allow 10 to 20 minutes for the interview.
4. Conduct the interview in a neutral manner. Check your verbal and nonverbal messages.
5. Use "I" messages when discussing the summary sheet. For example, "The following are the behaviors that I observed when you were working with residents and staff...."
6. Start with strong behaviors and compare with the nursing assistant's list. This creates a good mood.
7. Compare behaviors for improvement.
   a. Similar behaviors appearing on both evaluation forms can indicate insight into the problem. Both the nursing assistant and the practical/vocational charge nurse have noted similar behaviors in the clinical area.
   b. When the nursing assistant includes behaviors not noted by the practical/vocational charge nurse, this can indicate the value of self-evaluation. The charge nurse cannot observe everything.
   c. If the practical/vocational charge nurse includes behaviors not included by the

nursing assistant, this can indicate lack of self-evaluation by the nursing assistant.

8. Finish the evaluation interview with the plan for improvement for any behaviors that need to be modified. The nursing assistant's plan is especially valuable because it indicates personal thinking through of interventions needed for improvement.

9. Check feedback throughout the interview to ensure clear communication. Have the nursing assistant rephrase feedback to see whether your intended message was heard. Some people may distort the message. Clarify messages given by the nursing assistant for information not understood. Encourage questions about any areas on the evaluation that are not understood. For example, "What did you understand me to say regarding your areas of strength that I have identified?"

10. Have the nursing assistant sign and date both evaluations. You do the same. The signature indicates the forms were discussed and all questions were answered.

Your nonthreatening, objective approach to constructive evaluation will result in positive evaluation experiences for you and the nursing assistants on your team. Occasionally you may experience a situation in which a nursing assistant feels threatened and becomes defensive during evaluation. If the defensiveness begins to escalate or the person displays anger, terminate the meeting. Set a new time for another meeting. Have your supervisor present at this time. Such experiences are the exception, not the rule.

Empowering Team Members and Encouraging Personal Growth and Development of Confidence

It is rewarding to see the nursing assistants on your team increase their self-confidence and display career and personal growth. You can empower nursing assistants and **encourage** personal growth by your position as practical/vocational charge nurse because of the leadership skills you have developed. The nursing assistant must do the actual work to achieve confidence and growth. See Leadership Hint: Strategies to Increase Self-Confidence in Nursing Assistants and Leadership Hint: Strategies to Encourage Personal Growth in Nursing Assistants.

Leadership Hint

Strategies to Increase Self-Confidence in Nursing Assistants

1. Provide opportunities to be successful in new situations.
2. Praise beginning successes in new situations.
3. On clinical evaluation forms, include positive statements as well as negative statements.
4. With administration's support, plan educational opportunities for nursing assistants (e.g., seminars and in-service programs).
5. Include nursing assistants in planning meetings, in-service ideas, and so on.
6. Stand up for and support nursing assistants.
7. Actively listen to problems involving the clinical area.
8. Teach nursing assistants a new skill and/or how to improve an old one.
9. Provide challenging assignments.

Leadership Hint

Strategies to Encourage Personal Growth in Nursing Assistants

1. Display a balanced interest in personal problems of nursing assistants.
2. Encourage nursing assistants to solve their own problems.
3. Suggest referral when nursing assistants are unable to solve personal problems. Follow facility policies.
4. Think of nursing assistants as individuals. Clip and give pertinent cartoons, articles, and so on.
5. Be a mentor/coach/teacher.
6. Be a role model. Display a positive work ethic; demonstrate good clinical skills; get out from behind the desk and see what is going on with residents; display good grooming; give objective, specific feedback; address the problem, not people; and actively listen.

ADDITIONAL RESOURCES FOR THE LPN/LVN TO DEVELOP ORGANIZATIONAL, OCCUPATIONAL, AND HUMAN RELATIONSHIP SKILLS

There are various ways of adding occupational, organizational, and human relationship skills for survival in the workplace. Some of the following suggestions for additional learning for the practical/vocational charge nurse offer continuing education credits. See Leadership Hint: Sources of Learning Skills for the Practical/Vocational Charge Nurse Position.

Leadership Hint

Sources of Learning Skills for the Practical/Vocational Charge Nurse Position

1. Check with your local vocational/technical school for a practical/vocational nursing leadership course.
2. Ask your boss to consider in-service programs on leadership techniques, as well as updates on nursing skills. Suggest cosponsoring such in-services with the local technical college and making them available to a wide geographical area.
3. Form a network with other persons who fill first-line leadership positions. Be sure to go outside your institution, as well as the discipline of nursing. You will find that the leaders have similar problems regardless of the discipline.
4. Attend seminars relating to leadership topics as well as nursing topics.
5. Read books and articles that offer hints for leaders. Be sure your personal nursing library is up to date.
6. Enroll for certification courses to enhance your knowledge and skills. See Chapter 23 for tips on making your career grow.

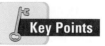

Key Points

- When the state's Nurse Practice Act allows, practical/vocational nurses are used as first-line leaders, especially in the nursing home/long-term care unit as charge nurse.
- The basic student practical/vocational nursing program offers students the opportunity to develop skills in nursing procedures, the nursing process, critical thinking, communication, time management, assertiveness, and stress control. These are skills needed for everyday practice, as well as leadership positions.
- Development of a leadership style is important in guiding nursing assistants to meet the goals of the long-term care facility.
- Established leadership styles range from the extreme of autocratic, with a pure emphasis on the task, to laissez-faire, which solely emphasizes concern with the employee.
- Situational leadership adapts a leadership style to the environment and situation at hand. It is the suggested way of leading in the twenty-first century.
- The five core skills of leadership involve the ability to (1) motivate team members, (2) communicate assertively, (3) problem solve effectively, (4) build a team of cooperative workers, and (5) manage stress effectively. These core skills lay the foundation for the development of other specific skills for leadership.
- Specific skill areas for nursing leadership include (1) occupational skills, (2) organizational skills, and (3) human relationship skills.
- No one chapter or course can teach you how to become a leader. The development of leadership skills is a process and evolves over time.
- In addition to training given by the institution, first-line practical/vocational nursing leaders need to educate and update themselves continually in the five core and three specific skill areas noted.

REVIEW ITEMS

1. Select the highest level of work motivator from the following list.

   1. Recognition and praise
   2. Job safety and security
   3. Social activities at work
   4. Policies, salary, and benefits

2. An LPN/LVN is interviewing for a charge nurse position in a long-term care facility. The employer questions the nurse about knowledge of situational leadership. Which of the following responses describes this leadership style?

   1. After report, tell nursing assistants the exact care to be given that shift and not to deviate from the care plan.
   2. In all situations, put nursing assistants before the policies of the nursing home and strive to be friendly and personal.
   3. To decrease workplace stress, seek suggestions from nursing assistants during a code for how to handle the situation.
   4. Evaluate the circumstances in the work environment and vary your leadership style to meet the needs of the situation.

3. Select the charting entry that is considered to be an objective entry describing the resident's response to the nursing intervention "force fluids."

   1. Nursing assistant spent much time forcing fluids from 8 AM to 11 AM.
   2. Resident drank a lot of fruit juice and Pepsi-Cola from 3 PM to 9 PM.
   3. Resident drank a total of 310 cc of liquids from 3 PM to 11 PM.
   4. Resident loves 7 UP, Coca-Cola, and orange juice without pulp.

4. Laura, a nursing assistant, has been absent four times this month, each absence occurring on the weekend. Which of the following practical/ vocational charge nurses is using problem solving to handle this situation?

   1. Focuses feedback on Laura's frequent absences for assigned shift.
   2. Downplays the importance of absences to make Laura feel better.
   3. Provides Laura with all the suggestions needed to correct the problem.
   4. Assumes being present for assigned shift is something Laura cannot do.

ALTERNATE FORMAT ITEM

A work-related conflict has surfaced between two nursing assistants on their shift at the long-term care facility, where a licensed practical/vocational nurse is charge nurse. Which of the following crisis intervention strategies does the charge nurse use to resolve the conflict? *(Select all that apply.)*

1. Develop a compromise solution to solve the conflict so that the two parties are satisfied with the solution.

2. To save time for resident care, limit the number of possible solutions offered to solve the conflict.

3. Instead of focusing on what each assistant wants for a solution, focus on why they want that specific solution.

4. Actively listen while each nursing assistant presents his or her side of the conflict and solutions.

5. Arrange to meet with the nursing assistants away from the site of the conflict to discuss the situation.

16 LPN/LVN Charge Nurse Skills: Management, Including Assignment and Delegation

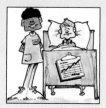

evolve http://evolve.elsevier.com/Hill/success/

Objectives

On completing this chapter, you will be able to do the following:

1. Using your state's Nurse Practice Act, identify the following as they apply to the charge nurse position for practical/vocational nurses:
   a. Requirements before assuming the licensed practical/vocational nurse (LPN/LVN) charge nurse position,
   b. Site of employment, and
   c. Scope of practice.
2. Review charge nurse job descriptions.
3. Identify specific institutional policies, regulations, and routines that the practical/vocational nurse needs to clarify when assuming a charge nurse position.
4. Collect a list of data that are needed before reporting a change of condition of a resident to a physician.
5. Discuss strategies for handling the following common LPN/LVN charge nurse problems:
   a. When nursing assistants bring problems from home,
   b. Encouraging nursing assistants to be accountable for learning skills, and
   c. Dealing with the demanding/complaining family.
6. Describe elements that need to be focused on when receiving and giving a change-of-shift report as charge nurse in the long-term care facility.
7. Discuss the assignment of tasks versus the delegation of duties with regard to the following factors:
   a. Your state's laws regarding the role of the practical/vocational nurse and the delegation of duties in the charge nurse position,
   b. Differences between assigning nursing tasks and delegating nursing duties,

   c. Legal aspects of assigning nursing tasks and delegating nursing duties, and
   d. The following criteria that need to be considered when assigning nursing tasks and delegating nursing duties:
      1) Right task,
      2) Right person,
      3) Right circumstance,
      4) Right direction/communication, and
      5) Right supervision (monitoring), feedback, and evaluation.
8. Using nursing process as a guide, discuss the method for assigning and delegating the following:
   a. Collecting data,
   b. Planning,
   c. Implementation,
   d. Evaluation,
   e. Putting it all together, and
   f. Reporting at the end of your shift.

Key Terms

Accountability (ă-KŎWNT-ă-BĬL-ĭ-tē, p. 288)
Assigning (assignment) (p. 286)
Change-of-shift report (p. 292)
Delegating (delegation) (DĔL-ĕ-GĀT-ĭng, p. 287)
Duties (p. 286)
Goals (outcomes) (p. 291)
Nurse Practice Act (p. 277)
Scope of practice (p. 289)
Tasks (p. 286)

Keep in Mind

"Effective leadership is putting first things first. Effective management is discipline, carrying it out."
Stephen R. Covey

Tricia was always a "saver," as her several well-constructed scrapbooks and boxes of books and papers from nursing school testified. Tricia looked at the carefully clipped classified ad she had saved from 5 years ago, when she had applied for her current nursing position. Five years ago her husband was transferred to the neighboring state of Oz. After 3 years' experience as an LVN in a nursing home, postgraduate courses in leadership at the local technical college, seminars, in-service programs, personal reading, and workshops, Tricia thought that she was qualified for a charge nurse position.

Tricia smiled as she pictured herself going in for the interview. That navy blue blazer sure paid off! And all her preparation for the interview served her well. What a sage Mrs. Kelly had been in Tricia's Personal/Vocational Issues (PVI) course, to recommend that a job applicant obtain a copy of the facility's mission statement before the interview. Although she did not have LPN/LVN charge nurse experience, she was sure her knowledge of the facility's emphasis and pride on providing quality care was a big plus in landing the job. Not to mention the enthusiasm and positive attitude she displayed to the interviewer about her willingness to learn and her confidence that she would be able to do the job. In addition, following the textbook suggestion to purchase the state of Oz's **Nurse Practice Act** before employment informed her of the ability of the LPN/LVN to delegate in the state of Oz and allowed her to ask delegation-related questions in the interview.

Five years had passed since she had gotten the job as LPN/LVN charge nurse. Tricia loved her job and smiled as she remembered many of the challenges she had faced early in her job as charge nurse. She began to page through that old sixth edition of her PVI textbook....

LPN/LVN

Full-time position available for an experienced LPN/LVN to join our long-term care facility as a charge nurse on the evening shift. Must have excellent communication and customer service skills, needs to be team-oriented, and must have current state of Oz license. We offer a competitive salary and full-benefit package. If you qualify, send résumé and cover letter to: Quality Care Home, 982 Brick Lane, Wayback, OZ 00005. For more information, contact Claudette Radant, DON at 987-123-4516.

(Before continuing, review Leadership Activity: Determining Your State's Requirements to Assume the Position of Practical/Vocational Charge Nurse, found in Chapter 15.)

Tricia looked at the job description the director of nurses gave her during her job interview. It all seems such a routine and comfortable part of her job, but Tricia remembers how overwhelming it was to read through the 12 areas of responsibility, along with the 15 duties of the charge nurse.

WHERE TO BEGIN? JOB DESCRIPTION FOR CHARGE NURSE

See Management Tool: Reviewing LPN/LVN Charge Nurse Job Descriptions.

Quality Care LPN/LVN Charge Nurse—LPN/LVN Job Description

QUALIFICATIONS

Licensed practical/vocational nurse with a current license to practice in the state of Oz under Chapter 747. The LPN/LVN should have a certificate of successful completion of an approved course in Medication Administration.

STANDARDS

The job of the LPN/LVN charge nurse is to ensure that residents receive nursing care, treatments, and medications that have been ordered by their physicians. The LPN/LVN charge nurse shall:

• Help coordinate resident care services (e.g., physicians, dietitian, activity director, physical therapist, and social worker).

Quality Care LPN/LVN Charge Nurse—LPN/LVN Job Description—cont'd

- Assist the Director of Nurses in the orientation of new employees.
- Evaluate work performance of nursing assistants.

RESPONSIBLE FOR

- Knowledge of residents' conditions at all times.
- Assigning actual nursing care tasks to nursing assistants.
- Providing nursing care according to physicians' orders and in agreement with recognized nursing techniques and procedures, established standards of care as described in Oz state statutes, and administrative policies of this long-term care facility.
- Recognizing symptoms: Reporting residents' condition, including changes, and assisting with remedial measures for adverse developments.
- Assisting physician in diagnostic and therapeutic measures.
- Administering medications and treatments as prescribed.
- Maintaining accurate and complete records of nursing data collection and interventions, including documentation on the residents' charts and Kardex records.
- Efficiency of execution of workload, including neatness and orderliness.
- Delegating duties, as appropriate, to nursing assistants.
- Maintaining a safe and hazard-free environment.
- Ensuring the residents' right to privacy.
- Maintaining the dignity of residents.

DUTIES

- Observes and reports symptoms and conditions of residents.
- Administers medications as prescribed by physicians. Gathers data about therapeutic response and side effects of medications.
- Takes and records vital signs when appropriate.
- Maintains charts and Kardexes, including residents' conditions and medications and treatments received.

DUTIES—cont'd

- Calls physician when necessary. Receives and records telephone orders.
- Calls pharmacist for prescription drugs as needed.
- Assists in maintaining a physical, social, and psychological environment for residents that is conducive to their best interests and welfare.
- Receives report at beginning of shift from offgoing personnel and assigns tasks to nursing assistants under the LPN/LVN charge nurse's supervision.
- Supervises, assists with, and evaluates delegated duties to nursing assistants.
- Evaluates the completion of nursing assistant assignments in a safe and timely manner.
- Provides report to oncoming shift.
- Evaluates nursing assistants in the performance of their job description and reports same to Director of Nursing.
- Attends supervisory staff meetings.
- Interprets state and federal guidelines to employees. Uses authority as LPN/LVN charge nurse to "follow code."
- Participates in orientation of all new employees assigned to LPN/LVN charge nurse.

 Management Tool

Reviewing LPN/LVN Charge Nurse Job Descriptions

Resources Needed:
- LPN/LVN charge nurse job descriptions of long-term care facilities

Review LPN/LVN charge nurse job descriptions of long-term care facilities at sites at which you affiliate during your student year.

The charge nurse job description might seem overwhelming at first, but it illustrates the reason state laws require that practical/vocational charge nurses have education, training, or experience beyond the basic practical/vocational nursing curriculum and documentation of such. It is difficult to prepare health care workers, in 1 year or less, to be able to function in this position immediately after graduation. After additional education, training, and experience, many LPN/LVNs become charge nurses, also called first-line managers, in long-term care units and nursing homes. They are doing an excellent job in that role. According to the 2006 practice analysis by NCSBN to gather data for content areas for NCLEX-PN®, 48.2% of LPN/LVNs stated they regularly had one or more administrative roles; 72.4% of those with administrative roles worked in long-term care; and 58% of those with administrative roles in long-term care indicated the charge nurse position as their administrative role (Wendt, 2007).

HOW LONG WILL IT TAKE ME TO PREPARE TO BE A CHARGE NURSE?

You are probably thinking, "How long will it take for me to get to this point in my practical/vocational nursing career?" The answer is individual to the person asking it. The law of some states specifically dictates that the charge nurse functions *in a nursing home* and under the direct supervision of a registered nurse. In these states the practical/vocational nurse could not function as a charge nurse in a medical clinic. Also, the LPN/LVN could not function under general supervision until after passing NCLEX-PN® examination. *Be sure to check your state's Nurse Practice Act.* Some practical/vocational nursing programs offer a postgraduate course that prepares graduates for an expanded role. The lawmakers of North Dakota have made practical/vocational nursing a 2-year program and focus on management in the second year. The answer to the question, "How long will it take for me to get to this point in my practical/vocational nursing career?" depends on your state's Nurse Practice Act, additional education, your motivation to learn the manager role, your ability to be a risk taker, and how you use your nursing experience.

HOW THIS TEXT CAN HELP YOU TO PREPARE FOR A FUTURE CHARGE NURSE POSITION

This text is unable to provide you with a concise recipe of how to function in the role of charge nurse as an LPN/LVN. This chapter begins with a discussion of areas of responsibilities, problems, and concerns that affect the LPN/LVN charge nurse in a long-term care unit or nursing home. Through active learning and an interactive format, this chapter also presents 12 Management Tools. These tools involve you with the many areas that need to be considered, understood, and investigated when assuming an LPN/LVN charge nurse position. The chapter also includes 10 Management Hints which provide concise information about concepts being presented. Seven critical thinking exercises present the opportunity to apply learning in the area of assignment and delegation.

Scenarios for three residents are interspersed throughout the nursing process guide for **assigning** and **delegating**.

You will be expected to be self-directed, to problem solve, and to think critically as you apply the information in Chapter 15. These are the very attributes employers expect of you as an LPN/LVN charge nurse. Reference is provided to specific resources needed to work through the Management Tools. You are encouraged to use the information from the entire text, your other classes, and your Learning Resource Center, as well as to work through the self-directed Management Tools. Your instructor is a valuable resource. Remember, also, the usefulness of peer group discussion.

At times we will flash back to Tricia, as she reminisces about her beginning days in the LPN/LVN charge nurse position. Her initial experiences and adjustment to the charge nurse role will show you the challenges and opportunities the LPN/LVN charge nurse role provides.

Tricia thought back to the orientation phase of her job. It seemed so overwhelming at the time. The thought of going through those thick manuals of policies, regulations, and routines was enough to give her a headache. However, they sure did contain valuable information. Mrs. Kelly gave the class the following sample checklist as a guide when reviewing these manuals.

A CHECKLIST OF POLICIES, REGULATIONS, AND ROUTINES FOR THE LPN/LVN CHARGE NURSE

Not all the areas included in this checklist are the responsibility of the LPN/LVN charge nurse in a nursing home/long-term care facility. However, LPN/LVN charge nurses need to have information for all the areas included so they can carry out their management **duties**. Because the LPN/LVN charge nurse has the responsibility to supervise nursing assistants, these personnel also need information about policies and routines. Orientation to your facility needs to include these items.

FACILITY ORGANIZATION/LEGAL ASPECTS

—Mission statement
—Organizational chart
—State statutes for all licensed persons on health care team
—Skills checklists for LPN/LVNs and nursing assistants
—Skills checklists for all cross-trained personnel
—Job descriptions and duties of RNs and LPN/LVNS
—Job descriptions and duties of unlicensed personnel and cross-trained personnel

FEDERAL, STATE, AND PRIVATE AGENCY REGULATIONS

—Inspection protocols
—Current federal (including HIPAA regulations) and state regulations
—Regulations of the Omnibus Budget Reconciliation Act of 1987 (OBRA)
—Regulations of the Centers for Medicare and Medicaid Services (CMS)
—Regulations of The Joint Commission (if facility seeks TJC accreditation)

PERSONNEL POLICIES

—Employee manual
—Time sheets—location and interpretation
—Vacation, holiday, sick leave policy
—Special request for time off, leave of absence
—Communication—reporting: on and off duty, sickness, absence, memos, bulletin board
—Meal and coffee break
—Smoking regulations
—Use of facility telephones and personal cell phones
—Uniform regulations

RECORDS AND UNIT ROUTINES

—General shift routine for days, evenings, and nights
—Duties of each of the three shifts
—Methods of reporting
—Procedure manual
—Facility policy manual
—Procedures specific to each division of the facility
—Nursing care plan system
—Nursing Kardex and Medix systems
—Routine for care planning conferences
—Routine for physicians' visits
—System of transcribing physicians' orders
—Location of reference books

UNIT ADMINISTRATION

—Admission, placement, transfer, and discharge of residents
—Care of clothing and valuables, including personal property list
—Routine for seriously ill residents
—Routine for death of a resident
—Autopsy permit
—Authorization procedure and forms for diagnostic tests and surgery
—Visiting hours
—Notary public

SAFETY POLICIES

—Side rails
—Restraints
—Fire regulations: reporting, evacuation plan, fire exits, location of fire extinguishers, preventive measures, fire drill procedure
—Use of oxygen

—Transportation of residents by cart, wheelchair
—Body mechanics and back safety policy
—Door alarms
—Standard precautions
—Security policies

HOUSEKEEPING, MAINTENANCE, AND SUPPLIES

—Linen: how supplied, extra linen
—Care of contaminated linens and dressings
—Unit cleaning procedure and responsibilities
—How to obtain supplies: drugs, sterile supplies, personal care items, kitchen items
—Maintenance and repairs requests
—Conservation of supplies, linen, and equipment

EQUIPMENT: HOW TO USE AND WHERE TO OBTAIN

—Oxygen
—Suction equipment
—Therapeutic beds
—Respiratory therapy equipment and services

FOOD SERVICE FOR RESIDENTS

—Ordering diets/diet changes
—Tray service
—Unit food stock items
—Special nourishments
—Policy for feeding residents
—Policy for dining room
—Policy for family trays

NURSING CARE PROCEDURES/ ASSISTING PHYSICIAN

—Bathing
—Mouth care
—Bed making
—Temperature (devices used), pulse, and respiration
—Blood pressure
—Catheterization
—Enemas
—Suppositories—rectal
—Recording intake and output

—Systems used for pressure ulcer care
—Collecting, delivering, and labeling specimens
—Assisting podiatrist with foot care
—Policies for sterile technique procedures
—Blood glucose monitoring
—Colostomy care
—Nasogastric and gastrostomy tubes: flushing, feeding, administration of medication
—Standard precautions
—Postmortem procedures

MEDICATIONS

—Medication system
—Policy for reordering
—Unit stock
—Ordering from pharmacy
—Review of metric system, proportions, abbreviations
—Drug errors: reporting, incident reports
—Narcotics count
—Sources of drug administration

DOCUMENTATION

—Method of documenting
—Computer system
—Forms used
—Flow sheets used
—Policy for phone orders
 Incident reports
—Lists for wanderers, hearing aid use, and so on
—Federal and state chart forms and requirements
—Private organizations' requirements

SPECIAL AREAS

—Emergency supplies
—Central supply area
—Physical therapy
—Occupational therapy
—Laundry
—Maintenance
—Break room
—Dining room
—Kitchen
—Business offices

—Social services
—Director of nurses
—Chaplain services/chapel area
—Staff educator
—Administrator of facility
—Conference rooms
—Activity department

MISCELLANEOUS

—Paging system
—Call light system
—Disaster plan
—Routine for residents who desire cardiopulmonary resuscitation
—Volunteer services
—On-call schedule
—Handling of wanderers
—Procedure for signing resident in and out of facility
—Hair care services

See Management Tool: Reviewing Policies and Routines.

Management Tool

Reviewing Policies and Routines

Resources Needed:
• Aforementioned checklist of policies, regulations, and routines for the LPN/LVN
• Your opinion and reasons (rationale)
   All policies, regulations, and routines of a health care facility are important. After reading the checklist, complete the following:
a. List the five items from Records and Unit Routines that you think are most necessary for effective running of the resident wings of the long-term care unit. Provide the reason (rationale) for your choices.

Item	Rationale
1.	
2.	
3.	
4.	
5.	

b. List the five items from Unit Administration that you think are most necessary for effective running of the resident wings of the long-term care unit. Provide your reason (rationale) for your choices.

Item	Rationale
1.	
2.	
3.	
4.	
5.	

Tricia came across a data list. Mrs. Kelly had stressed the importance of the LPN/LVN's assisting role in collecting data. Mrs. Kelly always said that what the LPN/LVN did with that data really separated the licensed nurse from unlicensed personnel. Mrs. Kelly had provided a helpful list of signs and symptoms to be aware of in various patient situations. She stressed it would not be a complete list but would be something to get us started. It had been some time since Tricia updated that list.

COLLECTING DATA AS A CHARGE NURSE

As LPN/LVN charge nurse, the **change-of-shift report** when coming on duty provides data for dividing the work of the shift among team members. Baseline data of residents for whom you are in charge also needs to be obtained. This involves a quick visit of each resident to compare the status of residents to the status reported at change of shift. You will also collect data periodically during your shift. The frequency of data collecting depends on patient condition. The following is a list of signs and symptoms that may indicate illness, exacerbation of a previous disease condition, injury, or decline in prior functioning.

Be observant with each resident interaction. When nursing assistants report that "something does not seem right," visit the resident to collect your own data. After collecting the data, record it on the proper form and report all abnormal observations according to agency policy. The actual data-collecting parameters given here are guidelines. Follow specific parameters given for the resident.

SIGNS AND SYMPTOMS

1. **Weight:** Increase or decrease of 5 to 10 lb in 1 week.
2. **Temperature:** Elevation over 100 °F orally or 100.6 °F rectally; temperature under 96.6 °F orally.
3. **Upper respiratory:** Head congestion, headache, sore throat, ear pain, runny nose, postnasal drip.
4. **Lower respiratory:** Acute onset or worsening of shortness of breath, dyspnea with exertion, orthopnea, cough (productive or nonproductive), wheezing or other abnormal sounds on inhalation or exhalation.
5. **Cardiac:** Blood pressure over 140/90 (new symptom); blood pressure below 80/50; irregular pulse (new symptom); chest, neck, shoulder, or arm pain; fatigue; increased frequency of angina; shortness of breath; orthopnea; peripheral edema; sacral edema or distended neck veins.
6. **Breast:** Lump found on palpation, discharge from nipple.
7. **Abdomen:** Localized or generalized pain, especially of acute onset; epigastric burning or discomfort; constipation; diarrhea; nausea; vomiting; bloody or tarry stools; loss of appetite.
8. **Musculoskeletal:** Swollen and tender joints, loss of strength in limbs, pain, loss of motion, ecchymosis, edema.
9. **Reproductive system:** Vaginal discharge, abnormal vaginal bleeding.
10. **Genitourinary:** Urgency, frequency, dysuria, nocturia, hematuria, incontinence. Male: Dribbling, inability to start or stop stream.
11. **Sleep and rest patterns:** Changes from normal routine, requirement of medication for sleep, nightmares or dreams.
12. **Appearance of skin:** Changes in color, turgor, contusions, abrasions, lacerations, rashes, lesions.
13. **Mobility and exercise:** Need for support in ambulation, changes in posture, weakness of extremities, changes in coordination, vertigo.
14. **Hygiene status:**
    a. *Mouth:* Condition of mucous membranes, gums, teeth, tongue, mouth odor.
    b. *Body:* Cleanliness, odor, especially of body creases and genital area.
    c. *Hair:* Grooming, distribution, scalp scaling, presence of disease.
    d. *Nails:* Color, texture and grooming of finger nails and toe nails.
15. **Communication:** Verbal, nonverbal, and affective, aphasia, level of understanding.
16. **Sensory-perceptual:** Ability to hear, condition of hearing aid; ability to see, condition of glasses; ability to feel in all extremities; ability to discriminate odors; ability to distinguish tastes.
17. **Cultural/religious:** Food preferences, wellness/illness beliefs, religious practices (e.g., rosary, prayer beads, Bible, religious readings, medals, icons, communion, clergy visits, confession, sacrament of the sick).
18. **Psychological status:** Level of consciousness, disorientation, intelligence, attention span, vocabulary level, interests, memory, affect.

Tricia remembered how Mrs. Kelly stressed the importance of getting to a room and personally collecting patient data, especially when there was a change of condition. Tricia found the example Mrs. Kelly gave so that members of the class could avoid the same situation.

THE REPORT THAT WASN'T

A nursing assistant (NA) reported to the LPN/LVN charge nurse (CN) that Mr. Jones "doesn't look too good to me." The charge nurse immediately called the physician.

Doctor Grimm:	What seems to be the trouble?
CN to NA:	What seems to be the trouble?
NA to CN:	I don't know. He just doesn't look right.
CN to Doctor:	He just doesn't look right.
Doctor:	How long has he looked like this?
CN:	I don't know. We just noticed.
Doctor:	What's his temperature?
CN:	Just a minute. I'll find out.
CN to NA:	Take Mr. Jones's temperature.
Doctor:	What are his other vital signs?
CN:	I don't know. The nursing assistant is going to check them.
Doctor:	How much fluid has he had?
CN:	Just a minute. (She puts the telephone down and goes to check Mr. Jones's IV.)
CN:	He's getting an IV now.
Doctor (with sarcasm in his voice):	Is he breathing? Never mind, don't send anyone to check. I will be over to check him myself. (The doctor slams the telephone down.)
CN to NA:	I don't know why he gets so upset every time I call him. What am I supposed to do?

See Management Tool: Reporting Change of Condition to the Physician.

Reporting Change of Condition to the Physician

Resources Needed:
- A checklist of signs and symptoms (earlier in this chapter)
- A medical-surgical textbook

List the data you would collect and any other pertinent information you would gather before notifying the physician of a "change of condition" in the following residents:
- Resident has history of compensated, left-sided congestive heart failure.
- Resident has cancer of the esophagus and uses a Duragesic patch for pain control.

Tricia began to think of the "people problems" she continually experiences in her job as LVN charge nurse. With each day that passes, handling these problems becomes easier and easier. Mrs. Kelly's basic advice, "Treat people as you would like to be treated," has saved the day on many occasions. That was good advice even for reporting change of condition to the doctor: "What information would I need if I was the physician and my patient had a change of condition?" As for dealing with doctors, residents, staff, and families, I sure remember situations that arose as clearly as if they happened yesterday.

COMMON PROBLEMS OF LPN/LVN CHARGE NURSE

Tricia recalled one morning during the second week of work after orientation to the charge nurse position. The nursing assistants were all tied up in knots. The babysitter for the three young children of Jenny, one of the nursing assistants, had quit the evening before, and when Jenny got up the next morning for work, her car would not start. All the nursing assistants were talking about Jenny's problems from the time they hung up their coats, straight through lunch and beyond. It was only the week before that Jenny found out she was overdrawn at the bank because she wrote checks before her paycheck was deposited by Quality Care Home and cleared by the bank. It seemed as though "things always happened to Jenny, and she was such a nice girl. It just was not right." All the nursing assistants were feeling guilty because all these problems happened to Jenny. Everyone was involved with how to get Jenny out of her current mess. Several of the nursing assistants forgot to do some of their tasks/duties, and Jenny needed a lot of assistance to get her assignment completed. As Tricia remembered that particular time, a picture flew through her mind. It was Mrs. Kelly standing in the front of the class with a stuffed toy monkey on her back.

WHEN NURSING ASSISTANTS BRING PROBLEMS FROM HOME

As an LPN/LVN charge nurse, it is important that you do not fall into the "monkey trap," as described by Blanchard, Oncken, and Burrows in *The One Minute Manager Meets the Monkey* (1989). You fall into the trap each time you take on a responsibility (monkey) that belongs to an employee. Once monkeys are adopted, they take a lot of time in their care and upkeep. LPN/LVN charge nurses can help nursing assistants become aware of this trap and be a role model for avoiding it.

Realize that you do not own any problems that nursing assistants experience. The nursing assistant owns the problem. Avoid feeling guilty because you cannot solve the problems of team members. Be supportive and express genuine concern and empathy, but realize that you do not have a license to counsel nursing assistants. Team members need to solve their own problems. Follow facility policies when personal problems interfere with work performance. Report the situation to your supervisor. Professional counseling in the community may be necessary. See Management Tool: When Nursing Assistants Bring Problems from Home.

Management Tool

When Nursing Assistants Bring Problems from Home

Resources Needed:
- Reading: The section "When Nursing Assistants Bring Problems from Home" (above)
- Creative thinking

  Pretend you are the LPN/LVN charge nurse the morning Jenny comes to work with her problems. Identify a way to handle the situation.

Tricia remembered Betty, a nursing assistant who had been employed at Quality Care Home for 6 months

when she told Kay, a nursing assistant on her wing, that she did not know how to use the new patient-lifting device. Kay stated she did not really have time, but Betty coaxed her to take the time to get the resident out of bed for her. Tricia had suggested to Kay a way of handling the situation that she had learned in PV class—a tip that would help Betty be more accountable.

ENCOURAGING PERSONAL RESPONSIBILITY IN NURSING ASSISTANTS

When nursing assistants cannot do something that is in their job description—for example, transferring a resident by a lifting device—it is their problem. Staff persons need to avoid assuming it is a staff problem. Be sure to follow the policy of the facility. For safety reasons, encourage nursing assistants to report to the charge nurse when they are having problems carrying out their assignment. This gives the charge nurse the opportunity to determine what staff member is skilled and available to assist in the situation. Encourage the nursing assistant to offer suggestions for learning to do the part of their job that they do not know how to do. Praise them for coming up with a plan, and add to the plan, if necessary. Write a note to your supervisor explaining the situation objectively and how you proceeded to remedy the situation. If necessary, request additional training for the nursing assistant. Learning who owns problems will help you control a large part of the stress you experience as an LPN/LVN charge nurse and help ensure the safety of resident care. See Management Tool: Encouraging Nursing Assistants to Be Accountable for Learning Skills.

Management Tool

Encouraging Nursing Assistants to Be Accountable for Learning Skills

Resources Needed:
- Reading: The section "Encouraging Personal Responsibilities in Nursing Assistants" (above).

  Develop a plan to encourage Betty to approach the lifting-device situation in a more accountable manner.

Tricia remembered instances in her student days and throughout her career when families had complained about care given to their relatives. These complaints troubled Tricia, who had high standards and prided herself on the quality of her nursing care. She would take the complaints seriously and investigate each criticism thoroughly. Sometimes nothing could be found out of order, and sometimes she began doubting her ability to self-evaluate. Once again, Mrs. Kelly offered insight into this common problem, which Tricia still uses today.

DEALING WITH DEMANDING/ COMPLAINING FAMILIES

A common problem in the nursing home is dealing with complaints of family members regarding care of their relatives. A common complaint involves physical care. Sometimes the family members become verbally aggressive, express concerns in an angry manner, and are very critical of the charge nurse. Others will be nonassertive and sarcastic. Remember the problem-solving process. First, collect data to determine the real problem. If there is a problem with physical care, identify and correct it. Sometimes when the problem is identified and solved, the complaints continue. Sometimes when no problem with physical care is identified, the family may continue the attack.

It is necessary to consider the situation in which the family finds itself. They are in a position of seeing their loved one progressively aging and deteriorating. This is a time of loss for the family. They may feel guilty about placing a relative in a long-term care facility or about not being able to continue care giving. They may have grieving issues to contend with. Lashing out may be their attempt at relief. To avoid personal issues, family members may unconsciously project blame onto nursing assistants and other members of the nursing staff. It is similar to looking at skeletons in other people's closets, so that you do not have to look at those in your own closet. This behavior may make a family feel better. It is important for staff to understand these issues to avoid hurt feelings. Avoid personalizing the situation.

Suggested interventions to deal with the demanding or complaining family are included in Management Tool: Interventions to Use for the Demanding/Complaining Family. When family complaints surface, investigate them, but remember to keep broad shoulders.

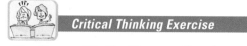

Management Tool

Interventions to Use for the Demanding/ Complaining Family

See Bauer and Hill's Mental Health Nursing (2000) for interventions for additional specific behaviors.

- Develop a sincere, nonpunitive relationship with the resident's family.
- Encourage the family to ventilate feelings about resident's placement in a nursing home, aging, and behavior.
- Try to identify the unconscious issue and address it.
- Determine needs the family is trying to fulfill through their demands, criticism, and complaints.
- Spend time with the family when demands or complaints are not being made.
- Establish rapport with the family to provide emotional support during this difficult time.
- Explain the resident's disease and expected behavior.
- Suggest joining a support group. These groups offer explanations for specific diseases, as well as a place to share feelings and frustrations.
- Encourage the family to stay involved with the resident and continue care giving and visiting.

See the following critical thinking exercise to practice dealing with the demanding and complaining family.

Critical Thinking Exercise

Dealing with the Demanding/ Complaining Family

Resources Needed:
- Reading: Chapter 15: Leadership Hint: Decision-Making Tree for Problem Solving on p. 258.

Mrs. Duffy, age 82, was admitted 2 weeks ago to Quality Care Home. You are an LPN/LVN charge nurse on her wing on the evening shift. Mrs. Duffy has osteoarthritis, short-term memory loss, and Parkinson's disease. In the past few days her family has been complaining about her hair care, mouth care, appearance, and missing items in her laundry.

- Develop a plan with specific interventions to investigate and alleviate these complaints.
- Despite modifications in Mrs. Duffy's care plan, the complaints continue. Plan specific interventions to handle the continuing specific complaints.

ASSIGNMENT AND DELEGATION

Tricia stopped at the topic of Assigning Tasks and Delegating Duties to Nursing Assistants. She remembered well the confusion she experienced in class in trying to understand the difference between assigning and delegating to nursing assistants. Like most of the students in her class, she thought assigning and delegating meant the same thing. They sure sounded the same. The fact that she went to school in a state that did not allow her to delegate to nursing assistants compounded her confusion in understanding these concepts. Mrs. Kelly, as usual, had the situation well under control. She said that although assigning and delegating had many similarities, there were differences that had legal consequences. The best place to start was to lay down the boundaries about what we were talking, define and describe the terms, and then go on from there. In case the students thought assigning and delegating were new concepts, Mrs. Kelly read the following quote:

> To be "in charge" is certainly not only to carry out the proper measures yourself but to see that everyone else does too. It is neither to do everything yourself nor to appoint a number of people to each duty, but to ensure that each does that duty to which he is appointed.

Florence Nightingale
Notes on Nursing, 1859

CHECKING YOUR NURSE PRACTICE ACT (NPA)

At this time, not every state in the United States allows practical/vocational nurses to delegate in their charge nurse positions. It is crucial that you check your state's Nurse Practice Act (NPA—the state law/statute that regulates your nursing practice) to determine whether you may delegate as an LPN/LVN charge nurse in your state. If you cannot clearly find an answer, contact your state's Board of Nursing (BON). Addresses and phone numbers of state boards of nursing are in Appendix A.

See Management Tool: Reviewing Your Nurse Practice Act for Authority to Delegate.

Management Tool

Reviewing Your Nurse Practice Act for Authority to Delegate

Resources Needed:
- Your state's Nurse Practice Act
  —Locate the section of your state's Nurse Practice Act that discusses your ability to delegate nursing duties as an LPN/LVN charge nurse.
  —In your own words, write that position.

If your state's Nurse Practice Act allows LPN/LVN charge nurses to delegate duties, you will have the authority to delegate duties to nursing assistants (unlicensed assistive personnel).

In 1994 the then-president of the National Council of State Boards of Nursing (NCSBN) stated, "Boards of nursing must clearly define delegation in regulation, promulgate clear rules for its use, and follow through with disciplinary action when there is evidence that the rules are violated" (Rachels, 1994). For this reason, some states may differ in their interpretation of delegation. This is one reason you need to check with the BON in your state for its interpretation of delegation. In addition to your state's Nurse Practice Act, be sure to review the following:

1. Rules and regulations of your state's BON.
2. Interpretations, guidelines, and memorandums developed by your state's board of nursing regarding delegation.

A state's NPA usually presents information in a general manner. Rules and regulations and interpretations of your BON are more specific statements. They make clearer the intent of the NPA and provide more specific details that describe your nursing practice.

Your state may give you permission to delegate as an LPN/LVN, but to delegate in your place of employment, your facility must also give permission for that function by including it in its written policies. For this reason, check facility policy regarding delegation of nursing duties by the LPN/LVN charge nurse.

The standards of nursing organizations are not legal statements, but they provide support to the legal decisions of your state. Be sure to review the standards of your nursing organizations that apply to delegation by the LPN/LVN. See Management Tool: Locating Positions of Nursing Groups and Employer on Delegation Function of LPN/LVN Charge Nurse.

Management Tool

Locating Positions of Nursing Groups and Employer on Delegation Function of LPN/LVN Charge Nurse

Resources Needed:
- Rules, regulations, interpretations, guidelines, and memorandums regarding delegation of your state's board of nursing
- Appendix B: NAPNES Standards of Practice and Educational Competencies of Graduates of Practical/Vocational Nursing Programs
- Appendix C: NFLPN Nursing Practice Standards for the Licensed Practical/Vocational Nurse
- Policies on delegation of employer
  Review the policies/rules and regulations/interpretations/guidelines/standards of the following agencies in regard to delegation:
- Board of Nursing
- National Association for Practical Nurse Education and Service, Inc.

- National Federation of Licensed Practical Nurses
- National League for Nursing
- Health care facility

GENERAL CONSIDERATIONS

Assignment and *delegation* are terms used in reference to allocating patient care activities to team members. Both terms refer to nursing actions or activities, but the terms do not have the same meaning. It is important to think about and use *assignment* and *delegation* in the way they are legally intended. **To help increase your understanding and decrease confusion, the terms** *assignment* **(assigning) and** *delegation* **(delegating) will be used in this text in the following way.**

—When discussing assignment, this topic will be used in reference to "tasks." Tasks are activities that are carried out by nursing assistants. Nursing assistants learn "how to" perform a task in their nursing assistant training and **these tasks are listed in their job description.**

—When discussing delegation, this topic will be used in reference to "duties." Duties are functions that are performed by LPN/LVNs because they successfully passed a licensing exam. The duties are included in the state's Nurse Practice Act. The duties are their **scope of practice**. The LPN/LVN learns "why" a duty is performed and "what" could go wrong during performance of a "duty."

Resident circumstances can change a "task" for a nursing assistant into a "duty" requiring the LPN/LVN to use the nursing process.

Whenever "charge nurse" is used, this title will be in the context of the LPN/LVN.

DIFFERENCES BETWEEN ASSIGNING AND DELEGATING
Assigning

Assigning is the method that work is distributed among team members for the shift. Assigning is a skill that every LPN/LVN needs to develop, if their state allows them to assume a charge nurse position. Distributing the workload by assignment is a routine part of the LPN/LVN charge nurse's job. Assignment always occurs at the beginning of every shift and as the need arises during the shift.

When LPN/LVNs make assignments to nursing assistants, they are allotting tasks that are in the job description of these health care workers. **The assigned tasks are tasks that nursing assistants are trained, hired, and paid to perform. The tasks are in *their* job description.** These unlicensed personnel have the responsibility to complete the assignment in a safe and timely manner. The LPN/LVN charge nurse shares responsibility with unlicensed personnel for the quality of the care delivered. In assigning situations, the LPN/LVN charge nurse needs to monitor the performance of the task and evaluate the quality and effectiveness of the care that was assigned. Management Hint: Assigning Tasks contains information to help understand assigning tasks.

Management Hint

Assigning Tasks

- The need to assign can occur at any time during the shift but *always* occurs at the beginning of the shift.
- The assigning of tasks is part of the LPN/LVN charge nurse's job.
- The LPN/LVN charge nurse assigns tasks to nursing assistants that are in *their* job description.
- Nursing tasks are tasks that nursing assistants are trained, hired, and paid to perform. See p. 292, Specific Tasks for Nursing Assistant Assignment.
- Because assignments involve allocating the tasks that are to be done by nursing assistants within *their* job description, these team members cannot refuse the assignment (Wywialowski, 2004).
- An exception to this is when nursing assistants decide they are unqualified to carry out the assignment.
- Nursing assistants assume responsibility and **accountability** for completing assigned tasks safely and in a timely manner.

Delegating

LPN/LVNs receive the authority to provide nursing care from the nursing license they receive after successfully passing the NCLEX-PN® examination. **When allowed by your state's Nurse Practice Act and facility policies,** delegating **duties in the long-term care unit involves transferring the authority to perform nursing duties that are in the job description of the LPN/LVN charge nurse (the person doing the delegating) to competent nursing assistants (unlicensed personnel, known as the delegate) in selected situations. These nursing duties are in *your* job description and "emerge" from your nursing license. These duties are in your scope of practice. Based on your scope of practice, the most important duty of LPN/LVNs is the assisting role in the nursing process.** See Table 16-1 for a comparison of assigning tasks and delegating duties.

Delegating is a complex skill requiring sophisticated clinical judgment. Delegation information, including scenarios, might be included in theory classes in your practical/vocational nursing program but opportunities to apply the information on clinical may be limited. To be effective, delegation is a skill that needs to be developed with a licensed nurse as a mentor after graduation (Grumet, 2005; Working with Others, 2005).

Delegating duties and assigning tasks are written in the job description of the LPN/LVN charge nurse at Quality Care Home. When allowed by your state's Nurse Practice Act and your facility, delegating is a voluntary function. You do not *have* to delegate because the facility allows it. Management Hint: Delegating Duties contains helpful information for delegating duties.

Management Hint

Delegating Duties

- When delegating duties, you decide to ask nursing assistants (unlicensed personnel) to do part of *your* job.
- Delegation involves the ability to share power with nursing assistants.

Table 16-1 *Comparison of Assigning Versus Delegating by the LPN/LVN Charge Nurse*

	ASSIGNING TASKS	DELEGATING DUTIES
To whom may tasks or duties be assigned or delegated?	Nursing assistants and other unlicensed personnel	Nursing assistants and other unlicensed personnel
Are tasks or duties in nursing assistant's job description?	Yes	No. The duties delegated are in the job description of the LPN/LVN. Specific duties are not listed. Delegated duties depend on the situation.
May nursing assistant refuse nursing task/ duty?	No, unless nursing assistant thinks he or she is unqualified for the assignment	Yes. In addition, the nursing assistant must voluntarily accept delegation function.
Who has accountability for nursing task/ duty?	The nursing assistant is accountable for safe care.	The LPN/LVN is accountable for delegating the right duty to the right person. The nursing assistant is accountable for completing the duty and in a safe manner.

- Delegation is *not* asking nursing assistants to do duties that the LPN/LVN dislikes doing.
- As LPN/LVN charge nurse, you are asking nursing assistants to help you perform some of *your* job description so that you may perform other responsibilities, with the ultimate goal of improving resident care and meeting resident goals (outcomes).
- **Because you are delegating part of *your* job as charge nurse, nursing assistants must give approval to the assignment.** Nursing assistants must voluntarily accept the delegation; they cannot be forced to accept the delegated duty.
- When delegating duties, the LPN/LVN charge nurse needs to provide the nursing assistant with the necessary information, assistance, and equipment to safely carry out the delegated duty.
- Employers may suggest that certain duties be delegated, but the LPN/LVN is ultimately responsible for the following:
  —Deciding *to* delegate a duty,
  —Deciding *what* duty to delegate,
  —Deciding *to whom* to delegate a duty, and
  —Deciding *under what circumstances* to delegate a duty.

WHY DELEGATING IS IMPORTANT

When allowed by your Nurse Practice Act and facility policies, learning to delegate duties from your job description to nursing assistants can have many advantages. Delegating can do the following:

—Can increase your effectiveness and efficiency as an LPN/LVN charge nurse.
—Can be instrumental in realizing patient goals (outcomes) in a cost-effective manner.
—May help nursing assistants increase and improve their job skills.

LEGAL ASPECTS OF DELEGATING

In the long-term care facility the LPN/LVN charge nurse, who is under the *general* supervision of a registered nurse (RN), is managing and directing the activities of nursing assistants (see Chapter 20). The RN might be in the building on days and evenings. On the night shift the RN might be at the other end of the telephone. When the RN delegates a duty to the LPN/ LVN charge nurse, and the charge nurse delegates to a nursing assistant, the legal principle of *respondeat superior* (see Chapter 20) comes into play. By that principle, the nursing act delegated is the act of the supervising nurse, the RN. The registered nurse is *ultimately* responsible for the supervision of nursing assistants. But the LPN/ LVN charge nurse assists in the supervision of these health care workers and shares accountability (meaning responsibility) with the RN for their actions.

Scope of Practice for the LPN/LVN

Never delegate what is in your legal scope of practice. Legal scope of practice is what you are able to do because you are an LPN/LVN (see Chapter 20). Your scope of practice includes the assisting role in the nursing process. The LPN/LVN charge nurse can delegate to nursing assistants the duty of checking a resident's intravenous (IV) site for intactness and dryness of dressing. However, nursing assistants are not trained in the basics of collecting data. If the resident complained of being cold at the site of the IV, nursing assistants might provide the patient with another blanket, turn up the heat, or turn down the air conditioning. They would not automatically check to see if the infusion device had come out of the resident's vein and was infusing fluid onto the bed sheets.

Although unlicensed assistive personnel obtain data while caring for residents, they do not have the nursing education to make a judgment about nor interpret that data. Therefore, nursing judgment cannot be delegated to or expected of nursing assistants. The LPN/LVN charge nurse needs to use his/her knowledge and experience to interpret data gathered by these members of the team.

Your license is at stake in the matter of delegating nursing duties. To be legally sound when delegating duties, see the suggestions in Management Hint: Suggestions for Legal Soundness When Delegating.

 Management Hint

Suggestions for Legal Soundness When Delegating

- Delegate only if allowed by your state's Nurse Practice Act and facility policies.
- Delegate duties for which nursing assistants have demonstrated ability.
- Provide specific, objective, clear-cut directions to nursing assistants for delegated duties.
- Provide assistance and instruction to nursing assistants when you delegate a duty.
- Monitor the activities of nursing assistants when they carry out delegated duties. Depending on the nursing assistant and the situation, this monitoring

can be as close as being "right there," to a periodic check.
- Intervene if correction is needed to maintain safety.
- On completion of the delegated duty, evaluate the safety and effectiveness of duties delegated to nursing assistants.
- If you delegated improperly and a resident was harmed, you are liable. This could result in a disciplinary action against your license and/or a civil suit (see Chapter 20).
- If you delegated properly, including monitoring, and the patient was injured, the nursing assistant is liable.

Tricia continued paging through her PVI text and notes. What memories they brought back! All those shifts of taking report and focusing on important aspects of each patient or resident on the clinical area had a purpose. Tricia remembered the first time she had taken report as an LPN/LVN charge nurse. Her new position of responsibility gave her a heightened sense of awareness of the data being given. Based on the data she received in report, she had to decide what to assign and what to delegate to nursing assistants for the shift.

USING THE NURSING PROCESS AS A GUIDE FOR ASSIGNING TASKS AND DELEGATING DUTIES

The nursing process will be used as the device to cover the various aspects that need to be understood and used when assigning or delegating:

- Collecting Data: Oncoming report, assessment of residents
- Planning: Establishing goals (outcomes) for the shift, setting priorities, and assigning/delegating,
- Implementation: Monitoring, assisting, being available, and intervening, and
- Evaluation: Two-way feedback.

COLLECTING DATA
Oncoming Report

Requirement 2E of TJC 2007 National Patient Safety Goals requires a standardized approach to communications (for example, change-of-shift report, which is sometimes called "hand off"), including an opportunity to ask and respond to questions during reports. If your facility has TJC accreditation, there may be a standardized form to use when receiving report. The 2007 National Patient Safety Goals of TJC are in Chapter 20 and can also be accessed at *http://www.jcrinc.com/13474/.*

Change-of-shift report allows the LPN/LVN charge nurse to collect data to determine how the work of the shift will be divided. Always keeping in mind patient goals (outcomes) for shift, report helps guarantee continuity in resident care.

Report When Starting Your Shift

Reports in long-term care units and nursing homes, as in other health care facilities, are a way to pass pertinent data to the oncoming shift. The report you receive when you are starting your shift will be your basis for collecting data about resident needs. This is legally necessary so that you can safely distribute the work of the shift to nursing assistants to provide care for specific residents by keeping in mind patient goals (outcomes). Report may be taped or oral, depending on TJC accreditation or agency policy.

When report is taped, offgoing personnel usually are still on duty. They answer call lights and attend to residents' needs while the oncoming shift listens to report. This enables the charge nurse to question unclear information after report. If facilities do not have a standardized report form, nurses develop personal ways of gathering data when they are taking report, including use of symbols and abbreviations. See Management Tool: Developing Your Personal Form for Collecting Data During Report.

 Management Tool

Developing Your Personal Form for Collecting Data During Report

Resources Needed:
- Method of gathering data during report that you have developed during the clinical year

- Sample of forms/method to gather information for report used by clinical sites where you have worked this year
- Your creativity

Develop a form that will help you gather the pertinent information needed to assume responsibility of taking charge of the residents on your wing(s). Include format, symbols, and abbreviations you find helpful and that will allow you to quickly and accurately gather the information. Compare your form with forms of classmates.

Assessment of Patients

Assignment/delegation of patients is usually done after report. Ideally, the LPN/LVN Charge Nurse makes rounds to personally assess each resident before making assignments. This baseline assessment allows the Charge Nurse to note any changes in condition of residents or discrepancies that may have occurred since report. If distribution of work for the shift is done before rounds and a change in assignment/delegation is required, the nursing assistant needs to be notified.

PLANNING

*"We may be very busy, we may be very efficient, but we will also be truly effective **only when we begin with the end in mind."***

Stephen R. Covey

Planning involves deciding goals (outcomes) for the shift, setting priorities of care, and then using specific directions, assigning/delegating the appropriate task/ duty to the nursing assistant who can safely and effectively complete the assignment/delegation.

Before Assigning Tasks/Delegating Duties to Nursing Assistants

Distributing the work to be done among nursing assistants follows change-of-shift report. Encourage nursing assistants to take notes and ask questions regarding the directions you give for assigned tasks/delegated duties. Resist the urge to think of work only as tasks to be completed and to just divide the work equally among team members. You know to what we are alluding—32 patients and 4 nursing assistants means each gets 8 patients. Take time to plan how work will be distributed. At first this part may seem tedious and time consuming, but planning becomes easier with practice and experience. This part of the nursing process is a good reason why the charge nurse position, by state law, requires experience beyond a new graduate.

Authors Hansten and Jackson (2004) state, "Fail to plan. Plan to fail." They provide the following suggestions to help nurses decide what to assign/delegate through effective planning:

—Identify resident goals (outcomes) and

—Set priorities.

Identifying Resident Goals (Outcomes). To be more effective in assigning/delegating and to make these functions more understandable, think in terms of resident goals **(outcomes)**. Goals are desired results in resident progress after nursing intervention. What should happen after nursing intervention by the nursing assistant? Why is the nursing activity being done? What is the goal (outcome) for each resident for the shift?

Critical Thinking Exercise

Formulating Goals/Outcome Examples for Residents

Formulate a goal (outcome) to be met at the end of the day shift for each of the following residents:

- **Harold,** an active 90-year-old with osteoarthritis, had a right total hip replacement and is completing his rehabilitation at Quality Care Home with the goal to go back to his apartment in assisted living. He is to walk x2 with stand-by assist and have one dry clean dressing change daily. His temp went to 100.4 °F last evening but he is not displaying respiratory symptoms.

  Goal (outcome) for Harold for day shift:
  Harold will maintain hip abduction when turning and getting out of bed to prevent hip dislocation. Harold will have causes of his elevated temp investigated.

- **Adelia,** age 76, and a two year resident of Quality Care Home, has type 1 diabetes and receives an intermediate-acting insulin injection each morning and capillary blood glucose monitoring ½ hour before meals with sliding scale short-acting insulin coverage. Adelia can be up ad lib and today is her shower day, which Adelia is looking forward to. The PM shift had trouble getting a blood sample and had to do **two** fingersticks to obtain a blood sample for testing.

  Goal (outcome) for Adelia for day shift:
  Adelia will have blood glucose monitoring done x2 with only one fingerstick required for each test.

- **Blake,** age 82, has resided at Quality Care Home for 3 years. He has arteriosclerotic heart disease (ASHD). He recently was hospitalized with a cerebral vascular accident (CVA) and is back at Quality Care Home. Blake has weakness on the right side of his body, is allowed up with the assistance of one, and uses a walker. He has dysphagia (difficulty swallowing).

  Goal (outcome) for Blake for day shift:
  Blake will eat breakfast and lunch without aspirating.

Setting Priorities. Set priorities among the goals (outcomes) for the shift. The priority (most important) care to be done can be evaluated according to the following criteria:

1. *Life-threatening situations—real or potential*
   a. A resident who has unrelieved chest pain that started on last shift. (Goal/ Outcome: Resident will be pain free at end of shift.)
   b. A resident who is dying. (Goal/Outcome: Resident will have a peaceful look on his face and lie still in bed without thrashing and picking at sheets because of comfort measures provided and presence of family.)
   c. A resident who is showing untoward effects to a newly ordered drug. (Goal/ Outcome: Resident will have stable blood pressure and respirations of 22 to 26 per minute. This requires frequent monitoring and reporting PRN to physician.)
   d. A resident attempted to flee the building several times on the last shift. (Goal/ Outcome: Resident will be present in building at end of shift, thanks to constant supervision.)

2. *Essential to safety.* This criterion pertains to residents and the nursing team.
   a. Which residents, because of their weight, require two persons to turn and position?
   b. Which residents, because of poor balance, need assistance to get out of bed, ambulate?
   c. Who is going to check special equipment (e.g., the stock of supplies used in emergencies) for shift?
   d. Does a resident require standard precautions that are infrequently used in the facility? Instruction may need to be given to nursing assistants.
3. *Essential to the medical/nursing plan of care.* Criteria include ordered treatments, facility routines for care, and interventions listed on the nursing plan of care; for example, dressing changes, administration of drugs, measuring vital signs, turning, transferring, ambulating, feeding and encouraging fluids, and monitoring of capillary blood glucose levels.

Criteria for Assigning/Delegating to Nursing Assistants

In 1995 the NCSBN prepared a position paper, "Delegation: Concepts and Decision-Making Process" (NCSBN; see Appendix G). This paper provides a decision-making process to be used by licensed persons in clinical settings as a guide for delegation of nursing duties. The position paper and additional National Council materials about delegation can be accessed online at *www.ncsbn.org* (type "delegation" in the search box).

NCSBN's position paper provides a checklist of five items to assist LPN/LVNs in making decisions about delegation. *The criteria to be followed for delegating also apply to assigning.* The checklist of rights includes right task. (When discussing delegation, the NCSBN uses the term task.) **Remember, to help differentiate and understand assigning versus delegating, we use the word "*task*" to apply to assigning and the word "*duty*" to apply to delegation of those functions that require the knowledge and judgment of your nursing license and experience.**

1. Right task (duty)
2. Right person
3. Right circumstance
4. Right direction/communication
5. Right supervision (Some states use the term *monitor* instead of *supervision* when the LPN/LVN performs this function.)

Right Task (Duty). A crucial legal consideration in dividing work among nursing assistants is nursing judgment. The LPN/LVN charge nurse needs to avoid real and potential harm to residents when allocating workload to nursing assistants. You are *legally liable* for improper assigning/delegating. Change-of-shift report and rounds for beginning of shift resident assessment gave you the opportunity, as LPN/LVN charge nurse, to collect data about the specific nursing needs of the residents for your shift and the complexity of those needs. Actual tasks/duties allocated depend on the following criteria:
—Laws in your state,
—Policies of the long-term care facility,
—Needs of the residents on your unit, and
—Training of nursing assistants.

Assigning Tasks. Assigning tasks involves dividing work that is in the job description of nursing assistants. Management Hint: Specific Tasks for Nursing Assistant Assignment contains specific tasks that could be assigned to nursing assistants.

Management Hint

Specific Tasks for Nursing Assistant Assignment

Routine:
- Personal care, including hygiene, dressing, toileting, grooming, and skin care
- Feeding and hydration
- Basic restorative *skills* including transfer, positioning, ambulation, and maintaining range of motion
- Measuring and recording vital signs, height and weight, and intake and output
- Assistance with elimination, including catheter care and enemas

- Maintaining safety factors, including fall prevention, application of heat and cold, and infection prevention
- Collecting specimens of urine and stool

Nursing assistants who have displayed an excellent work ethic, job performance, and skills may be offered additional, specialized training to become restorative aides. Additional training occurs for positioning, transferring, performing range of motion, using assistive devices, and preventing pressure ulcers.

Delegating Duties. Remember, delegating involves transferring the authority (the right) to perform a selected nursing duty (a duty your license gives you the right to do after attending a practical/vocational nursing program and passing a licensing exam given nationally). Delegation generally involves selected activities in patient care. A nursing assistant can receive an assignment, and within that assignment might be activities that need to be delegated. Avoid assuming that simpler duties may be automatically delegated. Management Tool: Criteria for Delegating Duties lists criteria for delegating duties to nursing assistants.

Management Tool

Criteria for Delegating Duties

The following are criteria for nursing duties that can be delegated for residents whose conditions are stable:

- The delegated duty must follow an unchanging procedure. (If this happens, then no.)
- The results of the delegated duty must be predictable.
- The potential for risk during performance of the delegated duty must be minimal (e.g., the patient with difficulty swallowing).
- The delegated duty should be necessary and routine in daily care.
- The delegated duty should not require nursing judgment (e.g., "I think the blood glucose level is normal").

- The delegated duty should not require frequent, repeated collection of data during performance of the duty.

The following suggestions include information to help decide what duty can be delegated.

- A question that can help the LPN/LVN make a decision as to what to delegate is, "What is the intended outcome (goal/desired result) of the nursing care in question?" In their article, "Delegating to UAPs—Making It Work," Hansten and Washburn (2001) use a bath given for several different reasons (goals/outcomes) as an example.
  —If the bath of a patient in long-term care, who is recuperating from total hip replacement, is being used as a teaching situation for family members to learn how to observe for signs of skin breakdown, then a licensed nurse needs to be part of the procedure.
  —If a resident who is recuperating from a stroke has a mobility issue, then a physical therapy assistant may be involved with range-of-motion training for the family during the bath.
  —The aforementioned two baths could be given as a team, with the nursing assistant bathing the resident while the licensed nurse points out pressure points susceptible to skin breakdown or the physical therapy assistant gives range-of-motion training.
  —If the desired goal of a bath is to have a long-term care resident bathed before being discharged, then the nursing assistant would be assigned.
- Given *specific* directions, nursing assistants can assist to collect, report, and document simple data, but not interpret that data.
- More complex skills to delegate depend on the following:
  —What is allowed by law in your state,
  —Resident needs of your unit, and
  —Further training of nursing assistants, for example, electronic blood glucose monitoring

A concise, across-the-board list of what nursing duties to delegate and what not to delegate does not exist. Management Hint: Why Lists of Duties to Delegate Do Not Exist contains the drawbacks of duty lists.

Management Hint

Why Lists of Duties to Delegate Do Not Exist

- A duty list for nursing assistants eliminates the need for collecting data of the needs of each patient.
- A duty could be on a list of acceptable duties to delegate to a nursing assistant, but the **patient situation** might indicate the duty would be dangerous or inappropriate for a nursing assistant; for example, feeding a patient with dysphagia (difficulty swallowing).
- The board of nursing has the responsibility to protect the patient. Licensed nursing personnel carry out this responsibility.
- A duty list for nursing assistants puts the control of nursing care into the hands of unlicensed persons who have had minimal training for patient care.
- *The exact duties delegated to nursing assistants are interpreted by each state's board of nursing and by each patient situation.*

It is somewhat easier to list what duties of the LPN/LVN **should** *not* **be delegated.** Management Hint: Examples of Duties Not to Delegate contains examples.

Management Hint

Examples of Duties Not to Delegate

- Sterile technique procedures: Nursing assistants do not have training in sterile technique.
- Crisis situations (you be there): Examples of crisis situations is a resident who develops chest pain.
- Initial patient education by an RN: in most states, LPN/LVNs may reinforce initial patient teaching given by the RN and provide information.

- Although nursing assistants can collect simple data, they have not been trained to make decisions about or interpret that data. For example, nursing assistants cannot evaluate results of capillary blood glucose monitoring and determine when vital signs need to be rechecked.
- Duties that are part of *your* legal scope of practice may *never* be delegated. Your legal scope of practice is your assisting role in the nursing process.

Critical Thinking Exercise

Delegating Duties

You practice in a health care facility that allows the LPN/LVN charge nurse to delegate nursing duties to nursing assistants. List two additional items to consider before actually delegating:

1.
2.

Right Person. The National Council's guidelines describe delegation as transferring the authority to perform a "selected nursing task" to a *competent* person. These guidelines also apply to assigning tasks to nursing assistants. According to NCSBN interpretation (Working with Others: 2005), a *competent* nursing assistant should be capable of the following, in addition to basic care:

- Communicate effectively,
- Collect basic subjective and objective data,
- Perform noncomplex nursing activities safely, accurately, and according to standard procedures, and
- Seek guidance and direction when appropriate.

The following suggestions will help you determine competence of nursing assistants.

Review Job Descriptions. Legally, you need to know the job descriptions of nursing assistants to whom you assign tasks. Check these job descriptions of the facility in which you are employed or on clinical affiliation as a student. See Management Tool: Reviewing Nursing Assistant Job Descriptions.

Management Tool

Reviewing Nursing Assistant Job Descriptions

Resource Needed:
• Job descriptions of nursing assistants
Make a list of the tasks nursing assistants can perform in various health care facilities.

Know Level of Competence. Know the level of clinical competence of nursing assistants you supervise. The following questions can help you determine the competency of nursing assistants on your team:
• Is the nursing assistant certified?
• How much nursing assistant training have they had?
• What skills are taught in their nursing assistant program?
• What is the nursing assistant's job description?
• Does the facility conduct yearly skills list updates? (Some LPN/LVNs keep a laminated copy of nursing assistant job descriptions and skills lists on their clipboards.)
• What clinical strengths have you observed?
• Have the nursing assistants demonstrated previous competency when performing the activity?
• What clinical weaknesses have you observed?
• Is orientation to your unit completed?
• What activities do nursing assistants say they feel qualified doing?
• What activities do nursing assistants feel unsure doing?
• Ask nursing assistants to describe what they would do in a specific situation. For example, "Tell me how you would get this resident with a total hip replacement out

of bed." If the nursing assistant hesitates or looks baffled, suggest that you will assist the nursing assistant when she gets the patient out of bed for the first time and use it as a teaching situation.
• Ask what the nursing assistant would do if a deviation from the normal procedure should develop. For example, "While getting this resident to stand up, what would you do if he got dizzy when attempting to stand?"
• Ask if the nursing assistant has done the procedure before. If nursing assistants misrepresent themselves by saying they know how to perform a nursing activity when they do not know how to perform the activity, they could be liable in a court of law. For example, if a nursing assistant tells you he or she could do a fingerstick test and then performed it incorrectly causing injury to the resident, he or she could be liable.

Refusing Assignment. If a nursing assistant does not feel qualified to safely perform an *assigned task* and refuses the assignment, the team member is then reassigned. It is a fine art distinguishing between "I don't want to" and "I don't know how to." If there is a training problem, follow the suggestion in Management Tool: Reviewing Nursing Assistant Job Descriptions. Make arrangements with the staff educator of your facility for this team member to receive the training necessary to safely perform the task(s). If there is an attitude problem, follow the suggestions in Appendix F. See Management Tool: Handling Refusal of Assignment by Nursing Assistants.

Management Tool

Handling Refusal of Assignment by Nursing Assistants

Resource Needed:
• Reading: "Refusing Assignment" above.
A nursing assistant on the team has refused your assignment to give a resident a whirlpool bath because he does not feel qualified to do the job safely. Write a brief note regarding this situation

to the staff educator of the facility. (In a real situation, also send a copy of the note to your supervisor.)

Once you work consistently with nursing assistants, they will prove their dependability and ability to pursue assigned tasks. Nursing assistants have the right to refuse a delegated duty. The LPN/LVN charge nurse then uses questioning to determine if the team member feels unqualified or simply does not want to do the activity. Feeling unqualified is a training problem; not wanting to do an activity is an attitude problem. Problems in attitude can interfere with a nursing assistant's growth as a member of the health care team.

Right Circumstance. NCSBN emphasizes that the setting and patient situation must be considered when delegating. The same criteria must be considered when assigning tasks. Assignment/delegation of duties would not occur if the following are true:

- Resident is unstable. The LPN/LVN would probably work as part of "pair caring" with the nursing assistant when a patient has difficulty swallowing, needs to be fed, and has a history of choking. The LPN/LVN would feed the resident and might use the situation as an opportunity to teach the nursing assistant techniques to use to avoid choking.
- The unit does not have equipment or supplies needed to safely carry out the procedure. The procedure would not be attempted until equipment and supplies were obtained.
- There are safety issues for the nursing assistant, including infection control issues.
- The staffing level is so limited that:
  — Supervision (monitoring) of assigned/delegated duties would not be adequate.
  — Assistance from the LPN/LVN might not be available when needed; for example, assistance when the nursing assistant has questions or needs directions.

Tricia chuckled as she thought about the time she asked a nursing assistant to force fluids for a resident with an elevated temperature. When the nursing assistant was approached during the shift, she kept reporting that she was forcing fluids. At the end of the shift, when asked for the volume of fluid taken by the resident during the shift, the nursing assistant replied that although she had forced fluids every hour, the resident took only 80 cc for the entire shift. Tricia thought that response served her right for not explaining the assignment objectively, as taught by Mrs. Kelly.

Right Direction/Communication. Using effective communication techniques is an excellent example of the leadership skills that are needed by LPN/LVN charge nurses. The LPN/LVN charge nurse's ability to communicate assignments effectively to nursing assistants for reaching patient goals depends on these skills.

As with all communication, assigning/delegating is a two-way process. The communication skills of LPN/LVNs and their management style are crucial for establishing a positive working relationship between charge nurse and nursing assistant. It is not only *what* you say, as LPN/LVN charge nurse, but also *how* you say it. **Inadequate communication, according to the National Council, is the most common reason delegated duties are not completed as expected.** The communication guidelines for delegating duties also apply to communication for assigning tasks. Communication skills need to be learned by studying and using the techniques. Review Chapter 9 regarding straightforward communication.

Do not just tell a nursing assistant what to do. Be sure to give the rationale for duties assigned or delegated. Explain *why* an assigned or delegated duty must be done first or at a specific time. Explain why you need the results at a specific time. Nursing assistants become frustrated and feel unsafe when expected to complete an activity when too little information is given. See Management Hint: Communication/Direction Responsibilities of the LPN/LVN Charge Nurse When Assigning or Delegating for communication guidelines that apply to assigning *and* delegating.

Communication/Direction Responsibilities of the LPN/LVN Charge Nurse When Assigning or Delegating

When assigning tasks or delegating duties, be sure to provide nursing assistants with the following information:

- Give objective, detailed, clear-cut verbal and written directions. Get to the point!
- Consider writing assignments in a concise, objective manner on a master assignment sheet.
- Explain what is expected at the nursing assistant's level of understanding.
- Be specific about the results you are expecting. Do not ask nursing assistants to "find out how the patient is." For example, have them ask the patient who has been itching because of a rash if the rash still itches.
- Provide guidelines for reporting after the delegated duty is completed. Provide the time you expect to be informed and why.
- Make sure your directions are specific and complete. Provide all the necessary information, including time, to get the task or duty done correctly and safely. For example, "Please report the numbers immediately after you measure Mr. Smith's blood pressure, pulse, and respirations. I need to know the numbers before his 0900 blood pressure medicine can be given."
- Given specific directions, nursing assistants can collect, report, and document simple data. However, they are unable to make judgments based on that data. For example, "Please report the results of Mr. Ettle's fingerstick immediately after you perform it so I can determine if he needs insulin."
- Tell nursing assistants when to consult with the charge nurse during the performance of an assigned/delegated duty. For example, "Let me know if you are having trouble getting the specimen."
- Clarify all messages by asking nursing assistants to tell you what it is you expect them to do.
- A "please" and "thank you" are in order as part of common courtesy.

Inform nursing assistants when you expect a report/rundown on activities. A suggested "routine" for reporting back to the charge nurse is before and after breaks and meals, and before going off duty. The exact number of reports depends on your familiarity with how the nursing assistant functions, the condition of the residents, and the nature of the assigned/delegated duty. Examples of delegated duties that need priority or more frequent reporting are blood pressure numbers when the resident is to receive blood pressure medicine and blood glucose monitoring with sliding scale insulin coverage. State **when** you expect to be informed, and **why**.

Review Chapter 15 for hints that can be used to motivate team members and the Leadership Activity: Using the Howlett Hierarchy in Leadership Situations.

Critical Thinking Exercise

Identifying Resident Goals/Outcomes

Using the information "Identifying Resident Goals/ Outcomes," p. 291, the reading "Subjective Versus Objective Charting," p. 262, "Signs and Symptoms" list on p. 281, and a medical/surgical text, write the following activities/observations to be assigned/delegated to nursing assistants in specific, objective, clear-cut terms. The directions need to be realistic, measurable, and time referenced.

1. Be sure to clean up Mr. Collar.
2. Make sure Mrs. Thren drinks today.
3. Mrs. Wall must get up today.
4. If Mr. Jones does not pass any urine, let me know.
5. Have Mrs. Neidert ready for her doctor's appointment.

Critical Thinking Exercise

Communicating Objectively to Nursing Assistants

This is your first month as charge nurse at Quality Care Home. Provide specific, objective, clear-cut data for the nursing assistant to be aware of while giving care in the following resident situations:

1. Resident has compensated right-sided congestive heart failure.
2. Resident is a poorly controlled diabetic who receives an intermediate-acting insulin each morning.

3. Resident has lost 5 lb in the past 2 weeks.
4. Resident has an order for a catheterized urine for residual.

Remember. When delegating, clarify that the nursing assistant has accepted the delegation. The nursing assistant's accountability in delegation includes accepting the delegated duty, in addition to safe performance in carrying out the duty.

Tricia Makes Assignments for the Nursing Assistants (see resident goals, p. 291)

- *Harold:* Tricia has worked with Jenny, CNA, for several years and assigns Jenny to Harry for personal care and assistance with ambulation as Jenny has had training as a restorative aid. Jenny verbally explains that she will make sure Harold gets up from the right side of the bed, does not cross his legs, or lean forward while getting up or sitting in the chair. Tricia assigns Jenny to care for Harold and set up for Harry's dressing change. Although Jenny is allowed to change clean dressings, she is to notify Tricia before she starts so Tricia can observe the surgical site because of Harold's temperature and lack of respiratory symptoms.
- *Adelia:* Lenore, CNA, has had training for capillary blood testing. Tricia has worked with Lenore for several months and thinks she has demonstrated proficiency in safely and accurately obtaining samples for glucose testing. Tricia assigns Lenore to Adelia and delegates capillary blood testing. When given information of the need for two fingersticks on the evening shift, Lenore explains she will identify the finger to be used for the fingerstick, warm Adelia's finger under warm water at the sink in the bathroom, and keep that hand down after Adelia sits before attempting to get the sample, Tricia reminds Lenore she needs the sample at 6:30 AM before breakfast and 11:30 AM before lunch trays so she can determine if she needs to administer

Adelia's sliding scale insulin coverage 1/2 hour before meals.
- *Blake:* Judy is a nursing assistant with 7 years experience, but is new to Quality Care Home. Judy has had restorative nursing training and does well with ROM, positioning, and transfers. Judy has generally been doing well feeding residents. However, last week Tricia saw a resident almost choke on a grapefruit segment while being fed by Judy. Tricia assigns Judy for the following care of Blake: Assist with AM care in bed, ROM, positioning, and assist with transfer from bed to chair. Tricia decides to be with Judy and "care pair." Tricia will feed Blake and use this as an opportunity to review with Judy hints and safety techniques for feeding residents with dysphagia.

IMPLEMENTATION
Right Supervision, Feedback, and Evaluation
The National Council defines supervision as "the provision of guidance or direction, evaluation, and follow-up by the licensed nurse for accomplishment of a nursing task delegated to unlicensed assistive personnel" (NCSBN, 1995). This definition is interpreted to include appropriate monitoring, intervention, and evaluation of the nursing assistant, as needed, while providing the delegated duty and feedback after the delegated duty is completed. The following suggestions also apply to assigning tasks. To comply with the National Council's guideline, the LPN/LVN charge nurse needs to carry out the suggestions found in Management Hint: Supervision and Feedback for nursing assistants regarding assigned tasks/delegated duties.

 Management Hint

Supervision and Feedback
- How often or closely the charge nurse monitors the nursing assistant carrying out the assigned task or delegated duty depends on the resident situation and the nursing assistant.

- The LPN/LVN needs to make himself or herself available for questions or concerns as they arise and to provide guidance when needed. Ask nursing assistant if assistance is needed.
- Determine if assigned tasks or delegated duties are being completed. If not, determine the reason for this (e.g., change of condition).
- If necessary, intervene in the situation to ensure carrying out the assigned task or delegated duty safely.

If you fail to supervise adequately and the resident is harmed, the situation could result in a civil suit in a court of law or disciplinary action against your license. See Chapter 20 for information about nursing and the law.

Assessment of residents and functioning of the team by the LPN/LVN charge nurse occurs periodically during the shift. Although clear communication with nursing assistants during assignment helps ensure that helpful information about residents will be collected during the shift, nothing can replace the charge nurse's contact with residents and judgment based on knowledge and experience.

Management Hint

Tricia Supervises the Nursing Assistants

At 7:30 AM and 11:30 AM Lenore reports, without reminder, Adelia's blood glucose levels. Lenore states she had no trouble getting the samples with one fingerstick. Tricia interprets that no sliding scale insulin is required.

Tricia sees Jenny and Harold as they walk to the dining room for breakfast and Jenny says Harold is very careful about getting up. Harold informed Jenny that "I need to keep that new hip in its socket" so he always gets up on the right side of the bed and never crosses his legs. Jenny notified Tricia after she set up for the clean dressing change and Tricia assessed the incisional line. There was no redness or edema at the area. Harold's lung sounds are clear and he denies coughing or congestion. Tricia asks Jenny to check Harold's temperature again at noon.

Judy sets up Blake for breakfast and notifies Tricia when his tray arrives. When Tricia enters Blake's room,

she notes that Blake is sitting up in bed. Tricia suggests that they have Blake sit in the chair for meals. When seated, Tricia reminds Blake to keep his head straight and not tilt it back while swallowing. Tricia turns Blake's head to the left (the unaffected side) and starts with a couple of spoonfuls of thickened liquids and explains this will moisten the membranes of Blake's mouth and throat to make swallowing easier. Tricia feeds one third of a teaspoon at a time of cream of wheat and scrambled eggs. Judy is attentive as Tricia continues with thickened liquids periodically. When done, Tricia arranges with Judy to be present while Judy sets Blake up and feeds him his lunch.

EVALUATION

You discovered in Chapters 1 and 15 that clinical evaluation is a two-way process. The information in those chapters applies to this part of the assignment/delegation process. See Management Hint: Evaluation and Feedback.

Management Hint

Evaluation and Feedback

Evaluation
- Check the completed duty that was assigned/delegated. Was the task/duty completed? Was the task/duty performed safely?
- Legally, the LPN/LVN charge nurse may not delegate a duty without checking the outcome of that delegation. Have resident goals (outcomes) been met?
- Has something unusual, undesirable, or unexpected occurred?
- Has the nursing assistant documented the activity?

Feedback
- Encourage the nursing assistant to offer input about the assignment/delegation. For example, "Dorothy, how did the bath go for Mr. Paul?" "Kyle, how do you think the day went? Was I available when you needed to question? What suggestions do you have that would make things flow more smoothly during the shift?"
- The LPN/LVN's leadership skills again come into importance during evaluation and feedback. Provide feedback as needed by the nursing assistant.
- Review and use guidelines for performance evaluation from Chapter 15.

Tricia's Evaluation of and Feedback from Nursing Assistants

Tricia thanks Jenny, Lenore, and Judy for their help and getting back to her with information and notifying her as quickly as they did. She asks each aide how they think the day went. Jenny and Lenore say the day went fine and that Tricia was available when they needed to report. Judy says the hints for feeding Blake, especially getting him up to eat and giving thickened liquids first to moisten membranes, were very helpful. All three say they hope to get the same assignment tomorrow and Lenore asks to watch Judy feed Blake so she can pick up some hints to use with patients with dysphagia.

PUTTING IT ALL TOGETHER

See the following critical thinking exercise.

Critical Thinking Exercise

Assigning Residents in Long-Term Care

Resource Needed:

- As LPN/LVN charge nurse and with available staff, make assignments for the day shift for wing 1 of the nursing home. Include the rationale (reason) for your assignment decisions. Assign and delegate as you feel is appropriate.

Staff available for the team

- Two student practical/vocational nurses who have completed half of their nursing program. Instructor makes assignments and is present on the clinical area.
- One nursing assistant who has worked at the facility for 10 years (on state directory).
- One nursing assistant who has 7 years' experience and has worked at your facility for 6 months (on state registry).
- One nursing assistant who was sent from a temporary agency to fill the position of a nursing assistant who has the flu. She completed a nursing assistant-advanced course 2 months ago (on state registry).

Tasks for day shift of Wing 1

- *Four showers.* Each of these residents transfers with the help of two. Each of these residents needs to be weighed, have blood pressure checked, and have a complete linen change on shower day. One resident scheduled for a shower says she feels dizzy and has a congested-sounding cough.
- *Sixteen partial baths.* Ten residents are able to wash their own face and hands when set up. Of the remaining six, one has developed a rash over his entire body, one needs electronic glucose-monitoring one-half hour before breakfast and lunch on day shift, and four are confused and incontinent of urine and feces. Each of these residents needs one assistant to transfer and ambulate.
- *One complex dressing change for a resident on a Clinitron bed.* (This resident is transferred by a patient-lifting device and requires total care.)
- *One PEG tube intermittent feeding with commercial tube feeding formula and drug administration at 8 AM and 12 noon on day shift.* (This resident is confused and requires two persons to ambulate.)

You have just completed assigning team members when one of the nursing assistants states she feels warm and then faints. As it turns out, she has a temperature of 102.2 °F and needs to be sent home. Reassign the residents on wing 1.

Critical Thinking Exercise

Delegating to Nursing Assistants

Resources Needed:

- Descriptions of recent clinical assignments for students in your clinical group
- Critical thinking

If your state allows LPN/LVNs to delegate, use Table 16-2 and the nursing process format in this chapter to practice assigning/delegating recent clinical duties for your clinical group to nursing assistants.

REPORTING AT THE END OF YOUR SHIFT

Giving report at the end of your shift requires planning. As the LPN/LVN charge nurse, you need reports from the nursing assistants before you can tape or give report. This is where the concise,

Table 16-2	*Delegation Decision-Making Tree for the Licensed Practical/Vocational Nurse*

Starting with question No. 1 below, if you answer "no" to a question, do not delegate. If you answer "yes," proceed to the next question.

1. Does your Nurse Practice Act give the LPN/LVN permission to delegate?	**No**	**Do not delegate**	**Yes**
2. Does the employing agency give the LPN/LVN permission to delegate?	**No**	**Do not delegate**	**Yes**
3. Is the duty to be delegated within the scope of practice of the LPN/LVN?	**No**	**Do not delegate**	**Yes**
4. Does the LPN/LVN have the education necessary to delegate nursing duties?	**No**	**Do not delegate**	**Yes**
5. Has the LPN/LVN collected data of the patient's needs?	**No**	**Collect data and continue**	**Yes**
6. Is the nursing assistant to whom a duty is being delegated competent to accept the delegation? (See pp. 293 and 295 for suggestions to determine competency.)	**No**	**Do not delegate**	**Yes**
7. Does the nursing assistant accept the delegated duty?	**No**	**Do not delegate**	**Yes**
8. Does the ability of the nursing assistant match the care needs of the patient?	**No**	**Do not delegate**	**Yes**
9. Can the delegated nursing duty be performed without requiring nursing judgment?	**No**	**Do not delegate**	**Yes**
10. Are the results of the delegated nursing duty reasonably predictable?	**No**	**Do not delegate**	**Yes**
11. Can the delegated nursing duty be safely performed according to exact, unchanging directions?	**No**	**Do not delegate**	**Yes**
12. Can the delegated nursing duty be safely performed without complex observations and the need for critical decisions?	**No**	**Do not delegate**	**Yes**
13. Can the delegated nursing duty be performed without the need for repeated data collection?	**No**	**Do not delegate**	**Yes**
14. Is the LPN/LVN who delegated the nursing duty available for monitoring the nursing assistant?	**No**	**Do not delegate**	**Yes→ May delegate**

Adapted by H. Howlett from *The Delegation Decision-Making Tree of NCSBN* [1997], which was adapted from the Decision Tree developed by the Ohio Board of Nursing.

clear directions that you gave to these team members during assignment/delegation will pay off. You will need to set priorities in deciding pertinent information to give to the next shift. Be sure to personally assess residents who have the following:

- Changes in condition,
- Current ongoing problems,
- New orders (and resident response to new orders), and
- Suspected side effects to medications.

Use the same sequence of data for each resident. This will make it easier for the oncoming charge nurse to take notes from your report. An example of a suggested sequence of data for reporting to oncoming shift for residents in a long-term care unit can be found in Management Hint: Reporting to Oncoming Shift.

Management Hint

Reporting to Oncoming Shift

Things to report:

1. Resident name, room number, and physician
2. New problems/concerns
3. Contact with physician and new orders
4. Progress of current, established problems
5. PRN medication—name of drug, time given, and reason for PRN medication; time follow-up is required
6. **Briefly** describe resident's behavior during shift; include any changes in resident's physical and mental status
7. Resident's voiding, bowel movement (continent versus incontinent)

Things to avoid during report include:

1. Meaningless chatter that has nothing to do with residents' nursing care and goals/outcomes
2. Routine nursing care, unless it has a bearing on current nursing problems
3. Personal opinions about residents' conditions
4. Value judgments, gossip about residents' lifestyles, behavior, or families

---

Tricia was very tired and began to put away her textbooks and scrapbook. The review of delegation in her old PVI text proved demanding for Tricia, but it also had been very pleasant reminiscing about her school days and early years as an LVN. She felt good with how far she had come since feeling insecure in those beginning days. At least, she now knew what to question and where to find the answers. It felt good to have a grasp of her LPN/LVN charge nurse position, especially the fine points of delegation of duties. Later, as Tricia was relaxing in a warm tub, a big smile came over her face. Tomorrow would be a big day in her life. Mrs. Kelly had strongly recommended membership in professional organizations. Tricia had been a member of the National Federation of Licensed Practical Nurses at the national, state, and local levels since graduation. Over the years she had assumed various committee assignments and officer positions at the local level of the organization. Tomorrow she would be installed as the first president of the organization at the state level from her local district! Tricia was proud to be of service to her career and looked forward to promoting and having a say in the direction practical/vocational nursing would take in the twenty-first century.

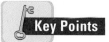

Key Points

- State Nurse Practice Acts specify requirements needed by LPN/LVNs to assume first-line manager positions.
- A common first-line manager position is charge nurse in long-term care units and nursing homes.
- Common charge nurse problems include nursing assistants who bring personal problems to work, the need for nursing assistants to be accountable for learning new job skills, and dealing with the residents' demanding/complaining family members.
- Oncoming shift report gives the charge nurse the opportunity to collect data about resident needs, identify resident goals (outcomes) for the shift, and assign nursing tasks to nursing assistants for resident care from *their* job description.
- Assessment of each resident after assignment/delegation identifies changes in condition/circumstances that may require a change in assignment/delegation.
- The charge nurse shares responsibility with nursing assistants for the quality of care that is given.
- Practical/vocational charge nurses routinely assign care to nursing assistants.
- Charge nurses, as part of their jobs, evaluate the thoroughness and safety of all tasks they assign.
- *If allowed in your state's Nurse Practice Act,* and included in facility policies, the LPN/LVN charge nurse may elect to delegate duties from the LPN/LVN job description to nursing assistants.
- Delegation gives the charge nurse time to focus on duties that cannot be delegated.

- Duties can be delegated, but the responsibility that goes with those duties remains with the registered nurse, under whom the charge nurse functions under general supervision. The LPN/LVN shares accountability in these situations.
- The charge nurse position is a complex role for LPN/LVNs. With additional education and experience, many practical/vocational nurses are doing an excellent job in this expanded role position.
- Your license is at stake in the matter of assuming the charge nurse position. Know your state laws regulating nursing.

REVIEW ITEMS

1. Select the defense mechanism that may be present in a family member who continually finds fault and criticizes the care given to a relative by nursing assistants.

   1. Projection
   2. Validation
   3. Introversion
   4. Conversion

2. Select the statement that indicates understanding of delegation.

   1. Nursing assistants cannot refuse a duty delegated to them by the practical/vocational nurse for any reason.
   2. Delegating duties depends on state law, facility policies, resident condition, and the LPN/LVN's desire to delegate.
   3. Any licensed practical/vocational nurse may delegate his or her role to a qualified, dependable nursing assistant.
   4. LPN/LVNs delegate duties to nursing assistants that are in the facility job description of the nursing assistant.

3. Alex, an LPN, has 2 months' experience in a nursing home. He is approached by his employer to perform nursing duties within the expanded role of the practical/vocational nurse as charge nurse. Alex knows the expanded role is allowed in his state, but he has not had a leadership component in the basic educational program. Select the best response in this situation.

   1. "I am unable by law to do this, and I could lose my license for functioning in an LPN expanded role."
   2. "I will not function in the expanded role because I did not study this in my student practical nursing program."
   3. "I need some time to contact my board of nursing to clarify state statutes for the LPN expanded role."
   4. "I will assume this role if you will train me for the duties I was not taught and document them in my file."

4. Cindy, LPN, is charge nurse on the evening shift at a nursing home. Select the priority action she will use in making assignments to nursing assistants.

   1. Cindy obtains feedback from the nursing assistants as to the type of procedures for which they feel competent.
   2. Cindy distributes the nursing tasks to be completed on the evening shift equally among the nursing assistants on the team.
   3. Cindy checks job descriptions and skills for nursing assistants to clarify who is competent to perform selected duties.
   4. After report when coming on duty, Cindy establishes patient outcomes for residents for the shift and sets priorities for care.

ALTERNATE FORMAT ITEM

Select from the following sources where permission for the LPN/LVN to delegate in long-term care can be found. *(Select all that apply.)*

1. BON
2. NCSBN
3. NFLPN
4. FACILITY
5. NAPNES

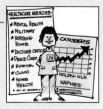

evolve   http://evolve.elsevier.com/Hill/success/

On completing this chapter, you will be able to do the following:

1. Compare public and private health care agencies according to the following criteria:
   a. Source of funding,
   b. Services provided,
   c. Examples of agencies in your geographical area, and
   d. Possible places of employment for practical/vocational nurses.
2. Differentiate between official and voluntary agencies.
3. Explain what is meant by private health care agencies as the usual entry into the health care delivery system in the United States.
4. Give an example of an:
   a. Official government public health care agency in your area,
   b. Official government public health care agency in your state, and
   c. Official government public health care agency at the federal level.
5. Identify the federal health care agency in the United States that is headed by an appointee of the president and advises the president in health matters.
6. List six agencies that make up the U.S. Public Health Service (USPHS).
7. Describe the responsibility of the World Health Organization (WHO).
8. Provide examples of two voluntary health care agencies in your area that are not listed in this chapter.
9. Explain the difference between proprietary and nonprofit health care agencies.

10. Discuss how primary care relates to family practice physicians.
11. Differentiate between general and specialized hospitals.
12. Explain the purpose of teaching and research hospitals.
13. Discuss the difference between ambulatory and acute care settings.
14. Define the term *freestanding*.
15. Describe free clinics as a source of primary care.
16. Explain the purpose of rehabilitation.
17. Explain what is meant by the following abbreviations:
    a. LTC,
    b. PAC,
    c. SNFSD,
    d. ALP, and
    e. CCRC.
18. Differentiate among the following types of facilities:
    a. Custodial care facility,
    b. Intermediate care facility (ICF),
    c. Skilled care facility (SCF), and
    d. Assisted care facility.
19. Discuss the major focus of community health nursing.
20. Explain the difference between community health nursing services and home health agencies.
21. List six possible nursing skills that a licensed practical/vocational nurse (LPN/LVN) might perform under registered nurse (RN) supervision, as a part of home health nursing.
22. Describe two circumstances for using adult day care.
23. List three examples of wellness centers in your area.
24. Explain the purpose of hospice.

Key Terms

Acute care (p. 308)
Adult care home (p. 312)
Adult day care center (p. 313)
Ambulatory care facilities (p. 310)
Ambulatory surgery centers (p. 310)
Assisted care (p. 312)
Board and care homes (p. 312)
Community health nursing (p. 312)
Community health nursing services (p. 313)
Continuous Care Retirement Community (CCRC) (p. 312)
Department of Health and Human Services (DHHS) (p. 306)
Free clinic (p. 310)
Free-standing (p. 309)
General hospitals (p. 308)
Group home (p. 312)
Home health nursing (p. 313)
Hospice care (HŎS-pĭs, p. 314)
Long-term care (LTC) (p. 311)
Nursing home (p. 311)
Official (government) health care agencies (p. 305)
Outpatient clinic (p. 309)
Post-acute care (PAC) (p. 311)
Primary care (p. 308)
Private health care agencies (p. 305)
Proprietary hospitals (for profit) (prŏ-PRĪ-ĭ-tĕr-ē, p. 308)
Public health care agencies (p. 305)
Rehabilitation (rē-hă-bĭl-ĭ-tā-shŭn, p. 309)
Residential care (rĕz-ĭ-DĔN-shŭl, p. 312)
Skilled care (p. 311)
Skilled nursing facility for severely disabled (SNFSD, p. 311)
Specialized hospital (p. 308)
Teaching and research hospital (p. 309)
Transitional care (p. 311)
United Nations (UN) (p. 306)
U.S. Public Health Service (USPHS) (p. 306)
Voluntary community hospital (p. 309)
Voluntary health care agencies (p. 305)
Wellness center (p. 314)
World Health Organization (WHO) (p. 306)

Keep in Mind

What is your passion? Choose carefully and make that first job worthy of you.

Health care agencies are not alike. They differ in size, focus, quality of service, and how they are financed. Do some research before making an application for work, so you can make an informed choice about employment after you graduate. Compose questions to ask during an employment interview. Refer to Chapter 21 for ideas.

Critical Thinking Exercise

Personal Vision of Working as a Nurse

What is your vision for working as a nurse after you complete nursing school?

PUBLIC VERSUS PRIVATE HEALTH CARE AGENCIES

For ease of understanding, the various health care services in the United States can be grouped into two general categories: (1) services delivered by the public sector, and (2) services delivered by the private sector.

Table 17-1 outlines the major differences between public and private health care agencies. As you read about public and private health care agencies, think of them as potential sources of employment for the LPN/LVN.

PUBLIC HEALTH CARE AGENCIES

There are two types of public health care agencies—official and voluntary.

- Official (government) health care agencies:
  - Government agencies that are supported by tax money
  - Accountable to the taxpayers and the government
  - Primary emphasis of government: the delivery of disease prevention and wellness promotion programs
  - Direct health care services sometimes provided
- Voluntary health care agencies:
  - Supported by voluntary contributions
  - Sometimes by a fee for service

Table 17-1 *Comparison of Health Care Agencies in the Public and Private Sectors*

| | PUBLIC | | PRIVATE |
	OFFICIAL (GOVERNMENT)	NONOFFICIAL (VOLUNTARY)	
Support	Tax money	Voluntary contributions and fees for service	Fees for service
Primary service	Programs of disease prevention and wellness promotion	Research and education	Curing disease and illness
Additional services	Sometimes direct service of health care	Offer direct health services	Disease prevention and wellness promotion
Accountability	Taxpayers and government	Supporters, boards, etc.	Owners
How programs determined	Mandated and nonmandated	Supporter interest	Defined goals of the organization

— Tuned in to public opinion, but are accountable to their supporters
— Activities determined by supporter interest, not legal mandate
— Primary emphasis on research and education
— May also offer direct health services to the patient

Some official and voluntary health care agencies operate at the local, state, federal, and international levels.

EXAMPLES OF PUBLIC HEALTH CARE AGENCIES
Official Government Agencies

Local. The official health agency at the local level is the city or county health department. These agencies have the following characteristics:
* They are funded by local tax money, as well as by subsidies from the state and federal levels of government.
* They carry out state laws (mandated) concerning community health.
* They carry out non-mandated programs, such as health promotion programs.

State. Each state has a state health department. This official health agency has the following characteristics:
* It is funded by state tax money.
* It sometimes receives money from the federal government.

Federal (National). The official health agency at the federal level in the United States is the Department of Health and Human Services (DHHS). DHHS has the following characteristics:
* It is funded by federal taxes.
* A person appointed by the president of the United States is head of the agency. This person advises the president in health matters.

The DHHS division that is concerned primarily with health is the U.S. Public Health Service (USPHS), which is made up of the following six agencies:
* Food and Drug Administration (FDA),
* Centers for Disease Control and Prevention (CDC),
* National Institutes of Health (NIH),
* Health Services Administration (HSA),
* Health Resources Administration (HRA), and
* Alcohol, Drug Abuse, and Mental Health Administration.

International. Health activities take place at the international level through the World Health Organization (WHO), an agency of the United Nations (UN).
* WHO is located in Geneva.
* The major objective of WHO is the highest possible level of health for people all over the world.
* WHO defines *health* as a state of complete physical, mental, and social well-being and not merely as the absence of disease or infirmity.
* WHO is funded through fees paid by member nations of the UN.

Learning Exercise

Local Health Care Agency

Identify an official and voluntary health care agency in your geographical area. What services does each agency provide locally?

VOLUNTARY HEALTH CARE AGENCIES

Voluntary or nonofficial health care agencies (Table 17-2) are so named because they are nonprofit. The health services they provide are complementary to **official health agencies**. They often meet the needs of persons with specific diseases (e.g., heart disease) and certain segments of the population (e.g., disabled). Although paid personnel work in voluntary health agencies, volunteers form a major part of their support system. Voluntary organizations are sites for volunteer service for practical/vocational nursing students and LPN/LVNs. Some examples follow. Refer to your local telephone directory for additional names and numbers of voluntary health care agencies.

Visiting Nurse Association

The Visiting Nurse Association (VNA) is a public voluntary agency that has the following characteristics:

* It provides home nursing care for persons with acute and chronic diseases. Care

Table 17-2 *Examples of Voluntary Agencies*

AGENCY	PURPOSE	CONTACT
American Cancer Society (ACS)	Cancer research, public information resource to patients, families, professionals	(800) ACS-2345, *www.cancer.org*
American Lung Association (ALA)	Research, professional education, resource for professionals and public	(800) LUNG-USA, *www.lungusa.org*
American Heart Association (AHA)	Research and education on heart disease and stroke	(800) 242-8721, *www.americanheart.org*
American Stroke Association	Research and education on stroke	(800) 553-6321, *www.strokeassociation.org*
Alcoholics Anonymous	Rehabilitation help and support to patients and families	Check telephone book's local listing, *www.alcoholics-anonymous.org*
ALS Society of America	Collects data on persons with amyotrophic lateral sclerosis (Lou Gehrig's disease) for research purposes; resource for public and professionals	(800) 782-4747, *www.alsa.org*
Easter Seals National Headquarters	Research and rehabilitative services for disabled children and adults	(800) 221-6827, *www.easterseals.org*
LaLeche League	Information and support for breast-feeding mothers; breast milk for infants because of health reasons but lack a source	(800)-LaLeche, *www.lalecheleague.org*
United Ostomy Association (UOA)	Education, information, and advocacy for patients undergoing intestinal or urinary diversion procedures	(800) 826-0826, *www.uoa.org*
American Diabetes Association (ADA)	Resource for type 1 and type 2 diabetes, nutrition information, referrals to doctors, and educational programs	(800) 342-2383, *www.diabetes.org*

includes health supervision, education, counseling, bedside care, and carrying out physicians orders.

- It visits mothers with newborn infants.
- It is engaged in health teaching.
- It frequently involves the family in the care of its own members.
- It assists with referrals for patients to other community services.
- It is staffed primarily by bachelor of science nursing (BSN) nurses and home health aides trained for specific tasks of personal bedside care.

Learning Exercise

Voluntary Health Care Agencies

Discover if there is a VNA or equivalent agency in your area. If so, do they employ LPN/LVNs? What are the skills that LPN/LVNs are able to perform with registered nurse (RN) supervision?

PRIVATE HEALTH CARE AGENCIES

You may be most familiar with **private health care agencies**.

- Entrance to the health care delivery system in the United States is generally gained through private health care agencies.
- Although some voluntary or nonprofit agencies are found in the private sector, private health care agencies are generally proprietary (i.e., for profit).
- They charge a fee for their services.
- Their primary emphasis has been on curing disease and illness, but a change in emphasis to include disease prevention and wellness promotion has occurred.

EXAMPLES OF PRIVATE HEALTH CARE AGENCIES

Private health care agencies have the following characteristics:

- They complement and supplement government agencies.

- In general, they are proprietary (for profit).
- Corporations that own a chain of health care facilities often own them.
- Occasionally, they are owned by an individual or by doctors who practice in the agency.

Compared with public health services, the greatest changes in health care services have been noted in the area of private health care agencies.

Family Practice Physicians

Primary care is the term used to describe the point at which an individual enters the health care system. Family practice physicians are a source of primary care. They provide diagnosis and treatment. The patient is billed a fee for these services. If further diagnostic evaluation is needed, the patient is referred to a specialist. Medical doctors function within the Medical Practice Acts of their respective states.

Private Practice Nurses

Specializing in primary health care, advanced practice nurses (APN) provide consulting and counseling services to groups of individuals. These nurses practice in all areas of health care. APNs fill an especially acute need in rural areas where physician services are sometimes difficult to obtain. The nurses function within the Nurse Practice Acts of their respective states. See Chapter 11.

TYPES OF HOSPITALS

PROPRIETARY HOSPITALS

Proprietary hospitals are for-profit hospitals operated for the financial benefit of the owner of the hospital. The owner may be an individual, a partnership, or a corporation. With good management techniques, the hospital can be run efficiently, and a profit can be realized. Today, when patients are admitted to the hospital, they are more acutely ill and require more skilled nursing care. This setting for health care is called acute care. There are more than 6000 general and specialized hospitals in the United States. Most are general hospitals, which are set up to deal with a full range of medical conditions experienced by patients. More than 1000 hospitals are set up to deal with a particular disease or condition (e.g., rehabilitation, cancer, orthopedics, mental illness). Specialized hospitals are limited to one type of patient, such as children, women, cardiac patients, etc.

For most conditions, a general hospital is able to accommodate a patient's needs. However, a general hospital may not have specialists with expertise for treating serious or unusual medical problems. The patient may need to be treated in a hospital center that has highly skilled specialists with advanced knowledge of the condition.

TEACHING AND RESEARCH HOSPITALS

Teaching and research hospitals can be private or public. They have a variety of goals, including the following:

- Treating patients, especially those with serious or unusual conditions,
- Training sites for physicians, nurses, and other health professionals, and
- Researching and developing treatments for disease conditions.

These hospitals are almost always affiliated with medical schools and have access to highly skilled practitioners.

PUBLIC HOSPITALS

Public hospitals include Veteran's Administration, state, county, and municipally owned and operated nonprofit hospitals. Hospitals for people with serious mental illness continue to be funded by federal, state, or county funds.

VOLUNTARY COMMUNITY HOSPITALS

Community associations or religious organizations operate voluntary community hospitals. These nonprofit hospitals provide short-term inpatient care for people with acute illnesses and injuries. Voluntary community hospitals are heavily dependent on gifts and donations to supplement sources of revenue. Ultimate responsibility for the hospital rests with the board of trustees, usually chosen from the community's business and professional people, who serve without pay. The board of trustees appoints a paid administrator to manage the hospital.

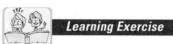
Learning Exercise

Hospitals

What kind of hospitals do you have in your area? Do they currently employ LPN/LVNs? If so, which nursing units employ LPN/LVNs?

_____

_____

AMBULATORY SERVICES

The continual rise in cost of inpatient care has resulted in the rapid development of a variety of ambulatory services. As a consequence, the number of inpatient days and the length of stay in acute care facilities have decreased. Ambulatory services offer less expensive care because admission to an acute care facility is avoided.

People who live in their own home, do their own care, or have care provided by family members generally use these settings. They come to these facilities for assessment, advice, monitoring, teaching, treatment, evaluation, and care coordination. *Private sector settings* are located in the following places:

- University hospital outpatient departments,
- Community hospital outpatient departments,
- Physician group practices,
- Health maintenance organizations (HMOs),
- Physicians' offices,
- Free-standing ambulatory centers (not attached to a hospital), and
- Nursing care centers.

Public sector settings include the following:

- Community health clinics,
- Indian Health Service, and
- Community and migrant worker health centers.

OUTPATIENT CLINICS

Outpatient clinics provide follow-up care to patients after hospitalization and have the following characteristics:

- They manage disease on an ambulatory basis for those who do not need to be hospitalized.
- They are a part of health care facilities or are **free-standing** (i.e., not attached to a hospital).
- They function by appointment only.
- They include specialty areas, such as diabetes, neurology, allergy, and oncology.
- The number of specialized clinics depends on the population of the area.
- They employ full-time staff.

URGENT CARE CENTERS

Services are available in ambulatory care facilities for walk-in patients who do not have an appointment. For some individuals, they replace doctor's offices. These facilities have the following characteristics:

- They make primary health care available, as an alternative to care by a family physician or care offered in a more expensive emergency room.
- People who do not have a family physician use them.
- Patients who desire faster service outside of regular office hours also use them.
- The names given to ambulatory care services reflect the type of care provided (e.g., convenience clinics, express care, quick care, urgent care).

ONE-DAY SURGICAL CARE CENTERS

One-day surgical care centers (ambulatory surgery centers) perform surgery at a scheduled date and time. Patients are discharged when they have recovered from anesthesia and are considered to be in stable condition. These surgery centers have the following characteristics:

- They eliminate the need and monetary charge for being hospitalized overnight.
- Their services are also known as outpatient surgery within an established hospital.
- Free-standing outpatient surgery centers provide outpatient surgery as their only service.
- Approximately 80% of surgical procedures are performed in this type of setting.

Learning Exercise

Ambulatory Care Providers

What are ambulatory health services in your area called? Do any of them employ LPN/LVNs? If so, what skills will the LPN/LVN perform under RN supervision?

_____

_____

FREE CLINIC

Some communities have established free clinics as an alternative means of providing primary health care. These free clinics have the following characteristics:

- Persons who cannot afford traditional health services or are reluctant to use more traditional services use the clinics.
- The environment is as free of red tape as possible.

TYPES OF CARE

WHAT IS SKILLED NURSING CARE?

- Registered nurses do wound care and change dressings after major surgery, or administer and monitor IV antibiotics for a severe infection.
- Physical therapists help to correct strength and balance problems that have made it difficult for a patient to walk or get on and off the bed, toilet, or furniture.
- A speech therapist helps to regain the ability to communicate after a stroke.
- An occupational therapist may also be needed on a long-term basis if the patient requires adaptive assistance using the upper body.

WHAT IS CUSTODIAL OR PERSONAL CARE?

Custodial care includes assistance with activities of daily living (ADLs) such as:

- Bathing,
- Dressing,
- Eating,
- Grooming,
- Getting in and out of bed,
- Walking around and
- Toileting (incontinence care).

OTHER TYPES OF FACILITIES

REHABILITATION SERVICES

After a patient has been stabilized following an acute illness or injury, a rehabilitation phase, lasting from days to years, may follow. Rehabilitation may take place in the following facilities:

- Rehabilitation centers,
- Long-term care facilities,
- Outpatient facilities,
- Group residential homes, and
- Patient's home. The focus, regardless of the setting, is the return of function and prevention of further disability. Nurses play an important role on the rehabilitation team.

 Learning Exercise

Rehabilitation Services

Where are the rehabilitation health services available in your area? What kind of rehabilitation is available? Do they hire LPN/LVNs? If so, what skills will the LPN/LVN perform with RN supervision?

LONG-TERM CARE FACILITIES

Long-term care (LTC) includes a range of medical services designed to help people who have disabilities or chronic care needs. All long-term facilities focus on promoting independence, maintaining function, and supporting autonomy.

NURSING HOMES

Nursing homes specialize in short-term or acute care, intermediate care, and long-term skilled nursing care. The basic differences in the nursing homes are the length of stay and level of care provided during the stay.

The care is paid for by:

- Private pay,
- Health insurance,
- Medicaid, or
- Medicare (Medicare will not pay when only custodial care is needed. Medicare pays when

skilled care is provided by licensed nursing personnel, under the direction of a physician, on a daily basis).

Skilled Nursing Facility (SNF)

A **skilled** nursing home offers 24-hour-a-day care for those who can no longer live independently. They can provide specialized care for those with severe illnesses; and help with activities of daily living (ADLs). The nursing home specializes in short-term or acute nursing care, intermediate and long-term skilled nursing care.

Short-Term or Acute Care. **Short-term care**, also called post-acute care (PAC), or transitional care, is for persons who have been hospitalized recently and typically have more complicated medical needs. It is provided by many long-term care facilities or hospitals. Included is rehabilitation service, specialized care for certain conditions such as stroke and diabetes, post-surgical care and other services associated in the transition between hospital and home. The goal is to discharge residents to their home or to a lower level of care.

Long-Term Skilled Nursing Facility. **Long-term care** (LTC) facilities provide a range of services for people with severe disabilities or chronic care needs. One such facility is known as a skilled nursing facility for severely disabled (SNFSD). It provides 24-hour-a-day care for persons with severe mental disabilities. Many of these facilities are locked or secure areas where residents reside for their own protection and the protection of others.

Intermediate Care Facility (ICF). An **intermittent care nursing home** provides 8 hours of care per day. The nursing home does not always have licensed nurses available. They provide medical, intermittent nursing care, dietary, pharmacy, and activity services.

ALTERNATIVES TO NURSING HOMES

These include:

- In-home care
- Retirement (assisted) care

- Residential care
- Hospice (end-of-life) care

IN-HOME CARE
Independent Living Apartments

Independent living apartments are not licensed or regulated. People living in these facilities are not there for personal or medical care, but like to live with seniors who share like interests. There generally are planned activities and trips and bus service for shopping.

Board and Care Homes

Board and care homes are also known as adult care homes, group homes, or family-type homes. The facilities offer temporary or long-term residential care, housekeeping, and custodial care (personal care services) for a small number of adults unrelated to the operator. Assistance with activities of daily living (ADLs), self-administration of medication, preparation of meals, special diets, and transportation are usually supervised and provided by the owner or manager. The residence may be a single-family home. The residence is licensed as an adult family home or adult group home. The department of social services oversees the operation.

Enriched Housing

Enriched housing is similar to adult homes, except seniors live in individual housing units. A minimum of one meal per day is usually provided. They are licensed by the State Department of Health.

RETIREMENT (ASSISTED) CARE
Assisted Living Programs

Assisted living programs (ALPs) provide "a home with services" (assisted care), which emphasizes a resident's privacy and choice. Living quarters are used by older adults who want to remain as independent as possible but cannot manage all of their ADLs. Residents typically have private, locking rooms and bathrooms (or apartments), shared only by choice. Living quarters are handicap accessible and are planned to accommodate the changing needs of residents as they age. Help with daily routine is available, but not 24-hour care. These services include bathing, dressing, daily activities, and health maintenance. Care management and skilled nursing services when needed, come from an outside agency. APLs accept private pay, Medicaid, and Social Security Supplemental Income (SSI) recipients. The facilities are family oriented, provide activities, and assist the resident with travel to outside appointments. The fee for one- or two-bedroom apartments includes utilities, weekly housecleaning, linen changes, and so on. An additional fee is charged for meals. The assisted-living facilities are often connected to a skilled nursing facility, and the resident can be moved into the skilled nursing facility if that level of care becomes necessary.

Continuous Care Retirement Community

A continuous care retirement community (CCRC) provides a continuum of living options from independent living, enriched living, assisted living, and skilled nursing home all on one campus. Residents can move from one level of care to another, as needs change.

 Learning Exercise

Long-Term Care Facilities

What long-term care facilities are located in your area? What level of care do they offer? Do they hire LPN/LVNs? If so, what skills will the LPN/LVN be expected to perform?

RESIDENTIAL CARE
Community Health Nursing Services

Nurses have always been at the forefront of community health nursing activity. The major focus of community health nursing is to (1) improve the health status of communities or groups of people through public education, (2) screen for early detection of disease, and (3) provide services for people who need care outside the acute care setting.

Community health nurses work with many different people and groups on prevention and modification of health issues. Among the many possible roles are advocate, caregiver, case finder, health planner, occupational health nurse, school nurse, teacher, and so on (Linton et al., 2000). Community health nursing services may exist as a part of an outpatient clinic service, a service attached to an HMO, or a freestanding private service.

Home Health Agencies

Home health agencies are public or private agencies that provide home health services, supervised by a licensed health professional in the patient's home, either directly or through arrangements with other agencies. Some examples of home health agencies include the following:

- Public, nonprofit (e.g., visiting nurse association),
- Public, nonprofit, freestanding (e.g., city, county (including county visiting nurse association), and state health departments),
- Private or nonprofit hospital-based (e.g., hospital home health agency), and
- Private, for-profit, freestanding (e.g., home health care owned by person or corporation).

Home health nursing differs from hospital and nursing home care by increased focus on family and the patient's environment. The purpose is to promote, maintain, or restore health or minimize the effects of illness or disability. An important role is to teach the patient and family self-care. Skilled services in home health care include the following:

- Skilled nursing,
- Physical therapy,
- Speech-language therapy,
- Occupational therapy,
- Medical-social services,
- Homemaker–health aide services, and
- Other therapy services may be offered.

Skilled nursing services are provided and directed by RNs. Basic nursing services are provided by LPN/LVNs under the supervision of an RN. *Depending on state regulations and agency policy,* LPN/LVNs are able to provide many home health services. Examples include, but are not limited to, the following:

- Teaching, supervising, or setting up medications,
- Injections,
- Ostomy care,
- Wound care and dressings,
- Finger sticks for blood glucose testing, and
- Catheter care.

Learning Exercise

Community Health Services

Are there community health nursing services or home care agencies available where you live? What services do they offer? Which of them employ LPN/LVNs? What skills are the LPN/LVN expected to perform under RN supervision?

Adult Day Care Centers

Hospital-based and freestanding adult day care centers provide services for individuals who need supervision because of physical or safety needs yet are not candidates for nursing home placement. Patients with families who are able to assist the person during evening hours and on weekends may prefer adult day care centers instead of nursing home placement.

The purpose of adult day care is to provide mental stimulation, socialization, assistance with some ADLs, and basic observation skills. Some typical services include transportation, meals, therapeutic activities, nursing interventions, and rehabilitation activities. The supervisor is often a social worker or RN. Certified nursing assistants (CNAs) and personal care assistants who meet state requirements assist with ADLs. Volunteers play a major role in some of the adult day care centers.

Adult Day Care Services

Is adult day care available in your area? Where are the centers located, what services are offered, and who staffs them? Do they employ LPN/LVNs? If so, what are the LPN/LVN's responsibilities?

Wellness Centers

An emphasis on promoting wellness continues to result in a multitude of services being offered in this area of health care. Not only have hospitals developed programs to detect disease in early stages, but they also have developed programs to promote wellness. Wellness center programs include nutritional counseling, exercise programs, stress reduction, and weight control. The private sector continues to be active in the wellness area. People have developed an interest in exercise and fitness clubs, weight-reduction programs such as Weight Watchers, smoking cessation classes, stress control, and parenting classes.

Learning Exercise

Wellness Programs

Choose one wellness program in your area. Find out what services it offers and the qualification of the staff that provides the information. Which programs employ LPN/LVNs?

HOSPICE (END-OF-LIFE) CARE

End-of-life services are available in many areas to persons who have been certified as terminally ill. The philosophy of hospice care is to maintain comfort as death approaches. The hospice may be in an institutional setting, such as the hospital or a freestanding agency. Hospice care is offered within the institution, especially if pain and symptom management is necessary, the family caring for the person needs respite, or for terminal care. Hospice home care is also available to those who wish to die in their own home. Because RNs, LPN/LVNs, home health aides, CNAs, and volunteers all staff a hospice, home care can be tailored to the person's needs.

Develop Your Own Style

Using clustering (concept mapping) shown in Chapter 4 as your guide, develop your own style/form to summarize the health care settings described in this chapter.

Critical Thinking Exercise

Has My Vision Changed?

Throughout your course of study, you will find that your interest in a particular area of nursing may change or be modified. Based on what you have learned from reading this chapter, what kind of health care setting is most appealing to you at this time?

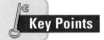

Key Points

- Health care services are delivered in public and private sectors.
- Public health care agencies are classified as official and voluntary.
- Official public health care agencies are supported by taxes.
- Official public health agencies are local, state, and federal agencies.
- FDA, CDC, NIH, HSA, HRA, and Alcohol, Drug Abuse and Mental Health Administration make up the USPHS.
- The public health care agency of the United Nations is WHO.
- Voluntary health care agencies are supported by contributions and provide complementary services to official health care agencies.
- Private health care agencies are generally proprietary (for profit).
- VNA provides home nursing care for persons with acute and chronic conditions.
- Primary care describes the point at which people usually enter the health care system.
- General hospitals deal with a full range of medical and surgical conditions.
- Specialized hospitals are limited to patients with specific diseases.

- Teaching and research hospitals offer treatment for serious or unusual conditions and usually are a training site for health professionals.
- Ambulatory health care services are available in both private and public sectors.
- Free clinics provide primary care for persons who cannot afford traditional health care services.
- Short-term care, also known as post-acute care, or transitional care provides rehabilitation services and specialized care as a transition between hospital and home.
- Long-term care facilities provide a range of services for people with severe disabilities and chronic care needs.
- Board and care homes, also known as adult-care homes, group homes, or family type homes offer housing and custodial care.
- ICF provides 8 hours of health-related care and services per day to residents who do not need acute or skilled nursing care.

- SNF provides 24-hour nursing care, specialized services, rehabilitation services, and other medical services.
- Assisted care residences are a "home with services."
- Continuous care retirement communities provide a continuum of living options as needs change.
- Community health, public health, and home health share many responsibilities. A major difference in home health is providing direct patient care.
- Adult day care centers provide socialization, mental stimulation, and assistance with ADLs, basic observation, and health referrals.
- Wellness centers provide nutritional counseling, exercise programs, stress reduction, weight control, etc.
- Hospice staff maintains comfort of the person as death approaches.
- Responsibilities of care agencies continue to be modified because of changes in the health care system.

REVIEW ITEMS

1. Which of the following is an official health agency funded by the UN?
   1. WHO
   2. CDC
   3. NIH
   4. FDA

2. How do official and voluntary agencies differ?
   1. Official agencies are proprietary.
   2. Voluntary agencies are tax supported.
   3. Official agencies provide primary care.
   4. Voluntary agencies emphasize research.

3. How will you explain the different levels of long-term health care to someone planning to seek placement for an elderly relative?
   1. Board and care homes provide "a home with services" added on, as needed.
   2. Intermediate care is suitable for persons who do not need acute or skilled care.
   3. Residential care provides 24-hour transitional care after hospitalization.
   4. Assisted care facilities offer 24-hour supervision and housing for 3 to 16 residents.

4. What quality would not be helpful when working with hospice?
   1. Knowledge of the physiological process occurring as death approaches.
   2. Ability to sit without the need for dialogue, if desired by the individual.
   3. Belief in the need to tell the individual your belief about life after death.
   4. Willingness to honor person's request for food, conversation, visitors, etc.

ALTERNATE FORMAT ITEM

What is the difference between community health nursing services and home health agencies? *(Select all that apply.)*

1. Home health agencies provide direct nursing service to people in their home.

2. Community health nursing services work on prevention and case finding.

3. VNA and County Health Department are examples of home health agencies.

4. Home health agencies have an increased focus on family and patient's environment.

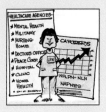

evolve http://evolve.elsevier.com/Hill/success/

Objectives

On completing this chapter, you will be able to do the following:

1. Describe two general methods of financing health care costs, as follows:
   a. Fee-for-service, and
   b. Capitation.
2. Explain the following methods of payment options for patients of health care:
   a. Personal payment (private pay),
   b. Nongovernment (private) health insurance, and
   c. Government-sponsored (public) health insurance.
3. Identify sources of funding for government health programs and private health insurance.
4. Discuss the following issues and trends that affect financing of health care:
   a. Cost of health care,
   b. Need for cost containment:
      1) Deficit spending
   c. Cost of health insurance,
   d. Cost of prescription drugs,
   e. Uninsured persons,
   f. Uncompensated care, and
   g. Government health insurance.
5. Give examples of comprehensive and incremental changes in health care.
6. Discuss the effect of the restructuring of the health care system on health care and employment opportunities for licensed practical/vocational nurses (LPN/LVNs).
7. Explain how the practical/vocational nurse participates in quality improvement.

8. Identify your reaction to change involving your nursing career and personal life.
9. Develop a personal plan to help you adapt to change in your nursing career and personal life.

Key Terms

Alliances (ă-LĪ-ăns-ĕs, p. 333)
Capitation (kăp-ĭ-TĀ-sŭn, p. 318)
Children's Health Insurance Program (CHIP/SCHIP [ess-chip]) (p. 324)
Coinsurance (p. 319)
Comprehensive method (p. 331)
Continuous quality improvement (CQI) (p. 336)
Copayment (p. 319)
Cost containment (p. 325)
Deductibles (dĭ-DŬK-tĭ-bŭlz, p. 319)
Deficit (DĔF-ĭ-s-ĭt, p. 322)
Diagnosis-related group (DRG) (p. 322)
Electronic Medical Record (p. 336)
Entitlement program (p. 320)
Fee-for-service (p. 318)
Gross domestic product (GDP) (p. 318)
Health care provider (p. 319)
Health maintenance organization (HMO) (p. 320)
Health Savings Accounts (HSAs) (p. 332)
Incremental method (p. 331)
Inflation (p. 318)
Managed care (p. 333)
Marketplace (p. 333)
Medicaid (p. 323)
Medicare (p. 320)
Out-of-pocket (p. 319)
Paradigm shift (păr-ă-DĪM, p. 333)
Patient-focused care (p. 335)

Preferred provider organizations (PPOs) (p. 334)
Premium (p. 319)
Private pay (p. 319)
Prospective payment system (PPS) (p. 322)
Restructuring (rē-STRŬK-chŭr-ĭng, p. 333)
"Seamless" systems (p. 333)
Service, quality, and cost control (p. 333)
Single-payer system (p. 332)
Third-party coverage (p. 319)
Total quality management (TQM) (p. 336)
Uncompensated care (p. 329)
Universal coverage (p. 331)
Unlicensed assistive personnel (UAP) (p. 335)

 Keep in Mind

Do you pay federal or state taxes? Then you help pay for health care for people without health insurance. Do you have health insurance? If not, who helps pay for your health care?

HEALTH CARE SYSTEM RANKINGS

THE UNITED STATES #1 AND #37!

The U.S. health care system has been described as "the envy of the world." Every year, patients from other countries seek medical care in the United States. This reflects the 2000 analysis of the world's health systems by a World Health Organization (WHO) survey that ranked the United States number 1 in regards to honoring the dignity of individuals, choice of **provider**, timely care, and confidentiality. Patients from other countries also value the expertise and availability of U.S. specialists, cutting-edge technology, and drugs that are researched and developed in the United States (World Health Organization Assesses the World's Health Systems, 2007).

The American health care system is a paradox. The U.S. health care system has also been described as a poorly designed, fragmented, and disjointed maze of services that lacks preventive care; wastes resources; is low quality, unsafe, and confusing. Because of these descriptors, the term *health care crisis* is used to refer to the current

state of health care affairs. Comments about the system may seem contradictory. The World Health Organization also ranks the United States number 37 in overall performance when relating outcomes to expenditures in health care. The United States has the highest health care spending (**deductibles, copayments, coinsurance,** and **premiums** for private health insurance) of industrialized countries. Yet, for all the spending on health care, the United States has lower life expectancy and higher infant and maternal mortality than most of the industrialized countries of the world (Kristof, 2007).

THE UNITED STATES #54!?!

The WHO places the United States number 54 out of 191 countries in fairness in financing health care. The United States spends $7026 per capita (per person) on health care. However, almost half of health care spending was used to treat just 5% of the population (Fast Facts, 2008). Many nations of the European Union scored better than the United States in the WHO's ratings because health care in these European countries is based on the premise that every resident is guaranteed the same quality of health care. Forty-seven million persons in the U.S. do not have health insurance (e-Alert/The Commonwealth Fund, 2007). Many people are unable to afford individual health insurance premiums, including premiums under a Consolidated Omnibus Reconciliation Act (COBRA) benefit (see p. 328). Some patients cannot afford prescribed drugs. Some cannot find a physician who will take a patient with a Medicare and/or a Medicaid card. Some employers have dropped health insurance benefits as part of their benefit packages to employees. Some individuals covered by a health insurance plan find themselves unable to afford deductibles, copayments, coinsurance, and/or complain of a decreasing quality in health care. Almost half of the one million personal bankruptcies in the United States are due in part to medical costs and crises (Hacker, 2007).

Canadian citizens have federally funded National Health Insurance (Canadian Medicare), whereas the individual provinces have responsibility for managing health care and partial responsibility for funding. This coverage is **portable** (not lost when a person moves), **universal** (all residents of Canada are insured), **accessible** (reasonably available), and **free from extra charges for core services** (physician and hospital care). Many Canadians have supplemental private health insurance to cover expenses not covered by Canadian Medicare. In 2005, Canada spent $142 billion on health care to provide core services to all citizens (Public vs. Private Health Care, 2006). Because of rising health care costs, increased waiting times for elective procedures, including surgery, and increased waiting times for diagnostic tests (especially tests involving radiology), the majority of Canadian physicians believe that reform is needed (Steinbrook, 2006). In looking for alternatives, leaders are rejecting the American market-driven system and its connection to powerful insurance companies and 47 million uninsured. Leaders are looking at the European system of mixed public and private health insurance. It is clear that even when people have access to health care through some type of health insurance plan, problems of quality, service, and cost arise. The basic information about health care settings (see Chapter 17) and the contents of this chapter will help you develop a better understanding of the health care system that will employ you.

Gross domestic product (GDP) is the combination of all goods and services produced in a nation's economy. The United States spends more of its GDP—approximately 16%—on health care than any other country in the world (Fast Facts, 2008). Canada, which insures all its citizens, spends approximately 10% of its GDP on health care. In 2004, health care spending in the United States was about 90% higher than in any other industrialized country (Fast Facts, 2008). Health care spending in the United States grows faster than inflation and personal income. (Inflation is a general rise in prices, usually persisting over several years and "allows you to live in a higher priced neighborhood without having to move" [Slavin, 1999]).

FINANCING OF HEALTH CARE COSTS

There are two major ways to finance health care services: fee-for-service and capitation.

FEE-FOR-SERVICE

The traditional method of paying health care bills is the system called fee-for-service. In this method, physicians are paid a fee by the patient for each service they provide. Under the fee-for-service system, if an attending physician has an agreement with the health insurance company of the patient, they are directly reimbursed for most ordered diagnostic tests and treatments for illness. If a physician does not have an agrcement with the health care insurer, the patient is reimbursed by the insurance company and then pays the physician. Some physicians now require patients to pay up front, and then the patient submits a claim to the insurance company and gets reimbursed. Under the fee-for-service system, some insurance companies do not reimburse the tests and treatments that could keep patients healthy or could identify illnesses in their early stages, when they are less expensive to treat. Over the years, insurance premiums soared under this type of fee system. To improve their margins of profit, insurance companies charge deductibles, copayments, and coinsurance.

CAPITATION

Capitation is an alternative to the traditional fee-for-service method of payment. Capitation involves a set monthly fee charged by the provider of health care services for each member of the insurance group for a specific set of services. If health care services cost more than the monthly fee, the provider absorbs the cost of those services. At the end of the year, if any money is left over, the **health care provider** keeps it as a profit. Suddenly, if a provider of health care services can keep a member of the insurance group healthy, that provider will make a profit! Study Table 18-1 for a comparison of the fee-for-service and capitation methods of payment for health care services.

Table 18-1 | *Comparison of Methods of Payment for Health Care Services*

	FEE-FOR-SERVICE	CAPITATION
Services covered	Each health care service claimed by the physician (e.g., diagnostic tests, treatments)	Health care services in group contract
Are preventive tests or treatments covered?	Depends on the plan	Wellness practices covered
Cost	Set fee per member of group	Set fee per member of group
How revenue is increased	Increase health care services Increase patient visits	Decrease health care services Increase number of persons served
Advantages	All tests and treatments for illness covered	Wellness encouraged No deductibles and copayments
Disadvantages	Emphasis on illness Deductibles and copayments keep patient from reporting illness in early stages	To realize a profit, needed tests may not be ordered

BASIC HEALTH INSURANCE TERMS

Before continuing, review the following health insurance terms to better understand the content that follows.

Premium: The monthly fee a person must pay for health-care insurance coverage.

Deductible: The yearly amount an insured person must spend out-of-pocket for health care services before a health insurance policy will begin to pay its share.

Copayment: The amount an insured person must pay at the time of an office visit, when picking up a prescription, or before a hospital service.

Coinsurance: Once a deductible is met, the percentage of the total bill paid by the insured person. The remainder is paid by the insurance company.

Health care provider: A licensed health care person, such as a physician, dentist, or nurse practitioner, whose health care services are covered by a health insurance plan.

HOW YOUR PATIENTS PAY FOR HEALTH CARE SERVICES

PERSONAL PAYMENT (PRIVATE PAY)

Payment directly by the patient (i.e., private pay) was the primary method of payment of health care costs before the 1940s. Although some patients may use this method of payment today, the cost of health care services discourages this method to be used by most of the millions of people in the United States who do not have health care insurance. Private pay patients may be able to negotiate a discount with some health care agencies.

HEALTH INSURANCE (PRIVATE INSURANCE)

Health insurance, like any insurance, spreads risk. The risk that is spread in health insurance is that the young and the healthy generally subsidize (support financially) the sick and older persons in the health insurance group. Those who are likely to have high medical bills are denied coverage. Administrative costs of private health insurance can run to 31% of premiums. These costs involve risk assessment of applicants, reviewing claims for reimbursement, profits to investors, and marketing.

Private Group Health Insurance

Group health insurance is a method of pooling individual contributions for a common group goal- protection from financial disaster as a result of health care bills. When insured, an individual is said to have third-party coverage (a fiscal middleman). This financial middleman pays the individual's health care bills. Employers offer most of the private group insurance in the United States.

No member of the group is denied coverage based on past medical history. In 2007, the average premium for family coverage was $12,106 per year, with employees contributing $3,281 per year (Kaiser Family Foundation: *2007 Benchmark Study Finds Health Insurance Premiums Continue to Rise Faster Than Wages*, 2007). Examples of private group health insurance include the following:

- Blue Cross and Blue Shield: Blue Cross covers hospital inpatient costs and Blue Shield covers inpatient physician costs. A major medical plan is available to include the cost of outpatient services.
- Health policies offered through commercial insurance companies. Many major insurance companies offer health insurance to individuals and groups.
- A health plan issued through a health maintenance organization (HMO). Regardless of how many services the HMO provides, it is paid an annual fee to maintain the health of each of its members (capitation). The healthier the patients are kept, the fewer treatments the HMO needs to deliver and the larger the profit margin for the HMO. For a fee, patients seek medical care at the first sign of symptoms. This is the time when health care is least expensive to deliver. See the section on managed care, later in this chapter.

Private Nongroup Health Insurance

Many major insurance companies offer health insurance to individuals who are not part of a group. Premiums are based on a person's health risk (if not denied coverage) and age. The cost for individuals is generally higher than for group plans.

GOVERNMENT-SPONSORED HEALTH INSURANCE (PUBLIC INSURANCE)
Medicare: A Program of Social Security

People of retirement age generally find themselves ineligible for group insurance plans because they are not employed. This inability to get insurance occurs at the very time when individuals are more likely to encounter medical costs because of chronic disease. If accepted in a private plan, many are unable to afford the plan. In 1965, Medicare was added to the Social Security Act. This federally sponsored entitlement program and public health insurance plan helps finance health care for all persons older than age 65 (and their spouses), who have at least a 10-year record in Medicare-covered employment and are a citizen or permanent resident of the United States. Coverage is also given to persons younger than age 65 who are permanently and totally disabled, persons with end-stage renal disease, and persons with Lou Gehrig's disease. No person is denied coverage based on past medical history. Forty-four million elderly and disabled persons in the USA are on Medicare (*Medicare: A Primer*, 2007). Administrative costs to run the Medicare program are approximately two percent. Money is saved by not having to work at screening out high risk patients. A current Medicare handbook can be accessed by typing National Medicare Handbook into *Google*.

Basic Components of Medicare (Original/Traditional Medicare).

Part A (Hospital Insurance). Medicare Part A helps pay for inpatient hospital care (Box 18-1). Part A is available without cost and is funded by a payroll tax. Money collected is put into a trust fund. In 2008, Part A had a deductible of $1,024 per benefit period and a coinsurance fee starting on the 61st day of hospitalization.

Part B (Medical Insurance). Medicare Part B is similar to a major medical insurance plan (Box 18-2). Part B is funded by monthly premiums. Premiums are income related. The 2008 monthly premium for Part B for incomes up to $82,000 (single) or $164,000 (couple) was $96.40. For annual incomes above these amounts, there are higher monthly premiums based on a sliding scale. The premium is deducted from the monthly Social Security, Railroad Retirement, or Civil Service Retirement payment. Part B required a $135 deductible in 2008. Part B pays 80% of most covered charges. The remaining 20% of charges are the patient's responsibility. Source: Medicare and You 2008 (CMS Publication Number 10050), Baltimore, MD: U.S. Department of Health and Human Services, Sept., 2007.

Box 18-1 | *Medicare Part A*

In 2008, Medicare Part A helped pay for the following types of situations:
- Inpatient hospital care (e.g., a semiprivate room, meals, drugs, supplies, lab tests, radiology, and intensive care units) and care in certified Christian Science sanatoriums,
- Twenty days' posthospitalization skilled nursing facility care (full cost) for rehabilitation services. The next 80 days are paid after a daily deductible of $124,
- Under certain conditions, home health care services with coinsurance charges for medical equipment, and
- Hospice care for terminally ill beneficiaries.

Part A does **not** pay for long-term care custodial services (e.g., patients only needing help with activities of daily living [including feeding]), private rooms, telephones, or televisions provided by hospitals, skilled nursing facilities, or Christian Science practitioners.

Source: Medicare and You 2008 (CMS Publication Number 10050), Baltimore, MD: U.S. Department of Health and Human Services, Sept., 2007.

Medicare Health Care Plans

The Original Medicare Plan (Traditional Plan/Parts A and B). This fee-for-service plan allows the beneficiary to go to health care providers or hospitals that accept Medicare patients. The health care provider gets paid for each Medicare-covered service provided. Medicare pays its share and patients pay their share.

Part C (Medicare Advantage Plan). Medicare Advantage Plans are government approved health plan options that are offered by private insurance companies. These plans are alternatives to original (traditional) Medicare plans. Coverage includes parts A and B and in some plans, Part D of the traditional plan. Generally, lower copayments and additional benefits (vision care, hearing aids) are offered in these plans but there may be a limit on where care can be obtained, which physician can be seen, and how often the beneficiary can see the physician. Benefits can change year-to-year. Different types of Advantage plans are described in Box 18-3.

Part D. Medicare drug legislation, passed in 2003, provided prescription drug coverage that helps to pay for brand-name drugs at participating

Box 18-2 | *Medicare Part B*

In 2008, Part B helped to pay for medically necessary (needed for diagnosis and treatment of a medical condition) services, which included the following:
- Physician visits and other medical services
- Outpatient hospital services (including emergency room visits) and outpatient mental health
- Clinical laboratory services and diagnostic tests (x-rays, MRIs, CT scans, EKGs),
- Ambulance transportation
- Durable medical equipment (wheel chairs, walkers, oxygen, hospital beds),
- Kidney supplies and services
- Some diabetic supplies,
- Physical, occupational, and speech therapy in a hospital outpatient department or a patient who resides in a Medicare-certified bed in a rehabilitation agency
- Limited chiropractic services,

- Preventive services: "Welcome to Medicare" physical exam in the first six months after enrolling in Plan B, cholesterol, lipid, and triglyceride blood levels once every 5 years, mammography every 12 months, Pap test and pelvic exam every two years, fecal occult blood test every year, screening colonoscopy every ten years, PSA test and rectal digital exam every year, flu shot once a year, pneumococcal vaccine once a lifetime, and bone mass measurements every 24 months, if at risk for osteoporosis, diabetic screening,
- Part B does **not** pay for most prescription drugs, routine physicals, services not related to treatment of illness or injury, dental care, dentures, cosmetic surgery, routine foot care, hearing aids, routine eye examinations, or routine glasses.

Source: Medicare and You 2008 (CMS Publication Number 10050), Baltimore, MD: U.S. Department of Health and Human Services, Sept., 2007.

| Box 18-3 | *Medicare Advantage Insurance Plans*

Shopping for Advantage Health Plans involves comparison of plans to find the right plan, at the right price, to meet personal needs. An online visit to *www.medicare.gov* can connect persons to sites that present health plan options in a specific area of any state.

- **Medicare HMO:** The Medicare patient can only go to doctors, specialists, and hospitals in this plan's network. A Point of Service (POS) option offered by **some Medicare HMO** plans allows the patient to go to doctors and hospitals outside the network for an additional fee.
- **Medicare PPO:** This plan has a network like HMOs but allows patients to go outside the network for an additional fee.
- **Medicare private fee-for-service plans (PFFS):** Any physician or hospital that accepts the plans payment can be chosen. The insurance company pays its share of doctor and hospital bills and the patient pays his or her share. The private insurance company, not Medicare as in the Original plan, decides how much the patient will pay.

Source: Medicare and You 2008 (CMS Publication Number 10050), Baltimore, MD: U.S. Department of Health and Human Services, Sept., 2007.

| Box 18-4 | *The Medicare Prescription Drug, Improvement, and Modernization Act of 2003 (MMA): Prescription Drug Benefit*

Participation is voluntary in the traditional Medicare plan and premiums depend on the private plan chosen. A Medicare Drug Benefit Calculator can be found online at *http://www.kaisernetwork.org/drugcalculator*. This calculator allows Medicare beneficiaries to enter their annual prescription drug costs and predict how Medicare Part D might benefit them.

Coverage for 2008
- Most plans have a coverage gap (the doughnut hole"). After the patient's s drug plan and the patient spend a specific amount for drugs, the patient must pay for drugs while in the gap till a specified limit is reached.
- For the remainder of the year, catastrophic coverage "kicks in", requiring only a copayment or coinsurance amount is required of the patient for prescribed drugs.

Source: Medicare and You 2008 (CMS Publication Number 10050), Baltimore, MD: U.S. Department of Health and Human Services, Sept., 2007.

---

pharmacies. See Box 18-4 for Medicare reform prescription drug benefits.

Because of the items Medicare does not cover, beneficiaries are encouraged to purchase private supplemental insurance in addition to Medicare, to cover copayments, deductibles, coinsurance, and limited-coverage situations that exist in the federal program. These policies are sold by private insurance companies. Enrollment in a Medicare prescription drug plan is also encouraged, if not included in the selected health care plan.

Diagnosis-Related Groups (DRGs) (Illness Categories). Payment for Medicare is a major item in the federal budget. In 2006, Medicare spending totaled $374 billion. Before 1983, hospitals submitted a bill to the government for the total charges they incurred for Medicare patients and were reimbursed for this amount. This was called a "retrospective payment" system because payment was based on actual costs.

Because the federal deficit (less money/revenue coming in than was needed to run all government programs) was consistently growing larger, the federal government was the first group to try to stop the skyrocketing cost of health care. On October 1, 1983, the Health Care Financing Administration (now the Centers for Medicare and Medicaid Services [CMS]) adopted a system of paying hospitals a set fee or flat rate for Medicare services, by telling hospitals in advance how much they would be reimbursed. Because the federal government announces to a hospital in advance what it will pay for health care costs, this system is called the prospective payment system (PPS).

Under the diagnosis-related group (DRG) system, a math formula is used to arrive at the fee the government will pay for hospitalization. This fee depends on the DRG category (illness) causing the patient's hospitalization. Hospitals receive a flat fee for each patient's DRG category regardless of length of stay in the hospital. Hospitals have an incentive to treat patients and discharge them as quickly as possible. If the hospital keeps the patient longer than the government's fee will cover and the patient cannot be reclassified in the DRG system, the hospital has to make up the difference in costs. If the acute care facility can treat the Medicare patient for less than the guaranteed reimbursement, the facility can keep the difference as profit.

Because Medicare patients, like all patients, are discharged sooner from hospitals than they were in the past (as a result of the PPS), extended care units are often used to continue convalescence. See Box 18-5 for an example of the amount out-of-pocket (i.e., amount paid by the patient) a Medicare patient pays for a hospital experience.

Medicaid (Medical Assistance)

The Medicaid program (Title XIX) was added to the Social Security Act in 1965. This program provides medical assistance for eligible families and individuals with low incomes and resources. Medicaid is a cooperative venture jointly funded by the federal and state governments. See Table 18-2 for a comparison of Medicare and Medicaid.

The federal government establishes broad, national guidelines for Medicaid. Each state establishes its own program services and requirements, including eligibility. For this reason, when eligible for Medicaid in one state, an individual is not automatically eligible in another state. Some states have additional medical assistance programs for indigent persons who do not qualify for Medicaid. These assistance programs do not receive federal funds.

Acts of Congress that have reformed the Medicaid system include the following:
- The Personal Responsibility and Work Opportunity Reconciliation Act (1996) reformed the nation's welfare laws. This act created a mechanism for temporary assistance for families in need. One of the primary goals

---

Box 18-5 | *What the Patient Pays When on Traditional Medicare Health Plan*

In December 2008, Miles, age 82 and a Medicare patient, required 3 days of hospitalization as a surgical patient because of a hip fracture. After discharge, he spent 20 days in an extended care unit for further physical and occupational therapy. The bills for this experience follow, with a breakdown of what Medicare pays and what Miles pays.

MEDICARE PART A
- Total hospital cost covered by Medicare Part A = $6000
- Deductible (paid by Miles) = $1024
- Medicare Part A payment = $4976

MEDICARE PART B
- Total for medically necessary services covered by Medicare Part B = $4000
- Deductible (paid by Miles) = $135
- Medicare Part B payment of 80% of $3865 = $3092
- Miles' 20% payment of $3865 = $773

EXTENDED CARE UNIT
- The fee for 20 days in extended care was paid by Medicare.

MILES' TOTAL CHARGES FOR THIS ILLNESS EXPERIENCE
- Hospital: Parts A and B = $1932
- Extended Care = $0
- Total = $1932

If Miles had supplemental health insurance, this insurance would pay Miles charges minus any deductibles and coinsurance required by his supplemental policy. If Miles did not have a supplemental policy, the $1932 would come out of his pocket.

---

of federal welfare policies is to move people from welfare to work. This goal becomes difficult when the unemployment rate increases and jobs are not available.
- The Balanced Budget Act of 1997 authorized welfare-to-work grants to states to create additional job opportunities for the hardest-to-employ of the recipients of the 1996 act. The goal was for successful progression of recipients into long-term unsubsidized employment. Once employed,

Table 18-2 | *Comparison of Medicare and Medicaid*

	MEDICARE	MEDICAID
Purpose of program	Health care for persons 65 years and older who are eligible for Social Security, the disabled, and persons with end-stage renal disease and Lou Gehrig's disease	Medical and health-related services for persons with decreased income and resources that meet eligibility requirements
Source of funding	Federal government (i.e., your tax money) An entitlement health care program. Congress must fund Medicare each year, as opposed to a discretionary program, in which funding must be approved yearly.	An entitlement program jointly financed by the federal and state governments (your tax money) Medicaid is a major expenditure in federal and state budgets
Who administers the program?	The federal government	Individual states. There is wide state variation in levels of eligibility and services provided.
Cost to individual to enroll	Part A: Hospital insurance for inpatient care. No cost for persons who meet eligibility requirements for Social Security. Part B: Medical insurance covering doctors' fees, etc. A premium or monthly fee is taken out of the monthly Social Security check when person registers for program.	No fee Must meet income eligibility requirements

Source: *Medicare: A Primer: 2007* and *Medicaid: A Primer: 2007.*

employees are eligible for employer health insurance benefits, if the employer offers these benefits.

- In 1997, Congress passed the Children's Health Insurance Program (CHIP) and authorized it for 10 years. This program is also referred to as SCHIP. This act provides health insurance for children in families who earn too much to qualify for Medicaid but cannot afford health insurance. All states participate in the program and are provided grants by the federal government to provide this coverage by expanding Medicaid or by expanding or creating a children's health program. SCHIP is credited with "catching" many uninsured children and providing health care coverage during economic downturns. In 2006, 6.6 million children were covered by SCHIP but over a million remain uninsured (Washington Health Policy Week in Review, 8/20/07). Although the program expired at the end

of September 2007, on December 31, 2007, CHIP received a temporary extension to March 31, 2009, without an expansion of the program to cover about 3 million additional children in low and moderate income families (Reuters, 2007).

ISSUES AND TRENDS IN HEALTH CARE FINANCING

Nursing organizations encourage nurses at all levels (LPN/LVNs and RNs from 2-, 3-, and 4-year programs) to be politically active. Political activism involves understanding and being involved in political and economic activities that can affect nursing and health of patients. Practical/vocational nurses can help shape health policy by educating their patients and state and federal legislators about issues in health care. To meet this expectation, practical/vocational nurses need to educate *themselves* about the cost of health care, how health care is funded, and the many issues and trends affecting health care today. Information about Congressional bills can be obtained at *http://thomas.loc.gov*. Basic information on how to identify and contact your elected representatives in Washington and your state can be obtained at *http://www.usa.gov/Contact/Elected.shtml* and at *www.nflpn.org*.

COST OF HEALTH CARE

Each year, the U.S. spends $2.2 trillion on health care. Some reasons for the high cost of health care are the costs of prescription drugs, medical malpractice lawsuits, and development of and increased use of medical technology.

See Box 18-6 to get a picture of what a trillion dollars looks like.

Need for Cost Containment

The driving force today in all public and private health care agencies is cost containment (the need to hold costs to within fixed limits) while remaining competitive in the health care marketplace. Pressure continues to be felt from the federal government, the insurance industry, employers, and consumers to reduce the cost of health care while maintaining high-quality care and service. Practical/vocational nurses need to remember that health care agencies are interested in improving their agency's "bottom line," by reducing waste and inefficiency. Practical/vocational nurses who identify wasteful practices and inefficient routines in their work settings while maintaining quality may in fact be saving their own jobs. See Box 18-7 for the role you play, as an LPN/LVN, in containing health care costs in your work setting.

Source of Revenue (Income) for Government Health Care

The federal government has two basic ways to raise revenue for running the government, including health care programs: (1) income tax, and (2) payroll tax. States raise revenue to run state governments, including health care programs, by state taxes and monies received from the federal government (Box 18-8).

Revenue to run federal programs is decreased by tax cuts and unemployment (if you do not have a paycheck, you cannot pay payroll or income taxes). This decrease in revenue can be offset by increasing taxes (increasing revenue) or by decreasing services (decreasing costs). Both of these options are unpopular with voters. Decreasing services may not be feasible or safe (e.g., decreasing funds for domestic security and the military). Be aware of the money you pay to run the federal and your state government.

Box 18-6 | *What Is a Trillion Dollars?*

- One **billion** of anything is a number with **nine** zeroes behind it (1 billion = 1,000,000,000).
- A **trillion** is a number with **12** zeroes behind it (1 trillion = 1,000,000,000,000).
- If you spent $1 million an hour, 24 hours a day, 365 days a year, it would take you 171 years to spend $1.5 trillion.
- In September 2007, Congress passed a new debt ceiling for the United States of $9.8 trillion. The debt ceiling is the total, cumulative (all combined debt) debt the government does not want to exceed.
- The federal deficit in June, 2008 was slightly more than $9 trillion. See the U.S. National Debt Clock at *http://www.brillig.com/debt_clock/* for the current debt, which changes daily.

Box 18-7 | *LPN/LVN Role in Containing Health Care Costs in the Work Setting*

- Follow facility policy for charging patients for all supplies used in their care.
- Follow facility policy for documenting patient care for reimbursement.
- Organize patient care for effective and efficient use of your time.
- Be efficient and effective in delivering patient care. If some aspect of care needs to be "redone," then you had time to do it right the first time.
- Ensure reimbursement plus decrease patient length of stay by implementing nursing care to help prevent complications.
- Meet the patients' needs, not your needs.

Box 18-8 | *Payroll Deductions*

- **Federal withholding tax:** This deduction provides general revenue for the federal government to carry out its programs. Examples of federal programs include education, defense, NASA, social programs (e.g., Medicaid, Children's Health Insurance Program [CHIP], Environmental Protection Agency, National Institutes of Health [NIH], and Centers for Disease Control [CDC].
- **FICA (Federal Insurance Contributions Act):** This deduction provides revenue for the regular Social Security pension program. A total of 12.4% of earned income, up to an annual limit ($97,000 in 2007), must be paid into Social Security. Wage and salaried employees contribute half the FICA bill (6.2%), and the employer contributes the other half (6.2%)
- **FICA medical:** This deduction provides revenue to run the Medicare program. A total of 2.9% of earned income must be paid into Medicare. Wage and salaried employees pay half (1.45%), and the employer pays half (1.45%). Monies from FICA and FICA Medical are placed in a trust fund to be used only for these programs. For this reason, the trust fund is referred to as the "lock-box."
- **State withholding:** This deduction provides general state revenue for state programs such as education, Medicaid, State Children's Health Insurance Program (SCHIP), benefits for state employees, state departments (e.g., public health, transportation, highway upkeep), prisons, etc.
- **Health insurance:** Your share of the health insurance premium for the insurance plan offered by your employer.

Learning Exercise

How You Support Government Services

1. Use a recent paycheck stub of your own or ask a friend to share one of theirs with you.
2. List the areas for which pay is deducted.
3. Using Box 18-8, identify the purpose for each deduction.

When Federal Spending Exceeds Revenue

When you spend more than you earn, you are engaging in deficit spending. Your options include the following:
- Develop a budget and stick to it.
- Work more hours.
- Get a second job.
- Use a credit card, pay the minimum due each month, continue charging until you reach your credit card limit, get another credit card, and so on until you cannot afford the minimum payment each month for all your cards.

Medicare and Medicaid are health care entitlement programs of the U.S. government. Those eligible because of age, disability, or economic status are entitled, by law, to the benefits of these programs. Costs for these programs keep increasing. In addition to payroll deductions, some revenue is required from the government's general tax fund to fund Medicare. Regardless of the cost of these programs, the federal government has to budget for and pay these benefits because they are entitlements. There are two ways to cut costs in these programs: (1) by passing new laws to change eligibility, and (2) by passing new authorization bills to alter funding. Authorization bills in Congress are bills that request and assign funding annually for government programs.

Health Care and the National Economy

American Heritage calls economics "the study of production, distribution, and consumption of goods and services." The national economy plays a great deal into health care economics. In the 1990s, the stock market was booming. In 2001, the federal government had a surplus of $344 billion. The terrorist attack of September 11, 2001, a recession (a downturn in the economy), corporate scandals, wars in Afghanistan and Iraq, unemployment, tax cuts, decreased revenue, and increasing health care costs have taken their toll on federal and state budgets. Physicians protest that Medicare reimbursement does not cover actual costs. The U.S. president promises millions of dollars to help combat the AIDS crisis in Africa. Nursing asks for increased money in the federal budget to combat the nursing shortage, including that of nursing instructors. Health insurance premiums keep rising yearly. The cost of health care continues to rise. "Baby boomers" are retiring, at a time when the number of younger persons paying into the Social Security/Medicare "lock-box" is declining. Billions more are needed to rebuild Afghanistan and Iraq.

Critical Thinking Exercise

What Government Services Are Justifiable?

1. List health care services, programs, and international aid you think justifies deficit spending by the federal government.
2. List domestic programs and services you think could be cut to avoid deficit spending.

COST OF HEALTH INSURANCE

The continual rise in health care costs has resulted in annual increases in health insurance premiums for employers. As noted previously, in 2007, the average cost of family health care coverage for an employer was over $12,000 per year. As a result, employers pass along the increasing cost of health insurance to workers, decrease benefits, or stop offering benefits. When employers offer health insurance benefits, premiums for the worker continue to increase at double-digit rates. In addition to increased premiums, workers face higher deductibles and coinsurance when health care is needed. For these reasons, plus decreased coverage and benefits, some workers drop employer-sponsored health plans. See Box 18-9 for additional issues and trends in health insurance.

Cost of Prescription Drugs

The cost of commonly prescribed drugs in the United States has risen twice as much as the rate of inflation (Freudenheim, 2006). Health care plans refuse to pay for medicines thought to be nonessential. Some health plans expect physicians to prescribe less expensive drugs and petition for approval of more expensive prescriptions. After decades of soaring drug prices, employers and

---

Box 18-9 | *Additional Issues and Trends in Health Insurance*

Health benefits for union members have become a principal issue in labor negotiations nationwide.
- Some employers are ending health benefits for workers who are already retired. Some employers are not offering health care benefits to current or new employees.
- Health insurance benefits for workers and their dependents and retirees of General Motors Corp., Ford Motor Co., and Chrysler Group add approximately $1500 to the cost of a new car and puts foreign competitors at an advantage because they do not have such costs (Zimmerman and Huffstutter, 2007).
- In 2006, 13.7 million 19- to 29-year-old young adults in the U.S. did not have health insurance. Some insurance companies offer extended health insurance policies for these adult children whose parents are holders of health insurance policies (e-Alert, 2008).

The common insurance plans offered are tiered plans. These plans give price categories for hospitals, doctors, and prescription drugs. The patient pays more when tiers 2 or 3 are selected. For example:
- Tier 1 represents the least expensive service (or generic drug).
- Tier 2 represents the more expensive service (or trade name drugs)
- Tier 3 represents services out of the established network (or a drug not on the insurance companies list of approved drugs for reimbursement). These services/drugs would require the insured person to pay the most out-of-pocket.

---

health plans expect employees to pay more for their prescriptions.

HMOs and other private health plans use their buying power to negotiate fairer prices through discounts for the drugs they purchase. People without prescription drug coverage and the uninsured pay much more than insurance companies for prescription drugs. The Medicare drug legislation of 2003 bars the federal government from using its power to negotiate lower prices from drug companies for the new drug bill. However, The Veteran's Administration negotiates lower drug prices for the VA system.

Drugs are expensive in the United States because drug companies can charge full price for the drugs, which includes the cost of research and development of new drugs. Cheaper drug prices exist in Canada because of Canadian government price regulation and the currency exchange rate. Canada's Patented Medicine Review Board must by law ensure that prices of patented drugs sold in Canada are "not excessive." Drug manufacturers set their prices within Canadian government guidelines (Barry, 2003). Refer to Box 18-4 for provisions of the Medicare prescription drug benefit.

 Critical Thinking Exercise

Buying Drugs from Foreign Sources

1. Discuss the positive and negative aspects of buying drugs from foreign sources.
2. Why are drugs from foreign sources less expensive than drugs manufactured in the United States?
3. Would you feel safe taking a drug from a foreign source?

THE UNINSURED

The 47 million Americans estimated by the U.S. Census Bureau to not have health insurance represent the largest increase in uninsured people in 10 years. The Census Bureau's numbers are widely used and are meant to identify persons not insured for the prior calendar year. Some economists and health policy experts suspect that it is difficult to count the uninsured because of the following factors:

1. People are continually losing and gaining coverage.
2. People do not understand the questions asked in government surveys.
3. There is no distinction made in surveys between long- and short-term health care coverage (Pear, 2003).

Traditionally, being uninsured was chiefly a problem of the poor and unemployed. In today's economy, there are two classes of employed uninsured.

- **Low-wage employees.** This class of people is employed in low-wage jobs that are less likely to offer insurance benefits. For this reason, you cannot assume that when the employment rate increases, the number of uninsured automatically decreases.
- **The middle class.** The problem of the uninsured has spread up the income ladder and into the ranks of the middle class. Some of these workers are priced out of the health care insurance market by rapidly rising health insurance premiums, including premiums for COBRA benefits (see p. 331). Americans who are too young for Medicare are finding themselves without insurance for the first time in their lives.

 Critical Thinking Exercise

Who Deserves Health Care?

1. Should all individuals in our society have access to health care?
2. Should health care be reserved for those who have private insurance or qualify for government programs?
3. Do you think health care is a right or a privilege?

COST OF LACK OF HEALTH INSURANCE

Leaving Americans uninsured does not mean wiping out the cost of their illnesses. The cost of needed health care becomes an issue when people are denied coverage, do not have health insurance as a benefit, cannot afford insurance premiums, lose health insurance, or refuse coverage. Alternatives to pay for health care include Medicaid (if they qualify), private pay (if they can afford it), charity care (if they can find it), or face medical bankruptcy.

A downturn economy increases the number of uninsured who are hospitalized and treated in the emergency room, where the bill is paid one way or the other by the community. (See the section on uncompensated care, later in this chapter.)

Lack of access to health care prevents individuals from receiving preventive care and seeking treatment when a health problem is developing. These individuals may seek treatment during the later stages of illness, usually at greater expense. Cancer is an example of a disease that is best treated and cured when diagnosed in its early stage. Another example is sinus infection. The most cost-effective means of diagnosing and treating a sinus infection would be an assessment by a family physician or nurse practitioner. However, this solution is not realistic if you do not have health insurance, your insurance company does not cover this type of visit, or you do not have the money to pay deductibles, copayments, coinsurance, or a retail clinic visit. When the sinus infection reaches the stage when it can no longer be tolerated, the individual might seek treatment at the local emergency department. Many people rely on emergency departments for all levels of health care due to lack of insurance (Mason, 2007). Emergency room treatment is intended for seriously ill or injured persons and not for less serious illnesses. Emergency department treatment is expensive for any condition.

Critical Thinking Exercise

Who Pays the Health Care Bill?

If a patient does not have health insurance or the ability to pay the emergency department fee, who pays the bill?

Hospital billing practices charge uninsured patients higher fees for services, including medications, than insurance companies for the same services. Big health plans provide bargain discounts for the patients they insure. Hospitals seek payment up front from uninsured patients. Uninsured persons may find it hard to buy an individual health insurance policy because of existing medical conditions, such as a history of sinus infections, allergies, irritable bowel syndrome, or a yeast infection. Growing federal and state deficits make it harder to find money to finance coverage for the uninsured through Medicaid. As employers cut back or drop health benefits, individuals are shopping for their own health insurance. Large insurance companies are part of the individual health policy market.

UNCOMPENSATED CARE

For many people, free hospital services are their only available form of health care, especially in times of crisis. These free services are known as free care, indigent care, and charity care. This uncompensated care results in huge yearly deficits for health care organizations. Uncompensated care includes services for which hospitals did not receive full payment and includes:

- **Free care:** Free services that hospitals provide to patients who show that they cannot afford to pay for their care.;
- **Bad debt:** Services that hospitals provide for which they expect to receive payment, but never receive it. For example, insurance companies or patients who do not pay their bills.
- The difference between what the hospital receives for treating Medicare and Medicaid patients and what it receives for treating privately insured patients.

There are laws that require hospitals to provide free services to those in need. These laws lack specific requirements and are vague as to the amount of free care hospitals must provide. Each hospital creates its own free care policy. Charitable physicians, community "free clinics," public hospitals, and private hospitals that offer free care do not replace health insurance.

Learning Exercise

Where Is Free Health Care Offered?

1. Investigate if your county or state has free care laws.
2. Inquire if the hospitals in which you affiliate have a free care policy.

GOVERNMENT HEALTH INSURANCE

Medicare and Medicaid, entitlement programs, continue to be major issues at the state and

Box 18-10 | *Additional Issues and Trends in Medicare*

- When 77 million baby boomers started to retire in 2008 and became eligible for retirement benefits, huge demands began to be placed on Social Security, including Medicare.
- Because Medicare reimbursement vacillates (fluctuates) between declining rates (sometimes not meeting the cost of service) and stable rates (squeezing profits), some doctors refuse to take new Medicare patients and threaten to drop existing patients in these categories. For example, some private fee-for-service providers will not accept new or threaten to drop Medicare patients. Physicians could get a small bonus in reimbursement if they report data on the quality of their care. Some health policy experts, politicians, and physicians are skeptical of pay-for-performance (Pear, 2006).
- The trust fund for Medicare Part A is predicted to deplete in 2019 because of the increasing cost of health care, increased use of health care services, and expensive new technology.
- The cost of premiums for Medicare supplemental health care plans and drug plans are increasing yearly, increasing out-of-pocket costs for patients.

- New and pricey treatments for common medical conditions that are a part of aging could benefit thousands of Medicare patients, but at a price.
- Uninsured adults with common chronic illnesses who become eligible for Medicare have 51% greater medical expenses and 20% more hospitalizations than Americans who had insurance prior to Medicare (Kolata, 2007).
- The Congressional Budget Office paid Medical Advantage Plans (i.e., insurance companies) 12% to 19% more than it would have cost for the same care in traditional Medicare (Pear, 2007).
- Starting October 2008, Medicare plans to no longer reimburse hospitals for the treatment of conditions, such as injuries caused by falls, infections caused by the improper use of catheters, and pressure ulcers developed in the hospital, that could have reasonably been prevented. Hospitals will not be allowed to bill the patient for any charges not covered by Medicare (Kaiser Daily Health Policy Report, 2007).

federal levels because of the increasing cost of health care. The Medicare program alone costs almost $374 billion a year (*Medicare: A Primer,* 2007). Some call Medicare a system out of control. Fifty-five million Americans received Medicaid in 2003 (*Medicaid: A Primer,* 2007). There is continued debate about possible changes in future Medicare and Medicaid benefits (Boxes 18-10 and 18-11).

Critical Thinking Exercise

What Services Should Medicare Offer?

1. Should Medicare pay for new technological procedures that are developed to treat common medical problems of the elderly?

2. Should cost-effectiveness enter the picture for treating Medicare patients?

Learning Exercise

How Has Medicare Changed/Evolved?

What changes in legislation at the federal level and at your state level have affected Medicare and Medicaid since the sixth edition of *Success in Practical/Vocational Nursing* was published?

Review the resources listed in Chapter 5 and the Internet resources in Appendix E for suggestions for finding information in the learning resource center (LRC) or your computer that can be used in obtaining up-to-date information for your nursing courses.

- Because of budget deficits and an economic downturn in 2008, some states consider cutting their Medicaid programs.
- Unemployment increases the numbers applying for government assistance after unemployment benefits run out.
- Because of reimbursement rates, some physicians and dentists refuse to take new Medicaid patients.
- Almost 30% of children eligible for SCHIP have not been enrolled (*Many Eligible for Child Health Plan Have No Idea*, 2007).
- Although the SCHIP program was extended in December 2007, a declining economy and new federal rules affecting Medicaid and SCHIP eligibility were hampering some states attempts to expand coverage in these programs.

REPAIRING THE HEALTH CARE SYSTEM

The major ways to accomplish health care reform are to do the following:
- Allow incremental changes in the marketplace, and
- Enact comprehensive changes at the federal level.

The health care system has been unraveling for years, getting stitched back together by temporary fixes. Incremental changes have not solved the problem of access of care for millions of uninsured persons. Although there is currently no organized attempt at the federal level to achieve a comprehensive method of health care reform, health care agencies, insurance companies, and individual states continue to initiate their own changes to attempt to control the cost of health care and the problem of the uninsured. This method of solving health care problems is called the incremental method. In this method, changes occur here and there without affecting the system as a whole.

Comprehensive changes affect the health care system as a whole and not in a piecemeal fashion. At the federal level, an example of comprehensive change would be the issue of universal coverage, which is coverage of all Americans with health care.

INCREMENTAL CHANGES

The following are attempts to increase coverage and decrease costs in a piecemeal fashion.

FEDERAL LEVEL
Health Insurance

In 1996, the issue of guaranteed coverage (i.e., the inability of an insurance company to drop a subscriber for any reason) was improved when the Clinton administration signed into law The Health Insurance Portability and Accountability Act (HIPAA; see Chapter 20). HIPPA amended the 1986 Consolidated Omnibus Reconciliation Act. Perhaps best known for its protection of privacy provisions, HIPAA also simplified administration procedures by reducing paperwork associated with health insurance reimbursement. Health insurance provisions of HIPPA are in Box 18-12.

However, the bill did not address the cost of this coverage. As health insurance premiums continue to rise, some COBRA monthly rates exceed $600 for individuals and $700 for families. Because of rising insurance premiums, many find the cost of obtaining health insurance under the COBRA law unaffordable.

Other federal incremental methods for providing health insurance are the CHIP (SCHIP), which has insured millions of children in families who cannot afford health insurance and the Medicare prescription drug benefit.

- Required renewal of a health insurance policy, regardless of the health status of any member of a group,
- Guaranteed access to health insurance for small businesses, regardless of the health status of an individual or family, and
- Guaranteed access to individual coverage for those who lose their job or change jobs. This coverage is without regard to health status. Renewal is guaranteed.

STATE LEVEL
The Uninsured

States are attempting to reduce their rising health care costs and cover their uninsured. Maine legislators passed a universal health care bill that was the first universal health insurance program in the nation and is trying to reform its original plan. Many states have proposed initiatives to increase health care coverage for their residents and lower premiums.

LOCAL LEVEL
Retail Health Care

Retail stores such as Wal-Mart, Target, and CVS have added clinics staffed by nurse practitioners or physician assistants to treat common health conditions such as sinus infections, allergies, and skin infections and give preventive care such as vaccines. Service is offered on a first-come, first-served basis for approximately $50.00 (*Retail Health Clinics on the Rise*, 2007). Wal-Mart and Target offer selected generic drugs at $4.00 per prescription per month in many states.

COMPREHENSIVE CHANGES

Ways of increasing health care coverage of Americans generally include two basic ideologies: (1) creating a system of universal coverage through a single-payer system, and (2) encouraging individuals to purchase private health insurance through tax break incentives as in Health Savings Accounts (HSAs).

Single-Payer System

In the single-payer system, payment for doctors, hospitals, and other providers for comprehensive health care for everyone regardless of past medical history comes from a single fund. Physicians and hospitals are private and negotiate for payment for services and are freely chosen by patients. Administrative costs are lower in this type of system. Medicare in the United States is an example of a single-payer system (*Health Care Reform in the US*, 2006). This type of system is not the same as socialized medicine in which health care providers are employees of the government and the government runs hospitals. The Veteran's Administration (VA) health care system is an example of socialized medicine.

People who favor universal coverage think it would be a more cost effective use of tax money that is already being used for health care by the uninsured and could be reallocated towards the cost of health insurance. Universal coverage would provide preventive care and catch some diseases in early stages when they are less costly to treat (Hadley and Holahan, 2004). Opponents of universal coverage object to the idea of tax money being used to insure all Americans.

Health Savings Accounts

Health Savings Accounts (HSAs) were created as part of the 2003 Medicare Drug Law. HSAs can be offered by employers or enrolled in on an individual basis (at a higher cost). This type of funding for health care involves a medical savings account that allows persons to save for medical expenses on a tax-free basis. The idea for HSAs is that patients will be more money-wise with how they use medical services if they must pay off the deductible of their annual health care bills from their accounts. These plans are linked with high deductible health plans (HDHPs) that have lower monthly premiums but higher out-of-pocket spending and are referred to as consumer-directed plans (Hoffman and Tolbert, 2006). Depending on plan, deductibles can be approximately $1100 for an individual or $2200–$5000 or more for a family. Monthly premiums range from $55 to $259 for a nonemployer individual plan (Yi, 2006). People tend to favor HSAs who are generally healthy and/or are in higher income brackets.

Fixing the problem of the uninsured takes a degree of social consensus and political will that our nation has not been able to muster (*Insuring America's Health*, 2004). We, the authors, have seen the importance and criticality of health care issues through six editions of this textbook. We have seen Congress debate and discuss the need for reform in Medicaid and Medicare and the problem of the uninsured. No comprehensive changes have come out of these debates and discussions. In the year before the presidential election of 2008, domestic policy and the economy, including health care, rated higher than Iraq on the public's priority list (The Pew Research Center, 2008).

Learning Exercise

Identify Changes in the U.S. Health Care System

Identify changes in health care policy that occurred after the presidential election of 2008.

_____

_____

RESTRUCTURING OF THE HEALTH CARE SYSTEM

The single word that describes health care in the United States continues to be *change*. The changes are dramatic, staggering, and continual. Some persons see the changes as chaos. Those who will survive see the changes as opportunities to improve the delivery of health care (*service*), increase the *quality* of that care, and decrease the cost of care.

A major change that continues to take place in health care services today is the restructuring of the health care system in the marketplace. This restructuring is a response to escalating health care costs. Strategies designed to decrease the cost of health care while maintaining service and quality require a radical shift in viewing how health care services are delivered, especially for those used to doing things the old way. These strategies require a "new lens" in the nurse's eye (paradigm shift). They do not reflect business as usual; and the word *business* is used intentionally. LPN/LVNs need to look at health care services from a business point of view. Business principles are running health care services. Service, quality, and cost control are attributes of health care that need to be understood and brought to all clinical situations by the practical/vocational nurse.

HEALTH CARE ALLIANCES, NETWORKS, AND CONSOLIDATION

Changes in the delivery of health care in the community involve new organization and structure of health care organizations. Alliances (partnerships) are formed among hospitals, clinics, laboratories, health care systems, and physicians. By joining together or **networking**, these alliances can coordinate the delivery of care and contain costs among providers of health care services. This system is a way to deliver health care services more efficiently in a climate of shrinking resources. All members of an alliance can buy supplies in quantity. They can share a computer system. Duplication of services and equipment is avoided.

Patient records can be more readily available on referral to another health care provider within the network. For this reason, alliances are called "seamless" systems. In a seamless system, a patient can move easily from health care service to health care service in the alliance without commotion and confusion. Alliances allow small, rural hospitals to continue to exist in a competitive market. Public-private partnerships continue to emerge. For example, public health agencies contract for services from private community nursing agencies. Such services control costs and continue to deliver quality care.

Consolidated systems of healthcare include hospital systems found nationwide. An example is the Aurora Health Care system that is a for-profit system of hospitals. Any profits realized go to the investors in a for-profit system.

Learning Exercise

Identify Restructuring of Health Care in Your Area

1. Identify health care alliances, networks, or consolidated systems that have formed in your area of the country.
2. Do these systems employ practical/vocational nurses?

_____

ALTERNATIVES IN HEALTH INSURANCE COVERAGE
Managed Care

Managed care is a health care delivery system developed to provide quality health care with cost and utilization (use) controls. Managed care tries to effect changes in the cost of health care by paying physicians to care for groups of patients for a set fee and limit services. Medical necessity and appropriateness of health care services are watched by a **utilization review** system. If physicians exceed an acceptable number of admissions to a health care facility or if patients exceed an acceptable length of stay, physician payment could be withheld (Cherry and Jacob, 2008). See Box 18-13 for examples of managed care plans.

REACTION TO MANAGED CARE AND HMOS

Some people were pleased with their treatment by HMOs. However, by 1999, there was a backlash of anger and frustration at managed care and HMOs by subscribers. HMOs originally came into existence to improve health care by allowing consumers to shape their own health plans with an emphasis on preventive care. Dissatisfaction with HMOs includes allegations and instances of delay in receiving needed diagnostic services and refusal of HMOs to approve procedures for various diseases and illness situations. Profits of managed care plans increased because of aggressive management of costs and double-digit increases in premiums. Because of rising health care costs, HMOs, known for their low-cost medical care, are losing consumers to PPOs, which are the least restrictive of managed care plans (Japsen, 2006).

The **National Committee for Quality Assurance** (NCQA) is a nonprofit group that provides objective nationwide assessment of managed care plans. This group issues report cards similar to *Consumer Reports* guides so that potential subscribers can evaluate a plan before they join. More information can be obtained at *http://web.ncqa.org*.

> **Box 18-13** | *Managed Care Plans*

HEALTH MAINTENANCE ORGANIZATIONS

- Are generally located in buildings that are used solely for HMO business, and all physicians working in the HMO are hired specifically for the HMO.
- Receive a prepaid fee to provide comprehensive care to members of the enrolled group.
- Encourage prevention of disease by the practice of preventive medicine.
- Discourage physicians from ordering excessive diagnostic tests and treatments.
- Patients may not have the option of choosing their physician each time treatment is needed. If a physician is chosen outside the HMO network, the cost has to be paid by the patient.
- Depending on the HMO, a member may go outside the HMO to see a desired physician with a point-of-service (POS) option. With the POS option the member pays an extra fee.

OPEN ACCESS PLANS

- Allow members to see specialist physicians within the network for treatment without need of a referral, as in traditional HMOs. This option may affect the subscriber's coinsurance.

PREFERRED PROVIDER ORGANIZATIONS

- **Preferred provider organizations** are an alternative to the strict utilization review system of some managed care plans.
- Fees are paid by fee-for-service and health insurance companies contract with physicians and hospitals and negotiate discount fees. These members of the network are "preferred" providers.
- Patients may choose to see any general physician or specialist in the network. If a patient chooses a preferred provider, a larger amount of the cost will be covered by the health care plan.
- Family practice physicians may be hired as members of a PPO. These physicians remain in the same office in which their family practice is located and continue to belong to the same physician group. Part of their day is spent treating patients in their own family practice, and part of the day is spent treating patients who are enrolled in the PPO under the rules of the PPO. Think of airline travel today. The person sitting next to you probably paid a different ticket price for the same service you paid for. The same may be true for the patient sitting next to you in the waiting room; these family physicians may have added a PPO service to their practice.

Identify Changes in Managed Care

Identify consumer-friendly changes in the policies of managed care that have occurred since the publication of the sixth edition of *Success in Practical/Vocational Nursing*.

CHANGES IN HEALTH CARE FACILITIES

Patients spend less time per admission to the hospital as the number of hospital inpatient days continues to decline. The acuity level of these inpatients is higher. More patients receive care in **ambulatory service (outpatient)** settings. Hospitals focus on needed services that are more profitable. The shortage of nurses, especially in specialty areas, including faculty in nursing programs, is alarming in number (see Chapter 11). When nurses resign or retire, it is difficult to fill their positions because of the nursing shortage. Other staff members are expected to assume the responsibilities of these staff persons. Reimbursement continues to be a problem for health care facilities.

Unlicensed Assistive Personnel

One survival strategy for acute care facilities continues to be the use of unlicensed assistive personnel (UAP) (see Chapter 11 for a review). UAPs can be found as patient care team members in all patient care units. Some business managers claim that many services and skills of highly educated persons can be delivered by less trained personnel without sacrificing quality. These skills include those performed by the practical/vocational nurse.

The assumption that these services and skills can be delivered in this manner without sacrificing quality continues to be challenged. Nursing research has demonstrated the financial benefit and positive clinical outcomes of care delivered by licensed nurses.

Cross Training

To decrease costs, some facilities **cross train** current staff to perform on units other than unit routinely assigned. This practice allows safe and effective use of staff when one's assigned unit has decreased census. Cross training also helps the nursing shortage. Cross training allows staff to be assigned from units with low census to units that have staffing needs caused by absences or increased patient census. Some staff members are cross trained for other hospitals in the system and are used under the same circumstances. Some health care workers are cross trained for specific tasks of other health care team members. Examples of this role shifting include nurses drawing blood and clerk receptionists bathing and feeding patients.

Minimum Nurse-to-Patient Ratios

California's safe staffing law took effect in January 2004. This law establishes minimum nurse-to-patient ratios on all hospital units. The law requires severity of patient illness and complexity of nursing judgment to be taken into consideration and units staffed accordingly. Mandating nurse-to-patient ratios is an attempt to improve quality and service.

Changes in health care continue to come fast and furiously!

Voluntary Versus Mandatory Overtime

Asking nursing staff (voluntary) and requiring (mandatory) nursing staff to work beyond an 8-hour shift has been the method some facilities use to attempt to provide patient coverage during the nursing shortage. A report from the Institute of Medicine indicated that nurses and nursing assistants who work more than 12 hours a day pose a serious threat to patient safety because of fatigue. The consequences of fatigue include: (1) slower reaction time, (2) a decrease in energy, and (3) diminished attention to detail. This report also poses some concern for voluntary overtime practices (Pear, 2003).

METHODS OF DELIVERING HEALTH CARE
Patient-Focused Care

The most dramatic change in the way health care is delivered has been the shift toward patient-focused care (see Chapter 11 for a review).

Procedures are simplified and made more efficient. One example is the charting method called charting by exception (CBE). In this charting system, normal events are charted merely by placing a check mark on a flow sheet. Only abnormal events or changes are charted in narrative form (see Chapter 20 for a review).

Electronic Medical Records

Electronic medical records involve recording all patient data in a computer and increase efficiency by reducing/eliminating the need for paper records, medical history forms, test request forms, drug prescriptions, written physician comments, etc. Such a transition would reduce medical errors, save lives, and save money. Patient records are available immediately to a specialist on referral.

Critical Pathways

Another example of efficient health care is the use of critical pathways (CPs). (See Chapter 11 for a review, including Figure 11-1 for an example of a CP.) This cost-effective method helps the patient reach discharge in the fastest time possible.

QUALITY IMPROVEMENT

The emphasis on quality assurance has been replaced by an emphasis on continuous quality improvement (CQI) and total quality management (TQM). Quality assurance stressed the identification of care that needed to be given to patients and evaluation of the results of that care. Quality improvement stresses the need to search continually for new ways to improve the process of patient care, prevent errors, and identify and fix problems. This makes the search for approaches to nursing problems a never-ending quest. Total quality management is the method by which CQI is carried out. Information about cardiac care and local hospital performance can be accessed at *http://hospitalcompare.hhs.gov*.

The Joint Commission (TJC) sets compliance standards for quality care and patient safety. Unscheduled visits by TJC are an attempt to make accreditation more focused on the continual process of providing safe and quality patient care. The emphasis of visits will be patient care. Instead of spending time, energy, and money getting ready for TJC visits, the emphasis will be on *always* being ready by consistently implementing quality standards for patient care and safety. Local hospitals accredited by TJC can be checked for safety and quality at *http://www.qualitycheck.org*.

A major way of improving the quality of patient care has been the formulation of nursing care plans by the RN, assisted by the LPN/LVN. This practice reflects TJC standard that the development of a plan of care be based on assessment data and be regularly reviewed and revised. Practical/vocational nurses have a responsibility to assist the RN with collecting data in patient care situations and offering input to the plan of care, whatever form it may take.

An important component of quality health care is that the providers of that care be able to demonstrate competency throughout their careers. Nursing licensure considers nurses from all levels of educational preparation minimally competent upon receiving the initial license, and continued competence is assumed throughout a career. Patients, lawmakers, employers, and professional organizations question this assumption. As this matter is debated and a method is devised to assure patients that their health care providers are competent and qualified, practical/vocational nurses need to update themselves continually in their area of practice.

Learning Exercise

Identify How You Will Stay Current in Your Career

Identify ways practical/vocational nurses can remain current in their areas of employment.

DEALING WITH CHANGE

If you had no prior experience in health care before entering the student practical/vocational nursing program, you may not be aware of the changes taking place in the workplace. If you had prior experience in the health care field, some of the changes you now observe in health care services may be obvious, whereas others may be subtler. Even new workers in a health career will see changes as their program of study progresses. How do you react to changes in your life? Whether changes occur in your personal life or career, it is important for you to remember that you have choices. Shuman (1995) describes how you can be a victim, a survivor, or a navigator of change.

Victims look at change in a negative way. Victims fear the worst will happen because of the proposed change and feel helpless in the situation. Victims do not willingly participate in the change process, allowing change to control them. Survivors resist change but go along for the ride. Survivors claim the change will never work, and if their prediction comes true, they will be heard to say, "I told you so." Navigators of change feel in control of the situation. They feel confident and excited about the possibility of being part of the solution to a problem. Navigators believe they have some control over change rather than being controlled by the change. When change is in the wind, are you a victim, a survivor, or a navigator?

In the twenty-first century, practical/vocational nurses need to define their role as more than the list of nursing tasks and duties they perform. Less trained, unlicensed persons on the health care team are also performing these nursing tasks and duties. *Practical/vocational nurses need to define their role in light of their assisting role in the nursing process.* Practical/vocational nurses are effective in noting new patient problems and collaborating with RNs in setting patient goals, performing nursing interventions, and evaluating the results of planning. It is these problem-solving and critical-thinking aspects of nursing that make practical/vocational nurses valuable members of the health care team.

Practical/vocational nurses need to present themselves in clinical situations as invaluable to the health care agency. Be self-directed, motivated, positive, and a problem solver in your daily work. Avoid being known as the staff person who always asks what needs to be done next. Identify what needs to be done, prioritize, and do it. Respond flexibly to changes that are presented. Identify tasks or protocols that could be done more efficiently. Use the critical thinking skills that were encouraged in your nursing program to devise innovative suggestions to make these areas more efficient and effective. Be a role model for practical/vocational nurses.

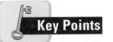

Key Points

- The cost of health care continues to increase. Cost is the driving force for change in the health care system.
- Traditional fee-for-service as a means of financing health care is being replaced by capitation.
- Insurance plans, both private and government-sponsored, are the major third-party payment systems in existence today.
- The national economy plays a role in financing health care.
- The number of uninsured is a major concern in health care.
- Comprehensive health care reform at the federal level has not occurred.
- Incremental health care changes at the federal level and in the marketplace center around attempting to decrease the cost of health care while improving service and quality of care.
- Changes in health care delivery, including patient-focused care, HMOs, PPOs, open access plans, health care alliances, electronic medical records, and quality improvement, address the issues of quality, service, and cost of health care.
- Practical/vocational nurses need to be self-directed, motivated, and positive problem solvers in their areas of employment.
- Changes in health care need to be approached with flexibility and viewed as an opportunity to improve the quality of patient care.
- Practical/vocational nurses need to ensure quality of patient care by keeping updated and current in their areas of employment.

REVIEW ITEMS

1. The driving force in health care today is:
   1. Controlling costs.
   2. Patient demands.
   3. Technological explosion.
   4. Labor negotiations.

2. Select the statement that best explains Medicare as a prospective payment system.
   1. Hospitals like the prospect of being paid by the federal government for health care services for elderly people.
   2. When the patient is discharged, the hospital calculates the bill and sends it to the federal government.
   3. Because of DRGs, the federal government tells the hospital in advance how much will be paid for an illness.
   4. The benefits covered by Medicare are changing rapidly because of new legislation by the federal government.

3. A patient tells the LVN about the new HMO that his employer has chosen to cover employees with health care benefits. Select the statement that indicates the patient understands the coverage of an HMO.
   1. "Each time I go to the doctor, I pay the charges as I leave the office and I send the bills to the HMO for reimbursement."
   2. "My annual physical is covered by the HMO, and I do not have to pay deductibles or copayments when I use the HMO."
   3. "The doctors hired by the HMO submit their bills to the HMO and receive reimbursement for the services they provided."
   4. "I must call the HMO each time I need to go to the doctor and obtain permission to be seen by a physician, or they will not pay."

4. You have been elected by your state as the first practical/vocational nurse to be a member of the US Senate. When you arrive in Washington, you find that the Senate's focus during your first year in office will be comprehensive health care reform. Each of the following projects would reform health care. Select which project would result in comprehensive health care reform.
   1. Reform Medicare and Medicaid to reduce fraud, waste, and inefficiency.
   2. Develop a plan for complete health care coverage for all the uninsured.
   3. Expand the Children's Health Insurance Plan to include their parents.
   4. Provide prescription drug coverage for all people on Medicare and Medicaid.

ALTERNATE FORMAT ITEM

Choose from the following list the source(s) of revenue that help finance state and federal government health care programs. *(Select all that apply.)*

1. FICA

2. FICA-Medical

3. Group Health Insurance

4. State withholding tax

5. Federal withholding

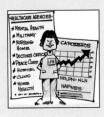

Objectives

On completing this chapter, you will be able to do the following:

1. List four current ethical issues of concern in twenty-first century health care.
2. Explain the differences among ethics, morals, and values.
3. Explain nursing ethics.
4. Identify ethical elements in your state's Nurse Practice Act.
5. Describe how the role of nursing has changed since the introduction of the nursing process and critical thinking into nursing curricula.
6. Discuss how nonmaleficence is more complex than the definition of "do no harm."
7. Differentiate between beneficence and paternal beneficence.
8. Explain the steps for an autonomous decision.
9. Describe how fidelity affects nursing care.
10. Discuss how a nurse applies the principle of justice to nursing.
11. Discuss the role of beneficent paternalism.
12. Differentiate between ethical and legal responsibility in nursing.

Key Terms

Autonomy (Ăw-TŎN-ŏ-mē, p. 347)
Beneficence (bĕ-NĔF-ĭ-sĕns, p. 346)
Beneficent paternalism (bĕ-NĔF-ĭ-sĕnt pă-TŬR-nă-līz-ŭm, p. 349)
Ethics (p. 340)
Fidelity (fī-DĔL-ĭ-tē, p. 348)
Justice (p. 349)
Morals (p. 340)
Nonmaleficence (nŏn-mă-LĔF-ĭ-sĕns, p. 345)

Nursing ethics (p. 341)
Privacy (p. 347)
Values (p. 340)

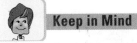

Keep in Mind

Nurses make decisions daily about right, wrong, good, bad, ought, and duty.

The twenty-first century presents numerous ethical issues in health care, as reflected in agency policies and medical procedures that create life, prolong life, cure chronic diseases, ensure a peaceful death, and end life. Additional ethical issues will arise as scientific research continues to explore possibilities, the procedures are discussed, and, if procedures are legalized, people press for their right to make autonomous decisions. Students in personal/vocational nursing classes identified the following current ethical issues in health care: in vitro fertilization, artificial insemination, surrogate motherhood, cloning, organ donation (including cadaver donations), child organ donors, procedures that use fetal tissues (stem cells) or organs from aborted fetuses, conceiving a child to produce tissue for a sibling, abortion, experiments that destroy a human embryo, euthanasia, assisted suicide, advance directives (including living wills and durable power of attorney), and insertion and/or withdrawal of feeding tubes. (For example, the patient has verbalized to the physician the wish to avoid further heroic means to stay alive. Two adult children have arrived and insist that all means be used to maintain life, but the three children already at the bedside do not agree. The patient lacks a living will and durable power of attorney and is unconscious at this point.) As you progress in your nursing program, add additional areas of ethical issues to this list started by your peers.

DESCRIPTION AND SCOPE OF ETHICS

Ethics is a system of standards or moral principles that direct actions as being right or wrong. Ethics is concerned with the meaning of words such as *right, wrong, good, bad, ought,* and *duty.* Ethics is concerned with the ways people, either individually or as a group, decide the following:
- What actions are right or wrong,
- If one *ought* to do something,
- If one has the *right* to do something, and
- If one has the *duty* to do something.

This basic definition is somewhat of an oversimplification. Ethics sounds like the words *morals* and *values,* but there are differences among them.

MORALS AND VALUES

Morals are concerned with dealing with right or wrong behavior (conduct) and character. The terms *ethics* and *morals* are difficult to define separately. *Morals* come from a Latin root, and *ethics* comes from a Greek root. Both words mean customs or habits and refer to the general area of rights and wrongs. The words are often substituted for each other. We will use *ethics* and *morals* in the same way in this chapter.

Values involve the *worth* you assign to an idea or an action. Values are freely chosen and are affected by age, experience, and maturity. A child usually embraces family values during childhood. The teen years are a time of trying out family values and either incorporating them or rejecting and replacing them with new values. Values continue to be modified throughout your lifetime, as you acquire new knowledge and experience. Based on changes in values, one's code of ethics/morals can be shifted (e.g., organ transplants after you have learned about or cared for a patient who receives a transplant).

Law is thought of as a minimum ethic that is written and enforced. As a licensed practical/vocational nurse (LPN/LVN), the Nurse Practice Act of your state is your final authority on what you are legally obligated to do as a nurse regardless of where you are employed (see Chapter 20 for more about nursing and the law). Have a thorough knowledge of the Nurse Practice Act of the state in which you are employed.

COMPARISON OF LEGAL ASPECTS OF NURSING AND ETHICS

Nursing ethics are similar to, but also different from, the legal aspects that regulate your nursing practice. Table 19-1 presents a comparison of legal aspects and nursing ethics.

Table 19-1	*Comparison of Legal Aspects and Nursing Ethics*	
	LEGAL ASPECTS	**NURSING ETHICS**
Definition	The state statutes that apply to licensed persons and the situations in patient care that could result in legal action	Set of rules of conduct
Focus	Rules and regulations	Ideal behavior of a group of licensed people
	Obligations under the law	Morality
		Higher standards
Applies to	Member of a professional/career group	Member of a nursing group
Participation	Mandatory	Voluntary
Source	Your state's Nurse Practice Act	NFLPN and NAPNES Codes, Florence Nightingale Pledge, PN Pledge

NURSING ETHICS

Nursing ethics, according to Miller-Keane, are "the values and ethical principles governing nursing practice, conduct, and relationships." Nursing ethics deal with the relationship of a nurse to the patient, the patient's family, associates and fellow nurses, and society at large. Nursing ethics attempts to look for underlying patterns or order in a large number of ethical decisions and practices of nurses, individually or as a group. Codes provide a guideline for what the LPN/LVN ought to do. However, codes do not carry the weight of law. It is interesting to note how many ethical items are actually found in the law, such as your Nurse Practice Act. Including ethical items in a legal document places emphasis on the importance of these items. It also gives the LPN/LVN a source to fall back on to defend the choices in behavior they make in regard to patients and families; it is then a matter of law.

ETHICAL CODES OF NAPNES AND NFLPN

Ethics that are adopted by nursing groups are in their codes of behavior. Both the National Association for Practical Nurse Education and Service, Inc. (NAPNES) and the National Federation of Licensed Practical Nurses (NFLPN) have an ethical code for LPN/LVNs (see Appendices B and C).

 Learning Exercise

Ethical Issues and Your Nurse Practice Act

Discover how your state includes ethical issues (what you ought to do as an LPN/LVN) in the law, which is your Nurse Practice Act (what you have to do as a licensed person).

- Read the ethical codes of the NAPNES and NFLPN.
- Use the NFLPN code as an example.
- Search for the elements of this ethical code in your Nurse Practice Act. Fill out the following worksheet.
- Summarize the ethical elements found in the Nurse Practice Act.

	Is this ethical area addressed in your state's Nurse Practice Act?	If "yes," cite section
1. Know the scope of maximum utilization of the LPN/LVN, as specified by the Nurse Practice Act, and the function within this scope.		
2. Safeguard the confidential information acquired from any source about the patient.		
3. Provide health care to all patients regardless of race, creed, cultural background, disease, or lifestyle.		
4. Refuse to give endorsement to the sale or promotion of commercial products or services.		
5. Uphold the highest standards in personal appearance, language, dress, and demeanor.		
6. Stay informed about issues affecting the practice of nursing and delivery of health care and, where appropriate, participate in government and policy decisions.		

	Is this ethical area addressed in your state's Nurse Practice Act?	If "yes," cite section
7. Accept the responsibility for safe nursing practice by keeping mentally and physically fit and educationally prepared to practice.		
8. Accept the responsibility for membership in NFLPN or the LPN/LVN organization of your choice, and participate in its efforts to maintain the established standards of nursing practice and employment policies that lead to quality patient care.		

YOUR PERSONAL CODE OF ETHICS

Practical/vocational nursing students and LPN/LVNs also have a personal code of ethics that provides personal guidelines for living. You ultimately chose what your personal code of ethics would include. Your personal code of ethics will influence your nursing ethics. Sometimes personal ethics conflict with the law (state's Nurse Practice Act). When personal ethics conflict with the law, you are obligated to follow the law. If you object to a medical procedure on religious or moral grounds, state this objection in writing. Present the statement to the employer *before* starting employment. The employing agency and *you* need to be clear in advance about your objection to procedures because of religious and moral reasons. For

example, you may be ethically opposed to abortion. Abortion in the United States is permitted under certain circumstances. You may ethically refuse to assist with the abortion procedure (and have stated this in writing at the time of employment), but post procedure you cannot refuse to give nursing care to the woman involved. "You may not abandon your patient," in the words of Sr. M. Antonette, former Director of Nursing at Sacred Heart Hospital in Allentown, PA. Abandonment is a legal matter. Your license is at stake. The best strategy is to seek employment in a health agency that does not participate in procedures/nursing care of which you do not ethically approve.

Some nurses have tried to opt out of caring for patients who have an illness that may be related to a lifestyle of which they do not approve. A nurse needs to separate personal ethics from nursing ethics. You are legally expected to care for a patient who has a lifestyle of which you disapprove. For example, when caring for an AIDS patient, use proper technique during care as with any patient with an infectious disease. You may not refuse to care for this patient. Ethically and legally this patient must receive the same level of care, with dignity and respect, as other patients do. *Nursing is not about giving care selectively to those patients you approve of and refusing care to others you see as less deserving.*

Critical Thinking Exercise

Personal Values

Write your personal value system regarding health and illness. Be concerned with content, not form. What you write will be an ethical code in progress. You may want to add or subtract statements after you have completed the chapter. It will also be a code you can modify as your experience with patients increases.

ROOTS OF NURSING ETHICS

Years ago, nurses saw themselves as doers, not thinkers. Nurses worked only to serve the physicians' wishes. Before nursing process and critical thinking were added to nursing curricula, those in the nursing profession did not see themselves as having something separate to contribute to patient care (in addition to the nurses' dependent role to physicians). Nursing ethics was primarily a modification of medical ethics and ethics of other professions at that time.

WHAT CHANGED?

The study of nursing was initially disease oriented. Nursing textbooks focused on the disease process, including cause, signs, symptoms, treatment, prognosis, and nursing care related to the treatment. Physicians did the medical assessment and wrote orders for the nurse to carry out. The nurse reported on patient progress, based on physicians' orders. Nursing assessments did not exist. Additional concerns the patient might have had (e.g., spiritual, cultural, emotional, sexual) were not routinely assessed. Patients were expected to follow physicians' orders without question. The nurse's job was to see that the orders were followed. The early nursing role was limited to the dependent relationship with the physician.

As nursing theories emerged, so did nursing process and critical thinking. Nursing textbooks mirrored the change to include nursing process and critical thinking. Nurses discovered that in addition to their dependent role to physicians, they had something special to contribute to the patient. Nursing discovered the patient. *The patient was a whole person, not just a disease.* With the help of nursing process, nurses had a way of identifying additional needs that could be responded to through nursing care. Rather than expecting patients to blindly follow orders because "we know what is wrong with you and we can fix it" (benevolent paternalism), patients were encouraged to be an active part in planning and implementing their nursing care plan (support of patient **autonomy**).

Changes in nursing did not happen easily. Many nurses were entrenched in their dependent role to physicians. Nurses thought nursing was being ruined by changes that were taking place. Nursing textbooks and curricula both had to change to reflect nursing process, critical thinking, and a focus on the total patient (not just the physically diseased portion of the patient). Adding nursing process and critical thinking changed the nursing role and changed nursing philosophy. This in turn influenced a change in nursing ethics.

Ethical principles in this chapter are about application of nursing ethics to nursing decisions and action. You are encouraged to look at both sides of an ethical principle. Recognize that no principle applies in the same way to all patients and their unique situation. No principle is absolute.

Review Chapter 6 on Critical Thinking. Critical thinking plays a major role in sorting out ethical choices and legal responsibilities in regard to the patient. The patient's knowledge of choices regarding care also affects ethical decision-making.

ETHICAL DECISIONS IN HEALTH CARE

ETHICS COMMITTEES

Health agencies such as hospitals have a medical ethics committee. This multidisciplinary team assists with difficult ethical decisions. Usually the discussions relate to new or unusual ethical questions. However, if you think the ethics committee makes all medical ethical decisions, you are only partially right. Patients arrive with their cultural- and/or their religion-based ethics. These were often established long before they were born. What the person can and cannot do in regard to their health care has already been established by the culture of which they are a part. See Chapter 13 to review spiritual needs, spiritual caring, and religious differences.

WESTERN SECULAR (NOT RELIGION OR STATE BASED) BELIEF SYSTEM

In the Western secular belief system the emphasis is shifted from duties to rights of the individual. This system has the following characteristics:
1. *Individual autonomy* means "self-rule." Individuals have the capacity to think, and based on these thoughts, make a decision freely whether or not to seek health care (the freedom to choose).

2. *Individual rights* mean the ability to assert one's rights. The extent to which a patient can exert their rights is restricted (i.e., their rights cannot restrict the rights of others). For example, the patient's right to refuse treatment can be at odds with the health professional's perceived duty to act always in a way that will benefit the patient (do good and prevent harm). An individual's right has become a central theme of health care.
   a. Right to consent to care
   b. Right to choose between alternative treatments
   c. Women's rights over their own bodies
   d. Right to consent or refuse treatment

Numerous bills of rights have been written. Fierce debates have taken place at state and national levels. The question of individual autonomy and individual rights is far from being settled. At the time of this writing, some laws based on individual autonomy and rights have been passed (e.g., Oregon Assisted Suicide Law, *Roe v. Wade*). However, there are attempts to have passed laws rescinded. *The question is:* To what extent do one's individual moral decisions (rights) get in the way of another's moral autonomy?

Critical Thinking Exercise

Personal Beliefs That May Affect Medical Decisions

What cultural or religious values do you hold that may affect personal health care decisions? Use your response to the critical thinking exercise on personal values to get started.

_____

_____

ETHICAL RESPONSIBILITIES OF NURSES

Sometimes, a problem arises that appears to be an ethical problem. It may instead be a problem of communication or trust or insufficient information (Soglin, 2005). Adding nursing process and critical thinking to nursing curricula changed nursing focus to the whole patient (not just the physically diseased area). The dependent role to

the physician remains, and responsibilities unique to nursing were added. The following responsibilities are both ethical and legal:
1. *Patient advocacy:* For example, the patient needs to be informed of what you will be doing with him or her (e.g., steps of a procedure). Find out what your role is in keeping the patient informed. In most states the LPN/LVNs role is to support teaching done by the registered nurse (RN) or the physician. If the patient has questions and you are unsure of whether it is within your role to answer, ask the RN. When the patient does make a decision, be supportive even though you do not agree with the decision.
2. *Accountability:* The word accountability means that you are answerable to yourself, to your assigned patient, to the team leader, to the physician, and to your instructor, who evaluates your work. As an LPN/LVN, accountability to the instructor is replaced by accountability to the employing agency. You are held accountable for all the nursing actions that you perform or are assigned to perform, and in a safe manner. The measures of accountability are the nursing standards of practice; that is, what a nurse with your education would do in a similar situation (see Chapter 20).
3. *Peer reporting:* Report peers for behaviors that are potentially harmful to patients (e.g., impaired at work because of alcohol and/or other drug use, stealing patient's medication, substituting water or normal saline for injectable narcotics, giving patients a cold shower).

PRINCIPLES OF ETHICS

As a nurse of the twenty-first century, you recognize there is something unique that a nurse has to offer patients beyond the dependent role to physicians. This realization places greater responsibility on practical/vocational nursing students (SPN/SVNs) to learn all they can during the nursing program of study. For example, now you can add knowledge of basic ethics to critical thinking as you assist the RN with nursing process. The data you collect will have an added dimension of ethics. It will make a difference in developing a quality care plan that considers the patient as a whole person, not just his or her physically diseased part.

At this level you incorporate a basic understanding of how SPN/SVNs and LPN/LVNs practice nursing according to nursing codes. Learning about ethics is more than being able to recite the definition to pass a test: it means being able to help make ethical decisions when ethical dilemmas arise.

The following ethical principles will be discussed in this chapter:

1. Nonmaleficence (do no harm),
2. Beneficence (do good),
3. Autonomy (free to choose),
4. Fidelity (be true), and
5. Justice (fair to all).

NONMALEFICENCE (DO NO HARM)

"It may seem a strange principle to enunciate as the very first requirement in a hospital that it should do the sick no harm. It is quite necessary nevertheless to lay down such a principle."

Florence Nightingale, *Leadership and Management According to Florence Nightingale,* by Ulrich B (1992) Appleton and Lange, Norwalk, CT, p. 22

The quotation by Nightingale refers to the ethical principle nonmaleficence. Nonmaleficence means *primum non nocere*: first do no harm. Nonmaleficence is the basis of many of the "rules" promoted by your instructors. Examples include the following rules:

- "Rule of 5" for giving medications,
- Checking the temperature of bath water,
- Checking the temperature of formula before feeding patient,
- Placing the bed to its lowest position after completing a treatment or preparing to leave the room,
- Raising side rails after care,
- Providing care for your patients when their ethical principles conflict with yours,
- Performing necessary procedures only, on patients, instead of unnecessary procedures to gain additional experience.

- Protecting those who cannot protect themselves; for example, mentally challenged, unconscious, weak, or debilitated patients.

If the principle of nonmaleficence is taken to the extreme, there are many nursing duties SPN/SVNs and LPN/LVNs could not perform. Few beneficial treatments are entirely without harm, including the following:

- Any time that you puncture the patient's skin with a needle, there is some tissue damage, a risk of infection, and the possibility of an untoward reaction to a solution if administered. All drugs have side effects: rare, serious, and not so serious.
- Any time you put a tube into a bodily opening (e.g., catheterization, irrigating a colostomy), there is some trauma to surrounding tissue. There is the possibility of introducing infection and penetrating the tissue wall.
- Many procedures hurt physically in the process of performing them (e.g., positioning a patient properly after surgery, cleansing the mouth of an elderly patient who has not had proper mouth care for a period, irrigating a pressure ulcer, moving a patient with osteoporosis from bed to chair to toilet and back).
- Giving a vaccination carries the risk of the patient experiencing a side effect, but the overall effect for most people is the prevention of serious diseases.
- When you monitor an IV, one thing to check is that the solution and additive, if any, are infusing, as compared to what the physician ordered. A common additive is KCl (potassium chloride). KCl within a narrow blood level range is necessary for proper heart functioning. If too little or too much is administered, it can result in heart dysfunction, sometimes resulting in death. (Jack Kevorkian, a physician who participated in several assisted suicides, used KCl as one of the drugs in his suicide machine.) KCl can save lives, but it can also kill.

Each of the procedures mentioned has the potential for doing good and doing harm. The question always is how to do the least amount of harm when doing something that is expected to result in good. The obvious answer is to never knowingly participate in any action that will deliberately harm the patient. The patient must also have agreed to the procedure verbally or in writing, depending on the procedure (autonomy). This is a reason for practicing procedures in the nursing lab; preparing for nursing care; reviewing your nursing care plan with the instructor; and reviewing action, side effects, and dose with the instructor before giving a medication.

The following are negative examples of nursing action meant to do no harm that result in harm:

- Putting down a patient's side rail without first checking that the patient's arm is not hanging between the rail and the bed. The patient who immediately comes to mind is a woman in her eighties whose arm was fractured and who received several skin tears and bruises. The staff person who put the rail down was irritated because of "a bad night shift" and was hurrying to get off duty.
- Rapidly feeding large spoonfuls of food to a patient who has a dry mouth as a side effect of medication. Because of the lack of liquid before beginning to eat, large spoonfuls of food, lack of adequate time to chew, and lack of additional liquid before the next bite, the patient aspirated some of the food that accumulated in his mouth. The patient survived but refused future attempts to eat when he saw the same nurse come in with his food tray.
- Placing a lap restraint incorrectly (the physician's order was for the patient to be restrained when up in a wheelchair). Because of improper placement of the restraint and lack of monitoring, the patient slid down and died as a result of hanging by the neck.

Learning Exercise

Procedures and Their Effects

Think about procedures with which you are familiar. Review the procedure. List two procedures that "do good" but also have the potential to do harm. State the good and potential harmful effect of each procedure.

BENEFICENCE (DO GOOD)

Beneficence means to "*do good*" with your nursing actions and is the basis of trust in nursing. It also involves preventing harm and removing harm. You have read how nonmaleficence and beneficence are often difficult to separate and may go hand in hand. There are two major nursing duties to the patient that are associated with beneficence:

1. *Put the patient interests first.* For example:
   - You do not go off duty until you hand over the care of the patient to equally skilled nursing staff to continue the nursing care. You are obligated to report to the nurse taking over the next shift what has transpired during the time you have been responsible for nursing care.
   - If you give the wrong medication, report it as soon as you recognize the error. Your ethical concern is to "do good" and "prevent harm." Beneficence is a greater good than concern for self in regard to the error.
   - You go to work even though you are tempted to call in sick, because you want to go visiting out of town for the weekend.
2. *Place the good of patients before your needs.* This is where interpretation of duty gets more complex. Does this mean that duty to the patient means utmost sacrifice? No, it does not. However, it does mean that you sacrifice something. For example:
   - *Patient needs* are *above organizational needs.* You may have administrative responsibility (perhaps as a charge nurse) that must be completed by the end of the day or meetings you are expected to attend

that day. If a patient needs your skill and expertise, as in an emergency situation, your first duty is to the patient.

- *Place the good of patients before your needs* does *not* mean that you begin to behave as though no one in the world can assume the nursing care you give to a patient. Do not stay past your scheduled hours when there is someone ready to assume responsibility for nursing care. This also means that you do not call the patient from home, accept calls in your home from the patient, or visit the patient after hours. If you are doing any of this, you have just entered an unhealthy codependent relationship with the patient.

 Critical Thinking Exercise

Ethical Obligations

When a patient is demanding, angry, or uncooperative and threatens to become violent, is the nurse obligated to put her or himself in danger of serious harm? Are nurses ethically obligated to perform heroic acts of self-sacrifice (Haddad, 2005)?

Volunteer (pro bono) work is a professional obligation of beneficence for nurses. For example, a nurse may decide to volunteer some hours a week at a free clinic or children's center.

AUTONOMY (FREE TO CHOOSE)

Autonomy does not mean that patients can do whatever they want. Autonomy means the following:

- *Thinking* through all the facts,
- *Deciding* on the basis of an independent thinking process,
- *Acting* based on a personal decision, and
- *Undertaking a decision voluntarily* without pressure, direct or subtle, from anyone else.

However, this does not mean that patients can do whatever they want. "Autonomy does not mean freedom to do as one wants or to act in accordance with one's desires. Autonomous

action is based on rational thought or reason. It embodies the notion of freedom and liberty, but only within the constraints of reason" (Rumbold, 2002). We expect people to respect our rights, and we respect their rights as long as their rights do not interfere with someone else's rights.

For patients to make an autonomous decision, they must have all the facts without leaving out information in order to influence the decision in a particular way. For example, the nurse may unintentionally (sometimes intentionally) influence the patient's decision by repeating what the physician has suggested is best for the patient ("The doctor would not have suggested the treatment if he [she] did not think it best for you." "The doctor knows what is best for you.").

There is also a fine line between autonomy and abandonment. Excessive control means interfering too much in a patient's life. Not interfering enough results in neglect of the patient. For example:

- The right of the elderly to make decisions about their treatment.
- A patient's right to be left alone or not treated.

More information is needed in both situations to determine if more or less interference is recommended.

Role of Privacy in Autonomy

Privacy is both an ethical and a legal issue. Autonomy includes a patient's right to privacy. This is the reason your instructor asks a patient directly for permission to allow SPN/SVNs to observe a particular treatment or to do a procedure. Similarly, the instructor checks with the patient before assigning a student to give nursing care. Privacy includes the right to choose care based on personal beliefs, feelings, or attitudes. It includes the right to decide what is done to their body (accepting or rejecting treatment or exposure of the body). As an SPN/SVN, you respect the patient's decision. When giving care, avoid exposing the patient needlessly in the course of care. *This is an invasion of privacy.*

Role of Culture, Religion, and Personal Values in Autonomy

Culture or a religion-based belief system may be contrary to the accepted medical ethics. Examples of decisions based on religion and culture include the following:

- The patient, a Jehovah's Witness, could benefit from a blood transfusion for severe blood loss. The adult patient has refused because a blood transfusion is forbidden by his religion (religion based).
- If the patient had been an underage child whose parents forbade the blood transfusion on religious grounds, the physician might decide to go to court to ask the court to overrule the parents' decision. The physician can do this because parents cannot give *informed consent* for the treatment of underage children. An underage child is too young to understand all the facts to make a decision required for informed consent. Parents can *authorize treatment* for what is appropriate for their children up to a certain age. In this case the physician has decided that the value of beneficence is greater than the value of respect for the parent's autonomy. The court is the greater authority and will decide if the physician can transfuse the child.
- A young woman is diagnosed with breast cancer. Her husband has received a complete explanation from the physician about her illness, alternatives for each treatment, anticipated effects, possible side effects, and prognosis with each treatment. Her husband will not permit any treatment to take place (culture based).

Personal values of the patient may also be opposed to accepted medical ethics. The following is an example of personal value–based decision:

- A man in his late sixties is diagnosed with advanced cancer of the colon. He has refused to have treatment, even though he understands that while not curative, the surgery could result in less discomfort for a period and more time to live (personal value based).

FIDELITY (BE TRUE)

Fidelity challenges each practical/vocational nurse to be faithful to the charge of acting in the patient's best interest when the capacity to make free choice is no longer available to him or her. This does not include rescuing behaviors and becoming paternalistic in making decisions for vulnerable patients (legal competency will be described in Chapter 20). As a nurse, you must *differentiate* between your feeling and choice on an issue and the feelings and wishes of the patient. These points are foremost in making a decision. Charting the patient's feelings and wishes as expressed, without your personal interpretation, provides information for the physician when important decisions need to be considered. Examples of breaching fidelity include the following:

- Discussing a patient in a public area such as the cafeteria, an elevator, at home, or with friends breaches fidelity. It isn't necessary to mention a patient's name for others to know who is being discussed. Fidelity and confidentiality (a legal term) have been compromised, as has the patient's dignity. The action says the patient has limited worth in the eyes of the nurse and chips away at the patient's self-esteem.
- You overhear LPN/LVNs speaking disrespectfully about an obese patient and complaining how difficult it is to move the patient. What will you do in response to this discussion? Explain why you will take the action you have chosen. Is it an ethical response?
- A student practical nurse shared a personal experience that sharpened her awareness of the meaning of fidelity. During her first day of the mental health rotation, she spotted her neighbor, now a patient, in the day room. The SPN's husband worked with the patient. One day the patient did not come to work. The boss offered no information about what happened. Being a close-knit neighborhood, the SPN's husband, other workers, and neighbors

speculated with great concern about the missing worker. Seeing him on the psychiatric unit was a shock and the SPN did not know how to approach him. The SPN asked her instructor for assistance. The instructor suggested that the SPN approach the patient and let him know that she recognized him. Most important was that the SPN reassure the patient she would not tell anyone he was hospitalized. The SPN was also to say to the patient that not telling anyone outside of the hospital was part of her nursing education and duty. That took care of the discomfort for both the SPN and the patient regarding his hospitalization. The class after the clinical day was about fidelity and confidentiality (a legal concern). The SPN was sure she would never breach her promise not to talk about patients, except to the health care team and her instructor. That evening at dinner with her husband, she decided he should know because of concern for his co-worker/friend. The SPN made her husband promise not to tell anyone what she was about to tell him. Her husband promised to do as she asked. Later that evening they went to pick up groceries. The SPN's husband was off in a different aisle when he ran into another co-worker. As she rounded the corner, the SPN heard her husband say, "My wife ran into Joe at the psych hospital this morning. He's a patient, but don't tell anyone." The SPN breached confidentiality, an ethical and legal matter. She also started a reaction of, "I'll tell you, but don't you tell anyone."

You alone make the decisions regarding what you do when away from the clinical area and immediate support and supervision of the instructor. In a sense, fidelity sits on your shoulder—to ignore or to embrace.

JUSTICE (FAIR TO ALL)

Justice means that SPN/SVNs and LPN/LVNs must give patients their due and treat each patient fairly. For example, each patient with the same diagnosis should receive the same level of care. Being fair does not mean giving every patient the same things. It means treating them all the same (i.e., with dignity and respect). As a nurse, you make daily decisions in order to give patients their "due." For example, the patients on your floor in the hospital represent different levels of wealth, social status, culture, religion, and moral and value systems. All are acutely ill. The newest patient has Kaposi's sarcoma, a defining component of acquired immune deficiency syndrome (AIDS). Do you classify AIDS as a life-threatening illness or as a retribution for behaviors you consider immoral? If your personal ethics interfere with the care you give, you may find yourself (1) giving this patient more time than needed and doing less than needed for other acutely ill patients, or (2) providing minimal care for the patient and lavishing attention on those who "deserve the care."

There are many daily issues related to justice that you have the power to decide on. Listen to your inner talk: "He's so young—so much living left to do; she's had a full life already; she's an alcoholic—never took care of her kids"—and so on.

Critical Thinking Exercise

Inner Talk

At the end of your next clinical day, take time to reflect on your reaction to patients and how it affected your patient care. Did the word *deserve* enter into your thoughts, or did you provide justice for all?

As an SPN/SVN, you report patients' comments regarding ethical matters to the RN. Final ethical decisions are not within the LPN/LVN scope of nursing practice. Recall also that ethics is what you *ought* to do; law is what you *have* to do.

ROLE OF BENEFICENT PATERNALISM

We are including beneficent paternalism because it continues to be confused with the ethic of beneficence (do no harm). Beneficent paternalism is a disrespectful *attitude* toward the patient and what the patient has to contribute to personal care and recovery. It is an "I know what's best for you" attitude that discounts the patient's knowledge of self. The following are examples of beneficent paternalism:

- When assisting to collect data, it is important to really *hear* what the patient is trying to tell you. If you have determined in advance that this patient fits into a "specific category," you will discount what the patient wants you to know.
- Assisting with developing the care plan without patient input will reflect the nurse's needs, not the patient's. Later on you will complain that the patient is noncompliant and will not cooperate with the plan of care. Ask yourself: Did the patient know what the alternatives were for treatment? Did the patient have the opportunity to offer input into the plan and agree to what the care plan would be? It is difficult for patients to cooperate when staff bruises their sense of autonomy.
- If the patient has agreed to the patient care plan, then coaxing the patient to do what has been agreed upon is beneficence. However, if you are influencing the patient into choosing one alternative treatment over another, it is paternalistic beneficence. If you find yourself saying, "I overheard the doctor saying he thinks you should choose this treatment," or "My husband chose the treatment and he is doing great," you are actively influencing the patient's decision (paternalism).
- Perhaps the patient asks your opinion for the choice, and you respond with your choice ("Well, if I were you, I would. ....") instead of saying, "The doctor explained the alternatives for treatment and the possible side effects of each, it is for you to decide what is best for you."

Beneficent paternalism is justified only in extreme circumstances and is most often a medical decision (e.g., a physician approaching the court to be allowed to do a potentially lifesaving procedure when parents have refused to sign an authorized treatment form for the child).

To avoid paternalism with new mothers, a lactation counselor at a public health nursing seminar presented the following method: "I wish all women would breastfeed their babies. The value to mother and child is a scientific fact. I present the facts and respond to their questions, but the final decision belongs to the mother. I respectfully support their decision."

PATERNALISM AND WOMEN'S HEALTH

The issue of paternalism toward women in medical research and receiving health care is slowly changing through the efforts of women themselves and the advocacy of nurses. The term *paternalism* is derived from a Latin word that means "father" (i.e., father knows best). In the health system it is interpreted, as "doctors know best because of their superior knowledge." Because the word is derived from the Latin word *pater* (father), men know better than women. Physicians define what is ill-health for women. Anything that is normally different from men is considered an illness and requires the physician's intervention. Because women are different from men biologically, medicine has defined what is normal for women as being abnormal. For example, menstruation, pregnancy, and menopause are defined as ill health instead of normal, healthy processes. Many of these same attitudes toward women continue in the health care system. Women are seen as victims of their own bodies who cannot help being sick. This sometimes leads to a patting-on-the-head approach. "You can't help it, but I can help you" is implied and is often followed by, "Just take these pills." Male physicians are just mirroring the attitudes of males toward females in society (Rumbold, 2002).

Your responsibility is to advocate for your female patient. Speak up when you see decisions being made on incomplete information (e.g., the female patient was not listened to by the physician or other health care worker). Review Chapter 14 regarding assertiveness and your responsibility. It reminds you that an aggressive, rude approach does not gain you anything except a bad reputation among your peers and patients. Practice assertiveness and remember that change will occur slowly. Many female patients are already experiencing a change, and assertively state their needs. Nurses who advocate for their female patients assist in this process of reducing a paternalistic attitude toward women—one patient at a time as the need arises.

 Critical Thinking Exercise

Do I Respond Differently to Male and Female Patients?

Keep track of the differences in your responses to males and females for 2 or 3 days. It is not necessary to record every contact. Just track the ones you can. Record your response, the sex of the person speaking, and what they said.

_____

_____

_____

When you think you have enough examples, review the data you collected. Use critical thinking to determine what differences you noted in your response to male and female patients. Because this is for your eyes only, be candid. Are there any changes that you recommend for yourself? If so, write them down.

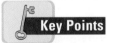 **Key Points**

- Ethics is concerned with the meaning of words such as _right, wrong, good, bad, ought,_ and _duty._
- Nursing ethics provide guidelines for making ethical decisions in nursing.
- Practical/vocational nurses need to be aware of the contents of their state's Nurse Practice Act regarding ethical issues.
- Ethics is something an SPN/SVN _ought_ to do. However, ethics themselves do not carry the weight of law.

- Content of the law (state's Nurse Practice Act) is something the SPN/SVN has to do.
- Both NAPNES and NFLPN provide an ethical code for SPN/SVNs and LPN/LVNs.
- SPN/SVNs and LPN/LVNs must know the nursing code of ethics and not confuse it with their personal code of ethics.
- Nursing role includes a dependent role to physicians and has progressed to include additional roles of:
  Providing nursing care to the whole patient, and being a patient advocate.
- Cultural and religious backgrounds and personal values may influence ethical decisions of patients seeking health care.
- Nonmaleficence means do no harm. Few treatments are entirely without harm.
- Beneficence means to do good with your nursing actions and is the basis of trust in nursing.
- Autonomy means respect for a patient's right to choose, as long as the patient's rights do not interfere with the rights of others.
- Fidelity means to be true. It challenges SPN/SVNs and LPN/LVNs to be faithful to the charge of acting in the patient's best interests, even when the capacity of free choice is not available to the patient because of their condition.
- Justice means that the SPN/SVN and the LPN/LVN must give the same level of care to all patients, with dignity and respect.
- If the LPN/LVN has ethical objection to procedures being done, a statement should be made in writing before beginning employment. Legal expectations identified in the state's Nurse Practice Act are not exempt. For example, a nurse must legally provide nursing care, even though he or she has not participated in the procedure, due to ethical objections as noted in writing, before beginning employment.
- Beneficent paternalism is justified only in extreme circumstances and is most often a medical decision.
- Paternalism in women's health care is changing slowly. Nurse's advocacy for women helps promote this change, one patient at a time.

REVIEW ITEMS

1. Which of the following defines *ethics*?
   1. Concern with practical issues of habits and conduct of persons or groups.
   2. The worth assigned to an idea or an action, freely chosen, affected by maturity.
   3. Concern with meaning of words such *as right, wrong, good, bad, ought,* and *duty.*
   4. Customs, habits, and behaviors in a society that are approved by that society.

2. Select the statement that **best** describes how nursing has evolved.
   1. Nursing discovered its unique role in nursing the whole patient, in addition to the diseased part.
   2. Nurses became upset by their dependent role to physicians and forced changes in the medical system.
   3. Nursing process and critical thinking promoted an easy change in how nursing is taught in schools.
   4. Nurses discovered that curricula and textbooks changed but not the work on patient care units.

3. How will you respond to the mother who has refused a blood transfusion for her 2-year-old son, but the doctor has asked the court to overrule her refusal?
   1. "In your son's case beneficent paternalism overrules respect for your autonomy."
   2. "In this hospital the doctor knows best because of his/her superior knowledge."
   3. "We have saved many children by ignoring parents' religious beliefs and doing what is best."
   4. "He is too young to understand and make his own choice in something this serious."

4. After seemingly successful treatment for depression and a serious suicide attempt, a patient will be in court this morning to find out if she will be released. The patient tells the SPN/SVN, "As soon as I get out, I am going to kill myself. Promise me you won't tell anyone." What course of ethical action should the SPN/SVN take?
   1. The SPN/SVN promises not to tell anyone. His personal ethic is to never break a promise when one is made.
   2. Psychiatric and nursing testimony is favorable to the patient. SPN/SVN reports the patient's comment to the judge.
   3. The SPN/SVN believes in waiting to see what will happen. He plans to do the same during the court hearing.
   4. The SPN/SVN keeps the promise made to the patient but convinces himself he is not meant to be a nurse.

ALTERNATE FORMAT ITEM

Which statement(s) **best** describe steps in making an autonomous decision? *(Select all that apply.)*

1. Voluntary without pressure

2. Fair to all parties involved

3. Doctor suggests solution

4. Ability to consider all facts

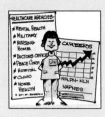

Objectives

On completing this chapter, you will be able to do the following:

1. Discuss the content of your state's Nurse Practice Act.
2. Describe the responsibilities of your state's board of nursing (or nursing regulatory board).
3. Explain the limits of nursing licensure within your state.
4. Define the nursing standard of care.
5. Differentiate between common law and statutory law.
6. Explain the difference between criminal and civil action.
7. Discuss the difference between intentional and unintentional torts.
8. List the four elements needed for negligence.
9. Review the steps for bringing legal action.
10. Differentiate between practical/vocational nursing student (SPN/SVN) and instructor liability in preventing a lawsuit.
11. Summarize the AHA's *The Patient Care Partnership: Understanding Expectations, Rights, and Responsibilities.*
12. Describe the major focus of the Health Insurance Portability and Accountability Act (HIPAA).
13. Explain the purpose of The Joint Commission (TJC) Patient Safety Goals.
14. Discuss the differences among general consent, informed consent, and authorized consent.
15. Differentiate between the living will and durable power of attorney.
16. Explain the difference between physician-assisted suicide and euthanasia.
17. Discuss the difference between a multistate compact and a border agreement.
18. Identify what is not included in an incident report.
19. Explain how you would legally deal with two difficult situations that might occur in a clinical setting.

Key Terms

Accountability (ă-kownt-ă-BĬL-ĭ-tē, p. 367)
Abandonment (ă-BĂN-dŏn-mĕnt, p. 381)
Advance directives (p. 375)
Assault (ă-SOLT, p. 360)
Authorized consent (p. 374)
Basic patient situation (p. 354)
Battery (p. 360)
Breach of duty (p. 363)
Border recognition agreement (p. 358)
Civil action (p. 359)
Common law (p. 358)
Complex nursing situation (p. 355)
Confidentiality (kŏn-fĭ-dĕn-shē-ĂL-ĭ-tē, p. 368)
Criminal action (p. 359)
Damages (p. 363)
Defamation (dĕf-ă-MĀ-shŭn, p. 360)
Delegated medical act (p. 355)
Depositions (dĕp-ō-ZĬSH-on, p. 363)
Direct supervision (p. 355)
Do-not-resuscitate (DNR) (rĭ-SŬS-ĭ-tāt, p. 376)
Durable medical power of attorney (p. 375)
Duty (p. 360)
End-of-life principles (EOL) (p. 378)
Euthanasia (ū-thă-NĀ-zhē-ă, p. 376)
Felony (FĔL-ō-nē, p. 359)
General (implied) consent (p. 374)
General supervision (p. 355)

Good Samaritan Act (p. 378)
Health Insurance Portability and Accountability
  Act (HIPAA) (p. 369)
Incident report (p. 379)
Informed consent (p. 359)
Intentional torts (p. 360)
Interstate endorsement (p. 357)
Institutional liability (p. 366)
Law (p. 354)
Liability (lī-ă-BĬL-ĭ-tē, p. 362)
Libel (LĪ-bel, p. 360)
Living will (p. 375)
Malpractice (professional negligence) (p. 361)
Misdemeanor (mĭs-dĭ-MĒ-nŏr, p. 359)
Multistate licensure (Nurse Licensure Compact)
  (p. 357)
Negligence (NĔG-lĭ-jĕns, p. 361)
Nurse Practice Act (p. 354)
Nursing standard of care (p. 358)
Oregon Death With Dignity Act (p. 377)
Patient competency (p. 373)
Patient Self-Determination Act (PSDA) (p. 375)
Personal liability (p. 366)
Preponderance (prĭ-PŎN-dĕr-ănce, p. 360)
Physician-assisted suicide (PAS) (p. 376)
Proximate cause (p. 363)
Slander (p. 361)
Statutory law (STĂCH-ū-TŎR-ē, p. 359)
The Joint Commission (TJC) (p. 358)
The Patient Care Partnership: Understanding
  Expectations, Rights, and Responsibilities
  (p. 368)
Unintentional torts (p. 361)
Vicarious liability (vĭKĂR-ē-ŭs, p. 366)

 Keep in Mind

Ethics and law drive the practice of nursing. When there is a dispute, law—the nurse practice act of your state—is the final authority.

"No employer/health care agency can give you permission to do something that your license/state's Nurse Practice Act does not allow you to do."
  Elizabeth Johnson
  Lead Instructor, Practical Nursing
  Northeast Wisconsin Technical Institute
  Green Bay, Wisconsin

Ethics in nursing deals with rules of conduct—what is right and what you ought to do in a particular situation. Ethical values, in turn, are the *basis* of nursing law. Law has to do with regulations that control the practice of nursing. Your state's **Nurse Practice Act** is your *legal* guideline in nursing.

Knowledge of your state's Nurse Practice Act will be valuable to you in making nursing decisions. Such knowledge also will help you protect yourself against acts and decisions that could involve you in lawsuits and criminal prosecution.

NURSE PRACTICE ACT

The state **Nurse Practice Act** defines nursing practice and establishes standards for nurses in your state. Ignorance of your state's Nurse Practice Act is never a valid defense against any legal proceeding regarding your license.

BASIC TERMINOLOGY

Basic terminology in a Nurse Practice Act remains standard in many states. As you study the scope of practice for licensed (or trained) practical/vocational nurses (LPN/LVNs) in your state, an understanding of the following terms is necessary.

- **Basic nursing care.** Nursing care that can be performed safely by the LPN/LVN, based on knowledge and skills gained during the educational program. Modifications of care are unnecessary, and patient response is predictable.
- **Basic patient situation.** Patient's clinical condition is predictable. Medical and nursing orders are not changing continuously. These orders do not contain complex modifications. The patient's clinical condition requires only basic nursing care. The professional nurse assesses whether the situation is a basic patient situation.
- **Complex nursing situation.** Patient's clinical condition is not predictable.

Medical or nursing orders are likely to involve continuous changes or complex modifications. Nursing care expectations are beyond those learned by the LPN/LVN during the educational program. The professional nurse assesses whether the situation is a complex nursing situation.

- **Delegated medical act.** During a delegated medical act, a physician's order is given to a registered nurse (RN), an LPN, or an LVN by a physician, dentist, or podiatrist.
- **Delegated nursing act.** In a delegated nursing act, an RN gives nursing orders to an RN, LPN, or LVN.
- **Direct supervision.** With direct supervision, the supervisor is continuously present to coordinate, direct, or inspect nursing care. The supervisor is in the building.
- **General supervision.** Under general supervision, a supervisor regularly coordinates, directs, or inspects nursing care and is within reach either in the building or by telephone.

CONTENT OF NURSE PRACTICE ACTS

The Nurse Practice Act of each state commonly includes the following content:
- Definition of nursing,
- Definition of LPN/LVN,
- Use of the title of LPN or LVN,
- Scope of practice,
- Elements of unprofessional conduct, and
- Functions of the state's board of nursing.

Learning Exercise

Get Familiar with Your State's Nurse Practice Act

Obtain a copy of your state's Nurse Practice Act (or occupational title act).
What does it state about the following topics?
1. Definition of licensed practical/vocational nursing in your state.

2. Use of the title LPN or LVN.
3. Specific functions of the LPN/LVN.
4. Elements of unprofessional conduct.

STATE BOARD OF NURSING (OR NURSE REGULATORY BOARD)

All states and provinces have examining councils that provide nursing examinations for licensure and review complaints that can lead to revocation of a license.

FUNCTIONS OF THE BOARD

State boards of nursing have committees or councils that decide whether specific activities are within the scope of LPN/LVN practice in their state. Because an activity is legal in one state, it does not make it legal in another state. See Box 20-1 for common Board of Nursing functions.

Some state nursing boards have developed a website and may offer a variety of services (e.g., license renewal, application for licensure by examination, verification of licensure status of a state nurse, change of address/phone number/e-mail address, download forms, links to continuing education courses, the state's Nurse Practice Act). It is important as a practical/vocational

Box 20-1 | *Common Board of Nursing Functions*

- Licensing and certifying nurses,
- Setting fees,
- Establishing standards for educational programs,
- Determining duration and renewal of licenses (some boards require continuing education credits for renewal of license),
- Maintaining inactive status lists,
- Carrying out disciplinary action for violators,
- Developing programs for impaired nurses, and
- Suspending and revoking licenses and dealing with the appeal process.

nurse to understand that you must limit your work to the area of nursing defined in the state's Nurse Practice Act.

In 2003 the National Association for Practical Nurse Education and Service, Inc. (NAPNES) issued a professional guideline for LPN/LVNs, "The LPN/LVN Fulfills the Professional Responsibilities of the Practical/Vocational Nurse" (see Appendix B). This is an example of a statement from an official nursing organization, but it does not carry the weight of law. These statements are useful as *guides* for behavior and may be used in a court of law as a point of reference.

The Nurse Practice Act of your state is always your final authority.

DISCIPLINARY RESPONSIBILITY OF THE BOARD

Each state's Nurse Practice Act lists specific reasons for which they seek to discipline a nurse. Eight general categories of disciplinary actions can be taken against nurses. "They are fraud and deceit; criminal activity; negligence; risk to patients because of physical or mental incapacity; violation of the nurse practice act or rules; disciplinary action by another board;

Box 20-2 | *Eight Categories of Disciplinary Actions Taken Against Nurses*

1. **Fraud and deceit:** Most often, fraud and deceit involves a person using fake means to get a nursing license (e.g., forging documents).
2. **Criminal activity:** Conviction of a felony, such as murder; or conviction for gross immorality, such as theft, fraud, personal misrepresentation, or embezzlement.
3. **Negligence:** The nurse does not do what a reasonable, prudent nurse would do in a similar situation. Negligence includes serious risk to the health, safety, or physical or mental health of a patient. (This may include patient injury.)
4. **Violation of the Nurse Practice Act:** Some state's Nurse Practice Acts spell out a specific violation in their state's Nurse Practice Act (e.g., unprofessional conduct, such as becoming personally involved with a patient).
5. **Discipline by another jurisdiction:** In the past it was difficult to find out if a nurse had been disciplined in another state. Now there are two national data banks that make it easier to track disciplinary action of LPN/LVNs in other states. However, it is not mandatory for the disciplining authority to notify a data bank. The data banks are as follows:
   a. *National Practitioner Data Bank* (NPDB). Established by federal law, it has been in operation since 1999. It contains information on final actions when guilt of a professional violation has been established or admitted. The NPDB primarily contains disciplinary actions taken against dentists and other health practitioners, including nurses. The

purpose of the data bank is to restrict the ability of incompetent professionals to move from state to state without disclosure of previous incompetence.
   b. *National Council of State Boards of Nursing Disciplinary Data Bank* (NCSBNDB) was established in 1990. It collects disciplinary information about nurses from, and distributes to all state boards of nursing. The state boards of nursing use this information for disciplinary and licensing purposes. Action by the Board can affect your license or certificate to practice in another state.
6. **Incompetence:** Examples include failure to meet generally accepted standards of nursing practice; negligence; and a nurse's mental disability that would interfere with patient safety.
7. **Unethical conduct:** Examples include a breach of nurse-patient confidentiality; refusal to provide nursing care for someone because of race, creed, color, national origin, disease, or sexual orientation; violation of the ethical code for LPN/LVNs; and failure to maintain nursing competence.
8. **Alcohol and/or other drug abuse:** Alcohol and other drug abuse by a nurse (e.g., diversion of drugs, often controlled substances, for personal use) is a threat to patient safety. Some nurses steal and sell diverted substances and equipment such as syringes and IV tubing, falsify patient records, and deprive patients of their medication, etc. The number of nurses disciplined for alcohol and/or other drug abuse is increasing.

incompetence; unethical conduct; and drug and/or alcohol use" (Brent, 2001). See Box 20-2 for Eight General Categories of Disciplinary Action.

DISCIPLINARY PROCESS AND ACTION

The disciplinary process is based on law and follows the rules of law. See Box 20-3 for the steps of a disciplinary process.

NURSING LICENSURE

It is nursing licensure that defines and protects the title of LPN or LVN. Some states (e.g., Minnesota) have amended their Nurse Practice

---

Box 20-3 | *Steps for Disciplinary Action*

- **Sworn complaint:** Filed against the LPN/LVN by a person, health care agency, or professional organization.
- **Complaint is reviewed:** The LPN/LVN receives a notice of the hearing, which will be before the State board of nursing or a state officer. Evidence of wrongdoing is presented to the nurse and board. The nurse and preferably the nurse's attorney, who understands nursing, present witnesses. The board makes a decision on findings.
- **Finding of not guilty:** No action is taken.
- **Finding of guilty of misconduct:** The board may issue a public or private reprimand, such as:
  - Continuing Education
  - Probation
  - Nonrenewal of license
  - Suspension of license
  - Revocation of license
  - If nurse is involved in alcohol or drug abuse, a diversion program may be an alternative. "Many states have developed Alternative to Discipline Programs for nurses with drug or alcohol dependencies that also meet certain requirements. These programs promote early intervention; support the treatment and recovery; and most important, monitoring when the nurse returns to work."

Information about the National Council of State Boards of Nursing can be obtained at *http://www.ncsbn.org/163.htm.*

Act to include the provision that only licensed practical or registered nurses may use the professional title "nurse."

On completion of a state-approved practical/vocational nursing education program, a graduate is eligible to apply for the national licensing examination in practical/vocational nursing (NCLEX-PN® examination). While awaiting examination results, the graduate may apply for a temporary permit to practice nursing. On successful completion of the examination, the graduate receives a nursing license. If the graduate nurse fails the NCLEX-PN® examination, the temporary permit is revoked. The graduate has an opportunity to retest at a later date for an additional fee. Until successful completion of the NCLEX-PN® examination, the temporary permit remains revoked and the graduate can work only as a nursing assistant.

WORKING IN OTHER STATES

States have arrangements for interstate endorsements for nurses who choose to work in other states. This means that it is possible to work in another state without repeating the NCLEX-PN® examination, after you meet that state's criteria for licensure by endorsement.

Some states are involved in multi-state licensure: mutual recognition model for nursing regulation. The NCSBN adopted the Nurse Multi-state Licensure Mutual Recognition Model in 1997. Utah was the first state to adopt the NCSBN compact language that took effect in 2000. The mutual recognition model allows a nurse to have one license in his or her state of residency and practice in other states, depending on each state's Nurse Practice Act and legislation. To become law, each state must pass the law as part of their state Nurse Practice Act. As of spring 2008, 21 states had mutual recognition compacts: Arizona, Arkansas, Colorado, Delaware, Idaho, Iowa, Kentucky, Maine, Maryland, Mississippi, Nebraska, New Hampshire, New Mexico, North Carolina, North Dakota, South Dakota, Tennessee, Texas, Utah, Virginia, and Wisconsin. A compact was pending in Rhode Island.

Learning Exercise

Compact States and the Nurse Practice Act

Obtain and read the Nurse Practice Act of a compact state by contacting that state's Board of Nursing. Addresses are available in Appendix A. If approved to work in a compact state, the LPN/LVN must know the contents of the NPA of the compact state.

The mutual recognition model is not the same as Minnesota's border recognition agreement (effective January 1, 2003), which allows nurses who have a license in the border states of Iowa, North Dakota, South Dakota, or Wisconsin to practice in Minnesota.

Learning Exercise

Interstate Agreement

Contact the board of nursing of the state in which you will be employed. Inquire if they have multi-state licensure or a border recognition agreement. If the state involved does not have such an agreement with other states, inquire what is needed for interstate endorsement.

VERIFICATION OF LICENSURE

Some boards of nursing are instituting online verification of nursing licensure. The board provides public information about nurses who have current licensure. The verification system enables potential employers to call and obtain a nurse's license number, registration expiration date, and whether any board action has taken place. The service is available 24 hours a day, 7 days a week.

Employers are able to use this option to comply with requirements for written verification of a nurse's registration by The Joint Commission (TJC).

UNLICENSED ASSISTIVE PERSONNEL

The use of unlicensed assistive personnel (UAP) to provide patient care has grown dramatically in recent years. (See Chapter 11.) It is expected that the trend will continue. These unlicensed persons are trained to perform a variety of nursing tasks. Licensed nurses need to be aware of specific training UAPs have had and facility job descriptions so that they may safely make assignments. Supervision of UAPs by the RN and the LPN/LVN charge nurse in long-term care to ensure safety of patient care is a major concern. There is concern that because of the lack of licensed nurses in an agency, duties might be delegated and/or assigned inappropriately to UAPs. It is the RNs and LPN/LVNs who stand to lose their jobs and licenses if the care provided by UAPs does not meet the standards of safety and effectiveness. The training program for UAPs does not provide the same in-depth education and experience that programs for student nurses provide. Licensed nurses are also accountable to both their employers and their state nursing boards.

NURSING STANDARD OF CARE

The nursing standard of care is your guideline for good nursing care. The phrase "you are held to the nursing standard of care" has important legal implications. The standard is based on what an ordinary, prudent nurse with similar education and nursing experience would do in similar circumstances. Resources for the nursing standard of care are found in Box 20-4. Note that unit routine ("I know you studied how to do this in nursing school, but this is how we do it here") is not on the list.

HOW THE LAW AFFECTS LPN/LVNS

COMMON LAW VERSUS STATUTORY LAW

The legal system in both the United States and Canada originates from English common law. Common law is called *judge-made law* because it originates in the courts. Common law is one way of establishing standards of legal conduct and is useful in settling disputes. Once the judge has made a decision, this decision *sets the precedent* for

Box 20-4 | *Resources for the Nursing Standard of Care*

- **Nurse Practice Act:** Identifies the minimum level of competency necessary for you to function as an LPN or LVN in your state.
- **Nursing licensure examination** (NCLEX-PN® examination): Tests for minimum competence.
- **Practical/vocational nursing programs:** Based on guidelines provided by the board of nursing, these programs guarantee a minimum knowledge base and the clinical practice necessary to provide safe nursing care.
- Curricula, textbooks, and instructors are resources for information about the standard of care.
- **Written policies and procedures:** The agency for which you work provides a standard of nursing care for you to follow. This is the reason why it is important for you to read the policies of the agency to find out whether verbal directions are supported by written policies. If a question about care ever comes up in court, a lawyer will use the agency's policy and procedure manual as one guide to expected behavior. Remember that policies and procedures do not overrule your state's Nurse Practice Act and educational preparation. However, institutional policies may be stricter than state law.
- **Custom:** An unwritten, usually acceptable way of giving nursing care. Expert witnesses, not your coworkers, would be called to testify to "the acceptable way."
- **Law:** Decisions that have been arrived at in similar cases brought up before a court (judge-made law).
- Statements from the NAPNES and NFLPN. See Appendixes B and C.
- Nursing texts and journals.
- Administrative rules of your board of nursing.

a ruling on a case with similar facts in the future. Informed consent and a patient's right to refuse treatment are examples of common law.

Statutory law is law developed by the legislative branch of the state and the U.S. Congress of the federal government. The Nurse Practice Act, which governs the practice of nursing, is an example of a statutory law. State boards of nursing can make nursing laws as long as the items in their laws do not conflict with any federal statutes.

CRIMINAL VERSUS CIVIL ACTION

The two classifications of legal action are criminal action and civil action. A criminal action involves people and society as a whole. It involves relationships between individuals and the government. A criminal action is classified as follows:

- **Misdemeanor:** A misdemeanor is the least serious charge and can result in a fine or prison for no more than a year. This criminal act might include taking a narcotic intended for the patient's pain relief and giving the patient another substance in its place.
- **Felony:** A felony is a serious offense with a penalty that ranges from more than 1 year in prison to death. For example, when the nurse injects a patient with a lethal drug to hasten death or removes life support before the patient has been pronounced dead by the physician.

Guilt on the part of the nurse needs to be established by producing proof **beyond a reasonable doubt**. Regardless of the outcome of the criminal case, when a criminal case is completed, it is possible to be sued in a civil court.

A civil action protects individual rights and *results in payment of money* to the injured person (e.g., a back injury was sustained during a fall because spilled urine was not wiped up. This injury caused the patient additional treatment time, including physical therapy, pain, suffering, and loss of time from work). A civil action involves a relationship between individuals and the violation of those rights. A **tort** is a civil wrong. The two kinds of torts are intentional and unintentional, which are described as follows:

- **Intentional:** An **intentional tort** is intended to cause harm to the patient (e.g., threat or actual physical harm).
- **Unintentional:** An **unintentional tort** did not mean to harm the patient. "I did not mean to hurt the patient" is no defense when you did

not use the "rule of 5" and gave the patient an incorrect medication, which caused injury.

Guilt on the part of the nurse can be established by a preponderance (majority) of the evidence. See Table 20-1 for a comparison of criminal and civil law.

INTENTIONAL TORTS

Tort law is based on the premise that in the course of relationships with each other there is a general **duty** to avoid injuring each other. A tort is a wrong or injury done to someone that violates his or her rights.

Intentional torts require a specific state of mind; that is, that the nurse intended to do the wrongful act. Assault and battery, false imprisonment and use of restraints, defamation that includes both libel and slander, and physical and emotional abuse are examples of intentional torts. Not all insurance companies cover intentional torts in their malpractice insurance policy. Check your policy.

Assault and Battery

Assault is an unjustified attempt or threat to touch someone. Battery means to cause physical harm to someone. When a patient refuses a treatment or medication, forcing the patient to take medication could result in an assault and battery charge against you. The patient gives *implied consent* (permission) for certain routine treatments when entering the institution. Patients retain the right to refuse any treatment verbally and may leave the institution when they choose, unless they are there for court-ordered treatment. Nurses can also protect themselves from assault by a patient, but can use only as much force as is considered reasonable for self-protection.

Treating a patient without consent is battery even if the treatment is medically beneficial. A physician might go to the court to attempt to get a court order to allow a blood transfusion for someone opposed on religious grounds. If the patient is fully competent, is not pregnant, and has no children, the court is likely to rule for the patient even if a blood transfusion would save their life. When faced with a similar situation, the practical/vocational nurse respects the patient's belief system and notifies the supervisor for further advice or interpretation.

Table 20-1 | *Comparison of Two Basic Classifications of Law*

	CIVIL LAW	CRIMINAL LAW
Who law generally applies to	Relationships between private individuals and infringements on individual rights	Relationships between individuals and the government (state) Society as a whole
Sources of law	U.S. Constitution, state and federal legislatures	U.S. Constitution, state, and federal legislatures
Punishment for breaking law	Payment of a monetary compensation	Death, imprisonment, fines, restrictions
How guilt is established	Proof by a preponderance of the evidence	Proof beyond a reasonable doubt
Examples of nursing liability	Contract Tort Unintentional Intentional Negligence	Murder, rape, larceny, homicide, manslaughter, assault and battery, embezzlement Felony/misdemeanor

Basic sources of law:

Common law—judge-made law. A trial judge's ruling lays down a legal principle and sets a precedent. These principles are used to decide future cases. This type of law is continually adapted and expanded.

Statutory law—formal legislative enactment. Law passed by Congress or enacted by state government. May be amended, repealed, or expanded by the legislature. Nurse Practice Act is an example of statutory law.

False Imprisonment and Use of Restraints

False imprisonment is keeping someone detained against his or her will. It can include use of restraints or seclusion in a room without cause and without a physician's order. Restraint by verbal threats of physical harm is also included in this category. **Chemical restraint** (with medication) is defined as administering a PRN medication with a sedating side effect every 4 hours to keep the patient tired and in his or her room. The intent is to keep the patient quiet and out of the way. The intended use of the medication has been circumvented to meet the nurse's need.

Defamation

Defamation means damage to someone's reputation through false communication or communication without their permission. Libel and slander are included in this category and are described as follows:

- **Libel** is defamation through **written** communication or pictures.
- Slander is defamation by **verbalizing** untrue or private information (gossip) to a third party.

The patient has the right to expect you to speak the truth. Additional unnecessary conversation with coworkers and those outside the agency can result in a charge of defamation. The same is true for taking unwanted photographs or showing a patient's injury, cancerous growth, gunshot wound, etc., to others, students included, without patient permission.

Consider also that you often are privy to information about the personal lives of other nurses, physicians, and other coworkers, and they are privy to information about you. Although the desire to repeat the information you hear may be tempting, it is best left unsaid.

Physical and Emotional Abuse

Physical abuse is generally easier to identify, although the victim may find creative ways to hide the injuries, for a period of time. Emotional abuse is often difficult to identify. The person doing the abusing may be very personable and attentive to the victim when they are in public. A former student described how everyone thought her husband loved her and how fortunate she was. When they were alone, he would tell her she was ugly, worthless, and no one else would ever want her or love her. When she became pregnant, he would always take her to her doctor appointment. He answered the questions for her and when she tried to speak, he would take over in gentle terms, doing the explaining. At no time was she alone with a doctor or nurse.

In the course of your career in practical/vocational nursing you will probably suspect or actually see the results of some type of abuse. As a practical/vocational nurse, you have a legal responsibility to report your suspicions or observations of abuse by following your facility's abuse policy. Note that a "suspicion" is a nagging doubt. Refer to your state's abuse laws for specific rules that govern your responsibility for reporting abuse. It is important to be empathetic (as opposed to sympathetic) so that your observations or reporting will be as objective as possible. Becoming a part of the patient's emotions may lead you to jump to conclusions or accept a particularly convincing but untrue explanation. Whether the patient is a child, woman, man, or elder, reputations are at stake. Once an accusation has been made, it is difficult to be truly free from it, even when proved groundless.

Follow your facility's policy for reporting abuse. The social services department can help you report abuse. Offer concrete, specific observations. Quote statements made and avoid offering a personal interpretation. Let the facts speak for themselves.

UNINTENTIONAL TORTS

An unintentional tort holds that the nurse did not intend to injure the patient. However, the nurse did not maintain the nursing standard of care and did not do what a prudent nurse with comparable education and skills would do in a similar situation. Negligence and malpractice (professional negligence) are examples of unintentional torts.

NEGLIGENCE

"**Negligence** is defined as conduct which falls below the standards established by the law for the protection of others against the unreasonable risk of harm" (Brent). A common type of negligence is personal injury. For example, your town has a law that states sidewalks must be shoveled within 24 hours after a snowstorm. Your sidewalk has not been shoveled within the 24 hours and your neighbor falls in front of your house and breaks an arm. The neighbor sues you for negligence. It is important to remember that in negligence the property owner did not intend to cause the injury to the neighbor, but knowing the risks and the law, he or she should have guarded against the injury. Good intentions do not enter in. It is your conduct, not your intent, which is the issue.

MALPRACTICE (PROFESSIONAL NEGLIGENCE)

Malpractice, the legal name for professional negligence, means negligence by a professional, in this case an LPN/LVN. The most common type of negligence in practical/vocational nursing relates to action or lack of action, not what you intended to do. See Box 20-5 for the most common sources of malpractice, according to O'Keefe (2001).

According to Zittel, senior manager of the New York Education Department's Office of the Professions, "I have told RNs that one of the reasons there are a lot more legal actions brought against LPNs is because you are abusing them.

Box 20-5 | *Some Common Sources of Malpractice*

- Medication and treatment errors,
- Lack of observation and timely reporting about the patient,
- Defective technologies or equipment,
- Infections caused or worsened by poor nursing care,
- Poor communication of important information, including change of condition, and
- Failure to intervene to protect the patient from poor medical care.

RNs are placing them in situations where LPNs have to make assessments and decisions when they are not supposed to." Zittel urged educators to advise students how to protect themselves and their license. For instance, LPNs who work in long-term care should have contact information of the RN on call and make sure that person will be able to respond to them within 15–30 minutes (*http://www.advanceweb.com/lpn*, May 21, 2007). This statement supports the need for LPN/LVNs to know their scope of practice and adhere to it.

All the charges of professional negligence (malpractice) listed could be avoided by good nursing practice (i.e., what a reasonable, prudent nurse would do in a similar situation).

Reminder: The student practical/vocational nurse is held to the level of a licensed practical/vocational nurse's performance.

There are occasions when the evidence is overwhelming and indicates the accused nurse is responsible for the patient injury. Such an occasion is called *res ipsa loquitur*, meaning the evidence speaks for itself. For example, a patient develops respiratory distress immediately after the nurse administered an improper medication to him or her.

MALPRACTICE INSURANCE FOR NURSES

More nurses are being named in lawsuits. Nurses assume liability for their own acts. Although the employing agency may assume responsibility for the nurse during a lawsuit, the agency can then turn around and sue the nurse. You can also be held responsible for the "neighborhood advice" you give—for example, telling a neighbor how to care for her sick child.

Each nurse must carefully consider whether it is necessary to purchase a malpractice insurance policy. Incidents of suing for malpractice continue, although your chances of being sued as an LPN/LVN are statistically small. Look carefully at the policy of the agency of which you are an employee. Some reasons for having your own malpractice insurance are found in Box 20-6.

| Box 20-6 | *Reasons for Your Own Malpractice Insurance* |

- The jury's award could exceed the limits of your agency's coverage.
- Your *employing agency* could pay out an award to a plaintiff and then counter-sue you.
- You acted outside the scope of employment, and the agency argues it is not liable.
- Your employer's policy covers you only on the job.
- An agency might carry a policy that covers you only while you are employed by that institution. A suit may come up years after you have stopped working for the employer. It is suggested that nurses purchase occurrence coverage if malpractice coverage is desired and not claims coverage. For this reason, occurrence coverage protects the nurse for each incident regardless of present employer.
- The agency may decide to settle out of court. Plaintiff could pursue a case against the nurse.
- Has your employer paid the insurance premium?
- After a settlement, *insurers* could turn around and sue the nurse.
- With your own coverage you will have your own lawyers, not the lawyers also defending the agency.

Learning Exercise

Malpractice Coverage

If you are currently assigned to a clinical area, find out what the agency policy is on malpractice coverage for practical/vocational nurses. Your instructor will be a good source in helping you locate this information.

FOUR ELEMENTS NEEDED TO PROVE NEGLIGENCE

Duty, breach of duty, damages, and proximate cause are the four elements that must be present to cause an action for negligence against the nurse. Each of the four elements must be proved by the patient to receive compensation. See Box 20-7 for the Four Elements Needed to Prove Negligence.

| Box 20-7 | *Four Elements Needed to Prove Negligence* |

1. Duty refers to the nurse's responsibility to provide care in an acceptable way. The nurse has a duty based on education, as well as the policies and standards of the place of employment.
2. Breach of duty means that the nurse did not adhere to the nursing standard of care. What was expected of the nurse was not done (omission) or was not done correctly (commission). An expert nurse witness establishes the standard of care.
3. Damages mean that the patient must be able to show that the nurse's negligent act injured him or her in some way. The patient must prove actual damage.
4. Proximate cause means that a reasonable cause-and-effect relationship can be shown between the omission or commission of the nursing act and the harm to the patient. Did the nurse's negligent act cause the injury in question?

STEPS FOR BRINGING LEGAL ACTION

Legal actions follow an orderly process. Remember that the nurse also has rights and is not considered guilty simply because someone filed a complaint. Steps for bringing a legal action by a patient are found in Box 20-8.

DEPOSITIONS

Depositions are used to gather information under oath (fact finding). Once the deposition is scheduled, provide information on where and how you can be reached. The depositions usually take place in an attorney's office. You may be able to request that it be in your attorney's office. (It will be helpful to have an attorney who understands nursing and is familiar with legal action against a nurse). Opponents' attorneys may also be present. However, only one of the opponent's attorneys should be permitted to ask questions so as not to "tag team," i.e., each fire questions at the nurse. A court reporter or stenographer will record your testimony.

■

| Box 20-8 | *Steps for Bringing a Legal Action by a Patient*

- The patient believes that the nurse has violated his or her legal rights.
- The patient seeks the advice of an attorney.
- The attorney has a nurse expert review the patient's chart to see whether the nurse has violated the nursing standard of care. If it is determined that a standard of care has been violated, a lawsuit is begun.
- The patient (the plaintiff) files a complaint that documents the grievance (violation of rules). This is served to the defendant (the nurse).
- The defendant responds in writing.
- The discovery period (pretrial activity) begins. Statements are taken from the defendant nurse, witnesses, nurse expert, patient (plaintiff), and other caregivers. Policies and procedures of the health care facilities are reviewed.
- During the trial, important information is presented to the judge or jury. A verdict (decision) is reached. The plaintiff (the patient) has the burden of proof (evidence of wrongdoing) during the trial.
- An appeal (request for another trial) can be made if either the plaintiff or the defendant does not consider the verdict acceptable.

Look professional as you would for a job interview. (See Chapter 21.)

Do your utmost to be calm and polite no matter how rude others, including the opposing attorney are to you.

HOW YOUR ATTORNEY WILL ASSIST

In preparation for a deposition, your attorney will:
- Provide a checklist of basic instructions for the deposition,
- Practice likely questions that may be asked and critique your responses,
- Prepare you for types of questions that may slant your testimony,
- Suggest appropriate ways to respond, but not tell you what to answer,

- Use a practice deposition video (usually, not always),
- Meet with you in advance, the day of the deposition to answer any last minute questions.

GIVING TESTIMONY

There are some basics to keep in mind during a deposition:
- It is important to tell the truth. Stick to the truth. Avoid being clever.
- A court reporter or stenographer can only record words, so questions must be answered verbally.
- Listen carefully to the question. If you do not understand the question, ask that the question be repeated or rephrased.
- Before answering, pause. This will give you an opportunity to consider the question. Think about what is being asked and how you will answer.
- Be specific in answering a question: if it is a "yes" or "no" question, then answer it that way. *Resist the urge to say more.* If you do not know the answer to a question, say so, and do not speculate. If you do not remember, say, "I do not remember."
- If your attorney instructs you to not answer a question, do not answer. Instruction to not answer a question is permitted under certain circumstances.
- Be careful not to reveal content of any conversation with your attorney.
- Ask for a break especially if you are tired or not thinking clearly. If there is a question pending, you will be expected to answer it before taking a break.
- You will not be permitted to take any notes during the deposition, nor will you be able to bring in notes, files, a calendar, note pad, or pen (Main and Todd, 2005).
- A few weeks after the deposition your attorney and you may be able to review the testimony and make corrections. You may be asked about the corrections during the trial.

GENERAL GUIDELINES FOR CHARTING

Charting (legal documentation) is part of your job as a nurse. It is not busy work. Legal documentation is required in all health care agencies. The forms and charting systems may be different, but the basics remain the same. The chart is a legal document and can be used in court. Review the charting procedure for your specific agency and adhere to it. Legal charting is also an opportunity for you to show that you have a legitimate knowledge base. It gives credibility to practical/vocational nursing as a vocation. Charting gives you the opportunity to show that you functioned within the standard of care.

Box 20-9   *A List of Charting Guidelines*

- Date and time should accompany each entry
- Each entry should be accurate, factual, specific, and objective. Nurses must constantly remind themselves to avoid subjective comments when charting. Subjective comments are judgments made by you. Avoid them. Eliminate the word "appears," except when it refers to a situation in which the patient is sleeping.
- Each entry must be legible, spelled correctly, and grammatically correct. A lawyer can question your ability to give competent nursing care if you do not have command of the English language. Print, if this is an agency policy, or if your handwriting is hard to read. Use correct punctuation, because the meaning of a sentence can change based on punctuation. Sloppy charting may be interpreted as sloppy or unsafe nursing care. It communicates that you did not take the time to write, and a lawyer could accuse you of not taking the time to care.
- Place entries on the chart as soon as possible after events occur. Chart entries are always entered in chronological order. This indicates when the event happened in the time column. If someone else charts before you are able to record an entry or if you have forgotten to record an entry, a late entry may be used. Put the actual charting time in the time column for the late entry and include the actual date and time of the events in the nurses' notes.
- For written entries, use permanent ink (no erasable pens) in the color identified in the institution's procedure manual. The trend is to use black ink and military time. Avoid using highlighters on any chart form. Many do not show up on photocopies or fax copies.
- Do not leave blank lines. If an item on a flow sheet does not apply, write in N/A (not applicable).

If other staff persons need to make an entry, do not save lines. They can make a late entry. Write your legal signature and title on the right. Use a line to fill in any empty space before your signature.
- Quotation marks to indicate "ditto" are never used.
- Use only approved abbreviations that are found in the institution's policy and procedure manual. Adhere to The Joint Commission 2005 official "do-not-use" list of abbreviations and those you learned in the classroom. The do-not-use list can be accessed at: *http://www.jointcommission. org/PatientSafety/NationalPatientSafetyGoals/07.*
- Document medical and nursing treatments performed and the patient's response to these treatments. If the patient refuses treatments, document the reason for refusal.
- When seeking help in difficult situations, document communication with supervisors by name and content of conversation.
- As an LPN/LVN, do not cosign for nursing students. If you must sign off a patient chart that is not for one of your patients, write, "I'm signing this to complete the record; I have no knowledge of the patient."
- Documenting another student's or staffs care that you did not witness or participate in leaves you liable for that person's errors. Additionally, this charting has limited creditability in the eyes of a court (considered secondhand information). It is prudent to refuse to do the charting for someone else.
- Do not add any notes once charting is complete, unless you use a late entry format.
- Do not delete notes or correct errors with "White Out" ink on written notes. When an error is made in charting, draw a single line through the error,

Continued

Box 20-9 | *A List of Charting Guidelines—cont'd*

write in the date and time, and sign. Do not write "error" above the entry; instead, write, "mistake in entry." A court may interpret the term "error" as indicating incorrect care.
- Record all abnormal observations, including changes in the patient's condition, and to whom these observations were reported.
- Record care actually given, not what will be given in the future.
- Each dated and timed entry must be signed using your full, legal title, as determined by your state.
- If you did not chart it, you did not do it, and a lawyer will surmise that you did not care!
- Avoid treating flow sheets casually. If you place a symbol indicating normal findings, be sure you have reviewed the health agency's parameters for normal findings. These can usually be found on the flow sheet.

- When doing computer charting, consider your sign-on code as equivalent to your signature. Use only your code and do not let anyone else use yours. Protect the patient's right to confidentiality by not leaving personal information available for viewing during charting or when you have completed your charting. Most computers are fitted with a computer screen that comes on quickly after use. With the new HIPAA (Health Insurance Portability and Accountability Act) rules, computers that previously faced the hall for the convenience of staff will no longer do so.
- Legally, it is important to document every intervention or patient instruction.
- If someone gives medication to your patient, they are responsible for doing all documentation including the data collection and the patient's response to the medication.

All formats, regardless of which method of charting is used by an agency, are adapted to the computer. Certain guidelines apply. See Box 20-9 for A List of Charting Guidelines.

LIABILITY

KINDS OF LIABILITY

Personal liability holds us responsible for our own behavior, including negligent behavior. This rule makes it impossible to completely shift responsibility onto someone else.

Vicarious liability means responsibility for actions of another because of a special relationship with the other. The term *respondeat superior,* Latin for "let the master speak," is based on vicarious liability. It is applied in the following two different ways:

1. **Borrowed servant doctrine** (e.g., the master/servant relationship between an employer [hospital] and an employee [nurse]). The employer (master) is assumed to be better able to pay for the injuries than the employee (servant). The employer may also be held responsible in a suit for the negligent acts of the employee performed during the time

of employment. This provides incentive for health care agencies to hire carefully, as well as orient and supervise the work of the employee.

2. **Captain of the ship doctrine** (e.g., in an operating room). A nurse becomes the temporary employee of the physician doing the surgery. This doctrine assumes that in this situation the surgeon exerts control of the nurse in relation to specific conduct that caused patient injury in the operating room.

Institutional liability is vicarious liability. It assumes that the health facility provides certain safeguards to keep the patient from harm. This includes a safe facility to prevent physical harm (e.g., adequate supervision of staff, adequate staffing, and safe equipment).

COMMON CAUSES OF NURSING LIABILITY

Many of the errors leading to common nursing liabilities can be avoided by following the guidelines you learned in nursing school. The major areas of liability (responsibility/accountability) can be categorized as lack of safety, knowledge, skill, observation and reporting, documentation, and acceptance of responsibility for nursing actions—

all of which are part of the usual clinical evaluation. The most common errors are drug errors, most of which can be avoided if you follow the guidelines you learn in basic nursing and practice in the clinical areas. One of the best defenses for prevention of legal liability is development of rapport with the patient. If you treat patients with courtesy and respect, they are less likely to sue (unless you provide care below the nursing standard of care). The very best defense is not to err in the first place.

RESPONSIBILITY AND ACCOUNTABILITY IN NURSING

Nursing demands that you be responsible. This means being reliable and trustworthy. At no time can you expect a peer, supervisor, or patient to say to you, "It's OK that you didn't come to work today because your car isn't functioning properly," or, "It's OK if we talk about your interests and problems today" (rather than those of the patients), or, "It's OK that you didn't do the work you were assigned because you're having a bad day." Nursing says, "I'm sorry that you have problems to cope with that are heavy, but it's up to you to deal with them because your priority in this vocation is the patient."

The word accountability means that you are answerable. As a nursing student, you are answerable to yourself, to your assigned patient, to the team leader, to the physician, and to your instructor, who constantly evaluates your work. As an LPN/LVN, accountability to the instructor is replaced by accountability to the employing agency. You are held accountable for all the nursing actions that you perform or are assigned to perform. The measures of accountability are the following nursing standards of practice:

- Nurse Practice Act of the state,
- NAPNES Standards and Educational Competencies of Graduates of Practical/ Vocational Nursing Programs (Appendix B),
- NFLPN Nursing Practice Standards for the Licensed Practical/Vocational Nurse (Appendix C)

They recommend minimal acceptable standards of nursing behavior for the SPN/SVN and the LPN/LVN.

LIABILITY OF STUDENT NURSES AND INSTRUCTORS

Student nurses are held accountable for the nursing care they give. They are held to the standards of a licensed practical/vocational nurse. This emphasizes *the necessity to prepare for providing care for assigned patients in the clinical area.* The instructor has the responsibility to make patient assignments based on the student's knowledge base and ability to give safe nursing care. The instructor is also expected to provide reasonable supervision for the care given by a student. A list of your responsibilities is found in Box 20-10.

FUNCTIONING BEYOND THE SCOPE OF PRACTICE AND EXPERIENCE OF AN LPN/LVN

As an LPN/LVN, you might be asked by an RN or physician to perform nursing duties beyond your scope of practice or experience. It is up to you to speak up. Box 20-11 contains examples of responses when asked to perform beyond your scope of practice.

When seeking employment check out the philosophy, mission statement, and policies of

---

Box 20-10 | *SPN/SVN Responsibilities for Patient Care*

- Prepare by reading the assigned patient's chart, patient profile, and plan of care, and develop your own plan of care for the patient to whom you are assigned.
- Look up action, safety of ordered dose, side effects, and nursing considerations for the assigned patient's routine, PRN medications, and IV additives.
- Review how to do ordered treatments.
- Compose a time sequence for care during your time with the patient.
- When you arrive on the clinical unit, review your plan of care with the instructor before you begin your nursing care.
- Identify a need for, and request additional help or supervision.
- Comply with agency and school of nursing policies.

| Box 20-11 | *Possible Responses When Asked to Perform Beyond Your Scope of Practice*

- "I am not legally able to do something beyond the LPN/LVN Nurse Practice Act."
- "I have never done this before. I will be glad to learn if you teach me, watch me demonstrate in return, and write a memo for my file that you have taught me to do this and watched a satisfactory return demonstration."
- "I was taught to do this while in school but did not have a chance to catheterize a real person. Please demonstrate and then watch me do a catheterization, before I catheterize a patient on my own."
- "My orientation here did not include how to make daily assignments according to skill level of staff. I need to be shown. Will you show me how to make assignments? I learn quickly, so it will be time well spent."
- "You have provided a detailed orientation, but I do not feel ready (or qualified) to assume a charge nurse position. I think I need more experience as a staff nurse, so I can function effectively and within my Nurse Practice Act."

your potential place of employment. Ask what is included in your job, the period of orientation you will receive, what the orientation will cover, and who will do the orientation. If you discover during your inquiry that your work will cover more than you have learned or tasks are beyond the scope of practice, say so. Listen also to your affective response: What is your intuition saying? Getting a job just to get a job may result in your being fired or losing your license. You may end up losing your job for what may not be your fault. The *ideal* of your ethics is that all share your ethics and are fair. The *reality* of ethics is sometimes quite different.

SPECIFIC PATIENT SITUATIONS

A professional relationship between the nurse and the patient is essential for the provision of nursing care. Legal precedent has established that the health care agency also has a responsibility to the patient. Patients have become increasingly concerned and vocal about the quality of care they expect to receive. Many of the issues are directly related to privacy, confidentiality, and safety. These are also concerns of health agencies and health care workers, including nurses.

PRIVACY AND CONFIDENTIALITY

Privacy in health care means the right to be left alone and free from intrusion, including the right to choose care based on personal beliefs, feelings, or attitudes; the right to govern bodily integrity (accepting or rejecting treatment or exposure of the body); and the right to control when and how sensitive information is shared. Confidentiality in health care refers to the nondisclosure of information regarding patients.

INFORMATION THAT MUST BE REVEALED

There are laws that require reporting of certain patient information without the patient's consent. The purpose is to protect the public. Patient information that must be revealed is in Box 20-12.

PATIENT'S RIGHTS

"Patient rights in all types of institutions are mandated by the U.S. Constitution and by state and federal laws. Legal rights might vary depending on the setting and the individual's competency" (Tyson, 1999).

The American Hospital Association (AHA) developed "The Patient's Bill of Rights" in 1972. It was revised in 2003, and renamed the "The Patient Care Partnership: Understanding Expectations, Rights, and Responsibilities." This is an ethical, not legal, document for hospitals recommending ways to guarantee patient rights. It is intended as a model for states to develop rights statements. Some state legislatures have adopted patient rights statements. Additional bills of rights have been developed for pregnant patients, nursing home residents, mental health patients, etc. Box 20-13 includes The Patient Care Partnership Recommendations.

Box 20-12 | *Patient Information That Must Be Revealed*

In all situations the supervisor, director of nursing, and policy set by the facility are resources.

- **Communicable disease:** To the local health department or the Centers for Disease Control and Prevention. This includes AIDS, but the nature of the disclosure varies according to state law.
- **Vaccine-related adverse reactions:** To the Department of Health and Human Services. (Reporting of some reactions is mandatory; for others it is voluntary. Call (800) 822–7967 for the Food and Drug Administration's reportable events table.)
- **Criminal acts:** All states mandate reporting of rape cases. Some mandate reporting of injuries by gunshot or sharp instruments. Some states require reporting of blood alcohol levels (BAL) beyond the legal limit. Clarify your state's specific mandates. The local police department is a good place to clarify what is reportable before an incident occurs.

- **Equipment-related injuries:** When use of a medical device results in injury or death, it is reported immediately to your supervisor and physician. If emergency first aid is called for, follow the procedure you have been taught.
- **When there is a clear and present danger:** HIPAA laws, for example, mandate reporting of patient mistreatment or professional misconduct. Report immediately to your supervisor or follow the policy manual for an emergency course of action.
- **Abuse and neglect of a patient or elderly person:** Report the incident immediately to your supervisor or director of nursing. They will usually follow up by reporting to police or social services.
- **Incompetence or unprofessional acts:** As defined by state law. Facilities have policies for how to report and to whom. Report immediately to your supervisor, to your director of nursing, or as directed in the facility's policy manual. Violation of nursing law will be reported to the State board of nursing.

Box 20-13 | *The Patient Care Partnership Recommendations*

- High quality hospital care.
- A clean and safe environment.
- Involvement in your own care
- Protection of your privacy.
- Help when leaving the hospital.
- Help with your billing claims (AHA, 2003).

Learning Exercise

Patient's Rights

Obtain a copy of your state or health facility's patient rights statement. Briefly explain what is meant by each of the main topics. Identify the topics that are a part of what you have already learned in nursing.

HEALTH INSURANCE PORTABILITY AND ACCOUNTABILITY ACT (HIPAA)

The U.S. Health Insurance Portability and Accountability Act (HIPAA) rules took effect on April 14, 2003, for health insurance companies, hospitals, clinics, doctors, pharmacies, and other health groups throughout the United States. The original intent of HIPAA was portability of employees from one job to the next. Portability is addressed in the law, but the main focus of the law is privacy. The law gives the patient rights over their health information. Basic HIPAA terminology is located in Box 20-14.

Basics of HIPAA

The following are the three basic parts of HIPAA:

1. **Protection of privacy.** HIPAA provides a guide for health-related facilities and individuals to establish privacy standards based on the HIPAA model. This is intended as a national privacy standard throughout the United States. When discussing privacy, HIPAA uses the term *protected health information* (PHI) when referring to patient information that should not be revealed.
2. **Administrative simplification.** The overall goal of administrative simplification is to reduce paperwork related to health care

Box 20-14 | *Basic HIPAA Terminology*

- **HIPAA:** Passed in 1996. Enforcement began April 14, 2003.
- **Portability:** Original intent of HIPAA (see Chapter 18) was portability of health insurance for employees from one job to the next.
- **Protection of patient privacy:** Main focus of HIPAA is protection of patient health information.
- **Covered entity:** Health facilities that provide, bill, or receive payment for health care as a normal part of business.
- **Health care:** Any care, services, or supplies related to care of a patient.
- **Privacy officer:** HIPAA requirement that all covered entities designate a privacy officer.
- **Notice of privacy practices:** Each covered entity must develop a document, written in plain language that explains the facility's privacy practices. It is distributed to all patients. The notice is also posted in a prominent place, to be read by all interested parties.
- **Department of Health and Human Services** (DHHS): The federal agency that oversees HIPAA.
- **Mandatory law:** Law that must be followed or penalties will be involved.

reimbursement (e.g., a goal is to develop a universal insurance claim form).

3. **Security standards.** The overall goal is establishing security standards for protection of electronic (computer and fax) transmission of PHI (e.g., password protection when using a computer is a HIPAA requirement).

 Critical Thinking Exercise

Patient Privacy

List examples of patient information that can compromise patient privacy if revealed.

_____

_____

_____

The Department of Health and Human Services is the federal agency that oversees HIPAA. It has emphasized reasonableness as a guide to applying HIPAA regulations. Depending on the facility with which you are involved, interpretation of HIPAA ranges from reasonable to very strict. HIPAA rules and regulations have been reviewed and updated yearly since 2003.

The Notice of Privacy Practices

The main focus of HIPAA is protection of privacy. Each covered entity must develop a written "Notice of Privacy Practices." The notice is made available to all patients, employees, and health-related companies with whom the facility does business (e.g., health insurance companies, medical equipment companies). The patient receives a personal copy to read and sign. Signing the copy denotes understanding of and agreement with the use and disclosure of PHI for treatment, payment, and facility operation. This is not the same as consent for treatment.

If the patient is incompetent, state laws are followed. This usually means that the patient's health proxy is treated as though he or she is the patient.

What the Notice of Privacy Practices Addresses

The Notice of Privacy Practices must address the following in plain language:

1. **Access to medical records.** Patients have a right to a copy of their medical record and to review the medical record upon request. The facility determines under what conditions the record can be reviewed. Generally this means reviewing the record with an RN or a physician present to translate medical terminology and answer questions. At no time does an SPN/SVN or LPN/LVN provide the record, or any part of it, to the patient. The request must follow the protocol set up by the facility. The Notice of Privacy Practices

must clearly state how to access the record. HIPAA provides up to 30 days for a facility to provide a medical record for a patient. However, Medicare regulations require that the record be made available to a Medicare patient within 24 hours.

2. **Amendments to the medical record.** According to HIPAA, patients have the right to request changes in their medical records. All covered entities must appoint privacy officers. It is the job of the privacy officer to process a request for change in a patient's medical record. The facility is obligated to consider the request and then notify the patient of the final decision.

3. **Restrictions on the use of protected health information.** Patients can restrict use of their PHI as long as the requested information does not interfere with activities related to treatment, payment, or facility operation. The privacy officer usually makes the final decision.

4. **Access to an accounting.** Patients can request a list of the people, companies, or agencies that have received their PHI. The Notice of Privacy Practices lists steps for requesting an accounting on written request from a patient.

5. **Confidential communications.** Patients may request that PHI be delivered in such a way that the sender cannot be identified. For example, the patient may request that blood test results be mailed in a plain envelope without the agency's return address.

6. **Complaints about violations of privacy.** Patients can file a complaint if they think their privacy has been violated. The Notice of Privacy Practices tells them how to contact the privacy officer, as well as how to file the complaint. The Notice also provides information on how to contact the Department of Health and Human Services (DHHS), the federal oversight agency for HIPAA. If a patient is not satisfied with the outcome of filing a complaint with the facility's privacy officer, they may choose to contact DHHS. If DHHS determines there is reason to investigate, they will do so and impose a fine on the covered entity if it has violated HIPAA law.

7. **Minimum necessary rule.** This rule assists you in making an on-the-spot decision about how much patient PHI you need to divulge. For example, if you are ordering a special bed for a patient, you will need to include the patient's height and weight. You will usually have no reason to include diagnosis, among other information.

8. **Telephone requests for PHI.** Nurses are often faced with telephone inquiries about a patient. It is difficult to identify who is really making the inquiry and for what purpose. "HIPAA suggests that whenever a caller asks for a patient, the provider can verify whether that person is in the hospital, but only if the caller asks for the patient by name. If the caller asks for specific information about the patient, the new guidelines recommend that only minimal information about general status be communicated. The caller should be directed to speak to the patient or family for further details" (Ecker, 2003). Exceptions to this rule include clergy who ask for all people of a certain faith or a patient who requests anonymity on admission. A parent, for example, may request anonymity regarding their child's hospitalization when there is concern of the child being abducted by the other parent.

9. **Email and faxes.** To reduce the possibility of error during electronic transfer of information, the "minimum necessary" rule applies. Perhaps you have experienced sending an email or fax to the wrong person. Think about the possible consequences of this happening with PHI. One safety feature is a disclaimer on an email or fax that identifies the mail as confidential and explains how to notify the sender in case of error.

Critical Thinking Exercise

Medical Records

Think of one or more reasons why a patient's removing or changing information in a medical record can affect a pending legal case.

Additional Concerns Not Addressed by HIPAA

Additional concerns not addressed by HIPAA include discarding PHI that is not meant for the patient's chart, and hallway conversation. See Box 20-15.

Learning Exercise

Maintain Patient Confidentiality

Keep confidential the conversations you overhear on the clinical area that include personal information about a patient and those that include more than the "minimum necessary" about a patient.

Box 20-15 | *Additional Concerns Not Addressed by HIPAA**

- PHI not meant for the chart includes daily patient assignments, nurse's personal notes about the patient (used as the basis for charting), and anything else with patient—identifying information that ends up crumpled and thrown in the wastebasket at the end of the shift. Many facilities are already dealing with this by identifying a specific disposal area where the notes ultimately get shredded.
- Hallway conversation remains a problem. For example, a conversation about a patient might not be overheard by the patient involved but is often overheard by other patients or visitors. The same is true with conversation in lunchrooms, nursing desk areas, waiting rooms, and elevators.

*Adapted from Ecker M. Protecting patient privacy: understanding the new federal HIPAA standards. *Midwest/Heartland Nurse Week*, Aug 18, 2003, pp. 20–21, and Anderson F. *Finding HIPAA in Your Soup*, February 2007.

Expect to find differences in interpretation of the law. Find a copy of the facility privacy policy during each clinical rotation and do the same with each job you have after graduation. Note the differences and adjust to them.

THE JOINT COMMISSION (TJC) NATIONAL PATIENT SAFETY GOALS

Nursing has always promoted safety first with patients, so TJC National Patient Safety Goals may seem too simple to make into hospital goals. Do not be fooled: TJC has been reviewing adverse incidents studies on causes of serious harm and death to patients since the mid-1990s. The results are startling. For example, the Institute of Medicine's 1999 study estimated that 44,000 to 98,000 Americans die each year as a result of medical errors. High on the errors list is medication error. Improper patient identification is often a problem in giving medication and also in doing wrong-site surgery. Nurses are often involved in the preparation for surgery and marking the site so that no confusion exists during the surgical process. Additional information is available at *http://www.jointcommission. org/PatientSafetyGoals*.

National Patient Safety Goals

TJC National Patient Safety Goals have been revised yearly since their conception. *There are gaps in numbering of the 2007 goals. Some original goals have been retired usually because the requirements were integrated into the standards. The number of the old goal is dropped and the numbering for new goals is continued. This is done so there will be no confusion about the content of a goal that is current.* See Box 20-16 for a listing of TJC 2007 Patient Safety Goals.

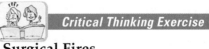

Critical Thinking Exercise

Surgical Fires

See Box 20-16. Goal 11 speaks of surgical fires. How do you prevent fires on a medical floor?

Box 20-16 | *TJC 2007 Patient Safety Goals*

- **Goal 1**. Improve the accuracy of patient identification. For example, before giving medication, have at least two ways to identify the patient (neither one can be the room number). The patient's wristbands, with identifying data, and the patient's chart, with matching name and patient number, are acceptable.
- **Goal 2**. Improve effectiveness of communication among caregivers. For example, use standard abbreviations and the 2005 TJC "do-not-use" abbreviation list. Check with your instructor if you are unable to read a doctor's order or other notes on the chart. Review the patient care plan you developed with your instructor before giving care.
- **Goal 3.** Improve safety in using high-alert medications. For example, prepare a medication such as insulin or a narcotic under instructor observation.
- **Goal 7.** Reduce the risk of health care–associated infections. Comply with current Centers for Disease Control and Prevention hand washing guidelines and other recommendations for preventing and transferring infection to the patient or your family.
- **Goal 8.** Accurately and completely reconcile medications across the continuum of care. Patient's current medication is compared with what was ordered while cared for in a health

facility. If the patient is transferred, a complete list of medications accompanies the patient. A complete list of medication is provided to the patient upon discharge from the health facility.
- **Goal 9**. Reduce the risk of patient harm resulting from falls. Follow the guidelines for fall reduction implemented at the health agency
- **Goal 10.** Reduce the risk of influenza and pneumococcal disease in institutionalized older adults through vaccination and identifying and reporting early symptoms.
- **Goal 11.** Reduce the risk of surgical fires.
- **Goal 12.** Implement TJC National Patient Safety goals as they apply to the health care agency. Know what goals the health agency is committed to and do your part.
- **Goal 13.** Encourage patient involvement in personal safety.
- **Goal 14.** Prevent decubitus ulcers. Follow unit protocols for decubital prevention.
- **Goal 15.** Identify patients with behavioral issues at risk for suicide or other self-destructive behaviors. Be aware of the patient's verbal, nonverbal, and affective communication. Avoid discounting what you hear and what you suspect. Report your concerns to the instructor or nurse in charge.

PATIENT COMPETENCY

You can expect to hear increased use of the term competency in both a legal and a clinical sense. The following details provide a brief framework to help you use this term correctly.

Patient competency has both a legal meaning and a clinical meaning. Some patients' rights issues are based on proof of competence or incompetence within the court system. *Legal* competency refers to a patient who is:

- Eighteen years old or older
- A pregnant or married woman
- A self-supporting minor (referred to as a legally emancipated minor)
- Competent in the eyes of the law (incompetence is determined by the court)

Clinical competency refers to a patient who is able to do the following:

- Identify the problem for which he or she is seeing the physician
- Understand the options for care and the possible consequences
- Make a decision
- Provide sound reasons for the option he or she chooses

PATIENT'S RIGHT TO CONSENT

The patient's right to consent to or refuse treatment is a significant example of patient autonomy (right to choose). It is advisable for a patient to be accompanied by someone he or she trusts whenever they go to a health agency for care. Patients are often stressed to the point that they do not "hear" what is being said to them. Words such as "cancer" and "heart attack" can cause sheer terror. Furthermore, some patients still are afraid to question the physician and therefore agree to procedures that they do not understand: "Whatever you think is best" is a frequent answer.

General (Implied) Consent

General (implied) consent for treatment is obtained on admission. It may be obtained by the LPN/LVN or by an admission clerk during a routine admission. The fact that a person has voluntarily sought admission to a health care agency and willingly signs a general admission form is an example of general consent. A patient may revoke this permission verbally or in writing (e.g., you walk into patient's room with a syringe and explain that the doctor has ordered Demerol for pain relief; the patient might say, "I don't want a shot, I'm going home").

 Critical Thinking Exercise

Resolve Consent Issues
What steps will you take in the situation just described?

Informed Consent

Informed consent must be obtained for invasive procedures ordered for therapeutic or diagnostic purposes (e.g., surgery). Informed consent means that the patient is told the following in non-medical language:

1. Diagnosis or suspected diagnosis;
2. Purpose and description of treatment (some surgeons are sending the patient home with a video that shows the surgery being performed before asking them to sign a consent form);
3. Expected outcome, expected benefits, possible side effects or complications;
4. Explanation of alternative treatments; benefits, possible side effects or complications;
5. Names and qualifications of the people who will perform the procedure (treatment):

6. Prognosis if treatment is not done (when known);
7. Answers to questions patient wants clarified;
8. An explanation that the patient has the right to revoke written permission at any time.

The patient must indicate comprehension (understanding) of the information. This means considerably more than just nodding the head. For example, have the patient explain in his or her own words what he or she thinks is going to happen, and the benefit and risk involved. Document the patient's understanding of the information.

Informed consent is the responsibility of the physician because he or she must explain the implications and complications of the procedure to the patient before written permission is obtained. *It is never the responsibility of the LPN/LVN.* If you are in the room when the physician is obtaining informed consent, you might be asked to witness the signing. "Being asked to witness a patient's signature on a consent form is no small responsibility. Your signature attests to three things: that the patient gave his consent voluntarily, that his signature is authentic, and that he appears to be competent to give consent" (Sullivan, 1998).

If the LPN/LVN is present when the treatment is being explained and the informed consent signed, the LPN/LVN may support the teaching that has taken place by the physician. Be sure to check your state's Nurse Practice Act. In some states LPN/LVNs may not teach at all.

Authorized Consent

Parents cannot give *informed consent* for the treatment of their children, but they can authorize treatment for their children up to a certain age (*authorized consent*). Courts of law recognize that parents generally authorize what is appropriate for their children. In most states, "minor" is defined as younger than age 18. Some states allow minors to give their own consent for substance abuse treatment, mental health problems, pregnancy, and sexually transmitted diseases (STDs). Emancipated minors are defined as those living on their own and managing their own finances or who are married and have children. They are competent to give their consent.

END-OF-LIFE ISSUES

PATIENT SELF-DETERMINATION ACT

The Patient Self-Determination Act (PSDA) is an amendment to the Omnibus Budget Reconciliation Act (a federal law). "The PDSA requires many Medicare and Medicaid providers (hospitals, nursing homes, hospice programs, home health agencies, and HMOs) to give adult individuals, at the time of inpatient admission certain information about their rights under state laws governing advance directives including:

- The right to participate in and direct their own health care decisions;
- The right to accept or refuse medical or surgical treatment;
- The right to prepare an advance directive;
- Information on the provider's policies that govern the utilization of these rights" (Patient Self-Determination Act at: *http://www.ascenionhealth.org/ethics/public/issues/patient_self.asp*).

ADVANCE DIRECTIVES

Two types of written advance directives are available to patients giving direction to health care providers about treatment choices in certain circumstances. The two types of advance directives are a living will and a durable power of attorney for health care. A good advance directive describes the kind of treatment that is desired by the person depending on how sick he or she is. Usually the advanced directive indicates what type of treatment is not desired. However, it can indicate that the person wants all possible measures used to prolong life. Information on advanced directives can be found by Googling Advanced Directives and clicking on familydoctor.org.

Living Will

The living will is a legal document that describes the kind of medical treatments or life-sustaining treatments the person would want if seriously or terminally ill. There are many issues that can be addressed including, the use of dialysis or respirators; whether the person wants to be resus-

citated if breathing stops; tube feeding; organ or tissue donation; hydration and other comfort measures, etc.

A living will does not let the person select someone to make decisions for them. An attorney is not required to draft a living will. The living will is filled out by the individual and witnessed by a person who will not benefit by the death of that individual.

Living wills are recognized as legal documents in 47 states in the United States, the District of Columbia, and Guam. They are not recognized as legal documents in Canada. The individual generally is advised to give a witnessed copy to the health care provider and a trusted friend or relation and to keep one copy in a location that is easily accessible. If a person is moving to or spending time in another state, he or she is advised to determine whether the living will is considered legal in that state. Otherwise, the person may discover too late that the written directive may not be honored. Blank forms are available from hospitals, other health care agencies, age-related organizations such as the American Association of Retired Persons (AARP), and attorneys' offices.

Durable Medical Power of Attorney

The durable medical power of attorney (DPOA) is a legal document that is valid throughout the United States. It names a health care proxy (any one at least 18 years old) to make medical decisions, if that person is no longer able to speak for him or herself. The DPOA is generally more useful than a living will. It becomes active anytime the person is unconscious or unable to make a medical decision. The DPOA may not be a good choice if the person has no one he or she trusts to make these decisions.

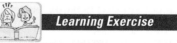
Learning Exercise

Legal Directives

Discuss the difference between the DPOA and the living will.

DO-NOT-RESUSCITATE ORDER

The do-not-resuscitate (DNR) order is an advance directive based on the Patient Self-Determination Act, which provides legal permission for a physician to write a DNR order. The physician may also write a DNR order for a patient who no longer has decision-making ability but does not have personal advance directives written and signed. Commonly called a "no-code" order, it is a legal order to not resuscitate a patient. The DNR order does not have to be updated unless the patient changes her or his mind. If a written DNR order does not exist and the nurse does not try to resuscitate the patient, the nurse is in effect making a medical decision. The nurse is practicing medicine without a license and may be subject to a lawsuit. There is no such thing as a partial or slow code. All caregivers must know when a written DNR order exists. Check your state and agency policies regarding DNR orders because there are considerable variations among states.

The role of the next of kin in making decisions about care for the patient differs from state to state. "The biggest challenge: no advance directive and family opposition. Only about 15% to 20% of patients have advance directives in the form of a living will or health care proxy. Although patients often express a preference to die at home, statistics show that 76% to 80% of people die in the hospital, 15% in hospice care and 5% to 9% in nursing homes" (Hanawalt, 2001).

Sometimes providers ignore patient advance directives. The instructions provided by the patient may be vague, or the physician might assume that the patient did not know about an available treatment or simply defers to the wishes of family members. Sometimes patients have not discussed advance directives with their physician, or a facility has a policy that a written physician's order of DNR must be in the chart to comply with the patient's wish. For your legal protection, know what your state and facility's policies are and whether the patient has a written advance directive that the physician is aware of. Do-not-hospitalize (DNH) orders may be more effective than DNR orders in limiting treatment and preventing unnecessary or unwanted patient transfer from a long-term care or to an acute treatment facility. Most important for you, as an LPN/LVN, is to know your agency's policy.

REMOVAL OF LIFE SUPPORT SYSTEMS

The physician must pronounce the patient dead and document this status before the nurse turns off the ventilator. If the nurse removes a life support system before the physician pronounces the patient dead, it can be considered an act of murder.

PHYSICIAN-ASSISTED SUICIDE AND EUTHANASIA

Physician-assisted suicide (PAS) and euthanasia are not the same. "Physician-assisted suicide refers to a physician providing the means for death, most often with a prescription. The patient, not the physician, will ultimately administer the lethal medication. Euthanasia generally means that the physician would act directly, for instance by giving a lethal injection, to end a patient's life." Information on Physician-Assisted Suicide can be found at: *http://depts.washington. edu/bioethx/topics/pas.html*. Both are different from a DNR order written by a physician, based on a decision made by the physician and patient or family. A DNR order is a passive action, with the goal of avoiding prolonging life unnecessarily, not actively ending it. See Table 20-2 for a comparison of active and passive euthanasia.

Some other practices different from PAS are:
- Terminal sedation that refers to sedating terminally ill persons to the point of unconsciousness and allowing them to die. If the person has made the decision to refuse further treatment the law and medical profession respect this.
- Pain medication that may hasten death relieves suffering for a terminally ill person has been held justifiable by courts as long as the intent is to relieve suffering.

"The American Nurses Association (ANA), as well as the American Medical Association (AMA) and the National Hospice Association, have issued position statements expressly declaring

Table 20-2	*Active and Passive Euthanasia**	
ACTIVE	**PASSIVE**
Actively end person's life	Avoid prolonging person's life
Initiate the dying process	Allow a deadly process that brings death to continue
Morally wrong	Morally permissible
Legally not allowed	Legally allowed
Forbidden by professional organizations	Approved by professional organizations
Actions that speed the process of dying	Do nothing to preserve life

*Euthanasia (Greek—good death, easy death, death without suffering).

opposition to nurse or physician participation in assisted suicide" (Daly et al., 1997).

Oregon's Death With Dignity Act

The Oregon Death With Dignity Act allows terminally ill Oregonians to end their lives through the voluntary self-administration of lethal medications, expressly prescribed by a physician for that purpose. Death With Dignity Act information is available at *http://www.Oregon.gov/DHS/ph/pas/faqs.shml*. The Death With Dignity Act legalizes physician-assisted suicide, but specifically prohibits euthanasia. The alternative is available only to Oregon residents.

According to the article "First Study on Patients Who Fast to End Lives," doctors note that one option is always legal: a sane, alert person can simply refuse to eat or drink. It is an option rarely taken, but now the first survey of nurses whose patients took the option to fast to end their lives has contradicted the popular assumption that such a death is painful and gruesome. Almost all of the 102 nurses surveyed said their patients who refused water and food had died "good deaths," with little pain or suffering, generally within two weeks. The patient most often becomes comatose: coma is the body's anesthesia. The lead author hesitated publishing the article because of the number of vulnerable patients, many with depression. It

is not for the LPN/LVN to tell patients of this option and/or to encourage its use. We include it here to dispel the often taught assumption that fasting always leads to a painful and gruesome death. Some cultures/religions are firm in their belief against euthanasia and assisted suicide in any form.

California, Washington, Michigan, and Maine's efforts to pass a death with dignity law have all been turned down by their voters. Thirty-nine states have specific laws that prohibit physician-assisted suicide and euthanasia. The Netherlands and Belgium are two countries that legalized euthanasia and physician-assisted suicide.

 Learning Exercise

Terminally ill Patients

With the permission of the instructor, divide into three groups. Choose a viewpoint about the terminally ill from the following descriptions. Be prepared to present reasons for the viewpoint. Choose a spokesperson to summarize the group views.

- Group 1: Terminally ill patients have the right to choose death by physician-assisted suicide.
- Group 2: Terminally ill patients must wait to die of natural causes.
- Group 3: The nurse's personal ethic conflicts with the decision of groups 1 and 2. Discuss the nurse's rights, roles, and responsibilities to the patient.

Refer to the critical thinking steps in Chapter 6 to assist you in making your decision.

ORGAN DONATION

Organ donations are voluntary. At this time organs cannot be bought or sold. Although many patients and families give permission for organ donation after death, the demand for organs far exceeds supply. You may have been asked to agree to personal organ donation at the time you got your driver's license. Many states participate in this effort. To increase the number of donors, it has been suggested that money be given to cover the donors' funeral expenses.

Body tissues that can be donated include skin, corneas, bone, heart valves, and blood. One example of a successful body tissue transplant was the transplantation of umbilical cord blood for a rare genetic bone disease at the University of Minnesota in Duluth in 1995. Approximately one cup of blood, taken from a newborn's discarded umbilical cord and placenta, was donated. Donated body organs include the heart, liver, kidneys, lungs, and pancreas.

Organ donation has raised both ethical and legal questions in some instances—for example, having a baby so that select organs or body tissues can be used to save a sibling.

END-OF-LIFE (EOL) CARE

There are numerous organizations and projects working on end-of-life principles. Numerous medical specialties including the American Medical Association and TJC have adopted or support core principles for end of life care. They accept the term palliative care to identify the wide range of clinical services available for patients whose disease is not responsive to curative treatment. Sample websites are included, if you are interested in pursuing information. An end-of-life movement article (Cox and Parkman, 2002) notes that "the EOL movement is not about relearning death and dying, it is about being proactive by increasing conversations and actions toward the preparation for better end-of-life journeys." A list of the principles for care of end-of-life patients can be accessed online at *www.milbank.org/endoflife/index.html*.

In 2001, Partnership for Caring: America's Voices for the Dying replaced the 62-year-old organization Choices in Dying. The best-known achievement of Choices in Dying was the development of advance directives, introducing the living will, in 1967. Partnership for Caring describes itself as "a national nonprofit organization devoted to raising consumer expectations for excellent end-of-life care and increasing demand for such care. It is the only end-of-life organization that partners individuals and organizations—consumers and professionals" Last Acts is a national coalition and campaign to improve the quality of life. Former First Lady Rosalynn Carter

is honorary chair. Information publications and articles on palliative, end-of-life-care, advance directives, and links to other resources can be accessed online at *http://www.lastacts.org*.

GOOD SAMARITAN ACTS

Good Samaritan Acts stipulate that a person who renders emergency care in good faith at the scene of an accident is immune from civil liability for his or her action while providing the care. All 50 states and the District of Columbia have enacted Good Samaritan laws (Brown, 1999). The state statutes are of special concern to nurses and physicians who provide emergency care outside of the agency that employs them. The statutes vary so check with your state's board of nursing or agency risk manager for information about your state's Good Samaritan laws. For example, in some states a nurse has a choice of whether to give aid to someone during an emergency outside of a health care setting. A few states obligate health care professionals to assist at a scene of an accident requiring medical help. If, for example, you provide pressure to stop severe bleeding and the patient develops complications, you will not be held responsible, as long as you acted without gross negligence. The laws also permit the nurse to give aid to a minor at a sports event or accident scene before getting authorized consent from the parents. The LPN must have permission to treat the person and verbal permission must be obtained from the victim. The person has the right to refuse. Once first aid is initiated the nurse is obligated to continue until the victim can be turned over to someone with comparable or better training (Christensen and Kockrow, 2006).

 Learning Exercise

Good Samaritan Act

Explain the protection that your state's Good Samaritan Act provides for the LPN/LVN.

SITUATIONS AND DOCUMENTATION

SITUATION: FORGOTTEN ENTRY

When you get home after the shift, you realize you forgot to chart, or you forgot to chart something important. There is no law against making entries out of order in the patient's medical record.

Documentation. If the information is very important, such as recording a medication that was given, call the nursing unit immediately. Speak to the nurse assigned to your patient and ask them to chart the information for you. As soon as possible, usually the next day, cosign the charting.

SITUATION: DOCUMENTING UAP CARE

Know the agency's policy. Many agencies have UAP checklists for routine care. The LPN/LVN follows up on the data as necessary. If you are documenting non-routine care, you want to be sure that you have either witnessed or verified that the care was given.

Documentation. Write in the name, followed with UAP. For example, "Shelley Hill, UAP, reported that _____." Follow with what you observed to verify that actual care was given.

SITUATION: DOCUMENTING SOMEONE ELSE'S CARE

If a nurse on the unit asks you to document care given by them that you did not witness and you do it, you could be at risk legally.

Documentation. This is quite different from having a staff member call in after he or she is off duty to ask you to make an entry. When the nurse is right there, refuse to do it. Offer instead to assist in completing their work so that they will be able to chart.

SITUATION: ILLEGAL ALTERATION OF A PATIENT'S RECORD

Tampering with a patient's record includes the following actions:

- Adding to someone else's notes,
- Destroying all or part of the record,
- Rewriting all or part of the record,
- Omitting important facts,
- Purposely writing inaccurate information, and
- Falsifying a date or time or adding a late entry without identifying it as a late entry.

Alteration can result in a person being charged with fraud. The usual reason someone tampers with a record is to cover up improper or ineffective care.

Documentation. When you discover a tampered entry, immediately contact your nursing administrator or risk manager. Avoid correcting the documentation. The risk manager will probably photocopy both your notes and the tampered entries. Continue to document honestly. You may be asked to write an incident report.

SITUATION: PERSONAL CRITICISM OF YOU IN PATIENT'S RECORD

This form of criticizing your patient care goes against accepted nursing standards.

Documentation. Once in the record, you may not alter the charting or add an entry to defend you. Notify your supervisor and speak to the nurse who made the entry. Perhaps they will be willing to complete a truthful incident report, noting only what they saw without blaming you or anyone else. If this problem is noteworthy, the administrator may choose to have an in-service program on proper use of nursing notes.

SITUATION: ILLEGIBLE PHYSICIAN'S ORDER

Ask for clarification. If you cannot reach the physician, contact your supervisor and they will follow a chain of command to obtain clarification. There may be another nurse on the unit who has no problem reading the physician's writing. If you find that you have problems reading certain physicians' orders, get used to checking the order with the physicians before they leave the unit.

Documentation. Document your attempts to reach the physician and the method used. A telephone logbook works well for this. When you finally have clear orders, write an entry on the physician's order sheet. For example, date, time, clarification of orders for date, time (of original entry), TO (telephone order), Dr. ___ , and your name and title.

SITUATION: TELEPHONE ORDERS

When used, physician's orders conveyed by telephone should be given directly to the nurse, who repeats the order back to the physician. Spelling of medications or treatments is checked if necessary. So many medications sound alike, and doses can be confusing. If it is a sensitive order, meaning one that carries special risk, two people should listen to the order. (This is suggested for all telephone orders.) Be sure to check the policy of your employer about the legality of an LPN/LVN accepting phone orders.

Documentation. The order is entered on the physician's order sheet as quickly as possible. Include the date and time of the order and that it was a telephone order (TO). Write your full name and credentials. If another nurse listened to the conversation with you, have him or her sign after your name. The order is then carried out the usual way. If the physician called the order in response to your data collection (assessment), write your reason in the nurse's notes for calling the physician, as well as the data you collected about the patient before the call. Once the order is carried out, collect data regarding the patient's response to the intervention ordered.

SITUATION: VERBAL ORDERS

Verbal orders should not be accepted, except in emergency situations. Written orders by the physician protect the physician, the patient, and the nurse. It is difficult to explain to a court why the physician, who has access to the chart, did not write the order. Verbal orders should be repeated for accuracy using the physician's exact words. Ask for names of medications to be spelled if any confusion exists.

Documentation. Record the order on the physician's order sheet as soon as possible. Include the date, the time, and that it was a VO (verbal order). Write your name and credentials. Example: Ellen A. Zaic, LVN, Charge Nurse, for Frederick Jones, MD. (Many agencies' policies require that the physician cosign the order within 24 hours.) Transcribe the order the usual way. Document data collection you have done before and after following the order.

SITUATION: QUESTIONABLE ORDER

A physician's written or verbal order is a legal order that the nurse must carry out. However, the nurse has the responsibility to recognize whether an order may harm the patient and can refuse to carry it out. Deal directly with the physician first. If this is unsuccessful, use the nursing chain of command, beginning with your immediate supervisor. If the problem is not resolved through the nursing channels, it must reach the physician chain of command quickly to avoid harm to the patient.

Documentation. Never change a questionable order on your own. The physician will usually rewrite the order or give a new telephone order. If not resolved at this point, document your refusal, your data collection as rationale, your discussion with the physician (include name), and whom you contacted.

For additional help, record the physician's response. Remember to note carefully the times of contact. A follow-up letter to the nursing administrator may be needed for the record. Be as objective as possible in discussing the event. Some agencies have special forms and procedures for documentation.

SITUATION: GIVING ADVICE

It has probably happened already that someone sought your advice for a remedy or the name of a competent physician. It probably even felt flattering. Be careful: You may have crossed the line into practicing medicine by suggesting something as simple as an over-the-counter medication. Giving the name of a specific physician may open you up to slander or libel. Give a list of physicians, if you must, rather than naming one (advice to your neighbors puts you in the same legal bind).

Documentation. In an agency setting, share the patient's questions with the head nurse or physician. Document the dates, times, and persons with whom you discussed the patient's concerns.

SITUATION: UNDERSTAFFED UNIT

"Floating" is working in an area that is not your usual work area. In 1991 TJC revised its nursing care standards, which are used as a basis for making accreditation decisions. One of these standards states that nursing staff should be competent to fulfill their assigned responsibilities. Directives from TJC include the need for timely and adequate orientation and cross training. LPN/LVNs need to receive adequate orientation, cross training, and education for float duty. You are responsible for informing supervisors if you do not feel competent to work in any assigned area.

Some agencies will fire you for not floating. Instead of refusing the assignment, negotiate with the nurse in charge regarding priorities of care. "Nice-to-do" tasks may have to be left undone. If you do not know how to do something, ask for instruction. Notify your supervisor if you are short-staffed. There is a legal concern regarding abandonment. You may not leave your place of employment until you can transfer the care of patients to your replacement.

Documentation. Follow this with a written statement about your concern in being assigned to an area in which you do not feel qualified to work. A memo is more effective than verbal notification alone. Keep a copy for yourself.

SITUATION: SIGNING A WILL

Nurses may witness the signing of a will if they do not stand to gain personally from the will. Check your agency's policy before doing so. Check with your instructor before you agree to witness the signing of a will.

Documentation. Document in the patient's record that you witnessed the signing of a will.

SITUATION: POSSIBLE NEGLIGENCE

Be sure you have all the facts before acting on your suspicions. Instead of gossiping, collect data from the patient, anyone who witnessed the behavior, the patient's chart, etc. Report possible negligence to the nursing supervisor.

Documentation. Fill out an incident report with facts only. Record events and patient and witness statements. Include names and titles of persons to whom you have made a report, with dates and times. In the nursing notes, describe any intervention you have taken to prevent further harm to the patient.

SITUATION: STANDING ORDERS

Some states do not allow standing orders, except in intensive and coronary care units. Because standing orders call for making judgments, the practical/vocational nurse must always check first with the RN before carrying out standing orders. If you are a charge nurse, request that the physician review standing orders on a regular basis and have the review dated and initialed.

Documentation. Document data collection that has caused you to be concerned about particular standing orders. Contact the RN and include the name of the RN, to whom you have expressed your concern, along with the date and time.

SITUATION: DISCHARGE INSTRUCTIONS AND PATIENT EDUCATION

The professional nurse, physician, podiatrist, or dentist initiates health teaching for patients. The practical/vocational nurse reinforces this teaching if permitted in your state's Nurse Practice Act. Teaching is the domain of the professional nurse, and LPN/LVNs play a supportive role in it, once the RN has started education. Discharge instructions are given verbally and in writing, with the patient signing a form indicating that he or she understands the information. Preprinted information forms are valuable and are available in many agencies. The practical/vocational nurse initiates patient teaching in the area of basic health care, such as cleanliness, how to avoid constipation, hand washing to prevent picking up or spreading illness, use of alcohol based hand sanitizer etc.

Documentation. All interventions, including patient teaching, whether reinforced or initiated, must be documented in the patient's chart. Be descriptive. Saying that discharge instructions or patient education was provided is not enough if there is a legal question after discharge.

TELEPHONE LOGS

Telephone logs can be used routinely to document the time, problem, and advice received or given. Also, attempted calls to physicians or supervisors should be logged.

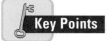

Key Points

- The state's Nurse Practice Act is the most definitive legal statute or legislative act regulating nursing practice. It governs what you can and cannot do as a nurse. Know it well.
- Student nurses are held to the standard of an LPN/LVN.
- Basic terminology in the Nurse Practice Act is standard in many states.
- Eight general categories of disciplinary action by the board of nursing include fraud and deceit, criminal activity, negligence, incompetence, violation of the Nurse Practice Acts or rules, disciplinary action by another board, unethical conduct, and alcohol and/or other drug use.
- Disciplinary action is based on rules of law. If guilty, the board may issue a public or private reprimand, such as probation, non-renewal of license, suspension of license, revocation of license, or instruction to enter into a voluntary diversion rehabilitation program, if the issue is alcohol and/or other drugs.
- After successful completion of the NCLEX-PN® examination, the LPN/LVN may practice in the state of licensure. Some other states accept licensure through interstate endorsement, multistate licensure compact, or a border recognition agreement.

- The Nursing standard of care is what an ordinary, prudent nurse with similar education and experience would do in a similar situation.
- Ethics deals with rules of conduct; law provides regulations that control the practice of nursing.
- Common law is judge-made law that is useful in settling disputes.
- The legislative branch of the state and federal government develops statutory law: The Nurse Practice Act is a statutory law.
- Civil action is related to individual rights; criminal action involves persons and society as a whole.
- Tort law has to do with a wrong or injury to someone that violates his or her rights.
- Intentional torts involve intended harm by the nurse, such as assault and battery; false imprisonment and use of restraints; defamation; and physical and emotional abuse.
- Unintentional torts mean no harm was intended by the nurse (e.g., professional negligence [malpractice]).
- Elements necessary for negligence are duty, breach of duty, damages, and proximate cause.
- Personal liability holds us responsible for our behavior, including negligent behavior.
- Depositions are used to gather information under oath.
- When giving testimony, take your time; say "yes" or "no" when possible, *without adding detail*; stick to facts; and correct mistakes and misconceptions.
- Documentation is a legal expectation in nursing regardless of the method used. If it was not charted, it was not done or it did not happen.
- Medication errors are among the most common errors related to nursing liability.
- Patient competency has both a legal and a clinical definition.
- Patient's right to consent is general, informed, or authorized depending on the situation.
- Patient rights include (1) the Patient Care Partnership: Understanding Expectations, Rights, and Responsibilities, (2) the HIPAA Privacy Rule, (3) the TJC National Patient Safety Goals, and (4) the Patient Self-Determination Act.
- The Patient Self-Determination Act involves advance directives (living will and durable power of medical attorney), written and signed by a patient to state his or her wishes for end-of-life care.

- DNR orders written by a physician are legal orders to not resuscitate a patient and are made possible because of the Patient Self-Determination Act.
- Nurses may not remove a life-support system until a patient is declared dead by the physician.
- Physician-assisted suicide involves a patient voluntarily ending his or her life by self-administering lethal medication prescribed by a physician, especially for that purpose. In the United States this is only legal in Oregon.
- Active euthanasia entails physicians directly administering a lethal medication to end a patient's life. This is not legal in the United States or Canada.

- The ANA and AMA oppose nurse or physician participation in assisted suicide.
- Organ donation has cultural, religious, legal, and ethical constraints. In the United States you can note on your driver's license if you wish to donate your organs.
- Good Samaritan Acts hold that a person who gives emergency care in good faith at the scene of an accident is immune from being sued. Some states have laws that make it mandatory to assist at the scene of an accident. A victim has the right to refuse aid.
- Incident reports should be legible, factual, specific, objective, and not worded to place blame.

REVIEW ITEMS

1. Which of the following is your legal guideline for all you can do as an LPN/LVN?

1. NFLPN and NAPNES
2. State board of nursing
3. Employee handbook
4. School of nursing

2. Which situation most clearly illustrates negligence?

1. The nurse became angry when the patient would not stop screaming and slapped the patient's face.
2. The nurse inserted the urinary catheter, even though the patient said she voided a large amount.
3. The nurse decided to restrain an elderly female patient to prevent her from falling out of bed.
4. The nurse forgot to lower the patient's bed after completing colostomy care and the patient fell.

3. How do you best respond to a teenage neighbor who is thinking about becoming an LPN/LVN "because it only takes a year and isn't hard like "real nursing'"?

1. "Surprise! Surprise! An LPN (or LVN) is a different level of nursing. There is a great deal of knowledge and nursing care skills that you are expected to learn in a short time. Even as a student you are held to the legal standard of a licensed nurse."
2. "You win the jackpot! Practical/vocational nursing is quicker and easier than becoming a registered nurse. Instructor expectations are not very high, and they are quick to forgive mistakes. The national examination at the end is a joke—so easy."
3. "It is, and it isn't! The trick at the end is to locate the state that has the least restrictions for what you can do. I've heard that some LPNs work as

RNs and the doctors don't know the difference! They start IVs and stuff right out of school."
4. "What an idea! They have already scared us with what the state board of nursing will do if we don't toe the line. Instructors make us learn a lot of extra stuff just in case the RN or doctor isn't available to answer patient questions and do their procedures."

4. How will you answer the lawyer's questions when asked to give testimony during a legal action?

1. Offer to tell what really happened when the wrong medication was given.
2. Avoid referring to any documents to show how well you recall the incident.
3. Fill in silences with information about the physician who ordered the medication.
4. Be specific, answering "yes" or "no" whenever possible, without adding details.

ALTERNATE FORMAT ITEM

Which of the following are legal patients' rights? *(Select all that apply.)*

1. The right to revoke a signed informed consent verbally on the way to surgery.

2. The right to take their medical records with them when they leave the hospital.

3. The right to designate who will make decisions for them should they become incapable.

4. The right to ask their physician to inject them with lethal drugs that will end life.

5. The right to file a suit for injury that they see as being the result of carelessness.

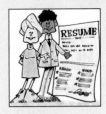

21 Finding a Job

CHAPTER

MICHAEL S. HILL, MS, CRC, ABDA, ACA, QRC

evolve http://evolve.elsevier.com/Hill/success/

Reference hierarchy (HĬ-ĕr-ăr-kē, p. 394)
Resignation courtesy (rĕz-ĭg-NĀ-shŭn, p. 415)
Résumé (RĔZ-ŭh-mā, p. 393)
Working the room (p. 389)

Objectives

On completing this chapter, you will be able to do the following:

1. List employment opportunities available to licensed practical/vocational nurses (LPN/LVNs).
2. Determine interpersonal styles and how to use them to achieve interpersonal rapport.
3. Describe and utilize individuals within your job search network.
4. Effectively participate in an informational interview.
5. Discuss how and where to best target job leads.
6. Role-play employer telephone contacts and respond positively to hard interview questions.
7. Practice filling out a job application, including a cover letter.
8. Develop a résumé, including a cover letter that will get an employer's attention.
9. Convey nonverbal messages at the interview.
10. Have insight into the cultural and age differences of the interviewer.
11. Discuss the importance of employer follow-up both at the time of application and after the interview.
12. Anticipate a successful pre-employment physical examination and drug screening.
13. Write an effective resignation letter with style.

Key Terms

Artful vagueness (VĀG-nes, p. 386)
Conditional job offer (p. 412)
Follow-up illusion (p. 413)
Hidden job market (p.393)
Illegal questions (p. 398)
Informational interviews (p. 390)
Interpersonal styles (p. 386)
Networking (p. 387)

Keep in Mind

All right, you've decided what you want to be when you grow up; now get out there and do it!

GRADUATION: CLOSER THAN YOU THINK

If you are reading this chapter, you are near graduation or may have graduated. Perhaps your expectation is that employers will be beating down your door. You may also be concerned about your career opportunities after investing so much money in your education.

You are to be congratulated for having become a member of a fast growing employment area: health services. In the *Occupational Outlook Handbook 2006-2007,* employment of LPNs is expected to grow about as fast as average for all occupations through 2014 in response to the long-term care needs of an increasing elderly population and the general growth of health care services. In 2004 it was noted that 27% of LPNs worked in hospitals, 25% in nursing care facilities, and another 12% in offices of physicians. Others worked for home care services, employment services; community care facilities for the elderly; public and private educational services; outpatient care centers; and federal, state, and local government agencies. Additionally, it was noted that one in five LPNs worked part-time.

Through 2014, competition for hospital jobs will be keen. As those jobs decline, LPNs will have better job opportunities at physicians' offices, outpatient care centers, home health care services, and nursing home/extended care facilities. Job growth and opportunities vary from region to region at different times. Employment opportunities vary according to each individual's tenacity, geographical location, and sometimes, just luck. Your job search will be more successful if you consider looking into areas such as those listed in Chapter 23.

WHAT DO I WANT TO DO?

Many job ads in newspapers, on the Internet, and in professional publications require the job candidate to have prior experience. By completing your program, you have gained practical experience. Now it is a matter of convincing the employer of the benefit to hire you. Think about what your education has provided you.

You have a distinct advantage if your educational program has included clinical (hands-on) nursing experience in the areas in which you are most interested. These nursing experiences include clinical rotations, special projects, computer work, or work with a temporary permit before taking the NCLEX-PN® examination.

Your practical work experiences will lead to clarification of your classroom instruction, help you hone your skills, and provide valuable work references. While completing your nursing education, the clinical rotations and work experience provide a significant step in your future job search. You have had an opportunity to learn about and develop skills that are valued in the major areas of nursing employment.

Learning Exercise

Consider the Following Questions:

1. What type of environment do I want to work in—direct health care, state/federal government, private duty, insurance-related, sales, industry, or other?

2. What population (i.e., type of client) do I find most rewarding to work with?

3. What kinds of nursing skills do I find most challenging and rewarding? Additionally, what new areas would I like to be involved in?

USING INTERPERSONAL STYLES TO YOUR BENEFIT

Mercer (2005) suggested there are seven ways to make a fantastic impression. He indicated the basic rule is, "humans crave to be around people who seem similar to them and, as a result, make a wonderful impression." Mercer suggested seven techniques:

1. *Forget the "golden rule"* of treating someone how you would like to be treated. Instead, he recommended, "treating other people the way they like to be treated, focusing on their likes, not yours."
2. *Reflect the other person's interpersonal style.* The four major interpersonal styles are results-focused, detail-focused, friendly-focused, and party-focused. Box 21-1 includes suggestions for reflecting each type.
3. *Mirror the interviewer.* Make your body language similar to the other's body language, vocal style, and attire. For instance, if the interviewer speaks slowly, then you should also.
4. *Listen attentively.* In doing this, the person being interviewed would paraphrase or repeat ideas the other person has said. This would also include asking questions about what was said and taking notes.
5. *Use artful vagueness.* Artful vagueness is responding to another's comment without implying that either of you is wrong. For instance, if a coworker said, "We should put all the patient mattresses onto the floor so we don't have to worry about patients

Box 21-1 | *Four Major Interpersonal Styles*

1. **Results-Focused**—Tell me how the patient is. (Speak rapidly and to the point about the patient's status.)
2. **Detail-Focused**—Tell me how your patient's day was. (Speak slowly and deliberately about every thing that happened with the patient.)
3. **Friendly-Focused**—How are we doing today? (Start off with small talk, such as, "The kids told me about a school project, which is due tomorrow so life is hectic as usual." Now for Mr./Ms. Jones here … then shift to a Results or Detail-focused patient report as needed.)
4. **Party-Focused**—Did Mr. Jones get his dinner yet? Hmmm, reminds me of the joke about the… (They like to tell jokes/stories and laugh before getting to the business of work.) Once they are done, they will shift to a Results-Focused or Detail-Focused style.

falling out of bed." A response of, "That's an idea" might be said or "You might be right," even if you were actually thinking, "what a stupid idea."

6. *Use the person's name.* We are drawn to people who use our names. Research has shown that high achievers tend to use the person's name one or two times in their conversation.
7. *Give compliments.* It has been found on average that high achievers gave out three compliments per day. Underachievers rarely gave out compliments…. Mercer went on to state that the above techniques might be viewed by some as "selling out." He then quoted a French saying to put it into perspective: "A car can go as far on square wheels as it can go on round wheels. The difference is that on round wheels the ride is much smoother." Go through life on round wheels.

NETWORKING YOUR WAY TO SUCCESS

Smart networking of influential people in your school and clinical work experiences can lead to finding new jobs, better pay, faster promotions, and greater job satisfaction.

NETWORKING FOR REFERENCES

- **Instructors** may be willing to write a positive recommendation if your work warrants it. Be sure to ask for permission before bringing in a form or giving out his or her name. Do not assume an instructor will give you a positive reference. Specifically ask, "May I list your name for a positive reference?"
- **Unit managers, supervisors, team leaders, staff registered nurses (RNs), and LPN/LVNs** are sources of information about job openings in their areas and can be approached for recommendations. Some students think they are "invisible" in the eyes of regular facility staff. Not so! Frequently staff members offer feedback to instructors and nurse managers about future employees.
- **School placement personnel** are a source of information when you register with the school's career service center, and can inform you about Job Service/WorkForce Centers and so on.

Listen carefully when feedback is passed on to you. You often have to work directly with primary nurses or team leaders. Identify the nurses whose work you admire and ask for their evaluations and suggestions about your work.

Before you complete a clinical rotation, *ask select nurses* whether they would be willing to write a positive reference letter for you. If the answer is "yes," write down the nurse's name (spelled correctly), job title, work address, and work telephone number. We encourage you to ask what he or she will say about you. When discussing references during an interview, it is to your advantage to allude to what they will say about you. If you do not ask what the person will say about you, you are risking the possibility that he or she will also discuss all your flaws.

A brief courtesy letter about your need for a positive reference letter should be sent at the time you begin your job search; follow-up telephone calls to reference persons 4 to 5 days after sending the letter will remind them of their promise to you. Your telephone contact might sound something like this:

"Hello, Ms. Anderson. This is Katelyn Bieser. I'm calling to follow up on the letter I sent you last week, to see whether you have had an opportunity to write the letter of recommendation we discussed at the end of the last rotation."

If the answer is "no":

Respond: "I know that you've been busy. Would it be best to follow up again some time next week? Or, **would it be easier if I drafted a possible** letter for your review and possible signature. What would you recommend?" Following their answer, say "Great, I will plan to": (1) "have a tentative letter to you with the next 2 days" or (2) "follow up with you on _____ (day) next week. Have a good day!" (A letter to the reference writer and a letter of recommendation might look like those in Boxes 21-2 and 21-3.)

NETWORKING FOR A JOB

When networking use previous contacts or be willing to meet new people who can help you, or use sources such as the following:

- **Family and friends with nursing contacts.** Let them know that you are looking for work. Ask for job leads and names of contacts. Follow up with these people every 2 weeks until you get the job you want. Remember to thank these people for all their help once you get the job. You may need their help again in the future. Job opportunities are often located not by what you know as much as by whom you know.
- **Former health care employers**. If you are interested in a nursing position, contact the employer.
- **Newspapers, nursing journals, the school alumni office, the Yellow Pages, the school's career placement office, state Job Service/WorkForce Centers, and local county agencies**

Box 21-2 *Sample Letter to Reference Writer*

May 12, 2009

Ms. Valerie George,
Surgical Care Charge Nurse
Veterans Hospital
1000 Veterans Lane
Minneapolis, MN 55402

Dear Ms. George,

Thank you again for agreeing to be a work reference. My experiences on the medical-surgical unit were both challenging and rewarding. I am pleased to now have the opportunity to use the skills you taught me.

I am actively seeking employment in medical-surgical units at hospitals within the metro area. A letter of recommendation from you is definitely an asset to my job search.

Knowing your busy schedule, I have enclosed a possible letter of recommendation for your review and signature. However, if you prefer to write your own letter, you may wish to mention my ability to work under pressure, ability to administer medication on time, communication skills with staff and patients, computer proficiency, and willingness to take on new assignments.

Your assistance in helping me secure employment is greatly appreciated. I plan to give you a call next week to let you know how my job search is going and answer any questions you may have regarding the letter. I look forward to talking with you soon.

Cordially,
Katelyn Bieser

2001 Putt Drive
Cottage Grove, MN 55016
(612) 555-2728

ENC: Reference letter

- There are **general career search sites** on the Internet that can be used/explored to find job opportunities. Box 21-4 lists several Internet sites for careers that will prove useful.

Box 21-3 | Sample Letter for Reference Writer to Complete and Place on Letterhead

May 18, 2009

Dear Employer:

Please accept this as a letter of recommendation for Ms. Katelyn Bieser, whom I supervised during her medical-surgical rotation. Katelyn was enjoyable to work with and displayed a high degree of skills as a student practical nurse.

Specifically, she learned new tasks quickly, attended to patient vital signs, was proficient on the computer, provided nutritional care, and administered medication promptly. Ms. Bieser was able to follow both physician orders and RN instructions and had a keen sense to know when to ask for help.

I believe that Katelyn will make a positive contribution to any hospital/company she chooses to work for. Should you have further questions about Katelyn's skills and abilities as a nursing professional, please feel free to contact me.

Cordially,
Valerie George, RN
Surgical Care Charge Nurse

Box 21-4 | Internet Sites for Careers

Career site suggestions include typing "practical nurse jobs" into your Internet search engine or visiting the following websites: ajb.dni.us; careerbuilder.com; careers.org; coolworks.com; degreehunter.com; job-bankusa.com; healthsource.com; nursefinders.com; monster.com; nationjob.com; hotjobs.yahoo.com; webcrawler.com; greatnurse.com; healthcare-jobbank.com; jobsonline.net; allhospitaljobs.com; 50statejobs.com; nursejobz.com; nursingcenter.com; afreserve.com; allnurse.com; medhunters.com; nurse-recruiter.com; medcareers.com; nurse-town.com; jobvertise.com; lpnjobs.com; lvnjobs.com; healthcareersource.com; employmentguide.com; govpot.com; licensed.practical.nurse.jobs.com; healthcareerweb.com; medicalexpress.com; if looking at opportunities in Canada, careerowl.com or globecareers.com. Also note that workingmother.com is a website that has identified companies they feel are women friendly.

Locally, consider checking to see if the facilities you wish to work for have websites of their own. This provides you with an opportunity to learn about job openings and the facility's mission statement. This can be done by typing in their name on an Internet search engine (i.e., using *http://www.google.com*, type in the name of the hospital) and/or contacting the receptionist at those facilities and asking for their Internet website address. *Hint:* When using the Internet, it will take time to locate job and career opportunity links. After entering the career/job area, try using the "search box" and type in "licensed practical (or vocational) nurse" as a possible shortcut. The beauty of the Internet is that you can search locally, by state, or in different countries.

Attend professional conferences or training sessions, "working the room." Before going, however, consider the color of the clothes you plan to wear to subtly influence the people you approach. Appold (2006) recommended if you wanted to appear authoritative, responsible, or knowledgeable, wear navy blue. For being successful, wear dark gray. To project dependability, being practical and stable, the color brown is used. Wear purple to represent intuitive, regal, and spiritual, and black for dignified and sophisticated. Once you have decided on your colors the author recommends that you:

- Arrive early to obtain your name badge and to see if you recognize the names on the other badges.
- Do not bring your "significant other" with you because he or she will expect your full attention or leave the room right away at the end.
- To begin working the room, strike up conversations at the name table, coffee/refreshment table, vendor booths, etc. An opening line might be, "Hi, I am ___ (your first name) from ____ nursing school. Who are you? What do you do?" Then, as people sit down for the conference, ask if you might join them. Do not sit at the table with other

students. Sit with people already working in the field, because their comments will be more pertinent and interesting.

- Identify the people who hire, by their more professional appearance and avoidance of eye contact with others.
- Sit down at the table and introduce yourself. An opening line might be, "Hi, I am _____ (first name). Have you been to one of these conferences before? Any idea who our first speaker is and what their background is?"
- Acknowledge that it was a pleasure to meet the person and request their business card, and/or pick up business cards on the tables, at the booths, etc.
- Avoid leaving these events early or immediately after the event ends. There are two types of people: Those who leave before the speaker's last words and those who mill around. Join the group that is milling around and talking about the conference. An initial statement might be, "I found Ms. Smith's comment about the _____ interesting. Is that your experience too?"

Learning Exercise

Networking for Jobs

Who is part of my job network? List these individuals in the spaces provided.

Name	Telephone
_____	_____
_____	_____
_____	_____

Networking should be a never-ending process, even after you have found your dream job. You never know when that dream job might come to an abrupt end because of reorganization or downsizing. Also, remember networking is a means to job satisfaction and advancement. Avoiding networking while you are in school or working is the worst mistake you can make.

As a rule, whether you are happily employed or looking for another job, the successful person is the one who makes a point of meeting someone new each day, either by telephone or in person. This includes:

- Displaying a positive affect with clients,
- Seeking your supervisor's input on how to build your career,
- Working on building relationships with key facility people where you work,
- Building positive peer relationships by being willing to lend a hand,
- Getting involved in facility and professional organizations, and
- Treating everyone as they would like to be treated. This will lead to access to other networks.

INFORMATIONAL INTERVIEWS TO CREATE FUTURE EXPECTATIONS

Chances are sometime during your educational program you will be asked to visit community health facilities. Your instructor will provide objectives to help make the experience worthwhile. Focus objectives or questions on the following areas:

- Purpose,
- Staffing patterns,
- Hours or shifts, and
- Facility specialty

Viewing this assignment as an informational interview will create an additional personal focus for you. The informational interview allows you to find out how the facility works firsthand, assists you in determining whether you would want to work there, and allows you to meet the employer before you actually seek a job.

To obtain an informational interview with an employer, it is important to practice with another individual prior to making the telephone contact. It may be tempting to make the phone call and read the example without practicing in advance. If you do this, remember that is exactly how it will sound—as though you are reading!

The following is an example of a telephone request:

1. Hello, my name is _____ (first and last name).
2. Who is in charge of hiring? (Emphasis is on first learning the name of the right person. DO NOT begin by asking, "May I speak to the person in charge of hiring?").
3. May I speak with Mr./Ms. _____?
4. Hello, Mr./Ms. _____. My name is _____ (first and last name).
5. I am a student practical/vocational nurse at (school's name).
6. As a part of my learning experience, I would like to visit your facility for an informational interview.
7. Would it be possible to set up an informational interview on _____ (day) at 9:00 AM or 2:00 PM, or another time?
   - *If the answer is yes:* Great! I'll see you on _____ (day). Thank you!
   - *If the answer is no:* Is there someone else whom you recommend I contact?

Learning Exercise

Practice Mock Interviews

List three persons with whom you can practice the informational telephone interview request.

With a peer, tape the above telephone request for information.

_____

_____

This is the time to concentrate on how your voice sounds to the employer with respect to pitch and intonation. There are several voice studies, self-help books, and companies devoted to helping people speak more clearly, making their voice more pleasant to hear, and keeping the person to whom they are talking interested. Spoken English has been broken down into five areas: Low-pitched (judged as more mature and truthful); Nasal (signaling low status and grating to the listener's ears); Monotone (boring and putting one to sleep); Loud (viewed as dynamic but shifty), and Whiny (lacking self-confidence—a turn-off).

Anderson (2007) recommended steps to develop a more powerful voice. They included:

- Take deep breaths without having your shoulders rise.
- Keep your back straight.
- Breathe in deeply and gently expand you abs and obliques, and say "Ah."
- Use your abs to expand your waist, and say "Ah" again in which your sound should get stronger.
- Let your throat be open and free of tension to prevent a high and squeaky voice.
- Practice the four "Ps" of vocal variety, including **pace** (too fast and you sound nervous, too slow and you're the village idiot), **pitch** (too low and no one will hear you, too high and you're nervous), **pauses** (use them sparingly, as too many suggest you're scrambling for thoughts), and **passion** (you should love your topic).
- Get rid of nasality. (If you are a whiner, try a yawn and feel your mouth open wide, resulting in a full resonate sound.)
- When your soft palate lowers, the air stream is blocked and the air can only pass out the nose, creating a nasal sound.
- Say the word "Ah" and feel your tongue as it peels down the roof of the mouth and allows the sound to lift.
- Modify your accent with the help of others to pronounce the most confusing words for you and model them face to face.
- Tune your tone to the occasion (learn to sound passionate even if you'd prefer to be someplace else).
- Be authentic (let your personality show).

Learning Exercise

Seek Critique of Mock Interviews

Find someone who will give you an honest opinion about how you sound on the above taped information interview.

Explain that you view the exercise as another learning experience toward achieving your goals.

_____

_____

There is usually no problem with speaking directly to top nursing management during an informational interview. Management wants to "get the word out" about what their facility really is like. However, do not make the mistake of turning this into a job interview. No one likes to be tricked, and management tends to have a long memory.

Look sharp during the informational interview. These are not "T-shirt, shorts, or jeans, and sandals" type trips. Consider them as future career opportunities. Keep a copy of the information you obtained with name, address, and phone number in a safe place (ask for their business card), for the time your job search begins. Follow up the informational interview with a thank you letter (Box 21-5).

HOW TO SEARCH FOR EMPLOYMENT OPENINGS

If you expect to work shortly after graduation, it is important to apply for employment approximately 2 months before graduation. Obtain a telephone answering machine, use a telephone "voice mailbox" service, or use your cell phone so you do not miss any calls from potential employers. Use a professional sounding message, such as "Hi, this is _____ (first name) and I am not available right now. Please leave your name, telephone number, day you that called, and what it is about. I look forward to talking with you soon."

Should your graduation be in December, do not fret. It is a myth that the November-December holiday season is the worst time to hunt for a job. The holiday season is among the best times to look for a job. Employers are already looking at staffing patterns for the New Year.

You need to do some homework in preparation for seeking employment. Find out all you can about the facility at which you wish to work. Facilities often provide websites or give out free pamphlets as part of their advertising. An easy way to locate company websites is to use search engines such as *Google.com, Yahoo.com,* or *MSN.com* and then type in the company name. Look for the facility's "mission statement"; determine the number of people they employ and annual

profits earned. Use the Internet to search for news stories/releases so you can work that into your interview and talk about how your skills relate.

Your school nursing program director may also have policy manuals for affiliated facilities. Ask to see those manuals and ask who does the hiring at each location. It is important to find out the name of the person who does the hiring or influences hiring. This is the person whom you will want to contact. You may be referred to another department, but there is a good chance your name will be remembered later.

Box 21-5 *Follow-Up Letter After Informational Interview*

January 22, 2009

Ms. Elizabeth Ekholm,
Director of Nursing
Lyngblomsten Health Care Facilities
1415 Almond Avenue
St. Paul, MN 55118

Re: Informational Interview

Dear Ms. Ekholm:

Thank you so much for meeting with me yesterday. The information you provided was both valuable and interesting. Your suggestions about what employers are looking for and which areas to focus my schooling on were very much appreciated.

I found that the variety of programs offered was progressive and individualized to meet the needs of the client and their families. The tour that followed supported your comments about positive interactions between staff and patients.

I can only hope to be fortunate enough to work at such a center after my graduation this June. Thank you again!

Sincerely yours,
Katelyn Bieser

2001 Putt Drive
Cottage Grove, MN 55016
(612) 555-2728 or *ktbieser@visi.com*

It is generally accepted that 75% to 85% of all available jobs are not advertised. Do not wait for an ad to appear before applying to an employer. The following are examples of sources of the hidden job market.

- Assistance from family and friends
- Employee recommendations at clinical site
- Submitting direct applications to employers
- Searching company websites, using terms such as "careers," "employment," "jobs," etc.
- State Job Service/WorkForce Centers
- Using Internet job sites (i.e., *Careerbuilder.com*)
- Using private employment or recruiter companies
- Searching state or federal government websites
- School placement offices, attending job fairs, etc.
- Volunteer activities, professional associations, etc.
- Contacting the state's nurses' union and asking about employers who are hiring
- Job fairs advertised in Sunday newspapers, Job Service/WorkForce Centers, on *Careerbuilder.com*, etc.

Apply directly to those employers, using website job applications, emails, or sending a cover letter and résumé. Make a follow up telephone contact to arrange an interview, or use it as a networking opportunity for additional job leads.

Often a brief, to-the-point letter, accompanied by a résumé, addressed to the director of nursing or nursing recruiter at the facility, is helpful. An example of a cover letter appears in Box 21-6. Avoid including a personal reference list or a photograph of yourself with the cover letter. Retain the reference list for your interview and provide it only on request. **Follow through by calling for an interview on the day stated in your letter.**

It is best to use Sundays and Mondays to research job opportunities and then contact employers from Tuesday forward. The best time to call employers for interview scheduling and making follow-up contacts has traditionally been after 9 AM. As a rule, employers no longer have the luxury of contacting every prospective job candidate, owing to time constraints and the demands

---

Box 21-6 | *Sample Cover Letter for Employment*

April 14, 2009

Ms. Jody Snyder,
Human Resources Director
Columbus Hospital & Clinics
2031 Lakeside Drive
Columbus, MN 55025

Re: LPN Staff Nurse Position

Dear Ms. Snyder:

I will graduate from the Rainy Lakes Technical College practical nursing program this June. While doing a medical nursing rotation at your hospital, I was impressed by the quality of client care, staff professionalism, and learning opportunities.

In addition to this rotation, my work experiences have included client care planning, plan review, direct client care, passing medications, computer entry, and team participation.

I am interested in obtaining employment at your hospital and being able to work with your staff again. I will contact you on Tuesday, April 21 to see whether you have received my résumé and to determine when we might arrange an interview. Should you wish to contact me before then, I can be reached weekdays after 3:30 PM. I look forward to speaking with you.

Cordially,
Katelyn Bieser

2001 Putt Drive
Cottage Grove, MN 55016
(612) 555-2728 or *ktbieser@visi.com*

---

of their own jobs. Those candidates who wait to be contacted should prepare to be disappointed when employers do not call.

If your resource for a job opening is the newspaper, call for an interview (unless the ad specifically states to write). The reason for this is that others are looking at the same ad, and in such cases, *"The candidate who hesitates is lost."* Ask to speak to the person in charge of hiring. Your conversation needs to reflect the following example:

1. Hello, my name is _____ (first and last name).
2. Who is in charge of hiring?
3. May I speak with Ms. _____?
4. Hello, Ms. _____. My name is _____ _____ (first and last name).
5. I will be graduating from the (school name) practical/vocational nursing program on _____ (date).
6. Do you have any practical/vocational nursing staff positions open?
   a. *If hiring:* Would it be possible to set up an interview on (date) at 9 AM tomorrow [pause for a moment]. *If no:* Would 2 PM tomorrow work? *If no:* What would be a better time and date? _____ Great! I will see you then.
   b. *If they are not hiring,* and you are told they are under a hiring freeze, catch your breath and don't be put off. An acceptable reply then would be:
      1) Oh, I hadn't heard that. I had thought this would be a very good facility to work at. Say, would it be possible to meet with you anyway? I would like to be the first person you consider when the freeze ends. *If yes,* see 6a. *If no:* Do you know of anyone who might be hiring?
      2) *If yes:* Would you also know the contact person and/or have a telephone number?
      3) *If no:* I appreciate your time. Thank you. Or, *if no:* Thank you for trying. Would it be possible for me to come in for an informational interview? *If yes,* see 6a. *If no:* Well, thank you again. Goodbye.

Deflect the employer's interview type of questions until the actual interview. The reason for this is there are employers who do not have openings, but feel it is kinder to ask you questions and then tell you that you're not what they're looking for. The second reason is that you do not want to be "washed out" by a telephone conversation if the employer does have a job.

If the employer begins to ask you questions about your background, education, or work experience, you might respond, "I have completed an accredited practical/vocational nursing program, have successfully completed the NCLEX-PN® examination, am licensed as a LPN/LVN, and have the required work experience. I would like the opportunity to discuss my qualifications during our interview." As in point 6a, say, "Would it be possible to set up an interview on Wednesday, etc.?"

The tone of your voice makes a significant difference on the telephone. If you smile while you are talking, you will project a positive tone. Practice the preceding format in advance with a friend. Write notes for your use.

Even if you are not ideally qualified for a job opening, apply if it appeals to you. Advertisements often describe the ideal candidate for the job, and the ideal is usually not available. If you do lack some skills that are required and you are able to obtain an interview, an employer will be impressed if you ask whether facility in-service programs, orientation, and continuing education courses are offered by the employer to enhance your job skills.

REFERENCES: A TIMELESS TREASURE

Prospective employers will be more interested in some work references than others. There is a *reference hierarchy* of individuals who act as references. Ranging from most to least important are: (1) Current or former nursing instructors, staff from clinical sites where you worked clinical rotations, and supervisors from past nursing-related work or volunteer experiences; (2) past employers or supervisor from non-nursing related jobs; and (3) personal references or friends. (Note: Employers generally don't bother to contact personal references and put little value in their opinions.)

Learning Exercise

Pick Your References

List the persons in your reference hierarchy, including the person's name, job title, address, and work telephone number. Three is the usual number of references requested. Pick and choose from your list of resources for maximum impression.

The statement "References on Request" can be placed at the end of your résumé. It is a matter of personal choice since the employer knows he will get them if interested. Letters of recommendation (preferred) or a reference list should be given to the interviewer if requested. References, however, are a "treasure." Avoid giving them out if you are not interested in the position and risk upsetting the reference.

RÉSUMÉS: THE CONTRIBUTIONS YOU WILL MAKE

Developing two versions (paper scannable and plain-text electronic) of your résumé is a must! It focuses on your work skills, experiences, and qualifications. Résumés are not used as a confession or "tell-all" script. They should not include such items as reasons for leaving past jobs, salary requirements, personal photographs, and personal data, including marital status, race, religion, height, weight, number or age of children, social club memberships, etc.

"Objective statements," located at the top of résumés, went out of fashion more than 20 years ago. Also, statements on "personal goals" or "health" are a waste of time and valuable space on your résumé.

Many résumés are never read because they are too cluttered, too wordy, or contain the aforementioned problems. Use short, bulleted sentences of no more than two to four words because *employers are comparing key words to the job description.* Employers are also reading résumés with the question, "What can you do for me?" So the bulleted sentences have to answer that question. Résumés may be varied according to the job you are seeking.

Essentially, all résumés have a format of profile/qualifications, education, work experience, licenses/professional memberships, and possible military experience. *It is recommended you stop and think about what specific classes or jobs you have performed and record them in your résumé.* Don't assume the employer knows exactly what you mean when you state in your résumé, "Performed nursing duties." It is recommended that military/work experience be listed in years rather than specific dates (i.e., 4 years). Older workers are encouraged

not to dredge up their entire work history; stop after the last 10 years. Also, avoid listing outdated experience or training (i.e., old computer programs, 1990 CPR class, etc.). *Remember, it is important that your résumé be truthful.* Employers may look for inconsistencies, work experiences that are too good to be true, or a résumé that appears purposely vague. Keep your résumé consistent and well balanced.

The initial impression made by the résumé is significant. Basic factors to consider for scannable/personal and electronic plain-text résumés are listed in Box 21-7. Three sample résumés, two typed (Boxes 21-8A and 21-8B) and one electronic (Box 21-8C), were found to be very successful.

COVER LETTERS: TAILORED TO FIT THE JOB YOU WANT

 Learning Exercise

Cover Letters

Why do cover letters need to be sent in with résumés?

It is essential to include a cover letter with each résumé. Cover letters may be submitted by computer, fax, mail, or dropped off with an application for the employer. Cover letters directly answer newspaper and Internet ad requirements. They also list qualifications or follow-up on the unsolicited phone calls you made inquiring about job openings. Cover letters also respond to direct inquiries, so remember to refer to a prior conversation with the hiring manager and/or to "drop" the name of the person who referred you. Neatness, correct spelling, and proper grammar are mandatory. Each letter should be one page, should be an original (never photocopied), should contain no errors or white correction ink, and should be typed in block letter format. If an employer asks for specific experience, be sure to list this in the cover letter, even if your experiences are not listed on the résumé.

Note: You may use the same cover letter you send out by post for your electronic mail. It is

---

Box 21-7 | *Basic Résumé Factors*

SCANNABLE/PERSONAL RÉSUMÉ FACTORS TO CONSIDER
• **Length:** Two pages maximum; one page is preferred. Paper: *Quality bond.* Stay with colors such as white, cream, beige, or gray. Use matching paper for the cover letter and envelope.
Typing: Absolutely no spelling or grammatical errors or extra marks. Type your résumé on a computer, use the spell check program, and use a laser printer, which is less likely to smudge. The computer allows for painless corrections. Updating is performed quickly. It is worth going to a quick print shop to make résumé copies. Standard copy machines provide poor-quality copies.
• **Faxing:** Copy your résumé onto white paper. By sending the fax on white paper, the transmission will be faster and the faxed copy will be clearer and easier to read.
• **Balanced space:** An uncluttered, balanced design is desirable so the résumé is easy to read.
Because most managers don't have time to read, a "bulleted" style is recommended when listing job skills and past duties.

• **Emphasis:** Depends on whether you have a strong or limited work history. Keep in mind to answer the employer's question, "What can you do for me?"

ELECTRONIC PLAIN-TEXT FACTORS TO CONSIDER
Criscito (2006) stated that with e-résumés, the more keywords and synonyms you are able to use, the better your chances of being selected in a keyword search. He also noted the general rule for new graduates was a one-page résumé and for those working one to two pages. With respect to résumé format, white space helps to define sections.
Electronic résumés should have no frills, so no word bolding, dot leaders, Italics, bullets, non-standard fonts, or underlining. The résumé should be typed onto a standard white background, so no special graphic backgrounds, speckled designs, etc. should be used. Also, remember if you chose to use two pages for your résumé to list the core of your skills on the first page because the employer may never bother to look at the second page.

---

recommended that you "paste" your résumé to the end of the electronic cover letter and send this out as a whole unit rather than as an attachment to the e-message. Depending upon the computer the employer has, she or he may be unable to open your attachment.

See Boxes 21-9A and 21-9B for sample cover letters to an employer contacted through an unsolicited telephone call and through a newspaper advertisement.

 Learning Exercise

Résumé
Develop a résumé and include a cover letter.

ANSWERS TO APPLICATION QUESTIONS

You will be asked to fill out an application either before or after an interview (see Box 21-10

for a sample application). It is important that you answer the questions truthfully. If you have had three or more jobs in the past 3 years, the employer will be concerned about this and expect you to supply good reasons for leaving the jobs. Reasons for leaving might include work interfered with school, a layoff, relocation, career exploration, job stagnation, etc. Employment gaps might be explained by responses such as laid off, job hunting, returned to school, travel, and family responsibilities.

If there are questions you wish to defer until the face-to-face interview, write "N/A" (for not applicable), "Will discuss," or leave the space blank. One such area might include expected wage and wages from former jobs. For current wage expected, write *"Open"* or *"Prevailing Wage"*; do not specify a dollar amount. With wages in former employment, leave the spaces blank if you know you were underpaid, or tell the truth if the wage was fair.

Note that if applying via the Internet, several companies use software job application programs that are set to reject applicants if all the data are not listed in the boxes. Some job experts recommend listing a

Box 21-8A *Sample Typed Résumé Starting with Work Experience*

KATELYN BIESER

2001 Putt Drive, Cottage Grove, MN 55301   ktbieser@visi.com   (651) 555-2728

PROFILE
- Medication Administration & Injections
- Bilingual English/Spanish Skills
- Direct Patient Care in Long-Term Facility
- Safety Focus on Patient Transfers
- Working Knowledge of Sterile Techniques
- Patient Observation & Condition Reporting
- Office Skills & Computer Proficiency
- Care Plan Monitoring & Reassessment
- Patient Family Education & Charting
- Worked in Fast-Paced Environments

PROFESSIONAL EXPERIENCE

Kesa Temporary Health Care, Inc. Contracted Services   **Licensed Practical Nurse**
Plymouth, Minnesota   2009 to present
- Personal Care Services
- Assisted Physicians w/Exams
- Patient Emergency Response
- Medication Administration/Injections
- Procedure & Diagnostic Scheduling
- Vital Sign Review/Documentation
- Assisted Medical Staff
- Quality Assurance
- Computerized Charting

Forest View Nursing Home Part-time to Attend School   **Certified Nursing Assistant**
Hastings, Minnesota   Two Years
- Served on Memory Unit
- Obtain/Chart Vital Signs
- Promoted Daily Living Skills
- Health Care Intervention
- Resident Feeding/Hygiene/etc.
- Worked w/in Team of 10 Staff
- Direct Patient Care
- Room Sterilization
- Duties As Assigned

The Small Town Café   **Waitress**
Bloomington, Minnesota   1½ Years
- Customer Base of 50
- Assisted w/Food Preparation
- Time Mgmt/Memory Development
- Customers Requested My Section
- Cashiering
- Cleaned Tables/Dishes

LICENSE/CERTIFICATIONS/MEMBERSHIPS
State of Minnesota Board of Nursing   Practical Nurse   **License**
St. Paul, Minnesota   2009 to present
American Red Cross   Cardiopulmonary Resuscitation   **Certificates**
St. Paul, Minnesota   2008 to present

EDUCATION
Rainy Lakes Technical College   Practical Nursing   **Diploma**
Minneapolis, Minnesota   2009
Cottage Grove High School   General Education   **Diploma**
Cottage Grove, Minnesota   2005

midrange salary in the box to position yourself to get the interview. We recommend listing $00.00 per hour and/or going to the employer's place and obtaining a paper application. Remember, lying on any application is typically grounds for termination.

Be aware that you do not have to answer questions about age, religion, marital status, children, physical data (unless they are specific require-

ments for the job), workers' compensation injuries, or criminal record (unless related to theft, assault, or use of drugs).

An employer's eyes will naturally gravitate toward any blank spaces. Therefore, answer every question, even if it does not apply to you (i.e., for military experience, write N/A in the space if you did not serve). Some employers view blanks or

Box 21-8B | *Sample Typed Résumé Starting with Education Experience*

KATELYN BIESER

2001 Putt Drive, Cottage Grove, MN 55301 ktbieser@visi.com (651) 555-2728

PROFILE

Direct patient care, medication administration & injections, time management, observation of patients and reporting, have a working knowledge of sterile techniques, performed care plan monitoring and reassessment, plus patient & family education. I also have bilingual English/Spanish skills, am office & computer proficient, and enjoy working in a fast-paced environment.

EDUCATION

| **Rainy Lakes Technical College** | Practical Nursing | **Diploma** |
| Minneapolis, Minnesota | | 2009 |

- Nursing Care Principles
- Professional Communication
- Nutritional Care Services

- Medication Administration
- Health Care Delivery
- Clinical Nursing

- Medical-Surgical Nursing
- Maternal/Child Nursing
- Psychosocial Development

| **Cottage Grove High School** | General Education | **Diploma** |
| Cottage Grove, Minnesota | | 2005 |

Emphasis on educational skills enhancement, including algebra, English, reading, spelling, and academic learning.

LICENSE/CERTIFICATIONS/MEMBERSHIPS

State of Minnesota Board of Nursing	Practical Nurse	**License** (In Progress)
St. Paul, Minnesota		2009 to present
American Red Cross	Cardiopulmonary Resuscitation	**Certificates**
St. Paul, Minnesota	First Aid Administration	2008 to present
NFLPN		**Membership**
Garner, North Carolina		2009 to present

PROFESSIONAL EXPERIENCE

| **The Small Town Café** | | Waitress |
| Bloomington, Minnesota | | 1½ Years |

- Customer Base of 50
- Assisted w/Food Preparation

- Time Mgmt/Memory Development
- Customers Requested My Section

- Cashiering
- Cleaned Tables/Dishes

| **Bieser Babysitting, Inc.** | Part-time due to school | **Child Care** |
| Cottage Grove, MN | | 2 Years |

- Personal Care Services
- Recreational Development

- Flexible Scheduling
- Cooking/Cleaning

- Nutritional Feeding/Care
- Safety Intervention

"will explain" as an automatic screen for someone they do not want to employ. Should you choose to answer illegal questions, the examples in Box 21-11 will be helpful. Do not attempt to falsify information, because this will provide grounds for dismissal after hiring. Personnel department will contact your references, schools, former employers, licensing board, etc., to verify the information on your job application and resume.

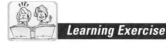

Learning Exercise

Job Application

Using the above suggestions, fill out a practice job application for a nursing position.

Box 21-8C | *Sample Electronic Plain-Test Résumé*

KATELYN BIESER

| 2001 Putt Drive, Cottage Grove, MN 55301 | ktbieser@visi.com | (651) 555–2728 |

PROFILE

Direct patient care, medication administration & injections, time management, observation of patients and reporting, have a working knowledge of sterile techniques, performed care plan monitoring and reassessment, plus patient & family education. I also have bilingual English/Spanish skills, am office & computer proficient, and enjoy working in a fast-paced environment.

EDUCATION

2009 Practical Nursing Diploma	**Rainy Lake Technical College**	Minneapolis, MN

- Nursing Care Principles
- Professional Communication
- Nutritional Care Services

- Medication Administration
- Health Care Delivery
- Clinical Nursing

- Medical-Surgical Nursing
- Maternal/Child Nursing
- Psychosocial Development

2005 General Education Diploma	**Cottage Grove H. S. System**	Cottage Grove, MN

Emphasis on educational skills enhancement, including algebra, English, reading, spelling and academic learning.

PROFESSIONAL EXPERIENCE

1½ Years Waitress	**The Small Town Café**	Bloomington, Minnesota

- Customer Base of 50
- Assisted w/Food Preparation

- Time Mgmt/Memory Development
- Customers Requested My Section

- Cashiering
- Cleaned Tables/Dishes

2 Years Child Care	**Bieser Babysitting, Inc.**	Cottage Grove, MN

- Personal Care Services
- Recreational Development

- Flexible Scheduling
- Cooking/Cleaning

- Nutritional Feeding/Care
- Safety Intervention

LICENSE/CERTIFICATIONS/MEMBERSHIPS

(In Progress)	LPN License	State of Minnesota Board of Nursing	St. Paul, Minnesota
2008 to present	Certificates	American Red Cross	Cardiopulmonary Resuscitation
			First Aid Administration
2009 to present	Membership	NFLPN	Garner, North Carolina

PREPARING FOR THE INTERVIEW

During an interview, you are also interviewing the potential employer (Box 21-12). If you have prepared adequately, you will be able to evaluate whether your job skills, physical abilities, and job interests match the objectives of the facility. Remember to bring a copy of your résumé, LPN/LVN license (if you have passed the NCLEX-PN® examination), CPR card, and medical records documenting tuberculosis skin tests, hepatitis B, and tetanus vaccinations, in case they should be requested (Anderson, 1997).

Interviews are stressful not only for you but also for employers. The employers have to fit interviews into their regular work duties, justify why one job candidate should be hired rather than another, and be on constant guard not to discriminate in matters of age, sex, race, and so on. Knowing that there are concerns on both sides— yours and the interviewer's—will help you be less

| Box 21-9A | *Sample Cover Letter: Unsolicited Telephone Call*

August 12, 2009

Ms. Chris Smekofske, RN
Director of Nursing
St. Helen General Hospital
8354 177th Lane
St. Paul, MN 55084

Re: LPN Staff Nurse Position

Dear Ms. Smekofske:

Thank you for taking the time to speak with me about the Practical Nurse position. As we discussed, I believe that my clinical work experiences and skills area a good match for the job.

In addition to two-plus years of Nursing Assistant experience, my education, job skills and abilities also include:

Direct Patient Care	Charting Observations
Communications	Exposure to a Variety of Patients
Orientation to Safety	Graduation from Accredited Program
Medical Staff Assistance	Personal Health Intervention
Willingness to Learn	NCLEX-PN® License (in progress)

I will plan to contact you on Tuesday, August 18, 2009, to see if you have had an opportunity to review my resume and to determine when an interview may be arranged. I look forward to speaking with you soon.

Cordially,

Katelyn Bieser
2001 Putt Drive
Cottage Grove, MN 55016
(612) 555-2728 or *ktbieser@visi.com*

ENC: Resume

---

defensive. It will also help you understand the meaning of the questions asked, so that you can answer them in an honest and reassuring way.

Part of your responsibility is to help the interviewer become comfortable with who you are and why you should be selected for the job. Yeager and Hough (1990) have suggested ways in which to deal with age and cultural differences encountered in an interview (Box 21-13).

INTERVIEW QUESTIONS AND ANSWERS: A CHALLENGING OPPORTUNITY

Often the first interview question, "Tell me a little bit about yourself," is an icebreaker designed to make you comfortable and determine what is important to you. Take advantage of the question. Put both you and the interviewer on even ground. Do not use the first question as an opportunity to talk about their illegal job application

---

| Box 21-9B | *Cover Letter: Newspaper Ad Response* |

August 12, 2009

Ms. Jennifer Abbinante, RN
Director of Nursing
St. Helen General Hospital
8354 177th Lane
St. Paul, MN 55084

Re: LPN Staff Nurse Position

Dear Ms. Abbinante:

Please accept my résumé as application for the Licensed Practical Nurse position advertised in the Minneapolis Star & Tribune. I believe that my work experiences through the Rainy River Technical College nursing program and at the nursing home are a good match for the position.

As a recent graduate of the Rainy River Technical College, I will be taking my NCLEX-PN® examination on September 27. My clinical work experiences include patient care planning, plan review, direct patient care, administering medications, and team participation. Additionally, I have worked as a Certified Nursing Assistant for 2 years at the Forest View Nursing Home in Hastings, MN, performing the aforementioned duties and more.

I will contact you on Tuesday, August 18, to see whether you have had an opportunity to review my resume and to determine when an interview may be arranged. I look forward to speaking with you soon.

Cordially,

Katelyn Bieser
2001 Putt Drive
Cottage Grove, MN 55016
(612) 555-2728
or *ktbieser@visi.com*

ENC: Resume

---

questions, your dysfunctional family, that you are having a bad day because of a fight with your spouse, etc.

Prepare for your interview by practicing the sample responses to typical interview questions given in Box 21-14. Do this as role-playing with another person in the role of the interviewer. For better preparation, ask the person to mix up the order of the questions. Have them include so-called illegal questions. This will prepare you to handle these questions effectively and make you appear confident when the actual interview occurs.

By being prepared you will not fall victim to the interviewer's most powerful tool: silence. Candidates will usually try to fill the void of silence by providing more information (often revealing details beyond their prepared answers) than they should. If this should happen to you, smile at the interviewer and wait for the next question. An example of "too much information" is, *Question:* Why did you leave your last job? *Answer:* As you know, I am a recent graduate and am looking for employment in my field of study *and I've never done anything before but work as a babysitter.* The italicized portion constitutes "too much information."

Box 21-10 | *Sample Job Application*

Position Desired _____

Dept./Area/Service Preferred: 1)_____

Full Time _____   2)_____

Part Time _____   3)_____ APPLICATION FOR EMPLOYMENT

Today's Date: _____

Date Available to Begin Work_____ ST. MICHAEL'S HOSPITAL

2004 Millennium Way, Forest Lake, MN 55025;
(651) 464–2004

PERSONAL (please print)   An Equal Opportunity Employer

Name _____

         Last   Other Last Name Known By   First   Middle

Address_____

         Street   City   State   Zip Code

Telephone Number (Home) (_____) _____   Business (_____) _____

Social Security Number _____/_____/_____   Date of Birth _____

Have you worked at St. Michael's before? _____ If so, what department?_____ Date?_____

What is your work schedule preference?_____

Will you work shifts? _____   Weekends? _____   Holidays?_____

Do you have the legal right to work in the U.S.?___Yes   ___No
(Final confirmation of employment with SMH is contingent upon timely completion of Employment Eligibility Verification
1–9 Form)

Have you ever plead guilty or "no contest" (nolo contendere) to, or been convicted of, violating any law, with
the exception of minor traffic violations (Please Circle) __Yes   __No

If yes, attach a description and explanation of your prior conviction history, including date of conviction, court
and details of each violation. Note: Disclosure of a criminal record does not automatically disqualify you from
employment consideration.

Have you ever been disciplined or involuntarily discharged for any reason by any employer? __Yes   __No
If yes, please explain.

EDUCATION

Name and Address of School	Circle Last Year Completed	Did You Graduate	Course or Degree
High School _____ Street Address _____ City, State, Zip _____	1 2 3 4	Yes or No	

Box 21-10 | *Sample Job Application—cont'd*

Nursing School _____ Street Address _____ City, State, Zip _____	1 2 3 4	Yes or No
College _____ Street Address _____ City, State, Zip _____	1 2 3 4	Yes or No
Trade/Business/Other_____ Street Address_____ City, State, Zip_____	1 2 3 4	Yes or No

If you did not attend high school, circle highest grade completed. 1 2 3 4 5 6 7 8 9

MEDICAL, TECHNICAL, AND PROFESSIONAL APPLICANTS

Current Number: _____

License _____ State _____ Occupation _____

Certificate _____ State _____ Initial License Date_____

Registration _____ Expiration Date _____

Has your license or registration ever been revoked and/or suspended ___ No ___ Yes   If yes, please
explain: _____

_____

List professional organizations to which you belong _____
List areas of special training or skills, equipment you operate, nursing units you've worked on, etc. _____

_____

_____

EMPLOYMENT—List your last four employers. Begin with your current or most Recent employer.

[1] Employer (company name): Job Title: _____ Your name at that time: _____
Dates of employment: Supervisor: _____ Telephone: (___)_____
     From_____ to _____
     Mth/yr.   Mth/yr.

Address:

Number of hours worked per week: ____   May we contact for   Reason for leaving or
                                          reference?   desire for change?

Description of specific duties (nursing applicants include specific units/departments worked in):

Continued

Box 21-10 | *Sample Job Application—cont'd*

[2] Employer (company name):   Job Title: _____   Your name at that time: _____

Dates of employment: Supervisor: _____   Telephone: (__)_____

      From_____ to _____

         Mth/yr.   Mth/yr.

Address:

Number of hours worked per week: _____   May we contact for   Reason for leaving or desire

                                        reference?   for change?

Description of specific duties (nursing applicants include specific units/departments worked in):

[3] Employer (company name):   Job Title: _____   Your name at that time: _____

Date of employment: Supervisor: _____   Telephone: (__)_____

      From _____to _____

         Mth/yr.   Mth/yr.

Address:

Number of hours worked per week: ____   May we contact for   Reason for leaving or desire

                                        reference?   for change?____

Description of specific duties (nursing applicants include specific units/departments worked):

EMPOLYMENT CONTINUED

[4] Employer (company name):   Job Title: _____   Your name at that time:

Dates of employment: Supervisor: _____   Telephone: (__)_____

      From_____ to _____

         Mth/yr.   Mth/yr.

Address:

Number of hours worked per week: ____   May we contact for   Reason for leaving or desire

                                        reference?   for change?

Description of specific duties (nursing applicants include specific units/departments worked in):

ADDITIONAL WORK REFERENCES—Do not list relatives or personal friends. List 2 work/education–related references who are in a position to evaluate your experience and qualifications.

Name	Occupation	Relationship	No. of years known

Address Phone:

                                        Home: (__)_____   Work: (__)_____

Name   Occupation   Relationship   No. of years known

Address   Phone:

                                        Home: (__)_____   Work: (__)_____

Box 21-10 *Sample Job Application—cont'd*

To assist us in evaluating your application, use the space below to summarize any additional information necessary to describe your qualifications or to address employment actions, criminal record, etc.

_____

_____

_____

_____

READ CAREFULLY BEFORE SIGNING

If employed by St. Michael's Hospital (SMH), I understand that in periods of low census or case load, I may be required to take time off without pay according to hospital needs, or I may be reassigned to another area of the hospital or to other tasks. I understand, agree to, and accept the requirement that I take such time off without pay or undergo such reassignments as a condition of hire.

I certify that the information I have provided in this application is true, complete and accurate. I understand and agree that any false statements or omissions will disqualify me from employment or cause the termination of my employment if such false statements and/or omissions are discovered after I have been hired. I hereby authorize SMH to investigate all statements and information included on this application, including but not limited to my employment record. I hereby release SMH and all educational institutions, employers, and personal references I have listed herein, their employees, officers, and agents, from liability for all claims or damages of any kind in connection with the release of information about me to St. Michael's Hospital pursuant to this authorization.

I understand and agree that if offered employment by SMH, I will be required to undergo a physical examination by a physician designated by St. Michael's Hospital and that any job offer made to me is contingent upon the results of such examination.

I also understand and agree that if I have applied for a position requiring direct patient contact, I will be subject to a criminal background check as required by state statute and this hospital. I understand and agree that if such criminal background causes me to be disqualified from direct patient contact, I will not be hired by St. Michael's Hospital, or if already hired, my employment will be terminated.

Employment at St. Michael's Hospital is at will, meaning that employment may be terminated by St. Michael's Hospital or the employee at any time, for any reason or no reason, with or without notice. I understand that if I am hired by St. Michael's Hospital, my employment will be at will unless the terms of a written contract applicable to my employment state otherwise.

_____
Applicant Signature

MAKING A LASTING IMPRESSION

Learning Exercise

Impression Counts

The kind of person you are is an additional concern to the interviewer. The impression you make includes everything that has been previously discussed plus your appearance and habits during the interview.

PERSONAL HYGIENE

- Bathe.
- Make sure hair is clean and arranged in a moderate style.
- Men's hair and beard should be neatly trimmed.
- Keep nails short, clean, and nicely manicured, with clear nail polish (*Note:* Research has identified long fingernails, fake nails, and nail polish as sites for harmful organisms. Some health facilities

Box 21-11 | *Sample Answers to Illegal Questions*

HAVE YOU BEEN HOSPITALIZED WITHIN THE PAST 5 YEARS?

Answer: I do not have any health problems that would interfere with fulfilling the described position.

HAVE YOU EVER BEEN ON WORKERS' COMPENSATION?

Answer: N/A (not applicable) (OR) I am able to perform all of the described job duties.

DO YOU HAVE A CRIMINAL RECORD?

Answer: I have gotten a speeding ticket, but have never been convicted of crimes involving drugs, theft, or assault. (OR) I have paid for that error in judgment, taken special classes, and am now wise enough not to repeat it.

Box 21-12 | *Sample Questions to Ask the Interviewer*

- Travel Nurse Depot (2003) suggested:
- What type of patients will I work with?
- How do you do your scheduling?
- Will I be floated to other units?
- What type of charting system is used?
- How big is the facility, and how many beds are in the unit?
- How long does orientation last?
- What is the nurse-to-patient ratio?
- What type of uniform is worn?
- Will overtime be available if I want it?
- Will I be able to request workdays?
- Will I be working every other weekend?
- Is testing required before going to the floors?

The author also recommends:
- Given my interests to work on a ___ unit, would it be possible to move to one if an opening became available?
- What opportunities does the facility offer for career development?
- Do you provide support or mentoring for new hires?

Box 21-13 | *Tips for Handling Differences between the Interviewer and You*

If the interviewer is younger than you statements such as, "I bring a lot of experience to this position" will have a more positive effect than, "I know I am older than the typical candidate, but...." If the interviewer is older than you statements such as, "I have always worked very hard and feel learning is a lifelong process" that will help establish your maturity.

With respect to cultural background, when there are differences between you and the interviewer, you need to remember that different groups have different norms concerning eye contact, personal distance, body language, joking/teasing, and other subtle aspects of communication.

To work through the differences, it is recommended you follow the interviewer's lead in the course of communication. Don't mime the interviewer's specific style, but allow her or him to establish some norms concerning how to communicate.

have been subject to litigation caused by infection and/or death traced to fingernail-related issues. These facilities have ruled that no personnel giving direct patient care are permitted to have long natural fingernails, have false nails, or wear fingernail polish of any shade.)

- If you are a smoker, remove yellow finger stains with bleach and water.
- Use an unscented deodorant.
- Recent mouth care is needed to remove bad breath. (Remember not to indulge in food or drink with a heavy unpleasant odor or food that may stain your teeth or tongue near the time of the interview.) Floss and brush your teeth, tongue, palate, and inner cheeks with a soft toothbrush. Use a breath freshener.
- Go easy on the aftershave or perfume, and don't sprinkle any on your clothing. Limit yourself to light perfume (a "clean" look and smell go a long way).
- Smell your clothes; don't go into an interview with your clothes smelling like you've been in a smoke-filled bar.

Box 21-14 | *Sample Interview Questions and Answers*

TELL ME ABOUT YOURSELF.

Answer: Would you like to know about my work history or personal life? *If work history*, provide a brief description of your schooling, past jobs, and goal to work as a staff/long-term care, etc. LPN. *For personal*, you might say, I have lived in this area all my life (or) my plans are to make this area my home. I recently graduated from Rainey River Technical College and am looking for a career I can grow in.

HAVE YOU EVER DONE THIS TYPE OF WORK BEFORE?

Answer: Yes, in fact some of my experiences include direct patient care during clinical rotations, volunteer work as a candy striper, experiences as a mother, and….

WHY DO YOU WANT TO WORK HERE?

Answer: The (facility name) has an excellent reputation in the community and job opportunities which, I am trained in. Additionally, your mission statement of _____ reflects my views on _____.

WHAT MOTIVATES YOU?

As a nurse I am motivated by work and its challenge of my skills on a daily basis. And, that with the right employer I will continue to learn new skills as medicine changes.

WHY DID YOU LEAVE YOUR LAST JOB?

Answer: As you know, I am a recent graduate and am looking for employment in my field of study. *Note:* If you have worked as an LPN/LVN: I am looking for a new position to expand my work skills, keep the job interesting, and provide better advancement opportunities.

TELL ME ABOUT YOUR LAST EMPLOYER.

Answer: I really enjoyed my work at _____, which has an excellent reputation for _____. But, now it is time to move on to new opportunities.

WHAT HAVE YOU DONE TO KEEP YOUR CLINICAL SKILLS CURRENT?

Answer: Well, in addition to participating in several clinical rotations during school, I recently joined the _____ (LPN professional organization) to keep abreast of new developments in nursing.

HOW DO YOU COMPARE YOUR VERBAL SKILLS WITH YOUR WRITING SKILLS?

Answer: Organizations are more dependent than ever on their employees' communicating well both verbally and in writing. I am constantly taking advantage of opportunities to develop in both areas by asking for feedback and utilizing the feedback I receive.

WHY SHOULD I HIRE YOU INSTEAD OF SOMEONE ELSE?

Answer: I think my references can best answer that question. I am sure when you contact them, they will agree I am hard working and dependable and get the job done correctly.

WHEN ARE YOU AVAILABLE FOR WORK?

Answer: Right away. OR: I would need to give my employer 2 weeks' notice. It will provide me time to tie up loose ends and my employer time to find a replacement.

Note: If the interviewer insists you terminate you job immediately, you are witnessing a power play. You need to ask yourself if you really want to work for this individual. This could be the tip of the iceberg for future power plays.

HOW IS YOUR HEALTH? ARE THERE ANY PARTS OF THE JOB YOU CAN'T PERFORM?

Answer: I have always been healthy. I see myself being able to perform all parts. I think the best approach to any job is to use common sense. If I need help, I am not afraid to ask for it.

WHAT ARE YOUR GREATEST STRENGTHS?

Answer: I would have to say that my strengths include (1) _____ , (2) _____, (3) _____, (4) _____, (5) _____.
Note: Your responses should be consistent with what your references say about you.

Continued

| Box 21-14 | *Sample Interview Questions and Answers—cont'd*

WHAT IS YOUR GREATEST WEAKNESS?

Answer: As you know, everyone has weaknesses. My greatest weakness right now is the various computer programs out there for charting on patients. Due to this, I prefer to be shown how to use the facility's program rather than be told to read the manual. I like getting things done right the first time.

WHAT ARE YOUR LONG-TERM GOALS?

Answer: Eventually, I would like to work as a Charge Nurse at this facility. Although my aim is not to replace the current Charge Nurse, it is my goal to learn all I can. This will help me better contribute to the team and you will feel confident that the work is being taken care of.

HAS AN EMPLOYER EVER FIRED YOU?

Answer: Before going to nursing school and getting my priorities straight an employer fired me for attendance problems. It was a valuable lesson that I learned from and will never repeat.

(*Note:* Do not start your response with "Yes"; address the issue.)

CAN YOU WORK UNDER PRESSURE?

Answer: Yes, I have experienced working under pressure for many years. This has meant meeting deadlines, dealing with difficult people, and developing employer confidence that the job will be done right.

WILL CHILDCARE BE AN ISSUE?

Answer: No, I have found a good daycare setting for my children. If they cannot go to daycare, I have worked out a system of alternating days with another provider or relative to take care of them so that work is minimally affected. *Note:* Although some individuals believe this is an illegal question, I contend the employer has a right to know. A stable staffing pattern is needed to maintain quality patient care.

WOULD YOU BE WILLING TO WORK OVERTIME?

Answer: Yes, if it will help the unit

MAY WE CONTACT YOUR CURRENT EMPLOYER?

Answer: Yes, but after a firm job offer has been made. I would appreciate it if before you contact my employer to allow me to talk with my supervisor first as a courtesy.

AREN'T YOU OVERQUALIFIED FOR THIS JOB?

Answer: I may be more qualified than other individuals you are considering, but this simply means that I will be able to make an immediate contribution. After learning your system, I hope to be eligible for advancement opportunities within the organization.

IS YOUR SPOUSE EMPLOYED? WILL THERE BE A CONFLICT?

Answer: Yes, my spouse has a job. No, I don't see that there would be a conflict. We are both looking forward to my working for you.

WHAT KIND OF SALARY OR WAGE DO YOU EXPECT?

Answer: What would a person with my background and qualifications typically earn in this position with your company? OR: I am ready to consider your best offer.

Note: If an employer insists you give a wage quote, give a wage using your bottom dollar and a realistic top wage. Possible salary resources include the Internet, labor market sites through your local Job Service/WorkForce Centers, or using *www.salary.com* and/or *www.bls.gov.*

Additionally, if you are considering relocation to another city/state, you are encouraged to use *www.home-fair.com* to determine how much salary you will need to maintain your current standard of living. For instance, during the year 2003 an individual earning $28,000 per year in Duluth, MN needed to earn $37,325 in Arlington Heights, IL.

Answer: I would think we could agree on a salary between $00.00 per hour and $00.00 per hour.

Box 21-14 | *Sample Interview Questions and Answers—cont'd*

DO YOU HAVE ANY QUESTIONS?

Answer: (See Box 21-13 for questions to ask the interviewer.) After your questions, ask if It would be possible to take a tour of the facility and ask about the date you might start. *Block & Betrus (2004) provided additional questions, which we have adapted and/or used for this section:*

HOW DO YOU DEAL WITH CRITICISM AND DESCRIBE A TIME YOU WERE CRITICIZED FOR POOR PERFORMANCE.

Answer: A person who doesn't make mistakes will never grow. Most recently, in school, I had problems with time management. Due to this I didn't do very well on a couple of tests and my teachers let me know they were disappointed because I hadn't done my best work. I agreed they were right and asked for assistance. One of my teachers then showed me how to improve my time management so the problem wouldn't happen again. And, it didn't.

HOW DO YOU VENT ANGER OR FRUSTRATION IF YOUR DAY HAS BEEN CHALLENGING OR STRESSFUL?

Answer: I am a walker and a talker. My first choice is to burn the stress off by walking/biking/ Health club, etc. I always feel better after exercising. If that is not available I will go outside on my break alone and talk out the problem and associated emotion. It is amazing what talking for 10 minutes will do for getting perspective back.

DO YOU HAVE A VALID DRIVER'S LICENSE?

Answer: I will use the city bus system to get to work. If the buses aren't running, there is always a taxicab available, plus I have a network of friends who can help me in a pinch. I have never been late to work.

IS THERE ANY TIME WHEN IT IS OKAY TO BREAK COMPANY RULES?

Answer: Yes, if someone's life was in physical danger.

ILLEGAL QUESTIONS/RESPONSES

(*Note: You don't have to answer these.*)

WHAT RELIGIOUS FAITH ARE YOU?

Answer: Religion certainly is a part of this great country of ours; but I prefer to separate religion from work. Don't you?

THAT'S A NICE NAME. IS IT JEWISH/MUSLIM/IRISH/ETC?

Answer: America is a melting pot. That's why it's the greatest country on earth. I feel we are all Americans first and foremost and that's the most important issue here. Don't you agree?

HAVE YOU EVER BEEN TESTED FOR HIV?

Answer: No, I have never had a reason to test for HIV, nor do I anticipate a reason to do so. (OR) No, has this facility had HIV problems?

WHAT IS YOUR SEXUAL PREFERENCE?

Answer: My friends and family call me _____ (first name). They support who I am and don't care one way or the other. Everyone who knows me, knows I do a good job and I provide excellent patient care. Now, isn't that what this interview is about?

CLOTHING

A nurse working in Hawaii indicated that it was acceptable to interview in Hawaii wearing dress shorts and a polo shirt or a muumuu. The nurse then postulated that the part of the country you live in dictates your interview wear. Mahan (2003) stated, "You'd be surprised at how many professional nurses come to an interview dressed inappropriately. Listen; jeans and a tee-shirt are never appropriate ... put on a professional looking attire." Zurlinden (2003) recommended conservative wear when applying for employment. He did indicate that "scrubs or your uniform are acceptable immediately after work, but only at the facility where you work." Zurlinden went on to ask why anyone would think about scheduling an interview on a workday, when they needed to be focused on the interview.

You can contact the human resources department of the prospective employer to ask about interview wear, or take the safe route of interviewing in conservative dress. When choosing clothing, both men and women should try on different suits or blazers to determine which fits best and hangs properly. There should be no overhang or tightness in the shoulder pad area. Poorly fitting suits look bad and wear out quickly. When buying clothing, the reality is students may not always be able to afford the ideal. You can always look your best in conservative clothes, which are clean and ironed, with polished shoes. Check out thrift stores and consignment shops; they are resources waiting to be discovered. Additionally, check out community organizations that loan clothing such as Clothes Closets (e.g., the YWCA). When looking for clothing, consider the following points:

MEN. Wear a long-sleeved white dress shirt, a solid or pinstripe navy blue or gray suit, and a medallion-patterned red or navy tie that is 3 inches wide and length down to your belt line. Dark shoes, "long" dark socks, and a belt that matches the color of your shoes are a must.

WOMEN. Choose solid or pinstripe navy, gray, or blue dresses, jacket dresses, or suits. Look for simple, straight or pleated skirts that reach at least knee level and are comfortable to sit in. (Save the sexy, short skirts, and/or lack of underwear for when you go out with your friends.) If wearing a skirt or suit, consider wearing a white, off white, or light blue cotton or silk blouse with a conservative neckline and buttons. For women

with prominent cleavage, a camisole underneath is recommended to keep the focus on your face. Wear dark, polished, low-heeled shoes with closed toes.

Women with larger hips may want to avoid wearing short jackets. Short jackets flatter women who are petite. Additionally, some women who wear gray jackets will want to keep the gray away from their faces by wearing a crisp white blouse or a soft beige sweater. From some, gray clothes worn too close to the face "drain away your fresh complexion."

MAKE-UP

Conservative make-up is always appropriate. Make-up should be kept to a minimum; wearing too much is the most common mistake. Remember: It is the confidence you display in the interview that makes you attractive to the interviewer.

ACCESSORIES

Wear simple jewelry or none at all. Simple necklaces such as a single strand of pearls, colored beads, or a silver or gold chain work well. Avoid drop, dangle, or chandelier type earrings and noisy charm bracelets that clank or have fake gems, etc. Remove piercings in nose, on tongue, etc. Cover tattoos. You will want to limit yourself to a small portfolio or briefcase that is large enough to hold any papers, resumes, etc. If you have a coat or umbrella, leave it in the car or politely ask where you can hang or lay it. The main point is to avoid holding items or balancing them on your lap. The fewer distractions, the more calm and focused you will be on the interview.

EYE WEAR

Don't wear the latest craze in eyeglasses, as they will only serve to distract the interviewer. Wear glasses that contrast the shape of your face. For a heart-shaped head consider glasses with a geometric frame that gives some width to the lower half of your face. A square-shaped head would benefit from a round or oval frame with some width. A round-shaped head should avoid dark frames and use angular and narrow frames—never a square or circle. If the head is oval shaped, then use a rectangular frame.

POSTURE

Walk tall and sit erect in the middle of the chair. Both feet should rest on the floor, and your head should be upright. Arms and hands should be in an open position and not crossed. (Remember, you have nothing to hide.) Keep your hands inactive. If you habitually fidget, consider bringing a paper clip to hold in your hands during the interview.

MANNER

Your manner should be assured. Do not interrupt the interviewer or rush the interview. Pause to think as needed, and then answer without hesitating. Ask for an explanation or repetition of any questions you do not understand. Eye contact is essential, especially when answering questions. If you are uncomfortable with making eye contact, two techniques can be used to correct this: (1) look at the person's nose, or (2) look at the space between the interviewer's eyebrows. Both techniques give the illusion of eye contact. Remember to look away periodically so that you do not appear to be staring. Avoid making negative statements about school, former bosses, jobs, current finances, personal problems, etc.

COURTESY

Arrive 5 minutes early and remember to shut off your cell phone; don't switch it to mute, as the interviewer will hear it. It is safe to say you will live for a half hour without talking to friends or family. When the employer enters the room, stand, smile, and extend your hand for a firm handshake. Do not use a "bone-crusher" grip or a limp, "dead fish" handshake. To get the handshake right, find someone to practice with before the interview. Additionally, if your palms tend to sweat, slide your hands alongside the top of your thigh when standing up. It will remove the moisture while appearing very natural.

With a handshake, say, "Hi, Mr. (Ms.) Smith, _____ (your name), I'm pleased to meet you." Similarly, when the interview is over, stand up, look the person in the eyes and offer your hand for a firm handshake. Address the employer by surname: "Mr. (Ms.) Smith, thank you for the opportunity to interview with you. I am very interested in the job. Would it be alright to call you next week to see if you have made a decision?" If you want the job, give the employer your work references or letters of recommendation. Lastly, ask the interviewer for his or her business card. The card will help you when sending your thank you letter (e.g., correct title, name, etc.).

HABITS

Do not chew gum or smoke while in the waiting room or during the interview. Also, don't smoke outside the building and then come in for the interview. Although the nicotine may make you feel calm, you will be bringing in the fresh smell of smoke. Cigarette smoke is often offensive to nonsmokers. Politely refuse an offer of coffee, tea, or cigarettes. In addition, do not attempt to read any materials on the employer's desk or computer screen.

DISCUSSING PREGNANCY ISSUES

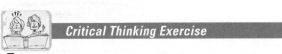 *Critical Thinking Exercise*

Pregnancy

If you are pregnant, what do you need to consider before talking with an employer about it? When do you tell a new employer that you are pregnant? Or, when do you discuss pregnancy so it doesn't interfere with career advancement?

Even if the Pregnancy Discrimination Act and/or Family and Medical Leave Act protects your job (FMLA applies if there are 50 or more employees with the company), these are tough questions. It has been this author's observation that women generally wait a couple of months before disclosing the pregnancy. In part this is to make sure it is a healthy pregnancy, financial concerns are addressed, and they are emotionally ready for all the attention.

When you are ready to talk about your pregnancy, be prepared to discuss (1) how long you plan to work, (2) how long you intend to be gone, and possibly (3) how your work will be covered while you are away. Then talk with your coworkers about the pregnancy and enlist their moral support. Expectant mothers will have both good and bad days during the pregnancy, and friends can be a great help.

Learning Exercise

Mock Interview

Enlist a peer to practice interviewing for a nursing position. Take turns in the role of a nurse seeking a job and the employer. Practice asking and answering questions to be anticipated during an interview. Using the suggestions in this chapter, including appropriate dress and behavior, stage a mock interview. Arrange with the media department of your school to videotape the interview. View the interview and self-evaluate and have peers evaluate your performance.

PRE-EMPLOYMENT PHYSICAL EXAMINATION, DRUG SCREENING, BACKGROUND CHECKS

More and more employers are requiring pre-employment physical examinations as part of conditional job offers. A conditional job offer states that you have been offered the job contingent on your passing a physical examination, drug screening/urine analysis, and/or background check. If you fail, the job offer is withdrawn.

PHYSICAL EXAMINATION

You will be required to meet with a doctor specified by the employer, who will perform an examination and can legally ask you about your past medical history. Think about any past surgeries, workers' compensation injuries, allergies, and family history, including cancer and heart trouble. Be prepared to provide the dates of these occurrences and the names of the physicians who provided treatment. If you have any personal concerns about the answers your physician might provide, call your doctor before the pre-employment physical examination. Discuss the prospective job and obtain his or her opinion.

DRUG SCREENING

If you are taking medications, be sure to notify the employer before the screening. You will want to reaffirm in the employer's mind you are taking a "medical prescription," physician recommended, that will not interfere with your work. You may need to provide a copy of your prescription.

Be aware that although drug-screening accuracy is improving, it is not 100% accurate. False-positive drug results may occur if medical conditions such as kidney infection/disease, liver disease, or diabetes exist. Common foods such as poppy seed foods, riboflavin in food (vitamin B_2 and hemp seed oil), or vitamin B_2 tablets may trigger false-positive results. Additionally, false-positive reactions occur with the following medications: Vicks NyQuil, Contac, Sudafed, and Dimetapp; Excedrin IB; Allerest; Robitussin Cold & Flu; Dexatrim; Acutrim; Vicks inhaler; Afrin; cough suppressants with dextromethorphan; asthma medications, including Marax, Bronkaid tablets, Primatene tablets; and prescription medications. If you are taking a prescribed medication, call your pharmacist and ask if the medication will trigger a positive drug result.

At this time, it is estimated there is a 5% to 14% error rate. Due to this, any positive drug screening test should be followed by a second and more rigorous test. Discuss with the employer that you are aware of reliability problems with initial drug-screening tests. State you would like to take another test, but with a different testing service. The employer can name the other service, date, and time for the screening. The key is sincerity; if you want the job, let the employer know you are willing to go the extra mile. If you fail a test and really want the job, you might consider discussing splitting or paying for the cost of the second test.

BACKGROUND CHECKS

Be aware that employers have begun to informally check online blogs to see whose names appear and what they have to say. They may also Google the person's name and email to see what pops up. Darrah (2006) stated, "It was not a good idea to do online blogging about yourself, people in your industry, coworkers or have a picture of yourself on your MySpace page." As an example, Darrah recounted a story about a man who had successfully participated in a job interview only to lose the opportunity when the employer found his web page, which included references to recreational marijuana use and his desire to "dance with the devil."

Employers are performing formal background checks on a more frequent basis. According to Krumrie (2003), background checks typically include "driving records, credit history, criminal records, court records, state licensing records, property ownership, education, and military records." Typically, employers will ask that a release of information be signed, which is either a part of the job application or on a separate form. Krumrie stated that to avoid inaccuracies, "job seekers could request their personal files from former employers once every six months." He recommended credit reports and criminal records be reviewed for accuracy and that education be correctly stated.

Gryskiewicz (2003) reported that, after a provisional job offer, companies such as hers hiring medical and other staff always used Employment Verification Firms (EVFs) to perform employee background checks. Employment background checks are viewed as a necessity because of statistics that indicate the following:

- Thirty-three percent of job applicants falsify employment applications,
- More than $15 billion is lost annually to employee theft,
- Approximately 3.2 million crimes and thefts occur at places of work, and
- Workplace violence costs employers more than $4.2 billion annually in lost work and legal fees.

EVFs check the accuracy of résumé employment dates, job tasks performed, education, accrediting licensure bodies, social security, date of birth, etc. Additionally, EVFs review credit history; criminal conduct, such as assault, theft, and drug use; and credit history. Gryskiewicz's advice is to be truthful! False, incomplete, or erroneous information is considered grounds for denying/terminating employment. As an example, Gryskiewicz reported how a job applicant applied for a job and listed her education as a master's degree. Through a background check it was learned the applicant had a PhD degree. Because of this job application falsification, the job offer was withdrawn. With respect to criminal records, Gryskiewicz indicated disclosure of a criminal record did not automatically reject applicants because some states have laws that a conviction cannot prevent a job offer unless a specific relationship is established between the crime and job requirements/environment. As such, all cases were individually reviewed.

AFTER THE INTERVIEW

Follow-up after a job interview is essential. It is a constant source of amazement to employers that 90% of the people who interview never follow up to see if they got the job. Recent graduates and even nurses who have been working in the field for some time are under the follow-up illusion that is the employer's responsibility to contact them. If you are not interested enough to follow up after the interview, why did you bother to interview in the first place?

Write a thank you letter to the interviewer the same day you interviewed. Write it while the information is fresh in your mind and before you become distracted by other projects. Remember, the more often the employer sees or hears your name, the better your chances of being hired. Don't be the person waiting for a telephone call. A thank you letter may be as simple as the one provided in Box 21-15.

Remember to follow up with the employer! Call the employer on the date stated in your letter. Make it a practice not to make follow-up contacts on Mondays. Mondays are traditionally full because of staff meetings, weekend concerns, staff discipline, paperwork catch-up, and other

| Box 21-15 | *Letter—Thank You for the Interview* |

August 12, 2009

Ms. Irene Fedun, RN
Director of Nursing
St. Helen General Hospital
8354 177th Lane
St. Paul, MN 55084

Re: LPN Staff Nurse Position

Dear Ms. Fedun:

Thank you for meeting with me today to discuss the LPN staff position. After our conversation about the job duties and the tour of the hospital floor, I feel that my work experiences and education are a good match.

Specifically, I look to work on the Memory Unit, as this is a special interest of mine.

Through our work together the patients will receive timely, quality care.

I remain very interested in the position. I will contact you on Tuesday, August 18th to see whether you have made a decision or whether a second interview will be arranged. I look forward to speaking with you soon.

Katelyn Bieser
2001 Putt Drive
Cottage Grove, MN 55016

(612) 555-2728 or *ktbieser@visi.com*

---

duties. The best times to make follow-up calls are after 9:00 AM. The key to a successful follow-up call is to be courteous but firm with the secretary. Ask to speak with the person in charge of hiring.

The following is a sample follow-up contact to an employer:

Secretary: Good morning, Human Resources (don't be surprised if no name is given).

You: Hi, I'm Katelyn Bieser. Is Ms. George available? I am following up on our previous meeting.

Secretary: One minute please. (Although the employer might be away from the office, or on another line, the secretary will probably

check to see whether your call should be taken.)

Secretary: I'm sorry, Ms. George is away from her desk/on another line/in a meeting, etc. May I take a message and/or would you like to leave a message on her phone?

You: Yes, thank you. Also, when is the best time to typically reach her?

You: (Transferred to message machine) Hi Ms. George, this is Katelyn Bieser and I am following up on our interview for the LPN staff position to determine if you have made a decision. I remain very interested in the job and can be reached at _____ (telephone number).

You: [If the employer is in] Hi Ms. George, this is Katelyn Bieser and I am following up on our interview for the LPN staff position. I was wondering if you have made a decision yet? Oh, you haven't. Would it be okay to follow up with you next Tuesday to see if you have made a decision? Great! I will call you then. (OR) Oh, you've decided on someone else. Would you keep me in mind if that person does not work out and/or another position becomes available?

 Learning Exercise

Thank You Letter

Compose a thank you letter after an employment interview for a nursing position.

RESIGNATION WITH STYLE

 Learning Exercise

Keep the Connections

Is there a difference between "burning bridges" and "untying the connection?" What is the value of recapping your accomplishments with a resignation letter?

Box 21-16 | *Sample Resignation Letter*

September 24, 2011

Ms. Sivia Hinkkanen
Director of Nursing
George County Hospital
1515 Rodeo Lane
Minneapolis, MN 55401

Dear Ms. Hinkkanen:

Please accept my resignation as Charge Nurse on Unit 3, to be effective on October 01, 2011. My association with the George County Hospital has been rewarding professionally and personally. It is satisfying to have been able to contribute to the positive reputation of client care.

I am especially pleased to have been a member of the Quality Assurance Committee, which furthered my professional growth. In addition, I remain appreciative of having been honored as "Employee of the Month."

Please accept my thanks for the support you have provided me during the past one-and-a-half years of employment. I wish the members of this hospital the very best.

Cordially,
Katelyn Bieser, LPN,
Alzheimer's Unit

In today's job market, employers continue to try to hold down their costs by limiting annual raises to 3% or less. However, in their desire to staff positions, some employers will offer job-hoppers (i.e., frequent job changers) 10% to 20% over their current wages, offer sign-on bonuses, and/or provide higher shift differentials.

If you are contemplating a change, it is recommended you look at how long you have been with the employer. If you have worked with the company less than 3 months, you can hop right away, remembering not to list the employer on your résumé. In the event you have worked longer than 3 months with the employer; it is recommended that you work a minimum of 1 year to obtain experience and demonstrate stability. (Contact your state board for length of time, as that may vary from state to state.)

If you have made the decision to leave your employer, it is important to leave the job with class. Perhaps the best expression I have heard is, "Untie, don't sever, the connection." You never know who may call your former employer as a part of their follow-up.

It is strongly recommended you have a position secured before leaving. Many employers today have what is called "at will" employment. Simply put, you or the employer can terminate your employment at any time, without advance notice or reason. As such, an employer may terminate your job the day you give notice.

That being said, we have found that several "at will" employers have personnel policies requiring a 2-week notice be given when resigning. The policies typically indicate that if a 2-week notice is given, the employee will be eligible for future rehire. It is resignation courtesy to give 2 weeks' notice whether there is a policy or not. This is a courtesy to your coworkers and to the employer so a new person might be hired and orientated before you leave.

Use a business format and plain paper, and type the letter. Even if you are leaving because of unhappy circumstances on the job, do not vent these feelings in the letter. As mentioned before, you may need this employer as a work reference in the future. Additionally, your current supervisor may also leave in the future, and all there is to remind the employer about you is your personnel file.

Because resignation is part of your permanent record, it provides you with an opportunity to recap your accomplishments or special recognition. The employer may refer to the letter when employers with whom you are seeking employment contact him or her. See the sample resignation letter in Box 21-16.

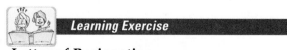

Learning Exercise

Letter of Resignation

Compose a letter of resignation from a nursing position.

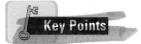
Key Points

- To be successful in your job, it is important to begin it with the first day of classes and continue from that day on.
- Opportunities present themselves to those who are willing to put forth a little effort and realize that the world does not owe them a living.
- The methods presented in this chapter have proved successful for graduates, people wishing to make career changes, or those wanting to institute a change in their work. Remember to treat your job search like a job.
- Make your contacts by telephone or computer, by forwarding résumés or cover letters, or by physically going to the employer to apply and schedule an interview.
- Explore the hidden job market via networking, the Internet, or using the telephone book and then calling employers, whether an ad has been placed or not.
- Dress for the job you want, not the job you have.
- Actively follow up on all interviews! Let the employer know that you are interested. Remember, the more often the employer hears or sees your name, the better your chances will be of getting hired.
- If you are hired, send thank you notes to those who helped you. You may need them again. Remember, you are responsible for making your own luck.

REVIEW ITEMS

1. What interpersonal style is representative of giving a "minute by minute breakdown of what happened that day?"
    1. Friendly-focused
    2. Detail-focused
    3. Results-focused
    4. Party-focused

2. Your employer has an employment policy of at-will employment. Which of the following reflects the meaning of this?
    1. The employer expects a 2-week notice before you leave their employment.
    2. The employer will determine the length or extension of probationary periods.
    3. The employer may terminate your job immediately without notice or reason.
    4. The employer will continue your employment indefinitely, provided the job requirements are met.

3. An interviewer asks you a question for which you do not have an answer. Which of the following would be an appropriate response?
    1. Ask the interviewer to please rephrase the question.
    2. Begin to answer and switch to a topic you know about.
    3. Smile pleasantly and say you don't know the answer.
    4. Take a key word from the question, and make up a response.

4. What criminal records would automatically preclude you from employment?
    1. Shoplifting offense
    2. Second-degree assault
    3. Possession of a crack pipe
    4. Graffiti/tagging property

ALTERNATE FORMAT ITEM

Which of the following uses of the Internet are helpful in job hunting? *(Select all that apply.)*

1. Perform online interview

2. Identify salary range

3. Complete job application

4. Locate job opportunities

5. Research facility information

22 The NCLEX-PN® Examination

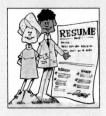

evolve http://evolve.elsevier.com/Hill/success/

Objectives

On completing this chapter, you will be able to do the following:

1. Explain the purpose of the NCLEX-PN® examination.
2. Research the requirements of your state board of nursing for eligibility to take the NCLEX-PN® examination.
3. Describe how CAT determines whether you pass or fail the NCLEX-PN® examination
4. Explain the process of endorsement.
5. Differentiate between a temporary work permit and licensure.
6. Discuss the proven way of preparing for the NCLEX-PN® examination.
7. Explain the legal implications of ignoring the NCLEX-PN® confidentiality clause and sharing information about the NCLRX-PN® content with others.

Key Terms

Authorization to test (ATT) (p. 421)
Candidate (p. 417)
Computerized adaptive testing
  (CAT) (p. 418)
Endorsement (p. 418)
Items (p. 418)
Mock examinations (p. 426)
NCLEX-PN® confidentiality clause (p. 418)
NCLEX-PN® examination (p. 418)
State board of nursing (p. 418)
"State boards" (p. 417)

 Keep in Mind

*Almost without exception, when student nurses are asked about their goal for the year, they respond by saying they want to pass **"boards,"** meaning, pass the National Council of State Boards of Nursing (NCSBN) practical/vocational licensure examination (NCLEX-PN®) to become a licensed practical or vocational nurse (LPN/LVN).*

BEFORE COMPUTERIZED ADAPTIVE TESTING

Initially, "state boards" were paper-and-pencil tests. Boards were given twice a year in most states at limited sites that remained the same year after year. Proctors chosen from instructors within the state monitored the examination. Most candidates were honest and did not attempt to cheat. Proctors tried to prevent cheating by those who were determined to pass using whatever means necessary. For example, occasionally a candidate would take an examination using another student's identity, wear a full skirt with "crib notes" written on the inside hem of the skirt, or have agreed on a system of coughs to assist a student who was not as prepared for boards. Although proctors attempted to be vigilant, there was no sure way of preventing all deception that occurred. Everyone took the same test, so students would collaborate to write down test questions they remembered. Some had a pre-planned meeting with an instructor to share the questions. Instructors would work the content of questions into their course.

Currently candidates' sign a NCLEX-PN® confidentiality clause prior to testing. Dr. Tom O'Neill, associate director, NCLEX Examination states that, "technically if students were to discuss the exam with an instructor they would be in violation of 'terms of confidentiality' they must agree to before they take the exam. These terms include not disclosing the content of the examination items before, during, or after the examination. Legal action could be taken against candidates that break the NCLEX-PN® confidentiality clause, including criminal prosecution and civil litigation as well as other administrative disciplinary actions" (2007).

The NCSBN decided a secure method of examination had to be developed. Since April 1994, practical/vocational nursing graduates (candidates) have taken the NCLEX-PN® examination by computer. This method is called computerized adaptive testing (CAT). All candidates will have different questions based on how they answer the previous question. The current testing service is Pearson Professional Testing (testing service for NCLEX-PN® examination). Testing centers are located across the United States and its territories, and testing is available year round (Pearson Professional Testing is referred to as Pearson VUE). Many types of examinations are administered at the Pearson testing centers. Some examinations require typing for essay-type responses. Earplugs may be requested of the Pearson staff if these typing sounds are a distraction to the nursing candidate.

WHAT IS THE NCLEX-PN® EXAMINATION?

The NCLEX-PN® examination is the National Council Licensing Examination for Practical/Vocational Nursing graduates. It is designed to test knowledge, skills, and abilities needed to safely and effectively practice nursing as a new entry level LPN/LVN. The NCLEX-PN®

examination results provide the basis for licenses granted to practical/vocational nurses by state boards of nursing. *Boards are the only agencies that can license a graduate of a practical/vocational program and release the test results to them. Do not contact Pearson VUE for test results, as they will not release the results directly to you.*

The NCLEX-PN® examination is given in the United States, American Samoa, the District of Columbia, Guam, the Northern Mariana Islands, Puerto Rico, and the Virgin Islands. This makes it possible to provide licensure by endorsement from one board of nursing to another. Endorsement means that an LPN/LVN may apply for licensure in a different state or territory without retesting. Taking the same examination in the United States and its territories facilitates endorsement from one nursing board to another.

As of January 2005, a pilot initiative was advanced by the NCSBN for international sites for NCLEX testing in Pearson Professional Centers for the purposes of licensure. The first sites are London, England, Hong Kong, and Seoul, South Korea. The NCSBN (2004) listed five top countries where nurses were educated outside the U.S. and took the NCLEX examination in hopes of obtaining nursing employment in the U.S. The countries are the Philippines, India, Canada, South Korea, and Nigeria.

There is concern about language proficiency and the NCSBN is discussing the possibility of English proficiency testing for foreign-born nurses as a part of licensure.

 Learning Exercise

Practicing in Other States

Research how to apply for licensure by endorsement in another state. Start by contacting the state board of nursing of a state in which you may be interested in applying for a job (Appendix A).

HOW THE NCLEX-PN® EXAMINATION IS KEPT UP-TO-DATE

The 2007 and 2008 (effective April 2008) NCLEX-PN® examination reflects the outcome of the *2006 Practice Analysis of Newly Licensed Practical/Vocational Nurse in the US*. Currently this survey is conducted every three years. In 2006, 6000 surveys were sent out to entry level LPN/LVNs. Not all LPN/LVNs could be found and others did not return their survey. Some LPN/LVNs had moved without notification of their change of address, did not give direct care as was required for the survey, or worked less than the 20 hours a week; 1045 responses were considered satisfactory for analysis.

The National Council prepares a test plan, which is helpful in explaining the general content areas of the test. The NCLEX-PN® examination is a secure examination, so no actual test items are included in the test plan. The document, *Test Plan for the National Council Licensure Examination for Practical Nurses*, is available from the National Council of State Boards of Nursing, 111 E. Wacker Drive, Suite 2900, Chicago, IL 60601; (312) 525-3600; or go to website *http://www.ncsbn.org* and type "NCLEX-PN" in search box.

CORE CONTENT

Four phases of the nursing process (see Chapter 8) are integrated into all areas of the NCLEX-PN® examination. The four phases are the basis for nursing care plans you developed for each patient assigned to you, prior to beginning nursing care on the clinical unit.

The four phases are:
1. Data collection (assessment),
2. Planning,
3. Implementation, and
4. Evaluation.

TYPES OF TEST QUESTIONS

The NCLEX-PN® examination contains items in the cognitive level of knowledge, comprehension, application, and analysis. Most of the items are at the application and analysis levels. These items require prioritizing and decision-making. See p. 83 in Chapter 6. There are two major types of test items: multiple choice and alternate format items.

Multiple Choice

The majority of test items are multiple choice. Each item describes a client or clinical situation. Four options are given from which to choose the correct response.

Alternate Format Item

As of 2003 the NCLEX-PN® examination includes alternate format items. Silvestri (2007) describes these items as:

- *Fill-in-the-blank*. Medicine and IV rate calculations, intake and output totals.
- *Multiple response*. Select **all** responses that pertain to the question with no partial credit given. For example, which of the following drugs are antihypertensives?
- *Prioritizing*. An ordered response is required. Options (nursing actions) are numbered as first, second, and third, etc. in order of priority or the mouse is used to drag and drop options in the ordered priority. For example, when doing the Heimlich maneuver, which of the following actions would you do first, second, third, etc?
- *Figure or illustration*. Questions are asked about a chart or figure. Either an answer is chosen from a list or the mouse is used to point and click a "hot spot" as the answer. For example, click the hypochondriac area.
- *Chart/exhibit questions*, A question is included with a chart or exhibit requiring use of the chart/exhibit to answer the question. For example, which lab result is normal?

An on-screen optional calculator is available for your use during the examination. Any item format, including standard multiple-choice items, might include charts, tables, or graphic images. A tutorial is provided on the computer screen regarding the operation of the computer and how to record answers. For general information about the NCLEX-PN® examination, call the NCLEX® Examination Department at 866-293-9600 or e-mail: *nclexinfo@ncsbn.org*.

Learning Exercise

What Is an Alternate Item Question?

Write an example of an alternate item format using problem solving.

_____

_____

TEST FRAMEWORK: CLIENT NEEDS

The content of the NCLEX-PN® examination is divided into four Client Needs categories. Client Needs provide an overall structure for defining nursing actions and competencies for a variety of patients in many settings and is in agreement with state laws and statutes. Two of the four categories are further subdivided. The percentage of test items assigned to each category and limited examples of content are included. Additional examples of content are found in the "NCLEX® Examination Test Bulletin" available at *ncsbn.org* and type NCLEX-PN in search box. The categories and subcategories are as follows:

1. Safe, Effective Care Environment
   a. Coordinated Care: 12–18%
      Examples: Advance directives, client rights, concepts of management and supervision, confidentiality, priorities, ethical practice, legal responsibilities.
   b. Safety and Infection Control: 8–14%
      Examples: Accident/error prevention, handling hazardous and infectious materials, medical and surgical asepsis, standard and other precautions, use of restraints, etc.
2. Health Promotion and Maintenance: 7–13%
   Examples: Aging process, ante/intra/postpartum and newborn care, expected body image changes, family planning, high risk behaviors, human sexuality, life choices, self-care.

3. Psychosocial Integrity: 8–14%
   Examples: abuse and neglect, behavioral intervention, crisis intervention, end-of-life concepts, mental health concepts, stress management, suicide/violence prevention, therapeutic communication.
4. Physiological Integrity
   a. Basic Care and Comfort: 11–17%
      Examples: Assistive devices, elimination, nutrition and oral hydration, palliative/comfort care, personal hygiene, sleep and rest.
   b. Pharmacological Therapies: 9–15%
      Examples: Expected effects, adverse effects, side effects, medication administration, pharmacological agents.
   c. Reduction of Risk Potential: 10–16%
      Examples: Vital signs, diagnostic procedures, laboratory values, therapeutic procedures, potential for complications of tests and surgery.
   d. Physiological Adaptation: 11–17%
      Examples: Basic pathophysiology, fluid and electrolyte imbalances, medical emergencies, radiation therapy, unexpected responses to therapies.

Critical Thinking Exercise

Client Need Categories

Provide a "real" example of a patient need for each of the categories and subcategories. Where in the scheduled studies of your program do you expect to learn what is needed for each subcategory? Relate information you give in pre-conference to the categories and subcategories.

_____

INTEGRATION OF NURSING CONCEPTS AND PROCESSES

Concepts and processes basic to the practice of practical/vocational nursing are integrated into the four categories of patient needs.

- *Clinical problem-solving process* (nursing process): A scientific approach to patient care. It includes data collection, planning, implementation, and evaluation (four phases of nursing process that apply to the practical/vocational nurse).

- *Caring*: Interaction with clients, families, and others in an atmosphere of trust and respect.
- *Communication and documentation*: Verbal and nonverbal communication with patient and those involved with care. Documentation (written or electronic) of all events and activities associated with the patient's care.
- *Teaching/learning*: Assist client to gain information, skills, and attitudes that lead to change in behavior.

Learning Exercise

Categories of Patient Care

Write a one-sentence example of how you might apply each of the four integrated processes in planning patient care.

OVERVIEW OF APPLICATION PROCESS

It is customary for the instructor to introduce you to the application process when it is time to apply to the state board of nursing (Board) for a license as an LPN or LVN. The process is as follows:

- Complete all eligibility requirements for licensure, as required by the board (starting with successful completion of the practical/vocational nursing program).
- Apply to the state board of nursing or territory in which you plan to be licensed for nursing. Follow your state board of nursing directions for licensure.
- Receive an "NCLEX® Examination Candidate Bulletin" from the board or the nursing program, or download it from *www.ncsbn.org*. This bulletin is useful because it includes information on application, registration, fees, scheduling an appointment, test security, rules during testing, sample testing, retesting, and more.
- The board notifies Pearson VUE if you have met all requirements and are eligible to take the NCLEX-PN® examination. You will be ready to register.
- NCLEX-PN® Examination registration is sent to Pearson VUE. Pearson VUE acknowledges your registration with a confirmation of registration by postal mail or email. If you provide an email address, you will receive your confirmation only by email. Otherwise, confirmation is by postal mail.
- Pearson Center sends you an authorization to test (ATT). The ATT contains the test authorization number, candidate identification number, and an expiration date. The period of time is set by the state boards and varies from 60 to 365 days. You must have the ATT before attempting to schedule an appointment to take the NCLEX-PN® examination.
- Make an appointment to test at any approved Pearson Professional Center (PPC). Pearson Professional Center locations and addresses are found on the NCLEX Candidate website (*www.pearsonvue.com/nclex*).
- Take the NCLEX-PN® examination on the scheduled day. Failure to arrive at the test site results in having the Pearson Center report you to the board and forfeiture of the registration and fee. You must go through the process again; that is, apply for registration and submit another fee.
- *Your state's board of nursing (not Pearson Center) notifies you of test results. DO NOT CALL.*
- All boards ask a candidate about previous criminal activity (felonies and misdemeanors—the board will decide if it influences your ability to be licensed). Be truthful.

Authorization to Test

Explain the significance of attaining the ATT before scheduling your appointment to take the NCLEX-PN® examination.

FEES AND OTHER IMPORTANT INFORMATION

- The fee for NCLEX-PN® is $200. There will be other fees required by the nursing board where you are applying. Fees vary. There is no refund of registration fee for any reason.

Fees

List fees required by your state's board of nursing (or by the jurisdiction where you are applying).

HOW TO REGISTER

Internet, mail, or telephone can be used to register. Pearson VUE will confirm receipt of registration and send an Authorization to Test (ATT) to the candidate. Once the ATT is received, schedule and test within the validity dates printed on the ATT.

Internet Registration

http://www.vue.com/nclex/.
Select the registration option.

- Answering all the questions on pages 4-7 in the candidate bulletin helps the candidate answer the questions regardless of the method used for registration.
- On the registration form, print your name exactly as it appears on your valid picture identification you will present at the Pearson testing center. The name on the Authorization To Test (ATT) you receive must match the name on the picture identification you present at the testing center.

- Pay for the registration (plus fees if required), using VISA, MasterCard, or American Express.
- If an email address is provided, correspondence will arrive by email only. This applies to all methods of registering.

Mail Registration

NCLEX Operations, PO Box 64950, St. Paul, MN 55164-0950

- A certified check, cashier's check, or money order made out to the National Council State Boards of Nursing has to accompany the registration. The board will determine what additional fees are required. Use a No. 2 pencil and fill in all the requested information. An incomplete registration form and/or incorrect fee will be returned. Use the envelope included with your registration form.

Telephone Registration

In the U.S.: 1-866-49NCLEX. For those candidates not registering in the US, numbers for other countries are found in front of the candidate bulletin.

- Fill out the registration form prior to making the call. The customer representative will ask the same questions that are on the registration form.
- Paying for registration when using the telephone is by credit card: Standard questions such as the name shown on the card, number, and expiration date are asked and the credit card is verified before the registration is processed.

AUTHORIZATION TO TEST (ATT)

If the ATT does not arrive within two weeks, call Pearson VUE at the appropriate number listed in the front section of the candidate bulletin (1-866-48NCLEX in the U.S.).

Time limit for all NCLEX-PN® examination registrations is 60 to 365 days. If you are not declared eligible within that time for taking the NCLEX-PN® examination, you forfeit the registration and the fee. To reapply, you must submit a new application and fee. Do not send another registration form before calling about your status. Duplicate registration fees are not refunded.

- Validity dates for ATT will not be extended for any reason. Once approved for testing the candidate must take the NCLEX-PN® examination within the approved time frame. The validity date varies from 60 to 365 days, depending on the time period specified by the state board.
- Schedule taking the NCLEX-PN® examination at a Pearson Center as soon as possible after receiving the ATT. Test centers may fill up quickly and attempting to make a last-minute testing appointment may result in missing the ATT validity deadline. Most Pearson Centers are open Monday through Friday, except on holidays, and you may test at any Pearson Center.

EXAMINATION SECURITY

The NCLEX-PN® examination ensures *minimal competency* to protect the public and because of this, strict rules for security have been established. For example:

- Arrive at testing center 30 minutes before the scheduled time. If you arrive 30 minutes later than the appointed time, you may be required to forfeit your appointment. Avoid bringing children, family, or friends to the Pearson Center. They will not be permitted to wait at the testing center.
- *Name*: Use your name in *exactly* the same form you used when applying for the NCLEX-PN® examination. If your legal name has changed since you applied, the only legal documentation acceptable the day of the test is a marriage license, divorce decree, and/or court action legal name change documents.
- *Proper identification*: Your ATT and a valid form of picture identification in English and signed in English are required. The only proper identification is a valid (not expired) U.S. driver's license; U.S. state identification, and passport. The only

acceptable identification in test centers outside of the US is a passport. The ATT contains your test authorization number, candidate identification number, and an expiration date.

ADDED SECURITY MEASURES

- You will be asked to provide your signature. A digital fingerprint and photograph will be taken. No hats, scarves, or coats may be worn while the picture is taken. Hats, coats or scarves may not be worn in the testing room. Exception is made for religious reasons. Your fingerprint, photograph, and signature accompany your examination results sent to the board and can be used to confirm your identity.
- Direct observation by staff and video and audio recording of the session occurs at all times during the examination.
- Personal belongings are kept in secure storage outside of the classroom during the test. The storage space is small, so plan accordingly. A Pearson staff person escorts you into a secure area. A similar process is followed when you prepare to leave the Pearson Center. At no time does any candidate walk into the secure area without an escort. (Visualize a system similar to accessing a safety deposit box at the bank.) All books, papers, unauthorized scratch paper, note boards, food, pens, purses, wallets, watches, beepers, cell phones, and other electronic devices are banned from the test room. The computer includes both a calculator and a time device that tells you how much time remains to complete the NCLEX-PN® examination.
- Erasable note boards are provided for use during the test and collected before you leave the room at the end of testing. Note boards cannot be taken outside the room.
- Leaving the room is permitted with permission only. You provide a fingerprint each time you leave and return to the testing area after a break.

Critical Thinking Exercise

Security Rules

Explain the significance of each of the security measures. Where will you put your car keys before testing?

Critical Thinking Exercise

Exam Results

Explain why the state board of nursing (rather than the Pearson Center) provides you with the results of the NCLEX-PN® examination.

TESTING TIME

Up to 5 hours is available for testing. This includes a short tutorial on the computer, which shows you how to register the answers to all items. There are two preprogrammed optional breaks, plus those you request. The computer notifies you of the optional breaks. You must leave the room for a break. All breaks count against testing time.

You may ask for assistance with the computer at any time if needed or if the computer does not seem to be functioning properly. Raise your hand for assistance, if you want to change note boards, or need a break. Remain in your seat, except when given permission to leave the room. Creating any disturbance can cause you to be dismissed from the room.

After you complete the exam, raise your hand. There will be a brief questionnaire on the computer for you to complete regarding the testing experience. You may also ask for a confidential comment sheet in order to write personal comments to the NCSBN. When all exam requirements are met, the test administrator (TA) will collect and inventory the note boards and dismiss you from the testing room.

REPORTING RESULTS OF EXAMINATION

Although the computer continuously computes the result of your answers, the Pearson Center does not release final results to you directly. The result is available only from the board approximately one month after testing. *Do not call the board, the NCLEX Candidate Services, the Pearson Centers, or NCSBN for results.* The results will reach you by postal mail from the state board of nursing.

OVERVIEW OF THE NCLEX-PN® CAT EXAMINATION

The NCLEX-PN® examination is a well-planned examination that takes into consideration differences in nursing regulations within states. The NCLEX-PN® examination is fair to each candidate and provides ample opportunity to demonstrate knowledge and ability as a beginning LPN/LVN. Important nursing content is included, regardless of the number of items chosen by the computer for a candidate.

You will find most of the items written at the application and analysis level of cognitive ability. For example, this could include prioritizing care for a number of clients, analyzing data to determine appropriate nursing action, etc. You use critical thinking, nursing process, and basic nursing knowledge as you do in the real world of nursing.

Previous knowledge about using a computer is unnecessary to take the test. The short tutorial includes sample items for practice. The items are clearly marked so you will have no problem recognizing when the actual examination begins. If you have problems using the computer during the test, you may raise your hand to receive help.

THE CAT METHOD OF TESTING

In the CAT method of testing, the computer selects the items you will answer while you are taking the examination. As you answer an item on the examination, the computer adapts the examination to your answer. This is possible because the computer has a large number of test items stored in its memory. As you answer the standardized items, the computer chooses the next best item to measure your competence. The practical/vocational nurse licensing examination decisions are not based solely on how many items a candidate answers correctly. It is also based on the difficulty levels of the items a candidate answers correctly.

"NCSBN increased the passing standard in response to changes in US health care delivery and nursing practice that have resulted in increased acuity of clients seen by entry-level PNs. The Board of Directors determined that safe and effective entry level PN practice requires a greater level of knowledge, skills and abilities than was required in 2002, when NCSBN established the present standard" (NCSBN, December 15, 2004).

Computerized adaptive testing administers items with difficulty levels so that each candidate will answer about half correctly. These items provide the most information. All candidates answer about 50% correctly because the computer presents them with questions to match their ability. The computer goes down a "pathway" or "branch," and no candidate has exactly the same test. Items that follow are based on the candidate's previous answer. This is why you *must* answer every item that shows up on the computer screen as they show up. You will not be able to go back and answer a previous question. The computer calculates each answer before it can choose the next item.

Testing stops when the minimum number of items is answered, if it can be determined with certainty that the candidate passed or failed. Otherwise, the process continues until it is clear (with 95% certainty) that the candidate's ability is above or below the passing standard.

All candidates answer a minimum of 85 items. The maximum number of items any candidate will answer during the 5-hour maximum testing period is 205. The computer indicates when the candidate has completed the test.

Note that each NCLEX-PN® contains twenty-five test items that are not scored because they are items being pretested for difficulty. These items might be used on future exams after they are analyzed. The candidate is unable to distinguish these items from regular test items.

If you run out of time before the examination is finished, passing will be based on having your final competence estimate above passing *and* having been *above the passing standard throughout the final portion of your examination.*

Critical Thinking Exercise

Computerized Adaptive Testing

Explain why the CAT method of testing provides a clearer picture of the candidate's competency than does the usual paper/pencil test.

_____

_____

APPLYING FOR A TEMPORARY PERMIT

Your instructor will assist you with an application for a temporary permit so you will be able to work as a graduate practical or vocational nurse (GPN or GVN). Once the result of the NCLEX-PN® examination is in, the temporary permit is automatically revoked. Passing the NCLEX-PN® examination means that you will work as a fully licensed practical or vocational nurse (LPN or LVN). If you fail the NCLEX-PN® examination, you will be required to surrender your temporary permit and work as a nursing assistant.

REDUCING ANXIETY BEFORE TESTING

Research had shown that if a person does not do well on tests, odds are that they (1) were less intelligent that the average student, (2) have poor study habits, or (3) have weak test-taking skills. The first reason does not apply or you would not have been admitted into the nursing program. The second reason probably does not apply if you had good study habits, having organized your study time as suggested in Chapter 3, and made use of study group time. If the third reason were an issue, you would have noticed it early in the program and sought help.

In many programs, instructors take time to review test questions and rationale for answers after a test. Sometimes having missed a question and then learning the correct answer fortifies the answer and rationale.

Normal anxiety is your friend. It is this "cause-and-effect" type of anxiety that actually makes you sharper and more alert during a test. Only when anxiety overwhelms you does it become your enemy. Accept the energy resulting from normal anxiety as your partner. Total personal comfort is not the key. Normal anxiety leaves you somewhere between too much relaxation and too much tension—perfect for testing.

Make the days before testing work for you through your daydreams and positive thinking. Think about what you think about. Are you in the habit of seeing yourself failing or just squeaking by? Because everyone daydreams and sets the stage for their reality, daydreaming is a natural way to practice being confident and successful. Visualization may be helpful. For additional ways to relieve anxiety, review suggestions provided in Chapter 10.

Spend the evening before the licensing examination doing what works best for you prior to a test. For some it is reviewing select notes. For others it is relaxing. Little will be accomplished by worrying or by last minute cramming. Read something light and entertaining, watch television, or do what you already know works for you.

Get a good night's sleep by going to bed at your usual time (whatever meets your sleep requirements). It is thought that sleep restores memories that were lost during a hectic day. Going to bed extra early and not falling asleep may just result in a new worry.

Follow through with your usual morning habits. Avoid forcing your system to adjust to a demand that is not a usual part of your routine.

Casual attire is appropriate. Think of comfort for sitting. Wear layers of clothing that can be adjusted to your comfort needs.

 Learning Exercise

Relax!

Make a *tentative* plan for what you will do the evening before the NCLEX-PN® examination.

A WORD ABOUT REVIEW BOOKS AND MOCK EXAMINATIONS

The major nursing publishing companies have developed new review books based on the NCLEX-PN® examination format. Each review book basically includes an outline of practical/vocational nursing content, items with explanations and rationale, and references for the answers. Items are intended to simulate the NCLEX-PN® examination format. Realize that the test items of the NCLEX-PN® examination itself are highly guarded and confidential. Actual NCLEX-PN® examination items are not included in any review book. Some review books contain computer disks with test items. These disks do not simulate CAT testing, but they do provide computer experience. L. Q. Silvestri's (2007) *Q and A for the NCLEX-PN® Examination*, (St. Louis: Elsevier/Saunders), contains 3000 NCLEX-PN® type questions and a comprehensive exam. It also includes a CD-ROM with 1500 questions from the text and 150 additional questions.

The best preparation is to study faithfully from the beginning of the program to its conclusion, on a regular basis, until you take the examination. Merely reading a review book at the end of the program, without studying the nursing content throughout the program, will rarely help you pass boards. The identified outcome of a nursing program is to learn, understand, and be able to apply basic nursing information in the care of patients on clinical during your student year and when you graduate.

Mock examinations are available. The NLN has a new diagnostic readiness test available online. The NCLEX-PN® Readiness Test provides the following benefits:

- Reports generate instantly and include a statement of a candidate's probability of passing NCLEX-PN®.
- The test is based on the NCLEX-PN® blueprint.
- Individual performance and class summary reports offer a comprehensive diagnostic profile, detailing areas of strength and weakness on multiple subscales related to the blueprint.
- Correct answer rationales for every item and a reference list are provided after the test is scored.
- Report summaries help educators formulate effective study plans for their classes and individuals and focus their review efforts.
- Provides individuals with valuable test taking practice.
- Both individual and class reports are available for download and can be retrieved for up to two weeks after the test is scored. Phone (800) 669-9656 or email at *CustomerHelp@nln.org.*

If you have an idea of your strong and weak areas, you can better focus your study efforts. Be sure to check publishers' offerings of mock examinations. Choose the one that most closely resembles the actual format of the NCLEX-PN® examination. As an SPN/SVN, you can benefit from tests during the year that encourage problem solving, application, and analysis of knowledge. Some publishers provide adaptive testing, as used by NCLEX-PN® examination. Use these experiences as additional means of preparing for your nursing licensure examination.

Good luck! Keep a positive mental attitude.

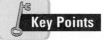
Key Points

- Lack of preparation of subject matter (poor studying skills and habits) and poor test-taking skills are the most common reasons for low test scores.
- Occasionally, fear and high anxiety are involved in low test scores. If this is an issue, do something about learning habits to reduce test-taking anxiety now.
- Graduate practical/vocational nurses (candidates) take the NCLEX-PN® examination (National Council Licensing Examination for Practical Nurses) to become licensed as an LPN/LVN.
- A computer administers the NCLEX-PN® examination, using the computerized adaptive testing (CAT) method of testing.
- Before scheduling the NCLEX-PN® examination, all practical or vocational nursing course work must be completed.
- Each candidate takes a different track (path) during the CAT method of testing. The zigzag track is based on the answer to the previous item.
- The NCLEX-PN® examination provides all candidates ample opportunity to demonstrate competency in practical/vocational nursing.
- Neither pass nor fail is related to the number of items answered by the candidate.
- The board of nursing to which you applied will provide results in approximately 1 month.
- NCSBN has expanded NCLEX testing to some foreign countries.

REVIEW ITEMS

1. Explain how CAT determines that a candidate has passed the NCLEX-PN® examination.

   1. The computer calculates accuracy or inaccuracy of a distracter chosen by a candidate.
   2. The computer subtracts the number of wrong from the number of right items to determine the score.
   3. The computer zigzags to find items that will indicate comprehension by the candidate.
   4. The computer determines that the candidate has 50% of the difficult items correct.

2. How is the NCLEX-PN® examination kept up-to-date with what LPN/LVNs are really doing in nursing?

   1. Each nursing school surveys its students during the first year after graduation.
   2. The state board of nursing requires a work survey as a part of license renewal.
   3. The NCSBN sponsors a job analysis of newly licensed nurses throughout the US.
   4. Each state board of nursing is required to do a work survey and submit questions.

3. A member of the class did not pass the NCLEX-PN® examination and is angry because the temporary work permit was revoked. The member asks, "Why do I have to work as an aide after completing school?" What is the correct response?

   1. "Any graduate who fails embarrasses the nursing school, and is punished for it."
   2. "The permit gives you one chance to function as a practical nurse without a license."
   3. "Go work in another state, where licensing laws are not as punitive as they are here."
   4. "If you can provide a 'hardship' excuse, the board will extend the work permit."

4. A candidate attempts to use study aids during the NCLEX-PN® examination. Which of the following is not a consequence of this action?

   1. Pearson Center notifies the NCSBN of candidate's action.
   2. Candidate is barred from taking the NCLEX-PN® examination in the future.
   3. Some state boards decide their response on a case-by-case basis.
   4. Pearson Center may dismiss or cancel testing result of candidate.

ALTERNATE FORMAT ITEM

Which of the following are required as security during NCLEX-PN® examination? *(Select all that apply.)*

1. Fingerprint

2. Observation

3. No. 2 pencils

4. Identification

5. Signature

23 How to Make Your Career Grow

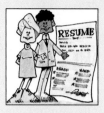

evolve http://evolve.elsevier.com/Hill/success/

Objectives

On completing this chapter, you will be able to do the following:

1. Identify areas of licensed practical/vocational nurse (LPN/LVN) employment currently available in your community.
2. Contact the state board of nursing to find out which certifications are accepted in the state in which you plan to seek employment.
3. Discuss three advantages of belonging to professional organizations.
4. Describe your postgraduate career goals. (Review your answer periodically.)
5. Investigate opportunities available to you for continuing education.

Key Terms

Career ladder programs (p. 447)
Certification in Managed Care (CMCN) (p. 446)
Long-Term Care Certification (CLTC) (p. 444)
Mobility program (p. 446)
National Association for Practical Nurse Education and Service, Inc. (NAPNES) (p. 440)
National Certification in Gerontology (p. 445)
National Certification in IV Therapy (p. 445)
National Federation of Licensed Practical Nurses (NFLPN) (p. 441)
National League for Nursing (NLN) (p. 440)
Pharmacology Certification (NCP) (p. 444)
Podcasting (p. 443)

 Keep in Mind

Have you developed an appreciation of nursing and the patients you work with? Does the role of LPN/ LVN fit for you and your dreams? Are you looking to continuing education in nursing? What is your personal goal?

NURSING OPENS THE DOOR TO A VARIED CAREER

Nursing opens the door to an entirely different world. You enter and touch the lives of many individuals and families. Patients trust you without having to prove yourself. They feel safe in the knowledge that you have pledged to do your best in providing care without judgment. Some patients and families will let you know their appreciation for your skill in doing nursing procedures; some will not let you know how deeply you touched their life and the lives of their loved ones.

Nursing challenges you throughout your career. As a student, you are expected to learn and use an entirely new language and yet always explain to a patient what you are doing in terms he or she can understand. The challenge continues when you graduate because you have only scratched the surface of knowledge in nursing. There are many more skills to perfect and a great deal more to learn from courses, in-services, workshops, and skilled nursing practitioners.

Every day will provide at least one answer to your question, "What did I learn today?"

Approximately one third of those who enter a nursing program do not complete the program for any number of reasons. A major reason is that the course of study demands a great deal of personal discipline, time management, and prioritization of needs (knowing the difference between "I want to" and "I need to"). Nursing changes you: You see and hear more in a short period than you ever imagined. Most of what you see and hear cannot be shared with anyone out of the immediate setting. Nursing is a maturing experience, often beyond your years. Both self-confidence and the ability to say, "I don't know, but I will find out," grow as your professional honesty is tested. Nursing opens doors for you in traditional and atypical careers. Be proud of choosing nursing as a career, and do not keep that information confidential!

2006 JOB ANALYSIS

The Job Analysis of Newly Licensed Practical Nurses is conducted every 3 years. The year 2006 participants were diverse in terms of their ethnic and racial background. 63.7% of participants were female and white non-Hispanic, 5.4% were Asian, 21.2% were African American, and 7.6% were Latino or Hispanic. 1.5% were educated internationally. The rest were educated in approximately 1200 state-approved schools. The average time of employment since licensure was 3.7 months. 63.4% had worked as nursing assistants for an average of 5 years.

Most of the nurse participants worked in nursing homes, long-term care facilities, and medical/surgical units, and a smaller number worked in rehabilitation units and other settings. Almost half worked the day shift. Almost an equal percentage worked the evening and night shifts. A small percentage worked rotating shifts.

The work of the newly graduated 2006 LPN/LVNs consisted primarily of safe medication administration, activities involved in safety and infection control, and activities related to basic care and comfort.

The 2006 newly licensed LPN/LVNs provided nursing care primarily to adult and elderly patients. Over half of these patients had a stable chronic illness. Almost half of the patients had behavioral/emotional problems. Approximately one third of LPN/LVNs worked with patients needing end-of-life care or acute care. An increased number of LPN/LVNs were working in long-term care and community-based settings. Approximately 48% of the LPN/LVNs noted that they had one or more administrative activities. The most frequent administrative activity was as charge nurse, primarily in the long-term care facilities. The next most frequent activity was team leader.

Approximately half of the participants had earned one or more certifications or completed additional course work. The most common certifications included basic life support, IV therapy, and phlebotomy. Forty-seven percent had no additional course work or certification.

If you are interested in reviewing the entire study, it is available online. Check *http://www.ncsbn.org* or Goggle by typing in "Report on Findings from the 2006 LPN/VN Practice Analysis: Linking the NCLEX-PN Examination to Practice." Use the exact title. The practice analysis can be downloaded free of charge.

LPN/LVN EMPLOYMENT OPPORTUNITIES AND SALARIES IN THE US

The Bureau of Labor Statistics, US Department of Labor, *Occupational Outlook Handbook* (2006–2007), reported that LPN/LVNs held about 726,000 jobs in 2004. Employment for LPN/LVNs is expected to grow as fast as average for all occupations through 2014. Projected need is approximately 282,000 LPN/LVNs. Hospital employment opportunities will continue to decline, but the need for LPN/LVNs in long-term care and home health facilities will continue to grow in response to needs of an increasing elderly population and rehabilitation needs because of early discharge from hospitals. Many LPN/LVNs will be leaving their job permanently and replacement will be a major source of employment. The average age of current LPN/LVNs is in the 40s.

Median annual earnings of LPN/LVNs in the United States during May 2004 were $33,970. Median wage means that 50% earn less than this amount and 50% earn more. LPN/LVNs in entry-level positions earn less than the median wage. The lowest 10% earned less than $24,830, and the highest 10% earned more than $46,270.

Home health care employment for nurses is also growing faster than average. As more treatments are possible in the home, more people are choosing to be cared for in their own surroundings. The home treatments are too complex and are not legally within the home health aide role. If the LPN/LVN does not already possess a treatment skill as part of practical/vocational education, the LPN/LVN can be taught by a registered nurse (RN) or physician to do any treatment legally within their scope of practice.

 Learning Exercise

LPN/LVN Wages

Search information on wages for the LPN/LVN position in at least two areas of personal interest in health facilities near you.

LPN EMPLOYMENT OPPORTUNITIES AND SALARIES IN CANADA

The Canadian Institute for Health Information (CIHI) reported in 2006 that the number of regulated nurses in Canada has increased slightly. The workforce included 64,951 licensed practical nurses. Just under half of the LPNs were employed full time. The average age of LPNs in 2004 was 44.4 years, with average age at graduation of 30.8 years. More practical nursing schools and postgraduate education and credentialing

courses have been developed in some areas of Canada. Examples include medication administration, intravenous therapy, psychogeriatrics, rehabilitation, or activation assisting.

The most frequent opportunity for practice is long-term care and, in some areas, hospital care. Other opportunities may include emergency room, palliative care, hospice care, operating rooms, and home support. The new areas of utilization were identified in the 2000 utilization study prepared for the Hospital Employees' Union in British Columbia (February 2003).

In Canada, there is considerable variation in LPN responsibilities in work facilities. Many competencies not being utilized are part of the practical nurse curriculum. Employees, patients, and other staff, unaware of current education requirements and regulatory framework required of the LPN, relate this to unfamiliarity. There is an effort to re-examine roles and assist in articulation between RNs and LPNs and empower all nurses to work within their scope of practice (*http://.cord. aacudiau.ca/neka*).

The CIHI (2005) reported that 9 out of 10 Canadian graduates currently work in the province from which they graduated. British Columbia (BC) and Ontario attract the greatest number of foreign-trained nurses. The overall rate for foreign trained nurses has remained fairly stable at 7%.

Average salaries vary depending on experience, health facility, certifications, and province. In BC for example, average salaries during 2001 were $32,754 annually (*http://www.workfutures. bc.ca/link.cfm?print=true&lang=end&noc=3233*). Jobs in other area were seen advertised at $17.91 to $23.45 hourly depending on experience and province.

 Learning Exercise

Areas of Interest

Is there a specific area you are interested in at this time? Know that you may change your mind based on classroom and clinical experience in a particular area.

WORK SITES AND NURSING CHARACTERISTICS

HELPFUL PERSONAL ATTRIBUTES

LPN/LVNs must be caring, have an empathic (not sympathetic) nature, and have a genuine concern for the welfare of their patients. Emotional stability is essential because work with sick and injured patients can be stressful. LPN/LVNs need keen observational, critical thinking, and decision-making skills and be able to communicate at a patient's level in order to be understood. A comfort level in doing basic nursing skills is absolute. If the LPN has been taught advanced skills that are within the state board's scope of practice for LPNs, then these skills need to be perfected. The condition of a patient may quickly change from stable to acute, and the nurse will have to respond to the situation without panic. LPN/LVNs work as part of a team and will be expected to follow orders and work under close supervision of an RN or physician. Assertiveness and patient advocacy are other important attributes. Since the LPN/LVN will often hear or see things that cannot be discussed with someone outside of the immediate area, confidentiality is a must. The LPN/LVN must also find healthy ways to relieve stress at the end of the shift that will not contribute to his or her personal health problems.

Learning Exercise

Personal Skills and Characteristics

Name some additional nursing skills and personal characteristics you have that enhance your ability to work in an area that currently appeals to you.

_____

_____

HOW OBRA RELATES TO SNF AND ICF

The Omnibus Budget Reconciliation Act (OBRA), 1987, was in large measure a response to evidence of mistreatment, abuse, and neglect of nursing home residents during the 1970s and 1980s. The Institute of Medicine set out detailed recommendations for improving care and these recommendations became the basis of OBRA, 1987. The Centers for Medicare and Medicaid (CMM) implemented the law over a period of years. Rules were not strongly enforced and by 1998, changes were made in the law. The change omitted language regarding nursing coverage for Skilled Nursing Facilities (SNF) and Intermediate Nursing Facilities (ICF). One year later, 1999, the language for nursing care was reinstated. It mandates that all SNFs and ICFs provide 24-hour licensed practical nurse care 7 days a week with at least one RN employed 8 hours a day, 7 days a week. Requests for waivers for LPN and RN coverage are reviewed and approved by CMM.

According to _Health Affairs_ (Nov/Dec 2001), some evidence exists of improvement in care. Identified improvements in care include:

- Declining use of physical and chemical restraints,
- Lower rates of urinary infections and use of catheters,
- Fewer hospitalizations.

Areas that lack change include:

- Pressure sore rates,
- Malnutrition,
- Dehydration,
- Other feeding problems,
- Bowel incontinence has risen slightly.

Learning Exercise

Availability of Leadership Course

Almost half of the newly licensed practical/vocational nurses who participated in the 2006 Job Analysis regularly assumed administrative responsibility, primarily in long-term care. Inquire whether a postgraduate LPN/LVN leadership/management course is available. Ask for details about the course.

_____

_____

EXTENDED CARE FACILITIES

The growing number of people age 65 and older has a positive impact on the availability of jobs for practical nurses. The nursing home population is made up of residents who are (1) completing recovery from surgery or trauma and are too well for the hospital but not well enough to go home; (2) elderly people who are unable to care for themselves because of medical or psychological impairment; (3) mentally retarded people who are unable to live independently or in group homes; (4) young to middle-aged persons with chronic debilitating disease or injuries from accidents; and (5) young, chronically mentally ill persons who need continual supervision and are not candidates for independent living or halfway houses.

LPN/LVNs hired for direct care measure vital signs, collect data, provide physical care and comfort measures, and give oral medications. Many state boards have flexible codes that permit more extensive use of LPN/LVN skills in nursing homes. Other codes are more restrictive. "Some states such as Louisiana, Montana, Maine, and Nevada, have detailed lists of tasks for the LPN. Other states such as Georgia, Alaska, Kentucky, and Oklahoma, have decision trees that are used to decide on appropriate tasks to be done. Connecticut has an extensive formula for decision-making that can be used regarding issues of practice. Washington has a decision tree that is used for making decisions and specifically states that there is no laundry list of approved and prohibited tasks. Some states such as Colorado and Nebraska use sections of the nursing care plan to detail work that can be done by different nursing personnel. South Carolina has developed extensive skills charts that are organized by body system job categories, and job experience within job categories. Neither Michigan nor Texas has a scope of practice or practice act for practical nurses" (*http://www.bhpr.hrsa.gov/healthworkforce/reports/nursing/lpn/c3.htm*).

There are still several points of contention in the scopes of practice for LPNs and RNs. Some points center around course names (e.g., mental health nursing instead of psychiatric nursing), on terms like *assessment*, *delegation*, and *decision making*. The difference in the terms *assessment* and *data collection* (the preferred term for LPN/LVNS) is difficult to define. Since critical thinking has been incorporated into the NCLEX-PN®, critical thinking is taught as a part of practical nursing

programs and is no longer a point of contention. As noted in the 2006 Practice Analysis, about half of the LPN/LVNs work as charge nurses, primarily in long-term care facilities: some work as team leaders. Many states and organizations offer postgraduate course and certifications. NAPNES offers certification programs in pharmacology and in long-term care (*http://www.napnes.org*). NFLPN offers national certifications in IV therapy and gerontology (*http://www.nflpn.org*). Wound certification is no longer available to LPN/LVNs in the same manner as before January 1, 2007. Some vocational and technical colleges offer postgraduate courses on being a charge nurse. Some states recognize postgraduate courses and certifications with an increase in salary and permit the LPN/LVN to make use of the skills they have learned in providing care. A major benefit of postgraduate information is knowledge gained for more effective patient care.

Extended care as an employment option may be available to you if you possess the following characteristics:

- Use solid nursing process skills in gathering data and use the care plan as a guide.
- Make use of critical thinking throughout the shift.
- Use therapeutic communication skills: differentiate between therapeutic and personal.
- Enjoy longer-term contact with people. (High turnover rates of staff have been associated with lower quality of care in some extended care facilities.)
- Provide excellent nursing care without immediate supervision of an RN or physician.
- Seek assistance or additional instruction as needed.
- Apply information about growth and development changes during illness.
- Willingly seek to learn new skills through continuing education and certification courses needed to take care of a varied population and age group.
- Listen to the patient regarding what they see as their needs for care.

- Treat patients of all ages and levels of growth and development with respect.
- Recognize when there is a significant personality clash with a patient to whom you are assigned and ask for a change in assignment (this statement assumes that you have already tried to talk over differences with the patient, and other staff is available to take over).

Other special qualities needed include patience; ability to see below the surface; willingness to listen; maturity; ability to determine priorities; ability to set limits; interest in working with people with disabilities; willingness to work with other health care givers, significant others, and family members; and a sense of security in regard to your personal value system. Prior experience on a medical/surgical unit is encouraged before working in an extended care facility.

LPN/LVNs who work in extended care are challenged to assist in providing a homelike atmosphere while dealing with immediate, long-term, and terminal health problems of the residents. The level of responsibility in extended care is great—the LPN/LVN often works in a charge nurse role, and although supervision is available from an RN, during some periods of the day, supervision may be general (i.e., at the other end of the telephone). Consequently, a solid knowledge and skill base are essential to know when to seek help and from whom. Nursing process and critical thinking provide the basis for skilled, compassionate care.

The charge nurse role also means the practical/vocational nurse is responsible for managing care given by other LPN/LVNs, certified nursing assistants, and trained feeding assistants. (Refer to Chapters 15 and 16 for more specific details on leadership and charge nurse skills.)

As the LPN/LVN in a nursing home facility, much of your work ultimately relates to assisting the residents to attain or maintain whatever capabilities they have in all areas of health. Through your efforts residents who are recuperating from surgery or trauma will realize their goal for recovery and discharge. For other residents, your role includes supporting them through the final step of the growth process—a dignified death.

HOME HEALTH NURSING

According to the US Bureau of Labor Statistics, faster-than-average growth is expected in home health services. This is in response to the number of older persons with functional disabilities, preference for home care, and technological advances that make it possible to do more complicated treatments in the home.

Because of shorter hospital stays, patients are receiving an increased amount of care in the home. The actual care given is under the supervision of an RN, who uses nursing process steps as a guideline to finalize a plan of care approved by the patient. Data from the LPN/LVN involved with care are essential to complete the care plan. Postdischarge (subacute) care fits in well with LPN/LVN basic education, thereby making LPN/LVNs invaluable in implementing the plan of care. LPN/LVNs' observation of physical and mental changes allows additions to the continuing data collection and evaluation of the plan of care. Because of difficulty in receiving payment from non-private sources, some home health agencies use LPN/LVNs for private-pay patients only. Others employ LPN/LVNs as home health aides to avoid restrictions. This is an unfortunate practice because the pay is lower and the LPN/LVN is always held to the standard of their highest license in legal situations. Because of need for the level of LPN/LVN skill, there is some hope the payment plan will be revised.

Helpful qualities for home health nurses include:

- **Flexibility**: You will have to improvise in the home, yet practice sound nursing principles. For example, this may include using makeshift equipment, determining how to clean the equipment, and using it to attain desired results.
- **Communication skills**: You are working in the patient's domain. You have to understand the patient's expression of needs and also make sure that you express yourself clearly and tactfully. For example, you may find yourself having to use words in the patient's vocabulary to be understood.

- **Self-confidence**: An air of insecurity or uncertainty will be picked up by the patient, resulting in lack of confidence in the LPN/LVN. This does not imply that you should fake confidence. Have knowledge and nursing skills that enable you to perform tasks efficiently. Do not ask for unnecessary reassurance from the patient when performing basic skills. Question away from the patient, unless an emergency exists. For example, you may be tempted to tell the patient, "this is only the second time I have changed a dressing on a foot without contaminating the dressing and I'm kind of nervous about it."
- **Sensitivity to physical and emotional changes**: Once the initial assessment is completed by the RN, it will be up to you to be alert to any changes of which the RN must be made aware. The RN must be able to depend on your observational skills, for safety's sake. For example, be tuned in to the person's affective communication as well as the verbal and non-verbal. Perhaps the individual is beginning to show signs of agitation that will need to be diffused before continuing the other work you have been assigned.
- **Ability to deal with emergencies**: Staying calm and following agency protocol is essential. For example, the patient may start to bleed from the wound you are dressing. Remembering what you learned to do in basic nursing and during first aid class is more effective than screaming that you can't stand the sight of blood! In an emergency, your motto is: "function now and shake later."
- **Nonjudgmental attitude**: This is a must because you work in the patient's home. You are providing a service. If you are comfortable with your own values, different values are not personally threatening. For example, the home may not be up to your standards in cleanliness.

MENTAL HEALTH NURSING

Mental health nursing facilities include psychiatric hospitals, community mental health centers, day treatment centers, and group homes for the recovering mentally ill. Many community mental health centers and group homes are staffed primarily with LPN/LVNs and nursing assistants, with RNs in a supervisory role. Many practical/vocational nursing programs have dropped the mental health nursing theory class and related clinical experience. Up to 14% of questions in the 2006 NCLEX-PN® examination were in the psychosocial integrity category.

In mental health nursing, LPN/LVNs are involved in performing treatments, administering medications, and tending to activities of daily living. Furthermore, LPN/LVNs perform a significant role in developing a therapeutic relationship with the patient and following through with the appropriate interventions, according to the patient's care plan. Mental health facilities practice a team concept in which everyone is expected to contribute to the patient's care plan, know the therapeutic guidelines in a patient care plan, and carry out the plan. A solid knowledge of mental health concepts and nursing process is essential.

Helpful qualities for working in a mental health unit include:

- Basic knowledge of dealing with psychiatric behaviors,
- Keen observational skills regarding behavioral change,
- Knowledge of basic self-defense (not offense),
- Experience with medical/surgical patients prior to working in a mental health unit,
- Calm and able to make quick decisions,
- Empathic rather than sympathetic,
- Good therapeutic communication skills,
- Separates personal and professional life,
- Nonjudgmental and respectful,
- Sound mental health,
- Excellent nursing process and critical thinking skills,
- Contributes to patient care plan,
- Follows established patient goals,
- Sets patient-centered limits assertively,
- Functions as a team member,

- Observes and reports patient changes,
- Does not take unnecessary risks with patients who are acting out and knows when to seek assistance.

MILITARY SERVICES

As a practical/vocational nurse, you will take basic training if you volunteer for military service in the reserves or for active duty. Contact recruiters for all branches of the military services including the National Guard. Compare the differences in available nursing careers to determine which branch best fits your needs. The US Army, for example, cross trains LPN/LVNs to be able to work in any area of the hospital. The benefits of military service also provide the financial means to continue education, and many LPN/LVNs have taken advantage of this benefit to become an RN and an officer. Some have gone on to get advanced degrees in nursing. Desirable qualities for military service nursing include the following:

- Interest in teamwork,
- Strong ego,
- Ability to cope with changing situations,
- Emotional stability,
- Good communication skills,
- Self-directed,
- Desire for adventure,
- Flexible,
- Adaptable,
- Empathetic (rather than sympathetic) with patients,
- Self-directed, but knows when to seek help,
- Healthy personal stress relieving habits.

A desire for a challenging career and an ability to adjust quickly to new situations are handy prerequisites for this kind of nursing.

HOSPITAL NURSING

The acute care experience in most practical/vocational nursing programs is found in the medical and surgical units of hospitals. In some areas of the country, hospital-based jobs have decreased and are available primarily to replace nurses who leave. In other areas of the United States, the nursing shortage has opened up employment in hospitals. Many of the ads for nurses are written for RN or LPN/LVN positions, so be sure to check that the job description is within the LPN/LVN scope of practice. Often the LPN/LVN is under-utilized in the hospital setting because the RN is not familiar with what the LPN/LVN is permitted to do legally. LPN/LVNs are often overheard complaining to each other that they do the same work as nursing aides. Your responsibility is to know what your scope of practice is within your state. Make this information, plus information on continuing education (including certifications you have earned), known to your RN supervisor. Some RNs do not trust LPN/LVNs primarily because they have never worked with them. Do your nursing care with skillful professionalism and help pave the way for other LPN/LVNs to be fully accepted in this important hospital-nursing role.

If you consider working in a specialty area, it is helpful to have both theory class and clinical experience, or additional education. Areas with complex nursing duties mean that additional postgraduate education such as in-service, workshops, or courses related specifically to the area are required. Previous nursing experience may also be listed as a requirement.

Refer to your state's Nurse Practice Act to see how performance of nursing acts beyond basic nursing care is handled. These acts are referred to as the expanded role of the practical/vocational nurse or performance of acts in complex patient situations (see Chapters 15 and 16).

Desirable qualities in hospital nursing include the following:

- Strong technical skills,
- Organizational skills,
- Nursing process and critical thinking skills,
- Strong ego,
- Copes well during emergencies,
- Teamwork: knows own and others' scope of practice, and
- Knows own limit and asks for help, as needed.

The anticipated pay scale is approximately two thirds that of the RN pay scale. Other benefits vary according to agency policy.

OUTPATIENT CLINICS, DOCTORS' OFFICES, AND CHIROPRACTIC OFFICES

Outpatient clinics and doctors' offices continue to provide jobs for many LPN/LVNs. Most clinics and offices are open Monday to Friday. The day begins later and, consequently, runs a little later. Assigned work varies but generally includes checking supplies, greeting patients, measuring vital signs, weighing patients, limited data collection about the purpose for seeing the physician, preparing the patient for an examination, assisting the doctor with the examination, and performing additional duties delegated by the physician. Cross training (learning to do jobs other than nursing) is expected in some of these facilities. For example, you might be expected to do basic lab tests, X-rays, and clerical work including answering telephones and making appointments.

If you are working as a private nurse for a physician, you can also expect to accompany the physician on hospital rounds and assist with examinations and treatments as needed. Because patients remain with the same physician, these nurses develop rapport with the patients, which is an asset to both the patient and the physician.

Desirable qualities include the following:
- Possesses good communication skills,
- Pays attention to detail,
- Enjoys routine,
- Possesses excellent organizational skills,
- Applies nursing process and critical thinking skills,
- Adapts and is self-directed when patient load is small,
- Treats all patients and their families with respect and empathy,
- Practices confidentiality and is respectful of patient's right to privacy,
- Maintains a sense of humor and uses it appropriately,
- Uses a well-modulated voice throughout the work period,
- Is flexible and willing to learn.

Previous work experience in a medical-surgical unit is advised to prepare you for data collection, administering medications, doing select treatments as assigned by the physician, and keeping records, as required.

OPERATING ROOM NURSING

Operating room (OR) technicians hired as OR nurses, for cost-cutting reasons, are not nurses. Technicians are not licensed and lack the extensive training that is required of LPN/LVNs. For example, technicians do not possess knowledge of the steps of the nursing process and critical thinking. Gathering data and skill in observation are not part of technician training. Technician training is limited to learning particular OR functions. LPN/LVNs who have worked in the OR for years describe their work as assisting the surgeon with instruments and equipment, collecting data, doing preoperative and postoperative patient care, and supporting postoperative education. They strongly urge that if you are interested in this line of work, stress your education and clinical skills as an LPN/LVN to your future employer.

In some states, LPN/LVNs can become trained to become an operating room technician. There is the combined value of being an LPN/LVN and operating room technician. If the operating room is your passion, it may be worth researching the possibility.

Desirable qualities for OR nurses include the following:
- Has good manual dexterity,
- Applies personal stress management skills,
- Separates personal and professional feedback from physicians and supervisors,
- Possesses a sense of self-worth,
- Accepts and follows directions,
- Uses nursing process,
- Maintains composure in a crisis,
- Differentiates between empathy and sympathy,
- Practices standard precautions: maintains sterile technique where needed,
- Maintains good personal health practices,
- Treats patients and their families with respect, and
- Maintains a willingness to learn.

VETERANS ADMINISTRATION (VA) CAREERS

Working with the nation's veterans in VA hospitals or veterans retirement homes are additional options for LPN/LVNs. You do not have to be a veteran to apply for employment. More LPN/LVNs are hired in veterans homes that are nursing homes than in the acute care veterans facilities.

Facilities generally provide new nurses an extensive orientation during duty hours regardless of the shift you are assigned. Veterans care includes medicine, surgery, spinal cord injury, alcohol/drug treatment, psychiatry, intensive care, hemodialysis, ambulatory care, and long-term care. Minimum qualifications include US citizenship, graduation or pending graduation from an accredited nursing school, and English language proficiency. Benefits are normally generous and based on civil service grades. LPN/LVNs with no experience start at GS-3 level. Salary rates are based on the grade, performance, and promotion to higher grades, overtime, and shift differential. If interested go to the "Job Search" section of the VA Careers website: *http://www.vacareers.va.gov/lpn.cfm*.

HOSPICE

Hospice care is for terminally ill patients of any age, in institutional settings or in their homes. The same qualities important in an extended care facility are important in a hospice setting. The nurse's role is to keep the patient comfortable and administer pain medication as ordered. In the past nurses sometimes withheld pain medication from the patient, even when ordered, in the mistaken belief that they might cause the patient to become addicted.

There is a first-person article in Advance for LPNs (12/18/06) "No Place Like It: Home Care Is Where the Nurse Is Proactive and the Patient Is King." Moore has been involved in hospice nursing for more than 10 years and writes of her experience with Vinnie (*http://www.advanceweb.com*). Moore was compassionate and innovative and Vinnie benefited from her approach until his death.

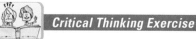

Critical Thinking Exercise

Medicating the Terminally Ill Patient

Think about the statement, "Withhold pain medication from a terminally ill patient so that he/she does not become addicted." Does that statement make sense to you? Explain your response.

OTHER JOB OPPORTUNITIES
Health Insurance Companies

Health insurance companies provide in-depth orientation for the work required. Some companies prefer to hire practical/vocational nurses immediately on graduation so the LPN/LVN is taught the company routine and does not have to unlearn previous practices.

Travel Nursing

There are a variety of ways to inquire about travel nursing as a career. Many health care–related websites include information on their site. Another option is to make your search selective. Use any search engine available to you on the computer and type in: travel nurse, travel nursing, travel healthcare, travel nursing career, or travel nurse information. Placing the words in quotes makes the search more selective.

Veterinary Clinics and Hospitals

For some LPN/LVNs, this is an opportunity to combine a love of nursing with a love of animals. In some states you may work as an assistant to the veterinarian in the care and treatment of animals. Other states, such as California, require a special training program and a passing grade in a state test to assist veterinarians.

Pharmaceutical/Medical Equipment Sales

Some pharmacies select LPN/LVNs to staff this particular area. For example, a former student practical nurse has become the colostomy care expert in her city and gives seminars on the topic to agencies, patients, and health professionals. She enjoys the backing of the drugstore management and a pharmaceutical company.

Coroner's Office

A former student practical nurse working with a coroner commented, "I never saw myself as doing this, but it is so interesting. I've learned a lot about people, pain, compassion, and myself. The doctor I work with is a born teacher and is always respectful of the person on whom he is doing the autopsy. He has helped me accept the life cycle."

Private Duty Nursing

LPN/LVNs have been employed for years as private duty nurses. This is frequently a long-term commitment on the part of an LPN/LVN. The most common responsibility is for ill, elderly individuals who wish to be cared for in their home rather than in an institution. It can also involve a child or adult with a long-term chronic illness. The LPN/LVN may be part of an around-the-clock care system with nurses on opposing shifts. Responsibilities vary according to the shift involved and include basic nursing skills. The LPN/LVN works under the general supervision of the patient's physician.

Parish Nursing

Some church parishes employ their own nurse to take care of basic health needs of the congregation. The work includes basic nursing skills such as measuring blood pressure, temperature, pulse, and respirations, and contacting a physician as needed. Foot care under the supervision of a podiatrist is sometimes included. Some parish nurses provide presentations on basic health care issues to the parishioners.

Temporary Help Agency

Temporary help agencies are listed under a variety of names. They supply nurses when requested by a health facility. Some provide temporary help exclusively for certain kinds of health facilities (e.g., long-term care). The need for help may be related to a shortage of nurses, lack of availability in the area, need for temporary coverage, etc. Assignments are intended to be short term. Sometimes the facility decides to hire the temporary nurse. Nurses who work for temporary agencies must be ready to "hit the floor running."

Consequently, the temporary agency rarely hires a newly licensed nurse. They prefer a nurse with at least 1 year of experience in a clinical hospital setting. The nurse must be competent in doing the required procedures. The temporary agency handles the contract for the health facility and for the nurse. Because of the immediate need for a nurse, the temporary agency usually pays the nurse a higher salary than usual. A former student used this method of nursing employment to pay for continuing education to become an RN. The ability to grasp information quickly, good nursing process skills, and good critical thinking skills are essential. Some temporary help agencies hire nurses for other countries and states.

Assisted Living Facility

Although adults who live in assisted living facilities do not need 24-hour skilled nursing care, they benefit from an LPN/LVN with good nursing process and critical thinking skills. The LPN/LVN is constantly gathering data on the medical and psychological condition of the client. A skilled LPN/LVN, for example, will be able to pick up soft signs such as an early cough before it goes on to become pneumonia. Assisted living facilities are often a part of a nursing complex. The RN in charge evaluates the needs of the resident at time of admission and assigns specific duties to the LPN/LVN. The RN also identifies the chain of command for the LPN/LVN should there be an emergency. If you like the human connection and function well with less supervision, this may be an area to consider.

Additional possibilities for employment to consider include:

- Residential treatment centers,
- Medical management companies,
- State, federal, or private prison systems,
- Corporate short- or long-term disability benefit administration case manager,
- Day care centers for adults and children,
- Weight loss clinics,
- Social service agencies,
- Ambulance and emergency medicine staff,
- Dentist office,
- Blood bank,

- Substance abuse clinics,
- Schools,
- Adult daycare,
- Welfare and religious organization,
- Specialized mobile units (e.g., blood mobile),
- Fitness centers,
- VISTA or the Peace Corps, and
- Certified Hearing Instrument Dispenser (additional education needed to attain certification).
- Other areas of interest to you we did not think about: Dare to apply!

 Learning Exercise

Area Job Opportunities

Investigate nursing job opportunities in your area. Add ideas to the aforementioned list.

_____

_____

PROFESSIONAL ORGANIZATIONS

Becoming a part of and participating in at least one professional nursing organization is essential for career development. Becoming an active member permits you to have a voice in the future of nursing. It is an opportunity to meet nursing leaders, learn about current issues that affect your career, and take part in education opportunities, as well as serve on committees that influence nursing policy.

NATIONAL LEAGUE FOR NURSING

The National League for Nursing (NLN) membership is open to all levels of nurses and anyone interested in nursing issues. One of the goals of the NLN is to lead in setting standards that advance excellence and innovation in nursing education. The NLN's "Excellence in Education Model" has relevance for all levels of nursing education programs from practical/vocational nursing to doctoral level nursing. The position statement urges nursing faculty to base their curriculum designs, teaching/learning strategies, and evaluation methods on research rather than on politically driven pronouncements (_http://_

www.nurseuniverse.om/Nursing-Job/2454.html). The NLN is available to help with changes with both workshops and individual programs.

In 1996, the NLN published "Competencies of Graduates of Educational Programs in Practical Nursing." Although these competencies have not been revised since 1996, the general categories around which they are organized are still relevant for twenty-first century LPN/LVN practice. Those general categories include the following: assessment, planning, implementation, and evaluation of patient care; serving as a member of the discipline of nursing; managing one's own actions and those of unlicensed health care providers; and political awareness.

The NLN Centers of Excellence in Nursing Education is designed to recognize schools of nursing that have achieved a level of excellence in specific areas. The application for accreditation is voluntary, has specific criteria, and requires fees. Contact information for the NLN follows.

NLN
61 Broadway, 33rd floor
New York, NY 10006
Phone: (800) 669-1656
Fax: (212) 812-0393
Website: _http://www.nln.org_

THE AMERICAN NURSES ASSOCIATION (ANA)

The American Nurses Association (ANA) only represents registered nurses (RNs). State affiliates of the ANA are altering bylaws to allow LPN/LVNs to join the association at the state level and pay dues but not have a voice or vote in the organization. **The ANA does not represent licensed practical/vocational nurses and has attempted to limit their scope of practice. In 1965 the ANA set policy to eliminate LPN/LVNs (Mahan, 2007) and attempted to do so again in the 1980s. See Chapter 7, p. 102.**

NATIONAL ASSOCIATION FOR PRACTICAL NURSE EDUCATION AND SERVICE, INC.

The National Association for Practical Nurse Education and Service, Inc. (NAPNES) was founded in 1941. The multidisciplinary composition of its membership includes LPN/LVNs, RNs, students, and schools of practical nursing, organizations, and public members promoting the ideals of NAPNES. It was the first organization dedicated to protecting practice and education and regulation of LPN/LVNs, nursing educators, practical nursing schools, and practical nursing students. Membership in NAPNES provides the following benefits:

- A year's subscription to *The Journal of Practical Nursing (JPN),* the oldest journal devoted entirely to practical/vocational nursing. This quarterly, peer-reviewed journal keeps you up-to-date with nursing articles, news about NAPNES, infection control, nursing law, and legislation and regulations affecting LPN/LVNs. The journal also includes feature articles about practical/vocational nursing, information about certification in pharmacology and long-term care, and other educational opportunities.
- The *eJournal of Practical Nursing* is also a publication of NAPNES. e-Members have all the rights and privileges of regular members, except they do not receive a printed copy of the *JPN.* Instead they access *eJPN* as a PDF download. Regular membership that includes the printed *JPN* is $75 and $25 for students. e-Membership is $35 per year and $10 for students. Because of savings to NAPNES through e-Membership, the savings is passed on to members. A vast majority of income for NAPNES is provided by membership dues.
- NAPNES has launched an online continuing education program called Continuing Education Record Keeping System (CERKS). This program is available to LPN/LVN and PN educators. Registration is free and includes an online record keeping system and instant certificate printing.
- The NAPNES website includes information about certifications, regulation news and updates, clinical articles, CEUs, podcasts, webinars, blogs, and jobs.

- The online bookstore offers members a 10% discount and free handling and shipping.
- Networking with other LPN/LVNs through the constituent state members throughout the United States.
- The NAPNES technology department has developed a tool for making nursing updates and education on line faster and easier.
- National representation and a say for the future of nursing.
- NAPNES Standards of Practice for LPN/LVN (see Appendix B).

For additional information contact:
NAPNES
1940 Duke St., Suite 200
Alexandria, VA 22314
Phone: (703) 933-1003
Fax: (703) 940-4989
Website: *http://www.napnes.org*

NATIONAL FEDERATION OF LICENSED PRACTICAL NURSES

The National Federation of Licensed Practical Nurses (NFLPN) was organized in 1949. It is the policy-making body for LPN/LVNs. NFLPN is made up of LPN/LVNs, SPN/SVNs, and affiliate members. Affiliate members receive all communications and may attend all meetings, but do not have the right to vote or hold office. NFLPN was formed by LPN/LVNs, who wanted an organization to work for and speak on their behalf. It is the only nursing organization governed entirely by LPN/LVNs. It is recognized by other national nursing organizations as the official voice of LPN/LVNs. The NFLPN motto is "The Spirit of Care—The Heart of Nursing."

NFLPN membership includes the following benefits:

- Complimentary quarterly subscription to *Advance for LPNs,* Special NFLPN Edition website *http://www.nflpn.org*
- National certification in IV therapy and gerontology (Educational Resources, Inc., is administrator of the program and may be contacted at (800) 292-2263)

- Tracking of your continuing education courses
- MBNA credit card
- NSO insurance discounts
- Annual convention and trade show offering CE courses
- Legislative watchdog on issues affecting LPN/LVNs
- Networking opportunities through your chapter meetings
- Student Honor Society for achieving PN students
- Monthly scholarship toward tuition for upward mobility through RUE Educational
- Bachelor of Science program for LPNs through Medical University of the Americas
- Annual LPN/LVN Recognition & Awareness Week (1st week in October each year)
- Discounted Convention Registration for members.

RUE Education in partnership with NFLPN is sponsoring websites for participating LPN associations. The websites make it possible to follow the work being done on your behalf. The quarterly *Visions* newsletter informs what is happening in regard to NFLPN and Rue Education opportunities.

See Appendix C for NFLPN Practice Standards for the Licensed Practical/Vocational Nurses.

For additional information, contact:
NFLPN
605 Poole Drive
Garner, NC 27529
Phone: (919) 779-0046
Fax: (919) 779-5642
Website: *http://www.nflpn.org*

CONTINUING EDUCATION

Historically, LPN/LVNs have a reputation for being apathetic in pursuing continuing education classes. This is difficult to believe because many LPN/LVNs have gone on to learn complex nursing skills after graduation. Continuing education classes are available through many agencies. If the education benefits the agency, they may be willing to pick up part or the entire fee. Some agency courses are free and are part of continuing service within the agency. Initial licensure is being questioned as providing competency for life. Your continued study helps keep you up to date and ensure competency as an LPN/LVN. Continuing education includes the following resources.

ORIENTATION TO THE FACILITY

Orientation provides an opportunity to learn about policies, regulations, routines, nursing care procedures, and variations in routine, plus a review of selected previously learned information and skills. Learning this information takes a period of time. Facilities generally have an education/in-service director who is in charge of orientation for new employees.

IN-SERVICE TRAINING

In-service training is information chosen to meet specific needs within a facility. Attendance at some in-service programs, such as a yearly update on blood-borne pathogens, is required. Offer suggestions for content to your employer. Usually a specified amount of time is required for in-service programs, such as 1 hour per month or three times per year, according to the agency policy. Depending on the credentials of the instructor, continuing education credits may be available.

WORKSHOPS

Workshops present information and an opportunity to practice what is being taught. Workshops provide opportunities to learn new skills. Workshop length varies according to content. Some agencies pay the workshop fee or expenses if the topic is specific to, and enhances, your nursing skills. Workshops are also a major source of continuing education credits that are required by many states as a part of continued licensure in nursing.

CONTINUING EDUCATION UNITS (CE OR CEUS)

Classes are often taught involving complex nursing skills such as intravenous therapy, physical assessment, LPN or LVN charge nurse (leadership/management), mental health concepts, nursing process for LPN/LVNs, and so on. Many vocational schools and community colleges will provide any course you are interested in, if you request it and enough people are available to make up the required minimum enrollment. Many of these classes provide CEUs, as opposed to course credit. You receive a certificate if you complete course work satisfactorily.

One of the most valuable benefits of continuing education classes is the opportunity to get together with other working LPN/LVNs. You discover similarities in challenges and satisfactions. Ideas are shared on how to deal with difficult situations in the work setting. It is a good idea to keep a running record of all in-service programs, seminars, and workshops taken, including dates, CEUs, and topics, for future reference. Ask for these records to be included in your file at your place of employment, and keep a copy for your own file. Some states require that you list the CEUs when you apply for license renewal. Other state boards of nursing want you to have the file available in case the board decides to check the accuracy of what you stated in your renewal application.

Continuing education contact hours are also available through your professional organizations. For example, RueCEU in association with NFLPN offers unlimited contact hours for 1 year for a one-time fee of $29.99 or $8.00 per contact hour (*http://www.RueCEU.com*).

INTERNET RESOURCES
Numerous sources are available online depending on what fits your need.
- *Advance for Nurses* (including *Advance for LPNs*) is available online with a free subscription (*http://www.advanceweb.com*). Current updates and nursing articles are available at the tip of your finger.
- Podcasts. This term is derived from the iPod from Apple Computer, Inc. The actual files are compatible with any MP3 player and are streamed from the Internet that allows users to listen directly through home computers. All kinds of information is available. Podcasts make an audio file available online for downloading via an automatic feed. You can then hear the podcast whenever you want from your own computer or a portable media player at you own convenience Look for this method of obtaining CEUs to be available for LPN/LVNs in the future. Currently, some podcasts offer CE credit for RNs. Depending on your areas of professional interests, it may be worthwhile subscribing. Check with your instructors for further information and availability of this learning tool.
- **Medscape** offers information on healthcare changes; new guidelines for care, emerging infectious diseases, sudden disasters, and more through daily summaries. Medscape offers partial CE hours through their Medscape Medical News service. Although the focus is primarily RNs, there is useful information for all nurses on a daily basis. The subscription is free through *http://www.Medscape.com*.

CERTIFICATION OPPORTUNITIES
Take advantage of knowledge available during certification seminars and self-study courses. Knowledge is the basis for improved nursing skills and safety in patient care. In many states/agencies, certification is also the basis for salary increases and advancement. Some states do not recognize the significance of the certifications. Avoid using this as an excuse to avoid certification. Enhancing your competence as a nurse increases both personal and professional satisfaction. Use the extended title you have earned and wear your pin(s) proudly. The 2006 practice analysis showed that of the 6000 LPN/LVNs, 53% earned certifications: basic life support (29.8%), IV therapy (21.4%), and phlebotomy (7.5%).

Some earned certifications in more than one area.

NAPNES CERTIFICATION PROGRAMS

NAPNES offers Long-Term Care Certification (LPN CLTC or LVN CLTC) and Pharmacology Certification (LPN NPC or LVN NPC). Both are offered online.

NAPNES Long-Term Care Certification (CLTC)

Long-Term Care Certification (CLTC) has replaced the previous Gerontology Certification program. Long-Term Care Certification is comprehensive and covers the entire life span of patients who are chronically ill in any age group. It is about excellence in nursing care with any age group.

To be eligible, the LPN/LVN must have a current license in good standing, have (documented) 2000 hours of long-term care practice within the previous 3 years, and receive a passing grade in the examination. PN/VN curriculum in most schools covers the information required to pass the examination. Optional study materials are available through NAPNES. Alternative certifications through other agencies are not recognized by NAPNES.

The examination consists of 150 multiple choice questions. The test is timed and automatically stops at the end of 2½ hours for scoring. The questions show up on the screen one at a time and cannot be printed. Keystrokes are counted and attempts to print the exam will result in failure.

Successful candidates receive an AFFIDAVIT online to print and sign before a notary public. The signed and notarized AFFIDAVIT is presented to NAPNES within 60 days for a certificate card that attests to having taken and passed the exam. The LPN/LVN may use the title LPN CLTC or LVN CLTC.

Recertification must be applied for in 3 years or the certificate expires 3 years from date of issuance. Directions for initial certification and recertification are available on *http://www.napnes. com*.

NAPNES Pharmacology Certification (NCP)

The NAPNES Pharmacology Certification (NCP) examination allows LPN/LVNs to measure their knowledge against a national test and offers a national credential, post-licensure, that many employers require. The candidate is tested on general principles of pharmacology, the role of the LPN/LVN with pharmacology, drugs affecting different systems, and nursing process for the patient receiving medications. Candidates also have the option of challenging the examination based on work experience and/or prior training. Certification equivalences are not accepted by NAPNES.

The NAPNES Pharmacology Certification is available to anyone who holds a current LPN/LVN license or a student who meets educational requirements to take the NCLEX-PN® (a program director signature is required on the application) and receives a passing score on the Pharmacology Certification Examination.

Fill out the application completely, sign, and enclose the fee made out to NAPNES. Some changes in requirements are in place as of January 1, 2007. Photocopies and faxes are not accepted. Non-members have a different fee from NAPNES members.

If the application is accepted, the candidate will receive a letter of approval, ID number, password, and written instructions on how to access the examination online. The approval letter, ID number, and password are valid for 60 days or until the examination is taken.

The online examination has 125 multiple choice questions. The 2-hour examination is timed, automatically stops, and is submitted for grading. Questions appear on the screen one question at a time. Keystrokes are counted and any attempt to print the examination results in automatic failure. Successful candidates receive an affidavit online to print out and sign before a notary public. The signed affidavit is presented to NAPNES within 60 days of the test for a Pharmacology Certification Certificate and the right to the title LPN NCP or LVN NCP. Recertification is required every 3 years from the date of initial certification.

Both the Long-Term Care Certification and the Pharmacology Certification have similar fees. Check the website for changes in application rules, fees for members and non-members, and fees for recertification. Currently, application forms, directions, and a study order form are available for download online. Registration and application can be made online (*http://www.napnes.org*). Fill out the application and mail to NAPNES at 1940 Duke Street, Suite 200, Alexandria, VA 22313. Sign and date your application. The initial fee of $100 is payable to NAPNES. NAPNES accepts money orders, Visa, MasterCard, and personal checks. Once the application is approved, you receive an individual ID number, password, and directions on how to access the examination online. The examination fee is payable online to Castle Worldwide, Inc. (the testing organization) and must be paid by MasterCard or Visa. The approval letter, ID, and password are valid for 60 days or until the test.

NFLPN CERTIFICATION PROGRAMS

NFLPN offers National Certification in Gerontology (LPN GC or LVN GC) and National Certification in IV Therapy (LPN IVC or LVN IVC). The cost of the 2-year National Certification is $175 and includes:

- One-year membership with the NFLPN
- Test content outline video
- Paper/pencil exam and answer sheet
- Scoring and diagnostic reports
- Certificate (upon passing)
- National registry
- Shipping and handling costs
- Earned titles IVC/GC
- Enamel lapel pin to signify certificate status (*http://www.nflpn.org/certification.html*)

There is a $55 discount for NFLPN members, and group discounts are available.

Both examinations assess knowledge base of IV or gerontology concepts, critical thinking skills, clinical application, and decision-making ability. Registration forms are available online at *http://www.nflpn.org/certification.html*.

The sponsoring facility administers the test in a secure setting and returns all test materials to Educational Resources, Inc. (ERI), the testing provider. They score the test and provide diagnostic scores and a certificate when the candidate passes. The LPN/LVN who completes the

exam successfully is placed in the NFLPN certification roster and earns the right to use the title after their name. Certification is effective for 2 years.

NFLPN IV Therapy Certification

A copy of the nurse's license and letter of endorsement that vouches for the nurse's clinical training and experience signed by the supervisor accompanies the registration form. A copy of school transcripts that shows successful passing of an IV therapy course is an alternative. The application is mailed to NFLPN with a sponsor letter and certification fee. If the application is accepted, the candidate receives preparation materials. Preparation is by viewing the exam outline video. The examination is sent to the nurse's sponsoring institution and a referral to the supervisor who will proctor the examination.

There are 99 questions on the IV therapy examination. It takes approximately 2 hours to complete the exam. Topics include:

- Fluid, Electrolytes, and Acid-Base Balance
- Fluid Administration
- Administration of Blood Products
- Administration of Total Parenteral Nutrition
- Medication Administration
- Special considerations including Legal, Pediatric, Infection Control

NFLPN Gerontology Certification

A specific course in gerontology is not required. A suggested reading list is included with the materials the candidate receives. The gerontology examination has 105 questions and takes approximately 2 hours. Gerontology topics include:

- Foundations of gerontology,
- Promoting health and wellness,
- Nursing care of the Elderly with Physical and Psychological Disorders,
- Special gerontology care issues, including Rehab and Restorative Care, Substance Abuse, Cancer, and Pharmacology,

All the other steps are similar to what has been previously described. For additional information contact:

ERI Educational Consultant
Phone: (800) 292-2273
Fax: (913) 362-4627
Website: *http://www.eriworld.com*

4435 Waterfront Drive, Suite 101
Glen Allen, Virginia 23060
Phone: (804) 747-9698
Website: *http://www.abmcn.org*

ABMCN CERTIFICATION IN MANAGED CARE

American Board of Managed Care Nursing (ABMCN) Certification in Managed Care Nursing is available to LPN/LVNs through a home study course. Order the course through ABMCN (*http://www.abmcn.org*). An option is to provide an affidavit of equivalency of a course taken elsewhere. The examination is provided through a proctor.

Options for eligibility include:

1. 1-year full-time employment as an LPN/LVN, or
2. 2 years acceptable employment providing direct or indirect care in an acute care facility, skilled nursing facility, mental health facility, or other healthcare organization, or
3. 1 year acceptable case management employment experience.
4. To be considered, employment must be verified, an official job description included and application signed by the employment supervisor.

Application and directions are available online. To be eligible, send in the following:

- Completed official registration form,
- Proctor agreement form,
- Copy of your current nursing license, and
- Registration fee—$295.

The examination includes basic knowledge of managed care, healthcare economics, healthcare management, and patient issues. Upon successful completion of the examination, the nurse is certified and may use the title Certification in Managed Care in Nursing (CMCN). Certification is valid for 3 years.

To inquire about managed care in nursing certification, contact:

American Board of Managed Care Nursing (ABMCN)
Contact person: Ann Patrick

MOVING UP

If you are an LPN/LVN who says, "I want to be an LPN/LVN. I have no desire to be an RN," you have obviously given careful consideration to your personal goals. Satisfaction in nursing, both for you and patients you care for, is closely related to clear-cut goals. If you decided you want to be an LPN/LVN, chances are you will be satisfied with your choice and will provide satisfactory care to your patients. If, however, someone else decided you should be a nurse, chances are you will never be entirely satisfied with the choice. This lack of satisfaction will be mirrored in care you give to patients. The same process is true in regard to making a decision to become an RN. If you do not want to become an RN, avoid letting anyone push you into it. Only when a goal is truly your own will you be motivated to do your best both in the educational process and in the care of patients.

If you want to enter an RN program, learn what programs of study are available. A major problem in developing upward mobility programs for LPN/LVNs is the belief held by some educators that a practical nursing course is terminal in nature; that some state boards of nursing will not permit upward mobility programs, nor will credit be given by some professional nursing programs. Although the same reasoning continues to be held in some parts of the country, other directors of nursing have successfully negotiated with state boards of nursing to develop progressive LPN/LVN-to-RN programs. Contact your state's board of nursing for a list of available professional nursing programs within your state.

EDUCATIONAL MOBILITY FOR NURSES

In *Career Ladder*, the author states, "I believe that historically the Helene Fuld School of Nursing at the Hospital of Joint Diseases and Medical Center (New York City) is the first program to demonstrate the belief that practical/vocational nursing is indeed a part of the nursing profession, and that a curriculum can be constructed that effectively articulates with one that prepares for registered nurse licensure with minimal repetition" (Ahl, 1975). The program, initially a 15-month course trimmed down to 47 weeks, was initiated in 1964. Justine Hannan, hospital director of nursing, worked with the board of nursing within New York State's Education Department. By 1968 the department granted full registration to the program. By 1970 it was accredited by the NLN. "The school has had an impact on the quality of nursing in its home hospital, and has sent graduates into dozens of other health care facilities throughout New York and fifteen other states. It has willingly shared its experience with educators who have made inquiries about its work, and has demonstrated that career ladder education is both valid and appropriate for a large number of persons who have the aptitude and commitment to such a goal" (Ahl, 1975).

Career ladder programs (seamless programs) are carefully planned to avoid duplication of content. "The curriculum is a Practical Nursing curriculum for the first year and an Associate Degree Nursing curriculum for the second. It is a totally new curriculum designed in terms of essential learning for beginning nursing competencies. It allows the student to be a competent practical nurse at the end of the program and a competent registered nurse at the end of an additional year" (Story, 1974).

Itasca Nursing Education Consortium (INRC)

A program approved by the Minnesota Board of Nursing is available through seven northern Minnesota technical, community, and 4-year colleges involved in the INEC. It was developed in 1982 to help the student move through the upper levels of nursing education. Students may enter the practical nursing program at four of the schools and participate as a full- or part-time student. On completion of the first year of the program, graduates become eligible to apply to take the NCLEX-PN® examination.

The second year is available at two community colleges. Admission requirements for the associate degree nursing program include completion of a practical nurse program; minimum cumulative GPA (grade point average) of 2.8; licensure as an LPN for the fall semester start or licensure within 10 weeks for the spring semester start; completion of pre-requisites (listed on website); all courses passed with a C grade or better; and pass the Nurse Entrance Test (NET) at or above the national standard for students enrolled in RN programs (*http://www.lsc.mnscu.edu/ Programs/Healthcareers/Nursing/ADHomePage/ Faculty.cfm*).

Upon completion, the graduate becomes eligible to apply to take the NCLEX-RN® examination. The nursing-associate degree RN may continue his or her education to receive a baccalaureate in nursing. This degree is available through two 4-year colleges that are members of the Consortium. For information contact:

Diane Kostrzewski
Director of Nursing Programs
Associate Degree Nursing Program
Lake Superior College
2101 Trinity Road
Duluth, MN 55811
Phone: (218) 733-7600 or (800) 432-2884
Website: *http://www.lsc.mnscu.edu* for general
    information about nursing programs

Sheridan College School of Nursing (SCSN)

Associate degree nursing programs vary in structure. For example, Sheridan College of Nursing Associate degree program in Sheridan, WY is considered an AD program. Student studies are based on associate RN needs. Students may opt to take the NCLEX-PN® at the conclusion of their first year and work as an LPN with successful completion of the examination. The LPN may choose to continue his or her studies an additional year with or without taking the NCLEX-PN®. Sheridan College of Nursing has also developed a partnership with the University of Wyoming for a BSN completion program. All courses and clinical experience are in Sheridan. The BSN completion program is flexible, geared to meet the student's need, and is approximately one year plus. For information about nursing programs contact:

Judith E. McDowell, RN, MS, CCRN
Director, Associate Degree Nursing Program
Sheridan College
3059 Coffeen Ave.
Sheridan, WY 82801-1500
Phone: (307) 674-6446
Website: *http://www.sheridan.edu*

Career ladder programs (seamless programs) exist in many areas of the country. Costs of programs vary considerably. Your state board of nursing is an excellent resource for information about programs in your area. See Appendix A for state board listings.

Minneapolis Community and Technical College (MCTC) Mobility Program

Minneapolis Community and Technical College has one of the oldest nursing programs in the country, and has continued to evolve with the times. Their major nursing program is a seamless program for nursing assistant/home health aide to practical nurse to associate in science (AS) degree RN. MCTC has an articulation agreement with Metropolitan State University and Minnesota State College and University (MNSCU) consortium, as well as many private institutions to progress to the bachelor of science in nursing degree. The program is accredited by the NLN and is approved by the Minnesota State Board of Nursing. For descriptions and requirements contact:

Carmen Franzmeier
Nursing Programs
Minneapolis Community and Technical
   College
1501 Hennepin Avenue
Minneapolis, MN 55403
Phone: (612) 659-6212 or (800) 247-0911
Email: *mctcinfo@minneapolis.edu*
Website: *http://www.minneapolis.edu/contactus.cfm*

Distance Learning Nursing Program at Excelsior College

Excelsior College (previously known as Regents College), of Albany, NY, is the first in the United States to have a distance-learning nursing program (online). The associate degree in nursing program began in 1972 and has been continuously accredited by the NLN. This has been an accrediting commission since 1975. There are no classes to attend, the student can study when convenient and take examinations when ready. Interest-free financing is available.

LPN/LVNs must apply for admission and be accepted to the School of Nursing before enrolling. Requirements are found on their website, *http://www.excelsior.edu*. Licensed LPN/LVNs are eligible to apply (exception of CA residents). The college is founded on the premise that what you know is more important than where you learned it. College faculty evaluates all previous credits you have earned. Possible credits include courses you have taken from other regionally accredited colleges and universities, military training, continuing education programs, and Internet-based programs. Generous learner support is made available to students from full-time advisors and nursing faculty. Students are able to study and prepare at their own pace while maintaining their jobs. Because there is no residency requirement, you will not have to repeat courses you have already taken. For information contact:

Admissions
Excelsior College
7 Columbia Circle
Albany, NY 12203-5159
Phone: (888) 647-2388
Website: *http://www.excelsior.edu*

NFLPN's iStudySmart.com. NFLPN has chosen **iStudySmart.com** as educational partners to assist LPN/LVNs continue their nursing education to become an ASN (associate in science RN) or BSN. *iStudySmart.com* helps you test out of college classes and receive college credit without attending class. You determine testing time when you are ready. Most local universities accept 30 to 45 semester hour of credit by exam. Fully accredited schools may accept more. Course work is available for purchase at *http://www. iStudySmart.com*. Course work is done online, in workbook format, or a CD-ROM. After purchasing the textbook, complete all the assignments.

Work through the practice exams and when ready, go to the local test site to have your examination for the course. Send the passing score to the university or college. To get started, go to the website and use the coupon code AR8R539 to receive a course discount. Call (800) 737-2222 for assistance or email info@istudysmart.com.

NONCREDIT RN PROGRAMS

Turf issues continue to exist in all levels of nursing: certified nursing assistant to LPN/LVN to ADN to BSN to MSN. Plan to be a part of the solution, not the problem, when you are in a position to make a difference. This is an area where you, as a member of your professional nursing organization, can have a voice in making a difference.

Some RN programs continue to not recognize the worth of practical/vocational education. These programs insist that LPN/LVNs start from the beginning and repeat all previously covered theory and skills courses, including basic nursing skills. The bottom line is that a number of programs are available throughout the country that can be used by the LPN/LVN to become an RN—if that is what is right for that nurse.

The state boards of nursing (see listing in Appendix A) are an excellent source for locating approved nursing programs. Many of the programs have websites that make it possible to get information about a program before inquiring directly. Request a list of board-approved professional nursing programs preparing for registered nurse licensure, which are open to the LPN/LVN.

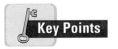
Key Points

- A majority of 2006 newly licensed LPN/LVNs work in long-term care facilities and a smaller number in rehabilitation units and other settings. Care was primarily for adults and elderly patients. Over half had chronic, stable illnesses. Almost half of the patients had behavioral/emotional problems.
- Employment of LPN/LVNs is expected to increase as fast as the average for all occupations through the year 2014, especially in long-term care and home health facilities.
- During the first quarter of 2004, salaries ranged from $24,830 to $46,240 annually in the United States.
- In 2004, approximately 726,000 LPN/LVNs were employed in the United States.
- Canada's workforce included 64,951 LPNs. Most opportunities for employment are in long-term care and some areas of hospital care. Salaries vary according to province, experience, and work area.
- In Canada, there is effort to examine roles and articulation between LPN and RN and empower all nurses to work within their roles.
- Desirable nursing characteristics for work areas vary according to the work involved. Overall, nurses must know how to think critically and problem solve, be emotionally stable, physically healthy, caring, and empathetic.
- Postgraduate certification courses are available for LPN/LVNs through NAPNES, NFLPN, and other organizations. Certifications increase knowledge and skill, and, in many states, the salary and position.
- LPN/LVN to associate degree programs in nursing are available throughout the United States. Contact your state board of nursing for a current listing of approved programs.
- Belonging to at least one professional nursing organization (e.g., NAPNES, NFLPN) provides benefits and, most important, a voice in the future of nursing.
- Turf issues continue in all levels of nursing: certified nursing assistant to LPN/LVN to ADN to BSN to MSN. When you are in a position to make a difference, plan to be part of the solution, not the problem.

REVIEW ITEMS

1. What is the current major area of employment for LPN/LVNs?

   1. Military
   2. Nursing homes
   3. Hospitals
   4. Clinics

2. Why become certified in nursing-related areas after becoming an LPN/LVN?

   1. The certifications are designed to increase your nursing knowledge and skill.
   2. You will gradually be able to assume the work of an RN without an RN license.
   3. Use of the extended title(s) will greatly improve your status among other employees.
   4. Unless your state board acknowledges the certification, it serves no purpose.

3. After a visit to an NFLPN meeting, you evaluate critically the major benefit to you as an LPN/LVN. Which benefit has long-term value to you and to nursing?

   1. Obtaining IV Therapy and Gerontology certifications through the organization.
   2. Working toward reform in nursing curricula and methods of teaching in nursing.
   3. Receiving reduced rates on insurance, continuing education, and credit cards.
   4. Being part of the policy-making body for LPN/LVNs, governed by LPN/LVNs.

4. As a charge nurse in a nursing home, which staff member will you assign to assist an elderly patient with complex eating or drinking problems?

   1. A patient who is able to coax other patients to do things.
   2. A certified nursing assistant who has received the required aide training.
   3. An assistant with 8 hours of training on feeding, who was hired by the home.
   4. No one. Do it yourself to evaluate the complexity of the patient problem.

ALTERNATE FORMAT ITEM

Using critical thinking, which of the following will enhance your career when choosing your first job as an LPN/LVN? *(Select all that apply.)*

1. Learn if the work you are expected to do is within your scope of practice.

2. Take the least-challenging job because you are just beginning your career.

3. Check availability of orientation, RN supervision, and instruction as needed.

4. Know the hours of work, salary, benefits, types of patients, in-service, and staffing.

State Boards of Nursing

(NOTE: Boards of nursing addresses, and some board of nursing websites in the United States, can be accessed online at *http://allnurses. com/nursingboards-a-k.shtml*, *http:// allnurses.com/nursingboards-l-o.shtml*, *http://allnurses.com/nursing boards-p-z.shtml*, and *www.ncsbn.org*. Addresses and contact numbers change periodically.)

Alabama

Alabama Board of Nursing
RSA Plaza, Suite 250
770 Washington Avenue
Montgomery, AL 36130-3900
Phone: (334) 242-4060 or
  (800) 656-5318
Fax: (334) 242-4360
Website: *http://www.abn.state.al.us/*

Alaska

Alaska Board of Nursing
550 West Seventh Avenue,
  Suite 1500
Anchorage, AK 99501-3567
Phone: (907) 269-8161
Fax: (907) 269-8196
Website: *http://www.dced.state.ak.us/ occ/pnur.htm*

American Samoa

American Samoa Health Services
  Regulatory Board
LBJ Tropical Medical Center
Pago Pago, AS 96799
Phone: (684) 633-1222
Fax: (684) 633-1869

Arizona

Arizona State Board of Nursing
4747 North 7th Street, Suite 200
Phoenix, AZ 85014
Phone: (602) 889-5150
Fax: (602) 889-5155
Website: *http://www.azbn.gov/*

Arkansas

Arkansas State Board of Nursing
University Tower Building
1123 South University, Suite 800
Little Rock, AR 72204
Phone: (501) 686-2700
Fax: (501) 686-2714
Website: *http://www.arsbn.org/*

California

California Board of Vocational
  Nurse and Psychiatric
  Technicians
2535 Capitol Oaks Drive, Suite 205
Sacramento, CA 95833
Phone: (916) 263-7800
Fax: (916) 263-7859
Website: *http://www.bvnpt.ca.gov/*

Colorado

Colorado Board of Nursing
1560 Broadway, Suite 1350
Denver, CO 80202
Phone: (303) 894-2430
Fax: (303) 894-2821
Website: *http://www.dora.state. co.us/nursing/*

Connecticut

Connecticut Practical Nursing
  Licensing
Department of Public Health
410 Capital Avenue, MS# 13PHO
PO Box 340308
Hartford, CT 06134-0328
Phone: (860) 509- 8000
Fax: (860) 509-7553
Website: *http://www.dph.state.ct.us/ Licensure/apps/PLIS/Nursing/LPN/ LPN_Home.htm*

Delaware

Delaware Board of Nursing
861 Silver Lake Boulevard
Cannon Building, Suite 203
Dover, DE 19904
Phone: (302)-739-4522
Fax: (302) 739-2711
Website: *http://dpr.delaware. gov/boards/nursing/*

District of Columbia

Health Professional Licensing
  Administration
Department of Health
717 14th Street NW, Suite 600
Washington, DC 20005
Phone: (877) 672-2174
Fax: (202) 727-8471
Website: *http://hpla.doh.dc.gov/hpla/ cwp/view,A,1195.Q,488526,hplaNav, %7C30661%7C.asp*

Florida

Health Professional Licensing
  Information
Mailing Address:
4052 Bald Cypress Way, BIN CO2
Tallahassee. FL 32399
Phone: (850) 488-0595
Fax: (850) 487-9625
Physical Address:
4042 Bald Cypress Way
Room 120
Tallahassee, FL 32399
Website: *http://www.doh.state. fl.us/mqa/*

Georgia

Georgia State Board of Licensed
  Practical Nurses
237 Coliseum Drive
Macon, GA 31217-3858
Phone: (478) 207-1300
Fax: (478) 207-1633
Website: *http://www.sos.state. ga.us/plb/lpn*

Guam

Guam Board of Nurse Examiners
Regular Mailing Address:
PO Box 2816
Hagatna, Guam 96932
Phone: (671) 735-7411
Fax: (671) 477-4733
Street Address (for FedEx and UPS):
651 Legacy Square Commercial
    Complex
South Route 10, Suite 9
Mangilao, Guam 96913

Hawaii

Hawaii Board of Nursing
Professional and Vocational
    Licensing Division
PO Box 3469
Honolulu, HI 96801
Phone: (808) 586-3000
Fax: (808) 586-2689
Website: *http://hawaii.gov/dcca/
    areas/pvl/boards/nursing*

Idaho

Idaho Board of Nursing
280 North 8th Street, Suite 210
PO Box 83720
Boise, ID 83720
Phone: (208) 334-3110
Fax: (208) 334-3262
Website: *http://www2.state.id.us/ibn/*

Illinois

Illinois Department of Professional
    Regulation
320 West Washington Street
Springfield, IL 62786
Phone: (217) 782-0800
Fax: (217) 782-7645
Website: *http://www.dpr.state.il.us/*

Indiana

Indiana State Board of Nursing
Professional Licensing Agency
402 West Washington Street,
    Room W072
Indianapolis, IN 46204
Phone: (317) 234-2043
Fax: (317) 233-4236
Website: *http://www.state.
    in.us/pla/bandc/isbn/*

Iowa

Iowa Board of Nursing
RiverPoint Business Park
400 SW 8th Street, Suite B
Des Moines, IA 50309-4685
Phone: (515) 281-3255
Fax: (515) 281-4825
Website: *http://www.state.
    ia.us/government/nursing/*

Kansas

Kansas State Board of Nursing
Landon State Office Building
900 SW Jackson Street, Suite 1051
Topeka, KS 66612-1230
Phone: (785) 296-4929
Fax: (785) 296-3929
Website: *http://www.ksbn.org/*

Kentucky

Kentucky Board of Nursing
312 Whittington Parkway, Suite 300
Louisville, KY 40222
Phone: (502) 429-3300 or (800)
    305-2042
Fax: (502) 429-3311
Website: *http://kbn.ky.gov/*

Louisiana

Louisiana State Board of Practical
    Nurse Examiners
3421 North Causeway Boulevard,
    Suite 505
Metairie, LA 70002
Phone: (504) 838-5791
Fax: (504) 838-5279
Website: *http://www.lsbpne.com/
    Faculty%20app%20and%
    20instructions.pdf*

Maine

Maine State Board of Nursing
158 State House Station
Augusta, ME 04333
Phone: (207) 287-1133
Fax: (207) 287-1149
Website: *http://www.maine.gov/
    boardofnursing/*

Maryland

Maryland Board of Nursing
4140 Patterson Avenue
Baltimore, MD 21215
Phone: (410) 585-1900 or (888)
    202-9861
Fax: (410) 358-3530
Website: *http://www.mbon.org/*

Massachusetts

Massachusetts Board of
    Registration in Nursing
Commonwealth of Massachusetts
239 Causeway Street, Suite 200
Boston, MA 02114
Phone: (617) 973-800
Fax: (617) 973-0984
Website: *http://www.mass.gov/
    ?pageID=eohhs2subtopic&
    L=5&L0=Home&L1=Provider&
    L2=Certification%2C+Licensure%
    2C+and+Registration&
    L3=Occupational+and+Professional
    &L4=Nursing&sid=Eeohhs2*

Michigan

Michigan/DCH/Bureau of Health
    Professions
BHP PO Box 30193
Lansing, MI 48909
Phone: (517) 335-0918
Fax: (517) 373-2179
Website: *http://www.michigan.gov/
    mdch/0,1607,7-132-27417_27529---,
    00.html*

Minnesota

Minnesota Board of Nursing
2829 University Avenue SE,
    Suite 200
Minneapolis, MN 55414
Phone: (612) 617-2270
Fax: (612) 617-2190
Website: *http://www.nursingboard.
    state.mn.us/*

Mississippi

Mississippi Board of Nursing
1935 Lakeland Drive, Suite B
Jackson, MS 39216
Phone: (601) 987-4188
Fax: (601) 364-2352
Website: *http://www.msbn.state.
    ms.us/*

Missouri

Missouri State Board of Nursing
3605 Missouri Boulevard
PO Box 1335
Jefferson City, MO 65102
Phone: (573) 751- 0293
Fax: (573) 751-0075
Website: *http://pr.mo.gov/*

Montana

Montana Board of Nursing
301 South Park
PO Box 200513
Helena, MT 59620-0513
Phone: (406) 841-2345
Fax: (406) 841-2305
Website: *http://mt.gov/dli/bsd/license/
    bsd_boards/nur_board/
    board_page.asp*

Nebraska

Nebraska Department of Health
    and Human Services System
    Department of Regulation and
    Licensure and Nursing Support
301 Centennial Mall South
Lincoln, NE 68509-4986
Phone: (402) 471-3121
Fax: (402) 471-1066
Website: *http://www.hhs.state.ne.us/crl/
    crlindex.htm*

Nevada

Nevada State Board of Nursing
License Certification and Education
2500 West Sahara Avenue, Suite 207
Las Vegas, NV 89102
Phone: (702) 486-5800 or (888)
    590-6726
Fax: (702) 486-5803

Nevada State Board of Nursing
Administration, Discipline &
    Investigations, and Discipline
5011 Meadowood Mall Way, Suite
    300
Reno, NV 89502-6547
Phone: (755) 688-2620 or (888)
    590-6726
Fax: (702) 688-2628
Website: *http://www.nursingboard.
    state.nv.us/*

New Hampshire

New Hampshire Board of Nursing
21 South Fruit Street, Suite 16
Concord, NH 03301
Phone: (603) 271-2323
Fax: (603) 271-6605
Website: *http://www.state.
    nh.us/nursing/*

New Jersey

New Jersey Board of Nursing
124 Halsey Street, 6th Floor
PO Box 45010
Newark, NJ 07101
Phone: (973) 504-6430
Fax: (973) 648-3481
Website: *http://www.state.nj.us/lps/ca/
    medical.htm*

New Mexico

New Mexico Board of Nursing
4206 Louisiana Boulevard, NE,
    Suite A
Albuquerque, NM 87109
Phone: (505) 841-8340
Fax: (505) 841-8347
Website: *http://www.bon.state.nm.us/*

New York

New York State Board of Nursing
Office of Professions
Division of Professional Licensing
    Services
Nurse Unit
89 Washington Avenue
2nd Floor West Wing
Albany, NY 12234
Phone: (518) 474-3817 ext. 280
Fax: (518) 474-3398
Website: *http://www.op.nysed.gov/
    nursecontact.htm*

North Carolina

North Carolina Board of Nursing
3724 National Drive, Suite 201
Raleigh, NC 27612
Phone: (919) 782-3211
Fax: (919) 781-9461
Website: *www.ncbon.org*

North Dakota

North Dakota Board of Nursing
919 South 7th Street, Suite 504
Bismarck, ND 58504
Phone: (701) 328-9777
Fax: (701) 328-9785
Website: *http://www.ndbon.org/*

Northern Mariana Islands

Commonwealth Board of Nurse
    Examiners
Public Health Center
PO Box 501454
Saipan, MP 96950
Phone: (670) 664-4812
Fax: (670) 664-4813

Ohio

Ohio Board of Nursing
17 South High Street, Suite 400
Columbus, OH 43215
Phone: (614) 466-3947
Fax: (614) 466-0388
Website: *http://www.nursing.ohio.gov*

Oklahoma

Oklahoma Board of Nursing
2915 North Classen Boulevard,
    Suite 524
Oklahoma City, OK 73106
Phone: (405) 962-1800
Fax: (405) 962-1821
Website: *http://www.youroklahoma.
    com/nursing/*

Oregon

Oregon State Board of Nursing
17938 SW Upper Boones Ferry Road
Portland, OR 97224
Phone: (971) 673-0685
Fax: (503) 673-0684
Website: *http://www.osbn.state.or.us/*

Pennsylvania

Pennsylvania State Board of
    Nursing
Penn Center
2601 North 3rd Street
Harrisburg, PA 17101
Phone: (717) 787-8503
Fax: (717) 783-0822
Website: *http://www.dos.
    state.pa.us/bpoa/cwp/view.
    asp?a=11048&q=432869*

Puerto Rico

Commonwealth of Puerto Rico
  Board of Nurse Examiners
800 Roberto H. Todd Avenue
Room 202, Stop 18
Santurce, PR 00908
Phone: (787) 725-7506
Fax: (787) 725-7903

Rhode Island

Rhode Island Board of Nurse
  Registration & Nursing
  Education
Three Capitol Hill
Providence, RI 02908
Phone: (401) 222-2231
Fax: (401) 222-6548
Website: *http://www.health.ri.gov/hsr/*
  professions/nurses.php

South Carolina

South Carolina State Board of
  Nursing
Synergy Business Park: Kingston
  Building
110 Centerview Drive, Suite 202
Columbia, SC 29210
Phone: (803) 896-4550
Fax: (803) 896-4525
Website: *http://www.llr.state.*
  sc.us/POL/nursing/

South Dakota

South Dakota Board of Nursing
4305 South Louise Avenue, Suite
  201
Sioux Falls, SD 57106-3115
Phone: (605) 362-2760
Fax: (605) 362-2768
Website: *http://www.state.*
  sd.us/dcr/nursing/

Tennessee

Tennessee Board of Nursing
425 Fifth Avenue North
1st Floor-Cordell Hull Building, 3rd
  Floor
Nashville, TN 37247
Phone: (615) 741-311
Fax: (615) 741-7899
Website: *http://health.state.*
  tn.us/Boards/Nursing/

Texas

Texas Board of Vocational Nurse
  Examiners
William P. Hobby Building, Tower 3
333 Guadeloupe Street, 3-460
Austin, TX 78701
Phone: (512) 305-7400
Fax: (512) 305-7401
Website: *http://www.bne.state.tx.us*

Utah

Utah State Board of Nursing
Heber M. Wells Building, 4th Floor
160 East 300 South
Salt Lake City, UT 84111
Phone: (801) 530-6628
Fax: (801) 530-6511
Website: *http://www.commerce.state.*
  ut.us/

Vermont

Office of Professional Regulation
National Life Office Building North
  Floor 2
Montpelier, VT 05620-3401
Phone: (802) 828-1505
Fax: (802) 828-2484
Website: *http://vtprofessionals.*
  org/opr1/nurses/

Virginia

Virginia Board of Nursing
Perimeter Center
9960 Maryland Drive, Suite 300
Richmond, VA 23233-1463
Phone: (804) 367-4400
Fax: (804) 527-4475
Website: *http://www.dhp.state.*
  va.us/nursing/

Virgin Islands

Virgin Islands Board of Nurse
  Licensure
Veterans Drive Station
St. Thomas, VI 00803
Phone: (340) 776-7397
Fax: (340) 777-4003

Washington

Washington State Nursing Care
  Quality Assurance Commission
Department of Health
HPQA #6
310 Israel RD SE
Tumwater, WA 98501
Phone: (360) 236-4700
Fax: (360) 236-4738
Website: *https://fortress.wa.gov/doh/*
  hpqa1/hps6/Nursing/default.htm

West Virginia

West Virginia State Board of
  Examiners for Licensed Practical
  Nurses
101 Dee Drive
Charleston, WV 25311
Phone: (304) 558-3572
Fax: (304) 558-4367
Website: *http://www.lpnboard.state.*
  wv.us/

Wisconsin

Wisconsin Department of
  Regulation & Licensing
Licensed Practical Nurse
1400 East Washington Avenue,
  Room 173
Madison, WI 53708
Phone: (608) 266-0145
Fax: (608) 261-7083
Website: *http://drl.wi.gov/prof/lpn/*
  def.htm

Wyoming

Wyoming State Board of Nursing
1810 Pioneer Avenue
Cheyenne, WY 82002
Phone: (307) 777-7601
Fax: (307) 777-3519
Website: *http://nursing.state.wy.us/*

NAPNES Standards of Practice and Educational Competencies of Graduates of Practical/Vocational Nursing Programs

These standards and competencies are intended to better define the range of capabilities, responsibilities, rights and relationship to other health care providers for scope and content of practical/vocational nursing education programs. The guidelines will assist:

- Educators in development, implementation, and evaluation of practical/vocational nursing curricula.
- Students in understanding expectations of their competencies upon completion of the educational program.
- Prospective employers in appropriate utilization of the practical/vocational nurse.
- Consumers in understanding the scope of practice and level of responsibility of the practical/vocational nurse.

A. PROFESSIONAL BEHAVIORS

Professional behaviors, within the scope of nursing practice for a practical/vocational nurse, are characterized by adherence to standards of care, accountability for one's own actions and behaviors, and use of legal and ethical principles in nursing practice. Professionalism includes a commitment to nursing and a concern for others demonstrated by an attitude of caring. Professionalism also involves participation in life-long self-development activities to enhance and maintain current knowledge and skills for continuing competency in the practice of nursing for the LP/VN, as well as individual, group, community, and societal endeavors to improve health care.

Upon completion of the practical/vocational nursing program the graduate will display the following program outcome:

Demonstrate professional behaviors of accountability and professionalism according to the legal and ethical standards for a competent licensed practical/vocational nurse.

Competencies which demonstrate this outcome has been attained:

1. Comply with the ethical, legal, and regulatory frameworks of nursing and the scope of practice as outlined in the LP/VN nurse practice act of the specific state in which licensed.
2. Utilize educational opportunities for life-long learning and maintenance of competence.
3. Identify personal capabilities and consider career mobility options.
4. Identify own LP/VN strengths and limitations for the purpose of improving nursing performance.
5. Demonstrate accountability for nursing care provided by self and/or directed to others.
6. Function as an advocate for the health care consumer, maintaining confidentiality as required.
7. Identify the impact of economic, political, social, cultural, spiritual, and demographic forces on the role of the licensed practical/vocational nurse in the delivery of health care.
8. Serve as a positive role model within health care settings and the community.
9. Participate as a member of a practical/vocational nursing organization.

B. COMMUNICATION

Communication is defined as the process by which information is exchanged between individuals verbally, non-verbally, and/or in writing or through information technology. Communication abilities are integral and essential to the nursing process. Those who are included in the nursing process are the licensed practical/vocational nurse and other members of the nursing and health care team, client, and significant support person(s). Effective communication demonstrates caring, compassion, and cultural awareness, and is directed toward promoting positive outcomes and establishing a trusting relationship.

Upon completion of the practical/vocational nursing program the graduate will display the following program outcome:

Effectively communicate with patients, significant support person(s), and members of the interdisciplinary health care team incorporating interpersonal and therapeutic communication skills.

Competencies which demonstrate this outcome has been attained:

1. Utilize effective communication skills when interacting with clients, significant others, and members of the interdisciplinary health team.
2. Communicate relevant, accurate, and complete information.
3. Report to appropriate health care personnel and document assessments, interventions, and progress or impediments toward achieving client outcomes.
4. Maintain organizational and client confidentiality.
5. Utilize information technology in support and communicate the planning and provision of client care.
6. Utilize appropriate channels of communication.

C. ASSESSMENT

Assessment is the collection and processing of relevant data for the purposes of appraising the client's health status. Assessment provides a holistic view of the client which includes physical, developmental, emotional, psychosocial, cultural, spiritual, and functional status. Assessment involves the collection of information from multiple sources to provide the foundation for nursing care. Initial assessment provides the baseline for future comparisons in order to individualize client care. Ongoing assessment is required to meet the client's changing needs.

Upon completion of the practical/vocational nursing program the graduate will display the following program outcome:

Collect holistic assessment data from multiple sources, communicate the data to appropriate health care providers, and evaluate client responses to interventions.

Competencies which demonstrate this outcome has been attained:

1. Assess data related to basic physical, developmental, spiritual, cultural, functional, and psychosocial needs of the client.
2. Collect data within established protocols and guidelines from various sources, including client interviews, observations/measurements, health care team members, family, significant other(s), and review of health records.
3. Assess data related to the client's health status, identify impediments to client progress, and evaluate response to interventions.

4. Document data collection, assessment, and communicate findings to appropriate member(s) of the health care team.

D. PLANNING

Planning encompasses the collection of health status information, the use of multiple methods to access information, and the analysis and integration of knowledge and information to formulate nursing care plans and care actions. The nursing care plan provides direction for individualized care, and assures the delivery of accurate, safe care through a definitive pathway that promotes the client's and support person(s)'s progress toward positive outcomes.

Upon completion of the practical/vocational nursing program the graduate will display the following program outcome:

Collaborate with the registered nurse or other members of the health care team to organize and incorporate assessment data to plan/revise patient care and actions based on established nursing diagnoses, nursing protocols, and assessment and evaluation data.

Competencies which demonstrate this outcome has been attained:

1. Utilize knowledge of normal values to identify deviation in health status to plan care.
2. Contribute to formulation of a nursing care plan for clients with non-complex conditions and in a stable state, in consultation with the registered nurse and as appropriate in collaboration with the client or support person(s) as well as members of the interdisciplinary health care team using established nursing diagnoses and nursing protocols.
3. Prioritize nursing care needs of clients.
4. Assist in the review and revision of nursing care plans with the registered nurse to meet the changing needs of clients.
5. Modify client care as indicated by the evaluation of stated outcomes.
6. Provide information to client about aspects of the care plan within the LP/VN scope of practice.
7. Refer client as appropriate to other members of the health care team about care outside the scope of practice of the LP/VN.

E. CARING INTERVENTIONS

Caring interventions are those nursing behaviors and actions that assist clients and significant others in meeting their needs and the identified outcomes of the plan of care. These interventions are based on knowledge of the natural sciences, behavioral sciences, and past nursing experiences. Caring is the "being with" and "doing for" that assists clients to achieve the desired outcomes. Caring behaviors are nurturing, protective, compassionate, and person-centered. Caring creates and environment of hope and trust where client choices related to cultural, religious, and spiritual values, beliefs, and lifestyles are respected.

Upon completion of the practical/vocational nursing program the graduate will display the following program outcome:

Demonstrate a caring and empathic approach to the safe, therapeutic, and individualized care of each client.

Competencies which demonstrate this outcome has been attained:

1. Provide and promote the client's dignity.
2. Identify and honor the emotional, cultural, religious, and spiritual influences on the client's behalf.
3. Demonstrate caring behaviors toward the client and significant support person(s).
4. Provide competent, safe, therapeutic, and individualized nursing care in a variety of settings.
5. Provide a safe physical and psychosocial environment for the client and significant other(s).
6. Implement the prescribed care regiment within the legal, ethical, and regulatory framework of practical/vocational nursing practice.
7. Assist the client and significant support person(s) to cope with and adapt to stressful events and changes in health status.
8. Assist the client and significant other(s) to achieve optimum comfort and functioning.
9. Instruct client regarding individualized health needs in keeping with the licensed practical/vocational nurse's knowledge, competence, and scope of practice.
10. Recognize client's right to access information and refer requests to appropriate person(s).
11. Act in an advocacy role to protect client rights.

F. MANAGING

Managing care is the effective use of human, physical, financial, and technological resources to achieve the client identified outcomes while supporting organizational outcomes. The LP/VN manages care through the processes of planning, organizing, and directing.

Upon completion of the practical/vocational nursing program, the graduate will display the following program outcome:

Implement patient care, at the direction of a registered nurse, licensed physician, or dentist through performance of nursing interventions or directing aspects of care, as appropriate, to unlicensed assistive personnel (UAP).

Competencies which demonstrate this outcome has been attained:

1. Assist in the coordination and implementation of an individualized plan of care for clients and significant support person(s).
2. Direct aspects of client care to qualified UAPs commensurate with abilities and level of preparation and consistent with the state's legal and regulatory framework for the scope of practice for the LP/VN.
3. Supervise and evaluate the activities of UAPs and other personnel as appropriate within the state's legal and regulatory framework for the scope of practice for the LP/VN as well as facility policy.
4. Maintain accountability for outcomes of care directed to qualified UAPs.
5. Organize nursing activities in a meaningful and cost-effective manner when providing nursing care for individuals or groups.
6. Assist the client and significant support person(s) to access available resources and services.
7. Demonstrate competence with current technologies.
8. Function within the defined scope of practice for the LP/VN in the health care delivery system at the direction of a registered nurse, licensed physician, or dentist.

As approved and adopted by NAPNES Board of Directors May 5, 2007.

NFLPN Nursing Practice Standards for the Licensed Practical/Vocational Nurse

"*Nursing Practice Standards*" is one of the ways that NFLPN meets the objective of its bylaws to address principles and ethics and also to meet another Article II objective, "To interpret the standards of practical (vocational) nursing."

In recent years, LPNs and LVNs have practiced in a changing environment. As LPNs and LVNs practice in expanding roles in the health care system, "*Nursing Practice Standards*" is essential reading for LPNs, LVNs, PN, and VN students and their educators, and all who practice with LPNs and LVNs.

NURSING PRACTICE STANDARDS FOR THE LICENSED PRACTICAL/VOCATIONAL NURSE

PREFACE

The Standards were developed and adopted by NFLPN to provide a basic model whereby the quality of health service and nursing service and nursing care given by LP/VNs may be measured and evaluated.

These nursing practice standards are applicable in any practice setting. The degree to which individual standards are applied will vary according to the individual needs of the patient, the type of health care agency or services, and the community resources.

The scope of licensed practical nursing has extended into specialized nursing services. Therefore specialized fields of nursing are included in this document.

THE CODE FOR LICENSED PRACTICAL/ VOCATIONAL NURSES

The Code, adopted by NFLPN in 1961 and revised in 1979, provides a motivation for establishing, maintaining, and elevating professional standards. Each LP/VN, upon entering the profession, inherits the responsibility to adhere to the standards of ethical practice and conduct as set forth in this Code.

1. Know the scope of maximum utilization of the LP/VN as specified by the nurse practice act and function within this scope.
2. Safeguard the confidential information acquired from any source about the patient.
3. Provide health care to all patients regardless of race, creed, cultural background, disease, or lifestyle.
4. Uphold the highest standards in personal appearance, language, dress, and demeanor.
5. Stay informed about issues affecting the practice of nursing and delivery of health care and, when appropriate, participate in government and policy decisions.
6. Accept the responsibility for safe nursing by keeping oneself mentally and physically fit and educationally prepared to practice.
7. Accept responsibility for membership in NFLPN and participate in its efforts to maintain the established standards of nursing practice and employment policies that lead to quality patient care.

INTRODUCTORY STATEMENT
Definition

Practical/Vocational nursing means the performance for compensation of authorized acts of nursing that utilize specialized knowledge and skills and that meet the health needs of people in a variety of settings under the direction of qualified health professionals.

Scope

Licensed Practical/Vocational nurses represent the established entry into the nursing profession and include specialized fields of nursing practice.

Opportunities exist for practicing in a milieu where different professions unite their particular skills in a team effort: to preserve or improve an individual patient's functioning and to protect health and safety of patients.

Opportunities also exist for career advancement within the profession through academic education and for lateral expansion of knowledge and expertise through both academic/continuing education and certification.

STANDARDS
Education
The Licensed Practical/Vocational Nurse
1. Shall complete a formal education program in practical nursing approved by the appropriate nursing authority in a state.
2. Shall successfully pass the National Council Licensure Examination for Practical Nurses.
3. Shall participate in initial orientation within the employing institution.

Legal/Ethical Status
The Licensed Practical/Vocational Nurse
1. Shall hold a current license to practice nursing as an LP/VN in accordance with the law of the state wherein employed.
2. Shall know the scope of nursing practice authorized by the nurse practice act in the state wherein employed.
3. Shall have a personal commitment to fulfill the legal responsibilities inherent in good nursing practice.
4. Shall take responsible actions in situations wherein there is unprofessional conduct by a peer or other health care provider.
5. Shall recognize and have a commitment to meet the ethical and moral obligations of the practice of nursing.
6. Shall not accept or perform professional responsibilities that the individual knows he or she is not competent to perform.

Practice
The Licensed Practical/Vocational Nurse
1. Shall accept assigned responsibilities as an accountable member of the health care team.
2. Shall function within the limits of educational preparation and experience as related to the assigned duties.
3. Shall function with other members of the health care team in promoting and maintaining health, preventing disease and disability, caring for and rehabilitating individuals who are experiencing an altered health state, and

contributing to the ultimate quality of life until death.
4. Shall know and utilize the nursing process in planning, implementing, and evaluating health services and nursing care for the individual patient or group.
   a. Planning: The planning of nursing includes:
      (1) Assessment/data collection of health status of the individual patient, the family, and community groups
      (2) Reporting information gained from assessment/data collection
      (3) The identification of health goals.
   b. Implementation: The plan for nursing care is put into practice to achieve the stated goals and includes:
      (1) Observing, recording, and reporting significant changes that require intervention or different goals
      (2) Applying nursing knowledge and skills to promote and maintain health, to prevent disease and disability and to optimize functional capabilities of an individual patient
      (3) Assisting the patient and family with activities of daily living and encouraging self-care as appropriate
      (4) Carrying out therapeutic regimens and protocols prescribed by personnel pursuant to authorized state law
   c. Evaluations: The plan for nursing care and its implementations are evaluated to measure the progress toward the stated goals and will include appropriate person and/or groups to determine:
      (1) The relevancy of current goals in relation to the progress of the individual patient
      (2) The involvement of the recipients of care in the evaluation process
      (3) The quality of the nursing action in the implementation of the plan
      (4) A re-ordering of priorities or new goal setting in the care plan
5. Shall participate in peer review and other evaluation processes.
6. Shall participate in the development of policies concerning the health and nursing needs of society and in the roles and functions of the LP/VN.

Continuing Education

The Licensed Practical/Vocational Nurse

1. Shall be responsible for maintaining the highest possible level of professional competence at all times.
2. Shall periodically reassess career goals and select continuing education activities that will help achieve these goals.
3. Shall take advantage of continuing education and certification opportunities that will lead to personal growth and professional development.
4. Shall seek and participate in continued education activities that are approved for credit by appropriate organizations, such as the NFLPN.

Specialized Nursing Practice

The Licensed Practical/Vocational Nurse

1. Shall have had at least 1 year's experience in nursing at the staff level.
2. Shall present personal qualifications that are indicative of potential abilities for practice in the chosen specialized nursing area.
3. Shall present evidence of completion of a program or course that is approved by an appropriate agency to provide the knowledge and skills necessary for effective nursing services in the specialized field.
4. Shall meet all of the standards of practice as set forth in this document.

GLOSSARY

Authorized (acts of nursing)
Those nursing activities made legal through state nurse practice acts.

Lateral Expansion of Knowledge
An extension of the basic core of information learned in the school of practical nursing.

Peer Review
A formal evaluation of performance on the job by other LP/VNs.

Special Nursing Practice
A restricted field of nursing in which a person is particularly skilled and has specific knowledge.

Therapeutic Regimens
Regulated plans designed to bring about effective treatment of disease.

Career Advancement
A change of career goal.

LP/VN
A combined abbreviation for Licensed Practical Nurse and Licensed Vocational Nurse. The LVN is the title used in California and Texas for the nurses who are called LPNs in other states.

Milieu
One's environment and surroundings.

Protocols
Courses of treatment that include specific steps to be performed in a stated order.

D Learning Exercises for Time Management

evolve http://evolve.elsevier.com/Hill/success/

Learning Exercise

Time Management: Sample Personal Roles and Activities

Following is an example of one person's listing of personal roles and activities. Using the blank page provided, list your personal roles and activities for each category. (Explanations for notations appear below, marked with an asterisk.)

School	Job	Family
*A Be at school 40 hours per week. A Be prepared to teach three courses each week (total of 25 hours in class and clinical)	A School is my job.	A Principal organizer for family of three. Ⓐ Spend time with son. Ⓐ Prepare dinner 7 evenings per week. Ⓑ Prepare one special breakfast on weekend. Ⓐ Do one load of laundry per day. Ⓐ Shop for groceries several times a week. Ⓑ Major housecleaning once a year. Ⓐ Perform errands as necessary. Ⓑ Attend PTA meeting. Ⓐ Attend Boy Scout activities.

Community

Ⓐ Lector at church.
Ⓑ Member of library board.
*Ⓑ Volunteer for Literacy Council.

Recreation

A Write a book.
A Attend concerts 5 times per year.
A Attend community theater 5 times per year.
B Attend movies and watch television periodically.
    Night out with husband.
A "Special" activities with son.
Ⓑ Selected activities that come up in community during year.

*A = priority items (These items have to be done.).
*B = nonpriority items (These items do not have to be done.).
Circled items = delegated items.

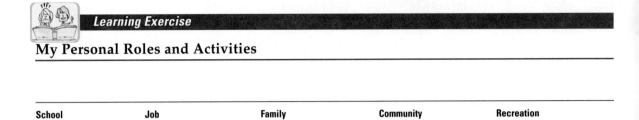

My Personal Roles and Activities

School	Job	Family	Community	Recreation

Use of Personal Time

To record personal time most accurately, be sure to pick a school day that includes usual activities. A blank page has been provided on page 464, so that you can record your activities in chronological order. When you add up the minutes spent in each activity, they should total 1440, the number found in each 24-hour day. A sample day's activity log follows. This example does not reflect how you actually spend your time. It merely reflects one person's use of time in a 24-hour period. You will see as many different one-day logs as there are students in your personal issues class.

Sample Personal Time and Activity Log for Monday

Time Span	Activity	Total Time
5:45–6:00 AM	Shampoo and blow-dry hair	15 minutes
6:00–6:30 AM	Eat breakfast and make "to do" list	30 minutes
6:30–6:45 AM	Dress	15 minutes
6:45–7:05 AM	Drive to school	20 minutes
7:05–7:30 AM	Prepare for first class	25 minutes
7:30–9:00 AM	Class	90 minutes
9:00–9:20 AM	Break	20 minutes
9:20–10:20 AM	Class	60 minutes
10:20–10:30 AM	Break	10 minutes
10:30–11:20 AM	Class	50 minutes
11:20–12:30 PM	Lunch	70 minutes
12:30–1:20 PM	Class	50 minutes
1:20–1:30 PM	Break	10 minutes
1:30–2:20 PM	Class	50 minutes
2:20–2:30 PM	Break	10 minutes
2:30–3:30 PM	Study	60 minutes
3:30–3:50 PM	Drive home	20 minutes
3:50–4:30 PM	Start laundry, dinner, "pick up" house	40 minutes
4:30–5:45 PM	Talk to son, study	75 minutes
5:45–6:15 PM	Dinner	30 minutes
6:15–8:00 PM	Read, prep	105 minutes
8:00–8:30 PM	Shower, set out clothes for tomorrow	30 minutes
8:30–9:45 PM	Read	75 minutes
9:45–5:45 PM	Sleep	480 minutes
		1440 minutes

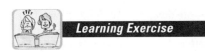
Learning Exercise

Personal Time and Activity Log for _____

(Day/Date)

Time Span	Activity	Total Time

Learning Exercise

Setting Personal Priorities

Review all the activities you have listed on p. 467 of this appendix under the five categories of roles you play in everyday life, and rank them according to the following directions:

1. Place an "A" beside the activities you have to do without question. Remember, "A" activities are those you have to do, not necessarily want to do. These are your priority activities. For example, you might not want to get up on rainy mornings and go to school, but you have to if you want to graduate.

2. Place a "B" beside those activities that do not have to be done. These are nonpriority items as far as your long-term goal and your well-being are concerned. You might want to do these activities, but you do not have to do them.

Many of you came to the practical/vocational nursing program while filling a variety of roles in your family and community. As much as you hate the idea, you will not be able to do everything you did before starting school. Are all the "A" activities really "A" activities? Can some

of them be moved to the "B" category while you are in school? This is like moving them to the back burner for now. Take a few minutes and review the "A" and "B" status of the roles you have listed. The sample roles and activity list on p. 466 has examples of setting priorities with activities.

Delegating Activities

Review your list of personal activities on p. 467, with the goal of determining whether the activity can be delegated to someone else while you are a student, and make the following notations:

1. Read over all your "A" activities (your "have to" activities).

2. Circle the activities that can realistically be delegated while you go to school.

Are the "B" activities still on your mind? Can any of these be delegated while you go to school? If so, circle them also. The "Sample Personal Roles and Activities" on p. 466. also has examples of activities that were chosen to be delegated. The only thing left to do is to contact the appropriate person to ask about delegating or assigning an activity.

Time Management: Weekly Schedule

Time	Sun	Mon	Tue	Wed	Thur	Fri	Sat
6–7 AM							
7–8 AM							
8–9 AM							
9–10 AM							
10–11 AM							
11 AM–noon							
Noon–1 PM							
1–2 PM							
2–3 PM							
3–4 PM							
4–5 PM							
5–6 PM							
6–7 PM							
7–8 PM							
8–9 PM							
9–10 PM							
10–11 PM							

Internet Resources

LEARN ABOUT THE INTERNET AND SEARCH TOOLS

www.learnthenet.com: Internet site for beginners, online etiquette, and more. In English, Spanish, and French.

www.google.com: Search plain and simple; no advertisements on search pages.

www.ask.com: Type in a question to be answered.

www.altavista.com: Search in 36 languages, including Spanish.

www.metacrawler.com: Searches several search engines at once.

www.webcrawler.com: Searches several search engines at once.

www.dogpile.com: Searches several search engines at once.

NURSING SITES

www.NewsForNurses.com: Site gathers "the best" from websites of interest to nurses.

www.advanceforlpns.com: Bi-weekly, up-to-the-minute clinical information and news. Sign up also for delivery to your email account.

www.nflpn.org: Home page for National Federation of Licensed Practical Nurses.

www.napnes.org: Home page for the National Association for Practical Nurse Education and Service.

www.nursingworld.org: The American Nurses Association; features current nursing news, articles.

www.nln.org: The National League for Nursing website.

www.minoritynurse.com: Provides articles and resources and information about education, career development, jobs, and minority health for minority nurses in the United States.

www.Nurse.com: Current news of interest to nurses, CEUs, jobs, plus.

www.nursingnet.org: forums, jobs, links, plus.

NURSING ORGANIZATIONS

www.ncsbn.org: National Council of State Boards of Nursing website; type NCLEX in quick links for NCLEX information.

www.nflpn.org: National Federation of Licensed Practical Nurses.

www.napnes.org: National Association for Practical Nurse Education and Service.

http://aamn.org: Purpose and objectives for The American Assembly for Men in Nursing. Provides a framework for discussion and factors that affect men in nursing.

http://www.nursingworld.org: *Nursing Insider* with the latest news for nurses.

LOCATING SPECIFIC INFORMATION FOR SPN/SVNS

GENERAL STUDY HINTS AND HELPS

www.nurseweek.com/calculators/: Calculators for oral liquid medications, pediatric doses using BSA (body surface area), and lots more.

www.learningext.com: The Learning Extension site of the National Council of State Boards of Nursing (NCSBN). Includes online courses for nurses, study hints for students, and an online review course for the NCLEX-PN® examination (fee involved).

www.bucks.edu/%7especpop/weekly-sch.htm: Blank for weekly schedule.

Note: Some websites listed in this section were used by the authors in the development of the chapters, but may have had specific periods in which they were active. Therefore some of them may not open.

www.cinahl.com: Cumulative index database. Does your school's learning resource center have an institutional membership?

http://www.ipl.org: Internet public library, including dictionaries, encyclopedias. A complete library.

http://nurseshift.com: Study tips. Study items for sale.

www.medscape.com/druginfo: This website contains drug information.

www.AlfaroTeachSmart.com: Critical thinking.

www.yoursurgery.com: Provides a description of common operations, anatomy of operative area, pathology, diagnostic methods, and postoperative care. Fee involved.

http://www.medi-smart.com/student.htm: Many study tips for your courses.

DIFFERENT CULTURES/RELIGIONS

www.adherents.com: Information about religions.

www.beliefnet.com: Spirituality and religion.

www.infoplease.com/ce6/society/A0851259.html: Wahhabi information.

www.culturediversity.org: Cultural concepts and case studies.

www.feng-shui-institute.org/yinyang.htm: Yin yang.

http://ethnomed.org/ethnomed/clin_topics/cambodian/ethno_wind.html#traditional: Information about cupping, coining, and pinching.

http://skepdic.com/evileye.html: Information about "evil eye."

www.tsha.utexas.edu/handbook/online/articles/CC/sdc1.html: Information about curanderos.

www.xculture.org: The Cross Cultural Health Care Program—cultural issues that affect the health of minorities.

www.minoritynurse.com: Provides articles and resources and information about education, career development, jobs, and minority health for minority nurses in the United States.

www.languageline.com: Subscribe to free monthly health newsletter regarding medical interpreters and communication in health care.

GOVERNMENT SITES

www.ahcpr.gov: Home page of the Agency for Health Care Policy and Research. Provides evidence-based information on health care outcomes, quality, and cost.

www.cdc.gov: Home page of Centers for Disease Control and Prevention.

www.fda.gov: U.S. Food and Drug Administration. Includes news, recalls, safety alerts, information for patients, health professionals, and more.

http://thomas.loc.gov: Source for legislative information for the U.S. House and Senate.

www.medicare.gov: Official U.S. government site for up-to-date Medicare information.

www.nih.gov: Home page for the National Institutes of Health.

www.census.gov/main: Data about the U.S. and economy.

www.MyPyramid.gov: The Center for Nutrition Policy and Promotion.

www.nlm.nih.gov: National Library of Medicine for the National Institutes of Health.

http://hospitalcompare.hhs.gov: Hospitals quality of care for heart attack and failure, pneumonia and surgery created by CMS and Hospital Quality Alliance.

www.qualitycheck.org: TJC hospital performance of 15,000 accredited health care organizations by city, name, or zip code.

www.usa.gov/Contact/Elected.shtml: Contact federal and state officials.

MISCELLANEOUS

www.rnweb.com: Access to select, current articles in *RN* magazine and CEUs.

www.exceptionalnurse.com: Website for nursing students and licensed nurses with disabilities. Includes Bablefish, a tool that translates site to other languages.

www.medscape.com: Provides a link to Medline, where you can search for nursing articles and read abstracts of selected articles; free CE, link to drug information, and more.

www.kaisernetwork.org: The latest news on health policy issues and sign-up for free email info.

www.malenursemagazine.com: YouTube videos about men in nursing.

http://www.guardian.co.uk/life/feature/story/0,13026,937913,00.html: Male and female brain.

www.nasw.org/users/skloot/ChangeStory.pdf: The brain and change.

http://www.jointcommission.org: The Joint Commission (TJC).

http://www.jointcommission.org/PatientSafety/Nationa lPatientSafetyGoals: TNC National Patient Safety Goals.

http://depts.washington.edu/bioethx/topics/pas.html: Ethics in Medicine.

http://www.Oregon.gov/DHS/ph/pas/faqs.shml: Oregon's Death with Dignity Act.

www.voicefortheuninsured.org: The American Medical Association's (AMA) proposal for covering the uninsured.

PERSONAL HEALTH

www.learningmeditation.com: Learn how to relax. Click on the text that interests you.

www.CBS.HealthWatch.com: Personal health management for men and women. Link to WebMD.

www.factsontap.org: Facts on tap: alcohol and drugs and your college experience.

www.DrWeil.com: Health advice from an MD who specializes in integrative medicine.

www.eatingwell.com: Good taste and good health, recipe, plus.

http://www.nlm.nih.gov/medlineplus/exercisean dphysicalfitness.html: Health topics, drugs, medical dictionary, medical encyclopedia, organizations for health info, Medline/PubMed, plus.

http://www.4women.gov/faq/exercise.htm: Physical activity info by DHHS.

www.healthywomen.com: Health, fitness, and more.

RESOURCES FOR PATIENTS

www.alz.org: Home page of the Alzheimer's Association.

www.arthritis.org: Home page of the Arthritis Foundation.

www.cancer.org: Home page of the American Cancer Society.

http://americanheart.org: Home page of the American Heart Association.

www.partnershipforcaring.org: Deals with end-of-life issues and provides state-specific living wills and advance directives.

www.efa.org: Home page of the Epilepsy Foundation of America.

www.lungusa.org: Home page of the American Lung Association.

www.ncadd.org: Home page of the National Council on Alcoholism and Drug Dependence.

www.nccam.nih.gov: Complementary and alternative medicine.

www.mayohealth.org: Drug information, healthy lifestyle, disease conditions, and much more.

www.aarp.org: Home page of the American Association of Retired Persons.

F The Howlett Style of Nursing Leadership

evolve http://evolve.elsevier.com/Hill/success/

The idea for this management style was found in the books *One Minute Manager* (Blanchard and Johnson, 1983) and *Putting the One Minute Manager to Work* (Blanchard and Lorber, 1998) and was originally written as *The Howlett Theory of Management for Nursing Instructors.**

1. Never assume employees know what is expected of them. Employees are informed of what is expected of them in their job descriptions. They are held accountable for these expectations. Expected performance needs to be stated objectively. This will make employees aware of the appropriate behavior to reach the institution's goals.

2. Reward employees for their "good" behavior (doing what is expected or going beyond the call of duty). This will encourage them to repeat good behavior. But do not ignore bad performance; to do so will have a negative effect. Most employees know what it is like to be caught doing something "bad." Surprise the heck out of them and catch them doing something good. Let them know how you feel about the "good" behavior. Praise them in someway (e.g., put their name on bulletin board,with a note indicating you caught them doing something "good," and list the behavior).

3. Employees, being human beings, will sometimes make mistakes; for example, they may not follow rules/policies. When these situations arise, determine whether it involves something the employee *cannot* or something he or she *will not* do. If the employee *cannot* do something, it is a training problem. Skill development is the suggested way of handling the situation. If the employee *will not* do something, it is an attitude problem. A reprimand may be in order, according to the policies of your institution (see No. 6).

4. Employees who feel good about themselves will produce good results. Let your employees know they are the best group in the world to work with because … (identify reason here). Wear an apron that says you work with the best staff in the world.

5. Written and oral feedback about behavior and its consequences, whether positive or negative, must be objective. Unemotionally, indicate what they did. Relate feedback as closely as possible to the event. Do not save feedback until clinical performance evaluation time. Point out the consequences of positive and negative behavior. For positive behavior, give praise in measurable terms, so the behavior can be repeated. Blanchard and Johnson suggest reprimanding negative behavior in such a way that the person will think about the *reprimand* after the episode and *not* the manner in which it was delivered. Offer praise at the end of a reprimand so that the reprimand is heard more clearly and does not ruin the impact of the praising. Focus reprimands on behaviors, not on the individual.

6. Sometimes employees do not respond to support or assistance and need to be disciplined or terminated. Refer to the policies of your institution.

The Howlett Style of Nursing Leadership has been used with practical/vocational nursing students. Its use has resulted in positive clinical evaluation experiences.

G REFERENCES

Blanchard K, Johnson S: *One Minute Manager*. New York: Penguin Putnam, 1983.

Blanchard K, Lorber R: *Putting the One Minute Manager to Work*. New York: Penguin Putnam, 1998.

---

*Amended 2008.

Delegation: Concepts and Decision-Making Process (NCSBN)

To meet the public's increasing need for accessible, affordable, quality health care, providers of health care must maximize the use of every health care worker and ensure appropriate delegation of responsibilities and tasks. Nurses, who are uniquely qualified for promoting the health of the whole person, by virtue of their education and experience, must be actively involved in making health care policies and decisions; they must coordinate and supervise the delivery of nursing care, including the delegation of nursing tasks to others.

Issues related to delegation have become more complex in today's evolving health care environment, creating a need for practical guidelines to direct the process for making delegatory decisions. Accordingly, this paper expands and builds on the National Council of State Boards of Nursing's (NCSBN's) 1987 and 1990 conceptual and historical papers on delegation, by presenting a dynamic decision-making process and practical guidelines for delegation (Hanstem and Washburn, 1992).

PURPOSE

The purpose of this paper is to provide a resource for boards of nursing, health policy makers, and health care providers on delegation and the roles of licensed and unlicensed health care workers. The paper emphasizes and clarifies the responsibility of boards of nursing for the regulation of nursing, including nursing tasks performed by unlicensed health care workers, and the responsibility of licensed nurses to delegate nursing tasks in accord with their legal scopes of practice. It provides a decision-making tool that can be used in clinical and administrative settings to guide the process of delegation. This paper also describes the accountability of each person involved in the delegation process and potential liability if competent, safe care is not provided.

PREMISES

The following premises constitute the basis for the delegation decision-making process.

1. All decisions related to delegation of nursing tasks must be based on the fundamental principle of protection of the health, safety, and welfare of the public.
2. Boards of nursing are responsible for the regulation of nursing. Provision of any care that constitutes nursing or any activity represented as nursing is a regulatory responsibility of boards of nursing.
3. Boards of nursing should articulate clear principles for delegation, augmented by clearly defined guidelines for delegation decisions.
4. A licensed nurse must have ultimate responsibility and accountability for the management and provision of nursing care.
5. A licensed nurse must be actively involved in and be accountable for all managerial decisions, policy making, and practices related to the delegation of nursing care.
6. There is a need and a place for competent, appropriately supervised unlicensed assistive personnel (UAP) in the delivery of affordable quality health care. However, it must be remembered that UAPs are equipped to assist—not replace—the nurse.
7. Nursing is a knowledge-based process discipline and cannot be reduced solely to a list of tasks. The licensed nurse's specialized education, professional judgment, and discretion are essential for quality nursing care.
8. Although nursing tasks may be delegated, the licensed nurse's generalist knowledge of patient care indicates that the practice-pervasive functions of assessment, evaluation, and nursing judgment must not be delegated.
9. A task delegated to an unlicensed assistive person cannot be redelegated by the unlicensed assistive person.

10. Consumers have a right to health care that meets legal standards of care. Thus when a nursing task is delegated, the task must be performed in accord with established standards of practice, policies, and procedures.

11. The licensed nurse determines and is accountable for the appropriateness of delegated nursing tasks. Inappropriate delegation by the nurse and/or unauthorized performance of nursing tasks by UAP may lead to legal action against the licensed nurse and/or UAP.

DEFINITIONS

Accountability: Being responsible and answerable for actions or inactions of self or others in the context of delegation.

Delegation: Transferring to a competent individual the authority to perform a selected nursing task in a selected situation. The nurse retains accountability for the delegation.

Delegator: The person making the delegation.

Delegate: The person receiving the delegation (known as delegate).

Supervision: The provision of guidance or direction, evaluation, and follow-up by the licensed nurse for accomplishment of a nursing task delegated to unlicensed assistive personnel.

Unlicensed assistive personnel (UAP): Any unlicensed personnel, regardless of title, to whom nursing tasks are delegated.

REGULATORY PERSPECTIVE: FRAMEWORK FOR MANAGERIAL POLICIES

Boards of nursing have the legal responsibility to regulate nursing and provide guidance regarding delegation. Registered nurses (RNs) may delegate certain nursing tasks to licensed practical nurses/vocational nurses (LPN/LVNs) and UAPs. In some jurisdictions LPN/LVNs may also delegate certain tasks within their scope of practice to UAPs. The licensed nurse has a responsibility to assure that the delegated task is performed in accord with established standards of practice, policies, and procedures. The nurse who delegates retains accountability for the task delegated.

The regulatory system serves as a framework for managerial policies related to the employment and utilization of licensed nurses and UAPs. The nurse who assesses the patient's needs and plans nursing care should determine the tasks to be delegated, and is accountable for that delegation. It is inappropriate for employers or others to require nurses to delegate when, in the nurse's professional judgment, delegation is unsafe and not in the patient's best interest. In those instances the nurse should act as the patient's advocate and take appropriate action to ensure provision of safe nursing care. If the nurse determines that delegation may not appropriately take place, but delegates as directed, the nurse may be disciplined by the board of nursing.

ACCEPTABLE USE OF THE AUTHORITY TO DELEGATE

The delegating nurse is responsible for an individualized assessment of the patient and situational circumstances, and for ascertaining the competence of the delegate before delegating any task. The practice-pervasive functions of assessment, evaluation, and nursing judgment must not be delegated. Supervision, monitoring, evaluation, and follow-up by the nurse are crucial components of delegation. The delegate is accountable for accepting the delegation and for his/her own actions in carrying out the task.

The decision to delegate should be consistent with the nursing process (appropriate assessment, planning, implementation, and evaluation). This necessarily precludes a list of nursing tasks that can be routinely and uniformly delegated for all patients in all situations. Rather, the nursing process and decision to delegate must be based on careful analysis of the patient's needs and circumstances. Also critical to delegation decisions are the qualifications of the proposed delegate, the nature of the nurse's delegation authority (set forth in the law of the jurisdiction), and the nurse's personal competence in the area of nursing relevant to the task to be delegated.

DELEGATION DECISION-MAKING PROCESS

In delegating, the nurse must ensure appropriate assessment, planning, implementation, and evaluation. The delegation decision-making process, which is continuous, is described in the following model:

I. Delegation criteria
A. Nurse Practice Act
1. Permits delegation
2. Authorizes task(s) to be delegated or authorizes the nurse to decide delegation
B. Delegator qualifications
1. Within scope of authority to delegate
2. Appropriate education, skills, and experience
3. Documented/demonstrated evidence of current competency
C. Delegate qualifications
1. Appropriate education, training, skills, and experience
2. Documented/demonstrated evidence of current competency

Provided that this foundation is in place, the licensed nurse may enter continuous process of delegation decision-making.

II. Assess the situation
A. Identify the needs of the patient, consulting the plan of care
B. Consider the circumstances/setting
C. Assure the availability of adequate resources, including supervision

If patient needs, circumstances, and available resources (including supervisor and delegate) indicate that patient safety will be maintained with delegated care, proceed to III.

III. Plan for specific task(s) to be delegated
A. Specify the nature of each task and the knowledge and skills required to perform it
B. Require documentation or demonstration of current competence by the delegate for each task
C. Determine the implications for the patient, other patients, and significant others

If the nature of the task, competence of the delegate, and patient implications indicate patient safety will be maintained with delegated care, proceed to IV.

IV. Assure appropriate accountability
A. As delegator, accept accountability for performance of the task(s)
B. Verify that delegate accepts the delegation and the accountability for carrying out the task correctly

If delegator and delegate accept the accountability for their respective roles in the delegated patient care, proceed to V.

V. Supervise performance of the task
A. Provide directions and clear expectations of how the task(s) is to be performed
B. Monitor performance of the task(s), to assure compliance to established standards of practice, policies, and procedures
C. Intervene, if necessary
D. Ensure appropriate documentation of the task(s)

VI. Evaluate the entire delegation process
A. Evaluate the patient
B. Evaluate the performance of the task(s)
C. Obtain and provide feedback

The Five Rights of Delegation provide an additional resource to facilitate decisions about delegation.

THE FIVE RIGHTS OF DELEGATION

- **Right task:** One that is delegable for a specific patient.
- **Right circumstances:** Appropriate patient setting, available resources, and other relevant factors considered.
- **Right person:** Right person is delegating the right task to the right person, to be performed on the right person.
- **Right direction/communication:** Clear, concise description of the task, including its objective, limits and expectations.
- **Right supervision:** Appropriate monitoring, evaluation, intervention, as needed, and feedback.

CONCLUSION

The guidelines presented here provide a decision-making process that facilitates the provision of quality care by appropriate persons in all health care settings. NCSBN believes that this paper will assist all health care providers and health care facilities in discharging their shared responsibility to provide optimum health care that protects the public's health, safety, and welfare.

REFERENCES
Hansten R, Washburn M. (1992) Delegation: how to deliver care through others. *Am J Nurs*, 92(8):87, 88, 90.

National Council Position Paper, 1995.

A

Abandonment Leave patient unit without a nurse of equal skill and education assigned to provide care for your assigned patient.

ABMCN Certification in managed care (CMCN). Offered by the American Board Managed Care Nursing. Certification valid for 3 years.

Accountability Obligation to answer for personal actions.

Acculturation Adopting the culture of a different group.

Active learning Taking charge of own education.

Active listener Listeners who are open-minded and curious and are always asking themselves questions about content.

Active listening Hearing sounds and searching for information relevant to those sounds, so that the sounds may be understood.

Acute care Higher level of care required for seriously ill patients.

Adult ADD Adult form of attention deficit disorder (ADD). Includes undependable memory and learning system.

Adult care home Assistive and health care services, provided in the home.

Adult day care center A service that provides mental stimulation, socialization, assistance with some activities of daily living (ADLs), and basic observation. Services often include transportation, meals, therapeutic activities, nursing interventions, and rehabilitation activities. The service is hospital based or freestanding.

Advance directives Written documents to state personal wishes regarding future health care.

Advanced practice Post-registered nurse (RN) degree, resulting in an expanded role (e.g., clinical nurse specialist, nurse practitioner, certified nurse midwife, nurse anesthetist).

Affective communication Sending or receiving information through feeling tone.

Aggressive An attacking type of behavior that occurs in response to frustration and hostile feelings.

Agnostic A person who holds the belief that existence of God can neither be proved nor disproved.

Allah Muslim name of the one supreme; God of Islam.

Alliances New partnerships among hospitals, clinics, laboratories, health care systems, and physicians. They coordinate the delivery of care, contain costs, and attempt to provide a seamless system.

Almshouses Homes for the poor and sick in the seventeenth and eighteenth centuries.

Ambulatory care facilities Primary health care services for walk-in patients. Also known as Urgent Care, Express Care, and Quick Care.

Ambulatory surgery centers One-day surgery centers that perform surgery at a scheduled date and time. Patient discharged home when recovered from surgery and is stable.

Analysis Break down complex information into its basic parts and relate it to the whole picture.

Anger management A way to deal with unjustified or inappropriately displayed anger.

Application Use learned information in new situations.

Artful vagueness Responding without implying either party is wrong. For example, saying, "You've got a point," or, "You may be right."

Assault An unjustified attempt or threat to touch someone.

Assertiveness A way of accepting responsibility for oneself by expressing thoughts and feelings directly and honestly, without blaming oneself or others.

Assigning (assignment) Allotting tasks that are in the job description of workers. Assigned tasks are those that these workers are hired and paid to perform.

Source: Chabner D.E. (2004). The language of medicine (7th ed.). Philadelphia: Saunders.

Pronunciation of Terms
The markings ˉ and ˘ above the vowels (a, e, i, o, and u) indicate the proper sounds of the vowels.
When ˉ is above a vowel, its sound is long, that is, exactly like its name; for example:

ā as in āpe; ī as in īce; ū as in ūnit; ē as in ēven; ō as in ōpen

The ˘ marking indicates a short vowel sound, as in the following examples:

ă as in ăpple; ĭ as in ĭnterest; ŭ as in ŭnder; ĕ as in ĕvery; ŏ as in pŏt

Assimilation Giving up parts of your own culture and adopting parts of the culture of the dominant group.

Assisted care Residences that provide "a home with services."

Associate degree nursing A 2-year community college or technical school program. The title RN is used after passing NCLEX-RN®.

Atheist A person who does not believe the supernatural exists and therefore does not believe in God.

Attitude Nonverbal expression of the way a person thinks or feels.

Audiovisual (AV) materials Films, videotapes, or CD-ROMs.

Auditory learner Talks to himself or herself or hears sounds when thinking. Learns best by hearing.

Authorization to test (ATT) Denotes that the graduate practical/vocational nurse has met the requirements for eligibility to take the NCLEX-PN® examination. ATT applied for and obtained from the testing center.

Authorized consent Parents cannot give informed consent for medical care of a child, but can give authorized consent instead.

Automatic responses Both passive and aggressive responses result from being caught by an emotional hook. These responses are not based on choice.

Autonomy Control over personal decisions.

Ayatollah A high-ranking religious and political leader in Islam.

B

Baccalaureate nursing program A 4-year college or university program.

Barton, Clara Founder of the American Red Cross.

Basic nursing skill Nursing procedure learned by the practical/vocational nursing student and suitable for providing nursing care to a patient whose clinical condition is predictable.

Basic patient situation Patient's clinical condition is predictable. Medical and nursing orders are not changing continuously. No complex modifications needed.

Battery Causing acute physical harm to someone.

Belittling Mimicking or making fun of person in some way.

Beneficence Doing good.

Beneficent paternalism Health care provider making decisions for the patient based on, "I know what's best for you." Discounts patient autonomy.

Biomedicine Belief that abnormalities in structure and function of body organs are caused by pathogens, biochemical alterations, and/or environmental factors.

Board and care homes Offer housing and custodial care. Also known as adult care homes or group homes.

"Boards" NCLEX-PN® examination.

Bodily/kinesthetic learner Learns best by touching, moving, and processing knowledge through bodily sensations.

Border recognition agreement Agreement among select states to permit licensed nurses to practice within their states, without additional criteria.

Breach of duty One of the elements needed to prove negligence. Means that the nurse did not adhere to standards of care.

Bridge program Associate-degree nursing program that admits LPN/LVNs to their course of study after they fulfill certain requirements.

Bucket theory Suggests that merely by lecturing, the teacher can transfer knowledge from the teacher's mind to the student's mind.

Buddha The enlightened one; Siddhartha Gautama, founder of Buddhism.

Burnout Negative attitude and behavioral change about one's career, working with patients, and self-care.

C

Call number Series of letters and numbers used to identify library materials and assist in locating materials.

Candidate Graduate practical/vocational nurse who will take (or is taking) the NCLEX-PN® examination.

Capability Ability or capacity.

Capitation Set fee for health care, paid annually regardless of the number of health services provided.

Career ladder programs Nursing programs planned to avoid duplication of content. The student may progress from a position as a nursing assistant to a practical/vocational nurse to an associate degree nurse to a baccalaureate nurse in approximately 4 years.

Case management method A method of patient care that uses care pathways or critical paths with an interdisciplinary staff. Focus is on quality, service, and cost.

Case method A method of patient care in which one nurse is assigned to give total care to one patient.

Case scenarios A printed or computer patient story that brings reality to theory in the form of a clinical situation.

CD-ROM Computer disk that contains information.

Centers for Medicare and Medical Services (CMS) Formerly Health Care Financing Administration (HICFA). Federal agency of Department of Health and Human Services. Certifies nursing homes for Medicare and Medicaid reimbursement.

Certification Certificate awarded to an RN or LPN/LVN after passing a comprehensive examination in a select area of practice.

Certification in Long-Term Care (CLTC) Postgraduate course offered by NAPNES. Replaces previous gerontology certification. Recertification is every 3 years.

Certification in Pharmacology (NCP) Postgraduate course offered by NAPNES. Recertification is every 3 years.

Change-of-shift report Report on patient condition at beginning and end of shift.

Chemical dependency Abuse of alcohol and/or other drugs.

Chiding Scolding.

Choice Act of choosing. For example, to speak assertively is to speak out of choice.

Christ Founder of Christian religion.

Civil action (related to individual rights) Involves the relationships between individuals and the violation of those rights.

Clerk receptionist Ward clerk. Assumes responsibility for many clerical duties in the patient care area.

Clinical pathway Blueprint for patient care. Includes time frame of significant events that are expected to occur each day a patient with a specific diagnosis is in the hospital.

Closed-ended questions Questions that require specific answers from a patient.

Codependency Situation in which a person allows another person's behavior to affect him or her and is obsessed with controlling that person's behavior.

Cognitive level Intellectual level of functioning.

Co-insurance Percentage of total bill paid for by insurance company once deductible is paid.

Commitment Pledge to do one's best.

Common law Judge-made law, which has its origins in the courts.

Communication blocks Stops meaningful conversation. Examples include chiding, belittling, probing, giving advice, and providing pat answers.

Community health nursing Nursing that focuses on improving the health status of communities or groups of people through public education, screening for early detection of disease, and providing services for people who need care outside the acute care setting.

Community health nursing services Nurses work with many people and groups on prevention and modification of health issues. Exist as part of clinic service, HMO, or is freestanding.

Community resources Include city library, museums, and health care facilities that offer programs and exhibits of interest to nurses.

Compensation Coping mechanism used to cover for real or imagined inadequacy by developing or exaggerating a desirable trait.

Complementary and alternative medicine (CAM) Focus is on assisting the body's own healing powers and restoring body balance.

Complex nursing situation Patient's clinical condition is not predictable. Medical and nursing orders are likely to involve continuous changes or complex modifications.

Comprehension Basically understand information, recall it, and identify examples of that information.

Computer-aided instruction An increasingly used teaching strategy in nursing education.

Computer simulation Learning activities on a CD ROM or floppy disc that makes use of an imaginary patient situation. The student uses the nursing process as he or she would in an actual clinical situation.

Computerized adaptive testing (CAT) Method by which NCLEX-PN® examination is administered to the candidate (nursing graduate who has fulfilled requirements for testing).

Conditional job offer Job offer contingent on passing physical, drug screening, and/or background check.

Confidentiality Not sharing patient information with anyone not directly involved in care without the patient's permission.

Conflict resolution A method of resolving differences in a peaceful way.

Constructive evaluation Critique directed toward performance and behavior; has no bearing on one's value as a person.

Continuous quality improvements (CQIs) Search for new ways to improve patient care, prevent errors, and identify and fix problems.

Continuum Continuous quality.

Cooperative learning Emphasis on individual accountability for learning a specific academic task while working in small groups.

Co-payment Percentage of the bill that is paid by a subscriber who is enrolled in a health insurance plan.

Copyright laws These laws permit a single copy of an article for personal use. Instructors may not make copies of articles, chapters, or books for distribution to each student.

Cost containment Holding costs within fixed limits.

Course outlines Up-to-date listings of what is covered in the course. Provided by the instructor.

Criminal action Involves persons and society as a whole; for example, murder.

Critical thinking Used to resolve problems and find ways to make improvements, even when no problem exists.

Cross training Health care workers are trained to provide specific skills outside their area of assignment/education, in an attempt to use workers more efficiently and reduce costs.

Cultural bias Unquestioned, unproved way of thinking.

Cultural competence The continuous attempt of practical/vocational nurses to gain the knowledge and skills that will allow them to effectively provide care for patients of different cultures.

Cultural differences Elements found in one culture may not be found in another.

Cultural diversity Differences in elements of culture in groups of people.

Cultural sensitivity Learning about other cultures and being respectful of their customs, rites, and beliefs.

Cultural uniqueness Differences such as family structure, food preferences, religious beliefs, concept of time, communication, education, economic status, wellness and illness beliefs, etc.

Cultural universality Similarities that all people share regardless of culture; for example, basic needs.

Culture The total of all the ideas, beliefs, values, attitudes, communication, customs, traditions, and objects that a group of people possess. Culture includes ways of doing things.

Customs Ways of doing things that are common to a group of people of the same culture.

D

Damages One of four elements needed to prove negligence. Means that patient must be able to show the nurse's negligent act injured the patient in some way.

Database Data gathered provides basis for developing and evaluating care plan.

Data collection Phase 1 of nursing process for practical/vocational nurses. Involves systematic gathering and review of information about the patient.

Decentralized The idea to locate centralized service departments, such as the x-ray department and the laboratory, on patient units. Health care workers are cross trained to provide a variety of services for the patient. The goal is patient-focused care.

Deductibles Amount the subscriber must pay before health insurance begins to cover costs.

Defamation Damage to someone's reputation through false communication or communication without permission.

Deficit Spending exceeds revenue.

Delegated medical act Physician's orders given to an RN, LPN, or LVN by a physician, dentist, or podiatrist,

Delegating (delegation) Generally, duties within the LPN/LVN job description that can be given to another worker to perform. Duties that are part of your legal scope of practice cannot be delegated. Check your Nurse Practice Act to confirm authority to delegate in your state.

Denial Coping mechanism that includes rejection of events as they really are. Eliminates need for anxiety.

Department of Health and Human Services (DHHS) Funded by taxes. Advises president on national health matters.

Dependent role With supervision. For example, the LPN/LVN functions in a dependent role to the RN, physician, or dentist.

Depositions Gathering information under oath. One of the steps in bringing legal action.

Desired patient outcome Observable result. Focuses directly on what the patient will accomplish (not what the nurse will do).

Diagnosis-related group (DRG) Prospective payment system. Specifies number of days for which Medicare will pay, based on illness category.

Differentiated practice System of assigning patients for care. Uses skill mix of nursing staff, according to patient needs.

Diploma nurse RN who has received his or her education in a 3-year hospital-based program.

Diploma program A 3-year educational program conducted by a hospital-based school of nursing.

Direct supervision Supervisor is continuously present to coordinate, direct, or inspect nursing care. Supervisor is in building.

Directed (or focused) thinking Purposeful and outcome-oriented thinking. Focuses on particular problem to find solution.

Discrimination Rights and privileges are withheld from those of another cultural group.

Discussion buddy Another student with whom you study and discuss the topic to comprehend the information.

Distance learning A course in which the teacher and student are separated by physical distance, using such tools as two-way television, videotapes, audiotapes, and the Internet.

Distracters Incorrect options for multiple-choice items.

Dix, Dorothea Lynde Appointed Superintendent of Nurses during Civil War in order to organize a corps of nurses to tend to wounded soldiers.

Do-Not-Resuscitate (DNR) Order written by physician. Patient recovery is beyond hope of recovery. Patient may have signed an advance directive regarding end-of-life care, which clarifies personal wishes.

Dual-eligibles The millions of Medicare beneficiaries who are also enrolled in Medicaid.

Durable medical power of attorney Identifies who will make decisions regarding future care, extent of treatment, and kinds of treatment if the person is unable to make his or her own decisions. Written while the person is mentally competent.

Duty One of four elements needed to prove negligence. Refers to nurse's responsibility to provide care in an acceptable way. As used in the text, responsibilities directly related to nursing licensure and scope of practice. Usually not delegated to someone with less education and nursing skill.

E

Effectiveness Choosing the most important thing to do, and doing it accurately.

Efficiency Getting tasks done in the shortest time possible.

Electronic Controlled by a computer.

Electronic medical record Patient records stored on a computer.

Emotional mind Site of positive feelings, such as love, caring, kindness, and compassion.

Emotional needs How people respond and deal with feelings of joy, anger, sadness, guilt, remorse, sorrow, love, etc.

Empathizer (empathiser) A person who intuitively figures out how people are feeling and how to treat them with sensitivity.

Empathy Respectful, detached concern.

Empower Enable, permit, and give power or authority.

Enculturation Process of learning your culture: the way your group does things resulting in a worldview.

Endorsement Agreement between states that nurses licensed in one state may become licensed in another if they meet the state nursing board criteria.

Entitlement program Those eligible because of age, disability, or economic status are entitled by law to benefits of certain programs. They must be funded.

Ethics Rules or principles that govern correct conduct.

Ethnic groups Cultural groups composed of people who are members of the same race, religion, or nation or who speak the same language.

Ethnocentrism The belief that one's own culture is best; the belief that one's way of doing things is superior/right/best.

Euthanasia Physician or other person administering lethal dose of medication to end life; illegal in the United States and Canada.

Evaluation Phase 5 of nursing process for LPN/LVNs. Compares actual patient outcomes to expected outcomes.

External distractions Interruptions in concentration from outside oneself, such as background sounds, lighting, peers, and so forth.

Extrovert A person who prefers action with others, talks more than listens, and learns by teaching others.

F

Facilitator Teacher who creates a learning environment by arranging for a variety of activities and experiences. The student is expected to participate actively in his or her own learning.

False reassurance Promising patient something you cannot deliver, such as saying, "You'll be just fine."

Feedback Response to sender's message as a part of meaningful conversation.

Fee-for-service Patient pays the physician a fee for each service provided.

Felony Serious offense, with a penalty that ranges from 1 year in prison to death.

Fidelity In nursing, to be faithful to the charge of acting in the patient's best interest when the capacity to make free choice is no longer available.

Fight-flight mind When feeling threatened, the mind is activated and person begins to defend self.

First Amendment Guarantees freedom of expression, as long as it is not at the expense of harming others.

Focused questions Questions that require definitive, precise information from a patient.

Follow-up illusion Irrational belief that it is the employer's responsibility to contact applicants after an interview.

Formal education Planned, organized learning, such as the nursing course of study.

Free clinic Used by persons who cannot afford traditional health care or are reluctant to use traditional services. The clinic charges a minimal fee.

Free-standing Health facility not attached to a hospital.

Functional method A method of patient care that is task-oriented and involves dividing the tasks to be done among staff members according to their abilities.

Fundamentalism A conservative form of a religion.

G

Gamp, Sairey "Nurse" character from Charles Dickens's 1849 novel, *Martin Chuzzlewit*. Provides negative portrayal of nurses and nursing care.

General hospitals Set up to treat a variety of medical/surgical problems.

General (implied) consent By entering a health facility voluntarily, a patient gives permission for treatment with noninvasive procedures. However, a patient may revoke this consent verbally and refuse to be treated.

General supervision Supervisor regularly coordinates, directs, or inspects nursing care and is within reach either in the building or by phone.

Generalization Broad, sweeping statements made about a group.

Gerontology Certification (GC) Postgraduate education in gerontology through NFLPN and ERI. Certification effective for 2 years.

Goals (outcomes) Realistic, measurable, time-limited statements of resolution of a problem or need.

Good Samaritan Act Stipulates that a person who provides emergency care at the scene of an accident is immune from civil liability for actions done in good faith. There is some variation of the law within states.

Gross domestic product (GDP) Combination of all goods and services produced in a nation's economy.

Group home Provides personal care services (custodial) to 3–16 residents. Provides help with ADLs, self-administration of medication, meal preparation, and transportation.

Guest speakers Nurses or other health professionals invited to present up-to-date information on areas of expertise.

H

Habits Established patterns of behavior.

Hard copy Data from a computer that is printed out to be read, rather than reading from the computer screen.

Hard wiring Biologically a part of brain development.

Health care provider A licensed health care person, such as a physician, dentist, or nurse practitioner, whose health care services are covered by a health insurance plan.

Health Insurance Portability and Accountability Act (HIPAA) Federal law Commonly called the Privacy Act. Steps and conditions for providing patient privacy in health care settings went into effect in 2003.

Health maintenance organization (HMO) A comprehensive care system of medical services based on a set, prepaid fee.

Health Savings Accounts (HSA) Funding for health care involving a medical savings account that allows persons to save for medical expenses on a tax-free basis. Carries lower monthly payments with higher deductibles.

Hidden job market Unadvertised jobs.

Home health nursing Provides health services supervised by a licensed professional in a patient's home. Examples include visiting nurse associations, health departments, home health agencies, etc.

Honesty To not deliberately deceive in order to present oneself in a better light.

Hospice care End-of-life care for the terminally ill. The philosophy is to maintain comfort as death approaches.

Howlett hierarchy Hierarchy of work motivators. Adapted from Maslow's Hierarchy of Needs.

Humor Communication characteristic to help "lighten up" a situation.

I

Idea sketches Representing a verbal concept with a picture.

Illegal questions Interview questions that do not have to be answered, such as age, marital status, number of children, and health problems, unless directly related to job.

Illiteracy Current definition is inability to comprehend meaning.

Impaired nurse One who is addicted to alcohol or other drugs.

Implementation Phase 3 of the nursing process for LPN/LVNs. Provides required nursing care to accomplish established patient goals.

Incident report Federally required brief narrative of incident, written by person who witnessed it. Purpose is in-house improvement of care.

Incremental method Changes that occur here and there without affecting the system as a whole.

Independent Function without supervision. For example, the RN role in the nursing process.

Inflation General rise in prices persisting over several years.

Informal education Obtained through school of life.

Informational interview By appointment, meet with an administrator to learn about a facility. This is not a job interview, although it is treated with the same courtesy.

Informed consent Obtained by physician for invasive procedures after physician has provided patient with facts about effects, side effects, alternative treatments, prognosis, etc. May be revoked verbally anytime, up to time of procedure.

Institutional liability Form of vicarious liability. Health setting sued for negligence of employee.

Intentional tort Intent to do a wrongful act.

Interdependent Collaboratively. For example, both RNs and LPN/LVNs carry out orders for treatments and medications written out by a physician.

Interlibrary loan services Allows libraries to borrow materials from other libraries that are not a part of their holdings.

Intermediate care facility (ICF) Recognized under Medicare program. Services for people who have physical or mental conditions, do not require acute or skilled nursing services.

Internal distractions Interruptions in concentration from inside oneself, such as daydreaming and boredom.

Internet Physical infrastructure that allows the electronic circulation of vast amounts of information to computer users. This information is unregulated and cannot always be taken at face value.

Interpersonal learner Learns best by sharing, comparing, cooperating, and interviewing.

Interpersonal styles Four major styles: (1) results-focused, (2) detail-focused, (3) friendly-focused, and (4) party-focused.

Interstate endorsement Agreement among states that licensed nurses do not have to repeat NCLEX-PN® examination if they meet criteria for working in the state.

Intrapersonal learner Learns best by working alone, self-paced instruction, and having own space.

Introvert A person who listens more than talks, concentrates; a reflective thinker who wants to understand the world.

Irrational thinking Based on Ellis (1994). Self-talk is often irrational thinking: Judgments are subjective and have no bearing on facts. Leads to negative emotions and stress.

Items Multiple-choice questions. Each item has a stem, distracters, and a key.

IV Therapy Certification (IVC) Postgraduate education on intravenous therapy, offered through NFLPN and ERI.

J

Justice Giving patients their due and treating them fairly.

K

Key Correct option for multiple-choice item.

Knowledge Repeat information exactly as read or told. Does not imply an understanding of the information.

L

Law Nursing law is based on each state's Nurse Practice Act.

Leadership Manner in which the leader gets along with co-workers, with the goal of producing workplace changes to meet the goals of the employing agency.

Learning resource center (LRC) The library.

Lecture-discussion strategy A strategy in which the instructor shares several ideas with the class and then stops to let the class discuss the ideas.

Left brain A person who is more orderly, logical, who reads and writes well, and excels at analytical thinking.

Liability Legal responsibility of a person to account for wrongful acts by making financial restitution.

Libel Damage to someone's reputation through written communication or pictures.

Librarian College-educated specialist in what the library has to offer.

Linguistic learner Learns best by reducing the number of words included in class notes.

Living will Written directive stating personal wishes regarding future health care. Not recognized as a legal document in every state or other countries.

Logical learner Learns best by using an organized method of study.

Long-term care Range of medical care to assist persons with disability or chronic care needs.

Long-term goal A general realistic statement of what one hopes to attain ultimately.

LRC holdings Library materials including books, catalogued materials, audio tapes, video tapes, etc.

M

Malpractice (professional negligence) A part of negligence that relates to lack of skill or misconduct by professional persons.

Managed care A system of controlling cost of health care by arranging health care at predetermined rates. An HMO is an example of managed care.

Management Organizing all care required for patients in a health care setting, for a specific period.

Manipulation An indirect way of dealing with issues that may be positive or negative. Negative (maladaptive) manipulation occurs if the feelings of others are disregarded or other people are treated as objects.

Map Care maps are a combination of care plans and critical pathways.

Mapping A form of note making in which information and its relationships are put in a visual pattern.

Marketplace Part of the economic system with least government intervention.

Medicaid Financial assistance provided by the federal government for states and counties to pay for medical services for eligible poor.

Medicare Federally sponsored and supervised health insurance plan for persons 65 years of age and older and persons under 65 years who are totally and permanently disabled.

Medicare Advantage Government approved health plan options to original Medicare offered by private insurance companies.

Medicare Quality Improvement Organizations (QIOs) Formerly known as peer review organizations. Under the direction of Centers for Medicare and Medicaid Services.

Melting pot The United States became known as the "melting pot" in the nineteenth century, when immigrants would assimilate into the dominant culture.

Mental imagery Uses the right side of the brain to generate pictures of an idea; the left side supplies the script.

Message The idea being conveyed or the question being asked.

Minitask Simple to do and takes no more than 5 minutes. An unpleasant, difficult, time-consuming task can be divided into a series of minitasks.

Misdemeanor Least serious infraction of the law. Can result in a fine or up to 1 year in jail.

Mission statement A statement that defines the purpose and goals of a health care organization.

Mississippi, 1914 First state to pass a law licensing practical nurses.

Mnemonic devices Memory aids such as rhymes or acronyms.

Mobility program Seamless program of study from NA to LPN/LVN to associate-degree RN.

Mock examinations Prelicensure and readiness tests in NCLEX-PN® examination format. Does not contain actual NCLEX-PN® examination questions.

Morals Ethical habits of a person.

Multiculturalism Mix of cultures.

Multistate licensure (Nursing Licensure Compact) Legislation in some states that renders a nursing license obtained in that state valid for practice in other states with multistate legislation. Each state's individual regulations must still be followed.

Musical learner Learns best by humming, singing, or playing an instrument.

N

NANDA North American Nursing Diagnosis Association.

NAPNES National Association for Practical Nurse Education and Service, Inc.

Naturalistic system Beliefs developed from the traditional medical practices of the ancient civilizations of China, India, and Greece.

NCLEX-PN® examination National Council Licensing Examination for Practical Nursing.

Negligence Conduct that falls below the standard of care established by law for the protection of others.

Networking Building relationships with instructors, employers, and peers, for the purposes of finding new jobs, better pay, faster promotions, and greater job satisfaction.

NFLPN National Federation of Licensed Practical Nurses.

NIC Nursing Interventions Classification.

Nightingale, Florence Founder of modern nursing, who is often known as "The Lady with the Lamp" because of her after-hours rounds with her lamp during the Crimean War.

NLN National League for Nursing.

NOC Nursing Outcomes Classification.

Nonassertive (passive) Fear-based, emotionally dishonest, self-defeating type of behavior. Gives message of "I don't count, you count."

Nonjudgmental Taking at face value. Accepting people as they are.

Nonmaleficence First, do no harm.

Nonverbal communication Sending or receiving information by facial expressions or body language.

Nurse Practice Act Governs the practice of nursing. Developed by most states and provincial board of nursing.

Nursing assistant Minimum 75-hour course prepares nursing assistant to give bedside care. Successful completion makes NA eligible for state registry.

Nursing diagnosis Summary, in nursing terms, from NANDA: Actual and high risk problems that nurses can respond to. Exclusive responsibility of RN in nursing process.

Nursing ethics System of principles governing conduct of nurses.

Nursing home Offers personal and skilled nursing care (if needed), 24 hours a day.

Nursing organizations Groups for nurses focused on nursing issues of importance.

Nursing process An orderly way of developing a plan of care for the individual patient. RN is responsible for developing the nursing diagnosis.

Nursing skills lab Resource that allows student nurses to practice and develop nursing skills.

Nursing standard of care Guideline for good nursing care. Standards are based on what an ordinary, prudent nurse with similar education and nursing experience would do in a similar situation.

O

Objective information Data that can be observed and verified. Data obtained by seeing, hearing, touching, smelling, tasting, measuring, counting, etc. Does not include subjective judgment.

Official (government) health care agencies Local, state, and federal health agencies supported by tax dollars.

Omnibus Reconciliation Act of 1987 (OBRA) Major federal legislation that addresses the quality of life, health, and safety of residents.

One-way communication When the sender controls a situation and offers no opportunity for feedback from the receiver; used to give a command.

Online catalog Computerized card catalog in the library.

Open-ended questions Questions that permit the patient to respond in a way most meaningful to him or her. These type of questions often begin with what, where, when.

Options Choices. For example, choices for answer in a multiple-choice item.

Original Medicare Part A (hospital insurance—no premium), and Part B (medical insurance) and Part D (prescription insurance). Plan B and D are optional and require a monthly fee.

Outcome Identifies the degree of progress made (or not made) by the patient toward reaching a goal.

Outpatient clinic Provides health care outside of the hospital setting. Staffed by physicians and nurses.

Outlining method Especially popular method of note making for left-brain dominant persons.

Out-of-pocket Fee a patient pays directly.

P

Paradigm A way of thinking.

Paradigm shift Change in the way of thinking.

Parish nurse Works in various church settings in a health ministry.

Passive learning Dependent on instructor to provide information, for example, through lecture.

Passive listener A person who receives sounds with little recognition or personal involvement.

Pastoral care team Members of the health team who assist nurses in meeting the spiritual needs of the patients.

Pat answers General responses. Communication block. Discounts patient as a person.

Patience Willingness to put up with waiting and being okay about doing so.

Patient Bill of Rights Mandated by federal and state laws. Spell out patient rights while hospitalized.

Patient competency Relates to ability to understand and make decisions. Has both legal and clinical meaning.

Patient-focused care Attempt to improve the quality of care by using hospital resources more efficiently to meet the patient's needs (e.g., decentralizing services).

Patient outcomes Focus on whether patient has accomplished what was desired during treatment. Does not focus on what the nurse did.

Patient Self Determination Act (PSDA) Basis for advanced directives. Federal law mandates that Medicare and Medicaid patients must be told of their right to execute advance directives.

Perceptual learning style Refers to learning by 3 main sensory receivers: vision, auditory, kinesthetic.

Performance evaluation Evaluation of clinical performance that involves both the teacher and the student.

Periodical indexes List of periodicals by author, title, and subject.

Periodicals Magazines published weekly, monthly, and quarterly.

Personal liability Holds person (nurse) responsible for own actions.

Personalistic system Belief that a deity, ghost, god, evil spirit, witch, or angry ancestor is punishing the sick person.

Phoebe Ordained deaconess during age of Christianity. Known as first visiting nurse.

Physician-assisted suicide Name tagged onto "Oregon Death with Dignity Law." Physician writes prescription for medication to end life but does not administer it. Patient self-administers lethal medication.

Planning Phase 2 of the nursing process for LPN/LVNs. Involves assisting the RN in development of the nursing diagnosis, goals, and interventions for the patient's plan of care and maintaining patient safety.

Podcast A digital recording of information on the Internet that can be downloaded to a personal media player or a computer.

Positive mental attitude Expectation to succeed combined with hard work.

Postacute care (PAC) Also known as subacute care or transitional care. Patient discharged from hospital to lower level, less expensive care. Will be discharged home when deemed ready.

PQRST method A method of reading to increase understanding by developing comprehension. (Stands for Preview, Question, Read, State, Test.)

Practical/vocational nurse A person who performs, for compensation, any basic acts in the care of convalescent, subacutely, or chronically ill, injured, or infirm persons, or any act or procedure in the care of the acutely ill, injured, or infirm under the specific direction of a registered nurse, physician, podiatrist, or dentist.

Preferred provider organizations (PPOs) Similar to HMOs, except that physicians maintain their own practice and continue to be part of their own physician group. Part of the day is spent treating patients enrolled in a PPO.

Prejudice The opinion that a person has about something, even though facts dispute the opinion.

Premium Monthly fee a subscriber must pay for health care insurance coverage.

Preponderance Evidence that is beyond a reasonable doubt.

Prig, Betsy Character similar to Sairey Gamp, from Dickens's novel, *Martin Chuzzlewit.*

Primary care The point at which a person enters the health care system.

Primary care method A method of patient care in which one nurse is responsible and accountable for care given to patients on all shifts from admission to discharge.

Priorities What is most important, as in determining priorities when planning patient care.

Privacy Both a legal and ethical issue. Patient's right to choose what is done to his/her body, based on personal beliefs, feelings, and attitude.

Private health care agencies Agencies that are generally proprietary (for profit) and that charge a fee for service. The primary focus is curing illness.

Private pay The patient pays out of pocket for services received.

Probing Pushing for information beyond what is medically necessary to know.

Problem solving A series of steps used to solve problems long before the nursing process was developed.

Problem-oriented thinking Focus on a particular problem to find a solution (e.g., planning your school, work, and home schedule).

Procrastination Putting off tasks that must be done.

Projection A coping or mental mechanism in which an individual attributes his or her own weaknesses to others.

Proprietary hospitals (for profit) For-profit hospitals.

Prospective payment system (PPS) A system in which the federal government announces to a hospital in advance what it will pay for health care costs.

Provider The organization providing health care services.

Proximate cause One of four elements needed to prove negligence. Refers to reasonable cause-and-effect relationship between omission and commission of nursing act and harm to patient.

Public health care agencies Made up of official and voluntary health care agencies.

Purpose Reason.

R

Rapport A harmonious relationship.

Rationalization A coping or mental mechanism in which the individual offers a logical but untrue reason as an excuse for his/her behavior.

Receiver Person receiving the message, idea, or question.

Recycled adult learner Adult person starting a new career by enrolling in practical/vocational nursing.

Reference hierarchy Ranking of references from best to least by employers: (1) current and former supervisors from work and volunteer experiences, unit managers, and teachers; (2) workers who have seen your work; and (3) personal references or friends.

Reference materials Includes medical and nursing dictionaries, almanacs, yearbooks, atlases, encyclopedias, handbooks, etc. Generally cannot be checked out, but needed material can be copied.

Referral Send or direct for help.

Reflective thinking Thinking about what you are thinking about.

Registered nurse A member of the nursing team who has gone to nursing school for 2, 3, or 4 years and has passed NCLEX-RN® to be registered. The person on the nursing team who functions independently in decision making regarding the nursing care of patients.

Rehabilitation After acute care is completed, treatment may continue in order to bring person up to maximum functioning.

Reincarnation Belief in rebirth of the soul in many bodies as many times as necessary to achieve enlightenment.

Religion Attempts to give form to spiritual beliefs by adopting specific beliefs and rituals.

Religious denomination An organized group of persons with a philosophy that supports their particular concept of God.

Repatterning Deliberately working to change a pattern that is not working. Pattern can be a way of thinking, feeling, or doing.

Research and teaching hospital Facility that treats patients with unusual or serious conditions. Training site for physicians, nurses, and other health professionals. Does research on illness and treatment. Develops new methods of treatment.

Residential care Broadly defined as 24-hour supervision of persons, for reasons of age or impairments. Falls between skilled care and intermediate care facilities.

Resignation courtesy A 2-week notice of ending employment is considered courteous even if not part of the contract.

Respect Consideration, regard.

Responsible Reliable and trustworthy.

Restructuring Changing something that is not working out as planned.

Résumé Summary of what you have accomplished— work, skills, education, experience, and sometimes personal achievements. Used to persuade an employer that you are the right person for the job. Limit to one or two pages.

Returning adult learner A learner in the age bracket of the mid-twenties or older who has entered an educational program and has not experienced formal education for a period of time.

Right brain The person shows more advanced spatial relationships, recognizes negative emotions more quickly, is less verbal, adds tone and inflection to voice, and sees total picture.

Rituals Religious practices that affirm believers' connection to a higher power.

S

Schedule A plan that identifies what needs to be done, who is doing it, and when it must be completed.

Scope of practice What the nurse is able to do legally.

Seacole, Mary Black nurse from Jamaica, West Indies. Helped Florence Nightingale during Crimean War. Used knowledge of tropical medicine, herbs, and natural plant medicines to treat soldiers with cholera, yellow fever, malaria, and diarrhea.

"Seamless" systems (1) Provide progressive nursing programs without the need to repeat courses, as the person goes from nursing assistant to LPN/LVN to associate degree RN; (2) Provide ease of movement from one health care service to another.

Self-directed learner Takes responsibility for own learning and performance.

Self-evaluation Objective look at personal performance with a plan for improvement.

Self-proclaimed nurse Informally trained persons who chose to or were appointed to care for people who were ill, injured, dying, or having babies.

Self-worth Sense of self. Crediting self for what you do well.

Semmelweis, Ignaz Philipp Hungarian physician credited with developing the first antiseptic method to combat death from "childbed fever by washing hands."

Sender Person conveying an idea or asking a question.

Sensitivity Awareness of what others are feeling. Tunes in on affective and nonverbal communication.

Service, quality, and cost control Major concerns in the area of providing health care.

Sexual harassment A form of assault. Abuse of power. Not about sex or passion.

Shi'ite An Islamic sect that believes that Muhammad designated a relative to be his successor.

Short-term goal A smaller, more reasonable and manageable unit of a long-term goal; that is, the small step toward attaining a long-term goal.

Simulation A learning activity that makes use of imaginary patient situations and mimics the reality of the clinical environment.

Single-Payer System Comprehensive health care for everyone regardless of past medical history. Payment comes from a single fund, e.g., the U.S. Medicare system.

Sisters of Charity Organized by St. Vincent DePaul to care for poor and the sick.

Skill mix Health care staff made up of workers with different levels of education and training.

Skilled care Trained medical professionals provide a higher level of care.

Skilled nursing facility (SNF) Patients with more serious problems need a higher level of care by skilled and well-trained staff.

Slander Damage to someone's reputation by verbalizing untrue or confidential information.

Socialization How a person of one culture learns how to function in another culture.

Spatial learner Learns best by studying diagrams, boxes, and special lists.

Specialized hospital Limited to one type of patient, such as women or children.

Spirit Life force that penetrates the person's entire body. Gives meaning to life.

Spiritual caring Recognize and support spiritual need of the patient in the health care setting.

Spiritual dimension That which gives insight into the person's meaning of life, suffering, and death.

Spiritual distress Observed in patients unable to practice their rituals or seen in those who experience conflict between their religious or spiritual beliefs and prescribed medical regimen.

Spiritual needs Requirements that arise out of the desire of human beings to find meaning in life, suffering, and death.

Spirituality Pertaining to the soul, one's life force.

Stacks Place in library where material that can be checked out is located.

Standards of care Used instead of care plans in some acute care agencies; include the priority nursing diagnosis for each patient, with appropriate assessments, nursing interventions, and expected outcomes (goals).

State board of nursing Develops and enforces Nurse Practice Act, which is the basis for nursing law. There is some variation among states.

Static mannequins Full-size body models or models of specific parts of the body made to be realistic.

Statutory law Law developed by the legislative branch of state and federal governments.

Stem First line of a multiple-choice item.

Stereotype Casting all people in a culture as being the same in regard to thinking, feeling, and acting.

Stress management Maintenance of stress at a moderate level. The reaction to both high and low levels of stress may be overwhelming.

Student nurse Person involved in a course of study to become a nurse.

Study group Peers who are actively involved in understanding information by discussing it in a small group.

Study skills lab A place where schools provide services to assist a student with academic problems.

Subacute care Short-term transitional care. Known as postacute care (PAC).

Subjective information Information based on a patient's opinion.

Subjective versus objective Subjective relates to patient's opinion about their condition (symptoms). Objective relates to what can be verified (signs).

Subungal zone Area in crook between the fingertip and the nail. Collects largest number of hand pathogens.

Sunni An Islamic sect comprised of the majority of Muslims. Sunnis believe that Muhammad did not designate a successor.

Support system Individuals who are available to assist patient when ill or dying, usually family and/or friends. Support may range from emotional to physical to spiritual. Also applies to personal support system.

Syllabus Up-to-date course document distributed at the beginning of a course. This document usually includes a course description, course objectives, course requirements, required text, grading scale, and instructor information.

Sympathy Feel the person's pain.

Systemizer (systemiser) A person who intuitively figures out how things work and what underlying rules control the system.

T

Tactual learner Learns best by doing.

Tasks Activities carried out by nursing assistants. As used in this text, basic skills the nurse has learned to do. For example, activities of daily living. Tasks can be assigned.

Teaching Originally thought of as lecturing to students. All responsibility was on the instructor. Current method equalizes responsibility between student and instructor and encourages a wide range of learning/teaching methods.

Teaching and research hospital Private or public hospitals that focus on treating patients; training physicians, nurses and other health professionals; and research and development.

Team building Working toward cohesion with staff so mission statement of health facility can be carried out in the course of patient care.

Team method A method of patient care in which small teams of nursing personnel are assigned to give total care to groups of patients.

The Joint Commission (TJC) Sets the standards of care for hospitals and long-term care agencies. Agencies receive accreditation if they elect to be reviewed and meet standards.

TJC National Patient Safety Goals 2003 federally mandated safety rules for health facilities.

Therapeutic Having healing properties, results of treatment.

Therapeutic communication Between the patient and the nurse. The focus is on the patient.

Thinking mind Creativity, reasoning, and analytical thinking occur in this part of the brain-the thinking cap.

Third-party coverage Health insurance.

Time management The effective use of time to meet goals.

Total quality management (TQM) A method by which continuous quality improvement (CQI) is carried out.

Traditional adult learner A learner who comes to an educational program directly from high school or from another program of study, usually in his or her late teens or early twenties.

Transitional care Subacute care at a lower level facility after acute (hospital) care is completed, but patient is not ready to go home.

Trust Rely on, depend on.

Tutoring Select study group. Student arranges for special help through instructor referral or self-referral.

Two-way communication When there is feedback or discussion between the sender and receiver; the usual form of conversation.

U

Uncompensated care Do not receive full payment for services because of free care, bad debt, or difference in what is charged and what insurance reimburses.

Understanding Comprehension. Able to recall and provide examples.

Unintentional torts Nurse did not intend to injure patient. Negligence and malpractice are examples.

Unit manager Has supervisor and management functions for patient units.

United Nations (UN) International organization that deals with world issues. Has representatives of many countries.

Universal coverage Health insurance coverage for all persons; usually paid through taxes.

Unlicensed assistive personnel (UAP) Trained by health care organizations to function in an assistive role to RNs and LPN/LVNs. Also known as patient care technicians, patient care associates, nurse extenders, and multiskilled workers.

U.S. Public Health Service (USPHS) Division of Department of Health and Human Services. Made up of six agencies.

V

Values Assigned to an idea or action. Freely chosen and affected by age, experience, and maturity.

Verbal communication Sending or receiving communication through the spoken or written word.

Vicarious liability Responsible for actions of another because of a special relationship with the other.

Virtual Simulated by a computer.

Visual learner Generates visual images; that is, thinks primarily in pictures. Learns best by watching a demonstration first.

Vocalization Verbalization.

Voluntary community hospital Nonprofit hospital operated by community association or religious organization.

Voluntary health care agencies Not-for-profit, nonofficial health care agencies that complement official health agencies and meet the needs of persons with a specific disease.

W

Wahhabism An ultraconservative form of Islam.

Wald, Lillian Began Henry Street Settlement visiting nurse service in New York in 1893 to care for indigent persons.

Wellness and illness Relative terms. Have different meanings for different cultures.

Wellness center Promotes wellness. Includes nutritional counseling, exercise programs, stress reduction, and weight control programs.

Working the room Identify and contact people in a position to hire you (e.g., during meeting or workshop breaks).

World Health Organization (WHO) International health agency of the United Nations, located in Geneva.

Worldview Shared by persons with same cultural background.

References and Suggested Readings

Chapter 1

Borysenko J. (2006, Sept). Conquer the five common fears that arise when you decide to return to class. *Prevention (online)*. Retrieved September 12, 2007 from http://www.prevention.com/cda/article/retrain-your-brain/a9c250lfa.

Chenevert M. (2006). *Mosby's tour guide to nursing school: A student's road survival kit*. St Louis: Mosby.

deWit S. (2007). *Saunders student nurse planner: a guide to success in nursing school*. Philadelphia: Elsevier Saunders.

Galbraith M. (2003). *Adult learning methods: a guide for effective instruction*. Melbourne, FL: Krieger Publishing.

Knowles M, Holton E, and Swanson R. (2005). *The adult learner: the definitive classic in adult education and human resource development* (6th ed.). New York: Butterworth-Heinemann.

Oblinger D, and Oblinger J. *Educating the net generation*. (2005). Page last updated 8/20/2007. Retrieved March 14, 2007 from www.educause.edu/educatingthenet.

Pauk W. (2006). *How to study in college*. Boston: Houghton Mifflin.

Sanoff A. (2005, May 8) Survey: High school fails to engage students. *USA Today*. Retrieved March 1, 2007 from http://usatoday.printthis.clickability.com/pt/cpt?action=cpandtitle=USATODAY.com+-+Survey%3A+High+school+fails+to+engage+studentsandexpire=andurllD=14.

Sherman R. (2006). Leading a multigenerational nursing workforce: issues, challenges and strategies. *Online J Issues Nurs*, 11(2). Retrieved June 29, 2006 from http://www.medscape.com/viewarticle/536480.

Skiba D, and Barton A. (2006). Adopting your teaching to accommodate the net generation. *Online J Issues Nurs*, 11(2). Retrieved March 8, 2007 from http://nursingworld.org/ojin/topic30/tpc30_4.htm.

Weston M. (2006) Integrating generational perspectives in nursing. *Online J Issues Nurs*, 11(2). Available at www.nursingworld.org/ojin/topic30/tpc30_1.htm.

Chapter 2

Barsch J. *Understanding your learning preference*. Ventura, CA: Ventura College Learning Disability Clinic.

Byrne M. (2001). Uncovering racial bias in nursing fundamentals textbooks. *Nurs Health Care Perspect*, 22(6), 299–303.

Chatterbean. *Are you a right-brain thinker?* Retrieved February 18, 2007 from http://www.chatterbean.com/right_brain_thinker/1/.

Clinton P. (2000). The crisis you don't know about. In *Book 4th anniversary issue*, pp L4–L11.

Eagleman D. (2007). 10 Unsolved mysteries of the brain. *Discover*. **PARS** International, pp 54–75.

Felder-Silverman Model. Learning styles. Retrieved April 11, 2007 from http://www.ncsu.edu/felder-public/Learning_Styles.com.

Felder R, and Soloman B. *Learning styles and strategies*. Retrieved April 11, 2007 from http://www.ncsu.edu/felder-public/lL.Sdir/styles.html.

Gardner, H. (1999). *Intelligence reframed: Multiple intelligences for the 21st century*. Basic Books: a member of the Perseus Books Group.

Gardner H. & Hatch T. (1990, March.) *Multiple intelligences go to school: Educational implications of the theory of multiple intelligences*. (Technical Report No. 4). New York Center for Technology in Education.

Gurian, M. (1997). *The Wonder of boys*. New York: Jeremy P. Tarcher/Putnum.

GSU master teacher program: on learning styles. Retrieved February 18, 2007 from http://www2.gsu.edu/~dschjb/wwwmbti.html.

Guardian Unlimited. *They just can't help it*. Retrieved February 18, 2007 from http://www.guardian.co.uk/life/feature/story/0,13026,937913,00.html.

ISD-Development. *Learning styles or, how we go from the unknown to the known*. Retrieved April 8, 2007 from http://www.nwlink.com/~donclark/hrd/learning/styles.html.

James E. Finding your learning style. *ADVANCE for LPNs*. Retrieved November 13, 2005 from http://lpn.advanceweb.com/common/Editoriall/Editorial.aspx?CC=57467.

Jensen, E. (1998). The learning brain. In *Teaching with the brain in mind*. Alexandria, VA. Association for Supervision and Curriculum Development.

Kelly K, and Ramundo P. (1993). *You mean I'm not lazy, stupid or crazy?!* New York: Scribner.

Lisa-Angelique L, and Cheong E. (2004, January). Learning Styles. *CDTL Brief* 7(1). Retrieved February 18, 2007, from http://www.cdtl.nus.edu.sg/brief/v7n1/default/html.

Miller M, and Babcock D. (1996). *Critical thiking applied to nursing*. St. Louis: CV Mosby.

Paul R, and Elder L. (2002). *Critical thinking: tools for taking charge of your personal and professional life*. Upper Saddle River, NJ: Financial Times Prentice Hall.

Note: Some websites listed in this section were used by the authors in the development of the chapters, but may have had specific periods in which they were active. Therefore some of them may not open.

Reis R. *Learning styles. Tomorrow's professor listserv.* Retrieved February 18, 2007 from http://sll.stanford. edu/projects/tomprof/newtomprof/postings/216.htm.

Springer S. & Deuttsch G. (1997). Attempts at applying asymmetry: Hemisphericity, education, and culture. In *Left brain right brain: A perspective on cognitive neuroscience* (5th ed). New York: W.H. Freeman & Co.

Wade N. Scans show different growth for intelligent brains. *The New York Times.* Retrieved March 30, 2006 from http://www.nytimes.com/2006/03/30/science/39brain.html.

Chapter 3

Alessandra T. (2005, April 13). Time management. *ADVANCE for LPNs.* Retrieved May 2, 2005 from HTTP://LPN.advanceweb.com/common/Editorial/PrintFriendly.aspx?CC=52647.

The basics of effective learning. (1997; updated 1999). Newtown, PA: Buck's Co. Community College. Retrieved from www.bucks.edu/%7especpop/weekly-sch.htm.

Chenevert M. (2006). *Mosby's tour guide to nursing school.* St Louis: Mosby.

deWit S. (2007). *Saunders student nurse planner: a guide to success in nursing school.* Philadelphia: Elsevier Saunders.

Kolberg J. (2006). *Conquering chronic disorganization.* Decatur, GA: Squall Press.

Lakein A. (1973). *How to get control of your time and your life.* New York: New American Library-Dutton.

Pauk W. (2006). *How to study in college.* Boston: Houghton Mifflin.

Self-help brochures: Time management. University of Illinois Counseling Center, Retrieved April 12, 2007 from www.couns.uiuc.edu/brochures/time.htm.

Silber L. (1998). *Time management for the creative person.* New York: Three Rivers Press.

Skloot R. (2007, Jan). Why is it so damn hard to change? *O, The Oprah Magazine,* 164–168, 213.

Chapter 4

Alfaro-LeFevre R. (2008). *Critical thinking and clinical judgement.* Philadelphia: Elsevier/Saunders.

Buzan T. (1991). *Use both sides of your brain.* New York: New American Library-Dutton.

Feller B. Study: Mindless reading has its costs. Green Bay Press Gazette, July 4, 2006.

Hancock O. (2006). *Reading skills for college students.* Englewood Cliffs, NJ: Prentice-Hall.

Hudson, R. (2005, April) Learning—that indispensable link to living. *Nursingmatters,* 17(4):13–14.

Kinser A. (2005, March 14) *Enhancing nursing student success through web-based remediation, part of a program titled Use of technology in nursing education,* Retrieved April 12, 2007 from http://ssti.confex.com/stti/bescience38/techprogram/paper_24561.htm.

Margulies N, Maal N, and Wheatley M. (2001). *Mapping inner space: learning and teaching visual mapping.* Tucson, AZ: Zephyr Press.

Mindless reading seen as fundamental. *Red Orbit,* 7/3/06, Retrieved March 8, 2007 from http://www.redorbit.com/news/science/55810/mindless_reading_see…

National Council of State Boards of Nursing. NCLEX-PN® Examination Test Plan for the National Council Licensure Examination for Licensed Practical/Vocational Nurses, effective April, 2005, Chicago: NCSBN.

Orlovsky C. (2007, March 6). *Nursing education in the virtual age.* Retrieved March 6, 2007 from NurseZone.

Paley A. (2007, Feb 23). *Test scores at odds with rising high school grades.* Retrieved March 1, 2007 from www.washingtonpost.com/wp-dyn/content/article/2007/02/22/AR2007022201781_pf.html.

Pauk W. (2006). *How to study in college* (7th ed.). Boston: Houghton-Mifflin.

Schemo D. (2006, Sept 2). At 2 year colleges, students eager but unready. *The New York Times,* Retrieved at New York Times.com on 10-8-06.

Silvestri L. *Q and A Review for the NCLEX-PN Examination.* St Louis: Saunders/Elsevier, 2007.

Chapter 5

Alfaro-LeFevre R. (2008). *Critical thinking and clinical judgement.* Philadelphia: Elsevier/Saunders.

Chenevert M. (2006). *Mosby's tour guide to nursing school: a student's road survival kit.* St Louis: Mosby.

Childs J, and Sepples S. (2006, May/June). Clinical teaching by simulation. *Nurs Educ Perspect,* 27(3):154–158.

Daunt T. (2004, Aug 24) *Etiquette revival: experts inject a little decorum into the rat race of rudeness.* Retrieved August 24, 2004 from http://www.chicagotribune.com/features/chi-0408240150aug24,1,2429375,print.story.

Delpier T. (2006, July/Aug) Cases 101: learning to teach with cases. *Nurs Educ Perspect* 27(4):204–209.

deWit S. (2006) Virtual clinical excursions—general hospital. *Fundamental concepts and skills for nursing.* St Louis: Elsevier.

Grady M, Yates VM. (2007, March/April). Portable media players in the skills lab. *Nurs Educ Perspect,* 28(2):62–63.

Levine J, Young, M, and Baroudi C. (2005). *The Internet for dummies.* Indianapolis, IN: Wiley.

National Council of State Boards of Nursing. *NCLEX-PN examiation test plan for the National Council Licensure Examination for licensed practical/vocational nurse.* Effective April, 2005. Chicago: NCSBN.

Pauk W. (2006). *How to study in college.* Boston: Houghton-Mifflin.

Silvestri L. Q and A for the NCLEX-PN Examination. St. Louis: Saunders/Elsevier, 2007.

Skiba D. (2007, March/April). Nursing education 2.0: You Tube. *Nurs Educ Perspect,* 28(2):100–102.

Staton T. (1962). *How to study* (5th ed.). Circle Pines, MN: Publisher's Building, American Guidance Service.

Chapter 6

Alfaro-LeFevre R. (2000). *Applying nursing process: promoting collaborative care* (5th ed.). Philadelphia: Lippincott.

Alfaro-LeFevre R. (2003, July). Improving your ability to think critically. *Healthcare Traveler,* 11(1):72–76.

Alfaro-LeFevre R. (2006). *Critical thinking indicators™.* Available at www.AlfaroTeachSmart.com.

Alfaro-LeFevre R. (2009). *Critical thinking and clinical judgment: a practical approach* (4th ed.). Philadelphia: WB Saunders.

Austhink Software Pty Ltd. Australia. *Augment mapping and critical thinking.* Retrieved February 18, 2007 from http://www.austhink.com/augmentmap/thinking/?gclid=CKnku92auYoCFQbmYAod0Te…

Bauer B, and Hill S. (2000). *Mental health nursing: an introductory text* (2nd ed., pp 69–70). Philadelphia: WB Saunders.

Christensen B, and Kockrow E. (2006). *Foundations and adult health nursing* (5th ed). St Louis: Mosby.

Ignatavicius D, and Workman ML. (2006). *Medical surgical nursing* (5th ed.). Philadelphia: WB Saunders.

A key to critical thinking habits of the mind: what are habits of the mind? Retrieved February 18, 2007 from http://hsc.unm.edu/consg/conct/habits%20of%20mind.shml.

National Council of State Boards of Nursing. (effective April 2008). *NCLEX-PN test plan.* Chicago: NCSBN, Inc.

National Council of State Boards of Nursing. *NCLEX Examination candidate bulletin* (2007). NCSBN at www.ncsbn.org.

National Council of State Boards of Nursing. *NCLEX-PN examination test plan for the National Council Licensure Examination for Licensed Practical/Vocational Nurses.* (1995). Chicago: NCSBN, Inc.

National Council of State Boards of Nursing. *NCLEX-PN examination test plan for the National Council Licensure Examination for Licensed Practical/Vocational Nurses.* (1998). Chicago: NCSBN, Inc.

National Council of State Boards of Nursing. *NCLEX-PN examination test plan for the National Council Licensure Examination for Licensed Practical/Vocational Nurses.* (2001). Chicago: NCSBN, Inc.

National Council of State Boards of Nursing. *NCLEX-PN examination test plan for the National Council Licensure Examination for Licensed Practical/Vocational Nurses.* Effective date: April 2005. Chicago: NCSBN, Inc.

National Council of State Boards of Nursing. *NCLEX-PN test plan for the National Council Licensure Examination for Practical/Vocational Nurses.* (2007) Chicago: NCSBN, Inc.

Potter P, and Perry A. (2003). *Basic nursing essentials for practice* (5th ed.). St Louis: Mosby.

Smith J, and Crawford L. (2003). *Report on findings from the 2003 LPN/VN practice analysis: linking the NCLEX-PN examination to practice.* Chicago: National Council of State Boards of Nursing, Inc.

University of New Mexico Health Sciences Center. *What is critical thinking?* Retrieved February 18, 2007 from http://hsc.unm.edu/consg/conct/whatis.shml.

Wendt K. (2007). *Report on findings from the 2006 LPN/LVN practice analysis: linking the NCLEX-PN examination to practice.* Chicago: National Council of State Boards of Nursing, Inc.

Chapter 7

ANA Report. (1944). Trained attendants and practical nurses. *Am J Nurs,* 44:7–8.

Backer B. (1993, March). The Nightingale pledge: a commitment that survives the passage of time. *Nurs Health Care,* 14:3.

Brown E. (1948). *Nursing for the future.* New York: Russell Sage Foundation.

Cherry B, and Jacob S. (1999). *Contemporary nursing issues, trends, and management.* St Louis: Mosby.

Christensen B, and Kockrow E. (2006). *Foundations and adult health nursing.* (5th ed.). St Louis: Mosby.

D'Antonio P. (1997). *Nineteenth century nursing. Reflections.* Indianapolis: Sigma Theta Tau, 3rd/4th Quarter, 3:3.

Deloughery G. (1998). *Issues and trends in nursing* (3rd ed.). St Louis: Mosby.

Deming D. (1944). Practical nurses—a professional responsibility. *Am J Nurs,* 44:36–43.

Donley R. (2002). *Revisiting the American Nurses Association first position on education for nurses.* 2002 *Online J Issues Nurs,* Retrieved May 31, 2002 from http://nursingworld.org/ojin/topic18/tpc18_1.htm.

Eyles M. (2001). *Mosby's comprehensive review of practical nursing for NCLEX-PN* (13th ed.). St Louis: Mosby.

Fahy E. (1993, March). Covering the history of nursing. *Nurs Health Care,* 14:3.

Florence Nightingale. Retrieved October 21, 2007 from *http://encyclopedia.tdf.com/p/Florence+Nightingale*

Frantz A. (1998, Oct). Nursing pride: Clara Barton in the Spanish-American War. *Am J Nurs,* 98(10).

Goldsmith J. (1942). New York's practical nurse program. *Am J Nurs,* 42:1026–1031.

Gosnell D. (2002). *Overview and summary: The 1965 Entry into Practice Proposal—Is it relevant today?* 2002 *Online J Issues Nurs.* Retrieved May 31, 2002 from *http://nursingworld.org/ojin/topic18/tpc18ntr.htm.*

James E. *Legacy lives on in advance for nurses.* Retrieved February 17, 2005 from http://Nursing.advanceweb.com/common/editorial/PrintFriendly.aspx?CC=49113.

Joel L. (2002). *Education for entry into nursing practice: revisited for the 21st century.* 2002 *Online J Issues Nurs.* Retrieved from http://nursingworld.org/ojin/topic18/tpc18_4htm.

Kalish P, and Kalish B. (1995). *The advance of American nursing* (3rd ed.). Boston: Little, Brown.

Kinder J. (1986, Nov). President NLN. Letter.

LeVasseur J. (1998). Plato, Nightingale, and contemporary nursing. *IMAGE: Journal of Nursing Scholarship.* Indianapolis: Sigma Theta Tau, 30(3).

Longfellow HW. (1975). *The political works of Longfellow,* Cambridge ed. Boston: Houghton-Mifflin.

McGuane E, and Bullough B. (1992, Dec). Proud history, promising future. *Pract Nurs,* 40–42.

Metules T. (1998, Dec). Pins and pinning-the traditions continue. *RN,* 12.

NLN Research and Policy. (1994). Practical nursing's role in a community-based health care system. *Prism: NLN,* 2:1–8.

Philips E. (1944). Practical nurses in a public agency. *Am J Nurs,* 44:974–975.

Pillitteri A. (1994, June). One nursing curriculum 100 years ago: a retrospective view as a prospective necessity. *J Nurs Ed,* 33(6):286–287.

Romanoff B. (2006, May). *Facts about Flo you may not know. Nurse Week,* 7(3):32–33.

Server S. (1998). The story of the lamp. *Am J Pract Nurs,* 5(1).

Seymour M. (2004, Oct 24). 'Nightingales': nurse's aides. *The New York Times*. Retrieved October 25, 2004 from http://www.nytimes.com/2004/10/24/books/review/24SETMOUR.html?8bu=8pageswanted=printandposition=.

Sigma Theta Tau International. (2006, Nov 5). *Helping nurses help others*. Indianapolis: Nursing Knowledge International.

Silvestri L. (2003). *Saunders comprehensive review for NCLEX-PN* (2nd ed.). Philadelphia: WB Saunders.

Thompson M. (1955). *The cry and the covenant*. New York: Signet Books.

Widerquist J. (1992). The spirituality of Florence Nightingale. *Nurs Res*, 41(1):49–55.

Chapter 8

Alfaro-LeFevre R. (2002). *Applying nursing process: promoting collaborative care* (5th ed.). Philadelphia: Lippincott.

ANA continuing education: nursing nomenclature and needed taxonomies for health care. 2000 Nursing Classification 1. Retrieved February 3, 2000 from http://nursingworld.org/mod7/cec1full.htm#accumulate.

Christensen B, and Kockrow E. (2006). *Foundations and adult health nursing* (Ch. 5). St Louis: Mosby.

Frederick J, et al. (2002). Speaking a common language. *AJN*, 101(3):2400.

Ham K. (2002). *From LPN to RN: role transitions* (Ch. 7). Philadelphia: WB Saunders.

Ignatavicius D, and Workman M. (2006). *Medical-surgical nursing: critical thinking for collaborative care* (5th ed.). Philadelphia: WB Saunders.

Johnson M, Bulechek G, and Dochterman J, et al. (2001). *Nursing diagnoses, outcomes, and interventions: NANDA, NOC and NIC Linkages*. St Louis: Mosby.

Johnson M, Maas M, and Moorhead S. (2000). *Nursing outcomes classification*. St Louis: Mosby.

Maslow A. (1943). A theory of human motivation. *Psych Rev* 50:370.

McCloskey JC, and Bulechek GM. (2000). *Nursing interventions classification* (3rd ed.). St Louis: Mosby.

MEDI-SMART. *Study tips from former nursing students*. Retrieved April 13, 2007 from http://medi-smart.com/study-tips.htm.

NAPNES. (2007, Summer). Standards of practice and educational competencies of graduates of practical/vocational nursing programs. *JPN*, 57(2).

National Council of State Boards of Nursing. Implementation of the 1999 NCLEX-PN test plan. (1998). In *Issues*. Chicago: NCSBN, pp 4–5.

National Council of State Boards of Nursing. *NCLEX-PN® test plan for the National Council Licensure Examination for Practical Nurses*. (2007). Chicago: NCSBN.

National Council of State Boards of Nursing. *NCLEX-PN® test plan for the National Council Licensure Examination for Practical/Vocational Nurses*. (2008). Chicago: NCSBN.

National Council of State Boards of Nursing. *NCLEX-PN® test plan for the National Council Licensure Examination for Practical/Vocational Nurses*. (2001, effective date April 2002). Chicago: NCSBN.

National Council of State Boards of Nursing. *NCLEX-PN® test plan for the National Council Licensure Examination for Practical/Vocational Nurses*. (1998, effective date April 1999). Chicago: NCSBN.

National Council of State Boards of Nursing. *NCLEX-PN® test plan for the National Council Licensure Examination for Practical Nurses*. (1995, effective date October 1996). Chicago: NCSBN.

Peseit DJ, and Herman J. (1998). OPT: Transformation of nursing process for contemporary practice. *Nurs Outlook* 46.

Chapter 9

Alessandra T. Sixteen common-sense listening tips. *ADVANCE for LPNs*. Retrieved March 3, 2005 from http://LPN.advanceweb.com/common/Editorial/Editorial.aspx?CC=4953.

Arnold E, and Boggs KU. (2003). *Interpersonal relationships; professional communication skills for nurses* (4th ed.). Philadelphia: WB Saunders.

Balzer-Riley JW. (2000). *Communications in nursing* (4th ed.). St Louis: Mosby.

Banotai A. Simplified strategies. *ADVANCE for LPNs*. Retrieved January 25, 2007 from www.advanceweb.com.

Bush K. (2001, March). *Do you really listen?* Retrieved from www.rnweb.com, 64:3.

Carey B. In the hospital, a degrading shift from person to patient. (10/16, 2005), *The New York Times*. Retrieved August 17, 2005 from http://www.nytimes.com/2005/08/16/health/16dignity.html?ex=1124942400anden=dlc1749…

Carson VB. (2000). The vehicle for healing: communication as part of a therapeutic relationship. In *Mental health nursing, the nurse-patient journey* (2nd ed., Ch. 10). Philadelphia: WB Saunders.

Federwische A. (2007). *RN and physician communication: from conflict to collaboration*. 2007 Spring Med/Surg Specialty Guide. www.nurse.com.

Fuimano, J. (2004, Dec 13) *Language matters*. *ADVANCE for LPNs*. Retrieved June 11, 2004 from http://www.advanceforlpn.com/common/editorial/PrintFriendly.aspx?CC=35819.

Gurian M. (1997). *The wonder of boys*. New York: Jeremy P. Tacher/Putnam.

Holman H. (2001, Dec). *Bottom line: providing age-appropriate care in healthcare organizations early through late adulthood*. NFLPN.

Holman J. (2001, May). *Providing age appropriate care in healthcare organizations: infancy to adolescence*. NFLPN.

Lauchnan R. (1999, June). Using email for effective and efficient communication. *Vitality*, 11.

London F. (2004). How to prepare families for discharge in the limited time available. *Pediatr Nurs*, 30(3): 212–214, 227. Retrieved August 13, 2004 from http://www.medscape.com/viewarticle/483097_print.

March A. (2002, April 1).: Are you really listening? *Bottom Line*, 23(7).

Sieh A. and Brentin L. (1997). *The nurse communicates.* Philadelphia: WB Saunders.

Tannen D. (1990). *You just don't understand.* New York: Ballantine Books.

Tokarski C. (2005). Better communication needed to reduce medical errors. *Medscape Medical News.* Retrieved February 4, 2005 from http://www.medscape.com/viewarticle/498276_print.

Ustun B. (2006, Oct). Communication skills training as part of a problem-based learning curriculum. *J Nurs Educ,* 45(10):421–424.

Chapter 10

ACE (2007). *Exercise you can't do without.* Retrieved 2/20/2007@ http://www.acefitness.org/fitfacts/fitbits_display.aspx?items=231.

Associated Press (2007, April 26). Study: *Overweight workers cost employers more.* Retrieved July 14, 2008 from http://www.usatoday.com/news/health/2007-04-23-overweight-worker-study_N.htm.

Baron, J. (2007). *Stress: A trigger for disease in advance for nurses.* Retrieved 2/24/2007 @ http://nursingadvanceweb.com/common/editorial/editorial.aspx?cc+84388.

Beattie M. (1992). *Codependent no more: How to stop controlling others and start caring for yourself.* Center City, MN: Hazelton.

Burnout: signs, symptoms, and prevention. Retrieved April 8, 2007 from www.Helppguide.org/mental/burnout_signs_symptoms.htm.

CDC. *General information on hand hygiene,* Retrieved April 8, 2007 from http://www.cdc.gov/nceh/vsp/cruiselines/hand_hygiene_general.htm.

Converso A, and Murphy C. (2004). Winning the battle against back injuries. *RN,* 67:2, 52–57.

Crocker E. *Learning to save your back.* Advance NewsMagazine for LPNs. King of Prussia, PA: Merion Publications. Retrieved August 1, 2006 from www.advanceweb.com.

Dunbar C. (2006, July 31). Infection squads. *Nurs Spectr.*

Dunbar S, and Levitt S. (2006, September 24), Freakonomics: selling soap. *The New York Times.*

Emery C. (2006). *Simple measures to reduce infections: Hopkins study finds catheter rules, clean hands aid hospitals.* Retrieved from http://www.baltimoresun.com/news/health/bal-te.infection 28dec28.0.7609251.story?coll=bal-home-headlines.

Girou E, et al. Efficacy of hand rubbing with alcohol based solution versus standard hand washing with antiseptic soap: randomized clinical trial. *BJM,* Retrieved April 8, 2007 from http://www.bjm.com/cgi/content/full/325/7360/362.

Goldman D. (2006). System failure versus personal accountability: the case for clean hands. *N Engl J Med,* 355(2):121–123.

Hand hygiene and multidrug-resistant organisms. (2004) *AJN,* 104(8):51.

Illustrated Health Encyclopedia (2007). Physical Activity. Retrieved 2/20/2007 @ http://stateman. com/health/healthfd/shared/health/adam/ency/article/001941.html.

McCaughey B. (2005, June 6). Coming clean. *The New York Times.* Retrieved June 7, 2005 from http://www.nytimes.com/2005/06/opinion/06mccaughey.html?th=andemc=thandpageswanted=print.

Mollard K. (2003). *Anatomy of a workout.* Duluth, MN: St Mary's Personal Fitness Center.

Nelson A, Fragala G, and Menzel N. (2003). Myths and facts about back: injuries in nursing. *Am J Nurs,* 103(2):32–41.

NIAAA. *A snapshot of annual high-risk college drinking consequences.* Retrieved May 2, 2007 from http://www.collegedrinkingprevention.gov/StatsSummaries/snapshot.aspx.

Rothrock J. (2006). What are the current guidelines about wearing artificial nails ans nail polish in the healthcare setting? *Medscape Nurses,* 8(2).

Tierro P. (2007). *Germ-fighting secrets: a leading microbiologist tells how to stay healthy.* Boulder, CO: Bottom Line.

University of Maryland Medical Center (2007). What are some specific stress reduction methods? Retrieved 3/25/2007 @ http://www.umm.edu/patended/articles/

USDA. (2005). *Anatomy of MyPramid.* Inside the pyramid. MyPyramid education framework. Why is physical activity important? Retrieved April 18, 2007 from www.MyPramid.gov.

U.S. Department of Health and Human Services (2003, May). *FDA Fact sheet on hand hygiene in retail and food service establishments.* Retrieved April 8, 2007 from http://vm.cfsan.fda.gov/~comm/handhyg.html.

Weiss B. (2005). Winning the battle with addiction. *RN,* 68(7):63–66.

Willett W. (2001). *Eat, drink, and be happy.* New York: Simon and Schuster.

Chapter 11

About us. Nurses for a healthier tomorrow. Updated 2006. Retrieved March 27, 2007 from http://www.nursesource.org/mission.html.

American Association of Colleges of Nursing. (2006). *Student enrollment rises in U.S. nursing colleges and universities for the 6th consecutive year.* Retrieved March 19, 2007 from http://www.aacn.nche.eduMedia/News/Releases/06Survey.htm.

American Association of Colleges of Nursing. (2007) *Nursing faculty shortage.* Retrieved March 19, 2007 from http://www.aacn.nche.edu/Media/FactSheets/FacultyShortage.htm.

American Association of Colleges of Nursing. (2007). *White paper on the education and role of the clinical nurse leader.* Retrieved February 27, 2007 from www.aacn.org.

American Association of Colleges of Nursing. *Nursing fact sheet.* Updated March 2007. Retrieved March 17, 2007 from http://www.aacn.nche.edu/MEDIA/FactSheets/nursfact.htm.

American Association of Colleges of Nursing (updated May, 20, 2008). *Support increased funding for Title VIII nursing workforce development.* Retrieved June 28, 2007 from aacn.nche.edu/Government/pdf/08 TitleVIIIFS.pdf.

American Association of Colleges of Nursing. *The essentials of doctoral education for advanced nursing practice.* Endorsed 10/30/06. Retrieved March 7, 2007 from www.aacn.org.

American Nurses Credentialing Center. (2007) *ANCC announces next generation nursing certification credentials.* Retrieved October 3, 2007 from www.nursecredentialing.org.

American Nurses Credentialing Center. (2007) *Certification and certification renewal.* Retrieved March 18, 2007 from http://www.nursecredentialing.org/cert/announce.html.

Auerbach D, et al. (2007) *Health Affairs,* 26(1):178–185.

Bureau of Labor Statistics, U.S. Department of Labor, *Occupational outlook handbook.* 2008–09 Edition, Licensed Practical and Licensed Vocational Nurses. Retrieved June 26, 2008 from http://www.bls.gov/oco/print/ocos102.htm.

The business case for nurse staffing. (2006). Washington, DC: Retrieved March 19, 2007 from www.academyhealth.org/connectingthedots/nursestaffing.pdf.

Chitty K, and Black B. *Professional nursing: concepts and challenges.* St Louis: Saunders/Elsevier. 2007.

Christensen B, and Kockrow E. (2006). *Foundations of nursing.* St Louis: Mosby.

Clinical doctorate in nursing: a newsmaker interview with Mary O'Neil Mundinmger, DrPH, executive summary from the nursing data review, academic year 2004–2005, baccalaureate, associate degree, and diploma programs. (2006, Oct) *Nurs Educ Perspect,* 27(5):267–269.

Hathaway D. *Introducing the doctor of nursing practice.* Posted on Medscape General Medicine on 4/7/06. Retrieved from www.medscape.com.

Henderson V. (1966). *The nature of nursing: a definition and its implications for practice, research and education.* New York: Macmillan.

Huber D. (2006). *Leadership and nursing care management.* Philadelphia: Elsevier/Saunders.

Lafer G, and Moss, H. (May, 2007). *A practical way to alleviate the nursing shortage.* A report prepared for the United Nurses of America, AFSCME, AFL-CIO.

LeMoult C. *Why so few male nurses?* Columbia News Service, April 18, 2006. Retrieved March 18, 2007 from http://jscms.jrn.columbia.edu/cns/2006–04–18/lemoult-malenurses/

Mason D. (2006, July). Mentored by an LPN. *Am J Nurs,* 106(7):11.

Men in nursing: still too few. (2006, Feb) *Am J Nurs,* 106(2):25–26.

National Council of State Boards of Nursing. *NCLEX-PN® Examination Test Plan for the National Council Licensure Examination for Licensed Practical/Vocational Nurses.* (effective April, 2005) Chicago: NCSBN.

National Council of State Boards of Nursing. 2008 *NCLEX-PN test plan.* Chicago: NCSBN.

Needleman J, Buerhaus P, Stewart M, et al. (2006). Nurse staffing in hospitals: is there a business case for staffing? *Health Affairs,* 25(1):204–211.

Nursing gets attention from philanthropists. (2007, Jan) *Am J Nurs,* 107(1):25–26.

Nursing shortage: no signs of relief. (2007, Winter) *Visions,* 113(1):1.

Nursing shortage update: a conversation with Peter Buerhaus (Fourth Quarter) *Reflections on Nursing Leadership,* 33(7). Retrieved December 31, 2007 from http:www2.nursingsociety.org/RNL/Current/features/feature2.htm.

Seago J, et al. (2004, Nov. 1) *Supply, demand, and use of licensed practical nurses.* Health Resources and Services Administration, Bureau of Health Professions, National Center for Health Workforce Analysis.

Seago J, et al. (2006). Can the use of LPNs alleviate the nursing shortage? *Am J Nurs,* 106(2):40–50.

Seago J, et al. (2007). How can LPNs ease the nursing shortage? *LPN2007,* 3(1):16, 18–19.

Smith A. (2005) An interview with Peter I. Buerhaus, PhD, RN, FAAN: on hopes and threats for nursing's future. *Nursing Economics,* 25(3): 183–185

Sorrentino S, and Gorek B. (2005). *Basic skills for nursing assistants in long-term care.* St Louis: Elsevier/Mosby.

Study examines LPN workforce. *NLN: Nursing Education Policy,* July 28, 2004.

Thieman L. (2006, July/August). To be or not to be . . . an LPN. *LPN2006,* 2(1):4–5

The truth, the whole truth, and nothing but the truth. (Winter 2006/Spring 2007). *The Jrnl of Pract Nurs,* 56(4): 5.

U.S. Department of Health and Human Services. *HRSA is the nation's access agency.* Retrieved March 29, 2007 from http://www.hrsa.gov/about/default.htm.

Wendt A. (2007). *2006 LPN/VN practice analysis: linking the NCLEX-PN examination to practice.* Chicago: National Council of State Boards of Nursing.

Yoder-Wise P. (2007). *Leading and managing in nursing.* St Louis: Mosby.

Zuzelo, P. (2007). *The clinical nurse specialist handbook.* Boston: Jones and Bartlett.

Chapter 12

Carroll R. The evil eye. *The skeptic's dictionary.* Retrieved on April 29, 2007 from http://skepdic.com/evileye.html.

Confessore N. (2006, June 4). A spoonful of foreign culture helps western medicine go down. *The New York Times.* Retrieved June 4, 2006 from New York Times.com.

Culver V. (1974). *Modern bedside care* (8th ed., pp. 374–384). Philadelphia: WB Saunders.

D'Avanzo C, and Geissler E. (2008). *Pocket guide to cultural assessment.* St Louis: Mosby.

deWit S. (2007). *Medical-surgical nursing: concepts and practice*. Philadelphia: WB Saunders.

Eggenberger S, et al. (2003, Jan 31). Culturally competent nursing care for families: listening to the voices of Mexican-American women. *Online J Issues Nurs*, 8(1). Retrieved April 26, 2007 from *http://nursingworld. org/ojin/topic20/tpc20_5.htm*.

Fadiman A. (1997). *The spirit catches you and you fall down*. New York: Farrar, Strauss, and Giroux.

Foster G. (1978). *Medical anthropology*. New York: John Wiley and Sons.

Goodstein L. (2007, April 15). For some Hispanics, coming to U.S. means abandoning religion. *The New York Times*. Retrieved April 15, 2007 from www.newyorktimes. com/2007/04/15/us/15hispanic.html?th=andemc.

Hall E. (1973 Reissue). *The silent language*. Westport, CT: Greenwood Press.

Hall E. (1966). *The hidden dimension*. New York: Doubleday.

Herndon E. and Joyce L. (2004, June 23). Getting the most from language interpreters. *Medscape*. Retrieved June 29, 2004 from www.medscape. comviewarticle/481334_print.

Honer D, and Hoppie P. (2004, Aug). The enigma of the Gypsy patient. *RN*, 67(8):33–36.

Jackson L. (1993). Understanding, eliciting and negotiating patients' multicultural health beliefs. *Nurse Pract* 18(4):30–32, 37–43.

Joyce E, and Villanueva M. (2004). *Say it in Spanish*. Philadelphia: WB Saunders.

Keefe S. Melting pot. (2005, Aug 29). *ADVANCE for LPNs: New York tri-state area*. pp. 10, 13–14.

Kutner M, et al. (2006). *The health literacy of America's adults: results from the 2003 National Assessment of Health Literacy*. National Center for Education Statistics. Retrieved September 16, 2007 from http://nces.ed.gov/ pubsearch/pubsinfo.asp?pubid=2006483.

Leininger M, and McFarland M. (2002). *Transcultural nursing: concepts, theory, research, and practice*. New York: McGraw-Hill.

Lipson J. (2006). *Culture and nursing care: a pocket guide*. San Francisco: UCSF Nursing Press.

Lobar S, Youngblut J, and Booten D. (2006, April 8). Cross-cultural beliefs, ceremonies, and rituals surrounding death of a loved one. *Medscape*, Retrieved April 15, 2007 from www.medscape. com/viewarticle/525639_print.

Minority Nurse.com. *The career and educational resource for the minority nurse professional*. www.minoritynurse. com/about/index.html.

Navarro M. For younger Latinas, a shift to smaller families." *The New York Times*, Retrieved December 5, 2004 from www.nytimes.com/2004/12/05/ national/05latina.htm?th=andpagewanted= printandposition=.

Ostrowski M. (2006, Sept). Say it in English. *RN*, 69(9):9.

Randall-David E. (1992). *Strategies for working with culturally diverse patients*. Bethesda, MD: Association for the Care of Children's Health.

Reinhardt E. (1995). *Through the eyes of others— intercultural resource directory for health care professionals*. Minneapolis: Hennepin County Medical Society, United Way Intercultural Awareness.

Rodriguez B. (1995, May 18). *Understanding and integrating cultural awareness and related issues into specialized health curricula*. Green Bay, WI: Seminar at Northeast Wisconsin Technical College.

Spector R. (2003). *Cultural diversity in health and illness*. Englewood Cliffs, NJ: Prentice Hall.

Srivastava R. (ed.). (2007). *The healthcare professional's guide to clinical cultural competence*. Canada: Elsevier.

Task Force, Junior League of Minneapolis, and University of Minnesota School of Public Health. *Transcultural nursing: basic concepts and case studies, 1997–2005*. Retrieved April 25, 2007 from www.culturediversity.org/.

Transcultural nursing: basic concepts and case studies, 1997–2005. Retrieved April 25, 2007 from www. culturediversity.org/.

U.S. Census Bureau. *Population Division, Population Projections Branch, 2004*. Retrieved April 25, 2007 from www.census.gov/ipc/www/usinterimproj.

U.S. Census Bureau. *WorldPOPClock Projection, Feb. 18, 2008*. Retrieved April 5, 2007 from www.census.gov/ ipc/www/popclockworld.html.

Varcarolis E, and Shoemaker N. (2006). *Foundations of psychiatric-mental health nursing* (5th ed.). Philadelphia: Elsevier/Saunders.

Chapter 13

Adler J. (2005, Aug/Sept). In search of the spiritual. *MSNBC /Newsweek Society*, August 29-Sept. 5 issue, 2005. Retrieved September 12, 2007 from http://www. msnbc,msn,com/id/9024914/site/newsweek/.

Aita J. (2006, June 21). Young Muslims work to improve Muslim-western understanding. *Washington File*. Retrieved April 29, 2007 from www.usinfo.state.gov.

Armstrong K. (2001). *Buddha*. New York: Penguin Group Penguin Putnam.

Armstrong K. (2000). *Islam*. New York: Random House.

Attwater D (ed.). (1997 [reprint]). *A Catholic dictionary*. Rockford, IL: Tan Books and Publishers.

Baha'ism. (2005). Retrieved May 8, 2007 from http:// www.infoplease.com/ce6/saociety/A0805751.html.

Banerjee N. (2007, April 23). Use of Wiccan symbol on veterans' headstones is approved. *The NewYork Times*. Retrieved April 24, 2007 from New York Times.com

Baptists. (2005). Retrieved May 8, 2007 from www. infoplease.com/ce6/society/AO856842.html.

Barrett D, Kurian G, and Johnson T (eds.). (2001). *World Christian encyclopedia: a comparative survey of churches and religions in the modern world*. New York: Oxford University Press.

Bauer B, and Hill S. (2000). *Mental health nursing: an introductory text*. Philadelphia: WB Saunders.

Beirich H. Radical powerhouse. (2007). *Southern Poverty Law Center: Intelligence Report*. Retrieved May 8, 2007 from www.splcenter.org/intel/intelreport/article. jsp?sid=397.

Bowker J (ed). (2005). *The Oxford dictionary of world religions.* Oxford: Oxford University Press.

Carson V. (1989). *Spiritual dimensions of nursing practice.* Philadelphia: WB Saunders.

Catechism of the Catholic Church. (1994). Liguori, MO: Liguori Publications.

Christian Science. (2005). Retrieved May 8, 2007 from http://www.infoplease.com/ce6/society/A0812103.html.

D'Avanzo C, and Geissler E. (2003). *Pocket guide to cultural assessment.* St Louis: Mosby.

Diamant A. (2007). *The red tent.* New York: Picador® USA.

Episcopal Church. (2005). Retrieved May 8, 2007 from http://www.infoplease.com/ce6/society/A0817503.html.

Esposito J. (1998). *Islam: the straight path.* New York: Oxford University Press.

Friends, Religious Society of. (2005). Retrieved May 8, 2007 from http://www.infoplease.com/ce6/society/A0819726.html.

Gellman M, and Hartman T. (2002). *Religion for Dummies.* New York: Wiley.

Gerardi R. (1989). Western spirituality and health care. In Carson V: *Spiritual dimensions of nursing practice.* Philadelphia: WB Saunders.

Gritsch E. (2002). *A history of Lutheranism.* Minneapolis: Augsburg Fortress.

Gyatso Tenzin (High Holiness the Dalai Lama). (2005). *Essence of the heart sutra.* Somerville, MA: Wisdom Publications.

Huels J. (1982). *The pastoral companion: a canon law handbook for Catholic ministry.* Chicago: Franciscan Herald Press.

Judaism. (2005). Retrieved May 8, 2007 from www.infoplease.com/ippa/a0001462.html.

Lawrence R. (2006, April 11). Faith-based Medicine. *The New York Times.* Retrieved from NewYorkTimes.com.

Leininger M, and McFarland M. (2002). *Transcultural nursing: concepts, theory, research, and practice.* New York: McGraw-Hill.

Lewis B. (2003). *The crisis of Islam.* New York: The Modern Library.

Lindner, EW. (2005). *Yearbook of American and Canadian Churches 2005.* Nashville, TN: Abingdon Press.

Lipson J, and Dibble S, (2006). *Culture and nursing care: a pocket guide.* San Francisco: The Regents of the University of California.

Mainline Protestant Churches No Longer Dominate NCC Yearbook's List of Top 25 U.S. Religious Bodies. News From the National Council of Churches, 3/30/05. Retrieved May 3, 2007 from www.nccusa.org/news/050330yearbook.html.

Mead F, and Hill S. (2005). *Handbook of denominations.* Nashville, TN: Abingdon Press.

Mennonites. Retrieved May 8, 2007 from http://infoplease./com/ce6/society/A0832697.html.

Nomani, A. (2005). *Standing alone in Mecca.* New York: HarperCollins Publishers, Inc.

Pentecostalism. (2005). Retrieved May 8, 2007 from http://www.infoplease.com/ce6/society/A0838204.html.

Pesut B. (2003, Nov/Dec). Developing spirituality in the curriculum. *Nurs Educ Perspect,* 24:6, 290–294.

Prayer and spirituality in health: ancient practices, modern science. (2005, Winter). *CAM at the NIH, XII(1).* Retrieved March 4, 2006 from http://nccam.nih.gov/news/newsletter/2005_winter/prayer.htm.

Proctor S. Beyond the veil. (2006, Sept 6) *ADVANCE for LPNs.* Retrieved November 10, 2006 online.

Prothero S. (2007). *Religious literacy: what every American needs to know—and doesn't.* San Francisco: Harper.

Religious Congregations and Membership (2000). *Glenmary Research Council, 2000.* Retrieved May 3, 2007 from www.glenmary.org/grc/RCMS_2000/findings.htm.

Religious Identification in the U.S. (2006, Dec 3). *Religious Tolerance Org. 12/3/06.* Retrieved May 3, 2007 from www.religioustolerance.org/chr_prac2.htm.

Rite of baptism. (1970). In *Rite of baptism for children.* New York: Corpus Publications.

Roman Catholicism. (2007). Retrieved May 8, 2007 from http://print.infoplease.com/ipa/aoo1466.html.

Schoenbeck S. (1994). Called to care: addressing the spiritual needs of patients. *J Pract Nurs,* 44: 19–23.

Seventh-day Adventists. (2005). Retrieved May 8, 2007 from http://www.infoplease.com/ce6/society/AO802573.html.

Smith-Stoner M. (2005, July 29). End-of-life needs of patients who practice Tibetan Buddhism. *Medscape,* Retrieved August 9, 2005 from www.medscape.com/viewarticle/508915_print.

Sumner C. (1998). Recognizing and responding to spiritual distress. *Am J Nurs,* 98(1):26–30.

Titus H, Smith M, and Nolan R. (1995). *Living issues in philosophy.* Belmont, CA: Wadsworth Publishing.

United Church of Christ. (2005). Retrieved May 8, 2007 from http://www.infoplease.com/ce6/society/A0850059.html.

United Methodist Church. (2005). Retrieved May 8, 2007 from http://www.infoplease.com/ce6/society/A0850064.html.

Wahhabi. (2005). Retrieved May 8, 2007 from www.infoplease.com/ce6/society/A0851259.html.

Chapter 14

American Nurses Association. *Position statements: physical violence against women.* Retrieved March 26, 2003 from www.nursingworld.org/readroom/position/social/scviol.htm.

Bast M. *Collaboration (vs. manipulation, coercion, or throwing your hands up in despair) Self-assessment.* Retrieved April 1, 2007 from http://www.breakoutofthebox.com/manipula.htm.

Bast M. Communicating Assertively. Retrieved April 1, 2007 from http://www.breakoutofthebox.com/assert.htm.

Belanger D. (2000). Nurses and suicide: the risk is real. *RN;* 63(10): 61-4.

California Department of Industrial Relations. *Guidelines for security and safety of health care and community service workers.* DOSH publications. Retrieved April 3, 2007 from http://www.dir.ca.gov/DOSH/dosh_publications/heworker.html.

Cancerline UK. (2002, May 14). *Violence against nurses "still a problem."* Retrieved March 26, 2003 from www.cancerlineuk.net/mainnav1/s_news_feed/s_news_archive/c_news_feed/id373511.pviolence00.htm.

Career planning, job burnout. Retrieved April 8, 2007 from http://careerplanning.about.com/od/workrelated/aburnout.htm.

Carrol, V. (March, 1997). Health and safety in workplace violence. *AM J Nurs* 99(3).

HealthyPlace.com. *Depression community. assertiveness, non-assertiveness, and assertive techniques.* Retrieved April 1, 2007 from http://www.healthyplace.com/Communities/Depression/suicide/assertingourselves.asp.

Improving communications. Assertiveness vs. passive and aggressive behavior. Retrieved April 1, 2007 from http://www.arthritis.ca/tips%20for%20living/communicating%20your%needs/develop%2.

International Journal for Quality in Health Care, Nurse Staffing and Patient Safety. *Current knowledge and implications for action.* Retrieved February 19, 2007 from http://inqhc.oxfordjounals.org/cgi/contents/full/15/4/275.

King S. (1996, August). *Top ten signs you are approaching burnout.* Retrieved February 8, 2007 from http://webpages.charter.net/stormking/topten.html.

Kurz J. (2002, July). Combating sexual harassment. *RN*, 65:7, 65–68.

Levine P, Hewitt J, and Misner S. (1998). Insights of nurses about assault in hospital-based emergency rooms. *Image J Nurs Schol*, 30(3): 9–10.

Lipson J. and Dibble S. (2006). *Culture and clinical care.* San Francisco: UCSS Nursing Press.

New York State Nurse Association. *NYSNA position statement. workplace violence.* Retrieved April 3, 2007 from http://www.nysna.org/programs/nai/practice/positions/position39.htm.

Nurse Advocate. *Violence against nurses: a silent epidemic.* Retrieved March 26, 2003 from www.nurseadvocate.org/silentepidemic.html. (First published in Workplace Violence Prevention Reporter, June 1998, James Publishing.)

Orr T. *Danger zone.* Retrieved November 2, 2002 from www.nurseweek.com/new/features/02–11/dangerzone_web.asp.

Pepin L. (2003). *violence against nurses in the workplace.* Retrieved March 26, 2003 from www.sen.parl.gc.ca/pepin/index.asp?PgId=688.

U.S. Department of Labor. (2004). *OSHA guidelines for preventing workplace violence for health care and social service workers.* Retrieved April 4, 2007 from www.osha.gov.

Chapter 15

Bates S. *Learning to lead.* (2006, May 15). Advance Online Edition for Nurses. Retrieved May 22, 2006.

Bennis W. (2003). *On becoming a leader: the leadership classic—updated and expanded.* Boulder, CO: Perseus Publishing.

Blanchard K, et al. (1985). *Leadership and the one minute manager.* New York: Morrow.

Blanchard K, et al. (1991). *The one minute manager builds high performance teams.* New York: Morrow.

Blanchard K, and Bowles S. (2001). *High five! The magic of working together.* New York: HarperCollin Publishers.

Blanchard K, and Johnson S. (1993). *The one minute manager.* New York: Berkeley Publishing.

Blanchard K, and McBride M. (2003). *The one minute apology.* New York: Harper Collins.

Department of Health and Human Services. *Quality improvement organizations: overview.* (2006). Baltimore: Centers for Medicare and Medicaid Services. Retrieved May 22, 2007 from http://www.cms.hhs.gov/QualityImprovementOrgs/.

Department of Health and Human Services. *Quality improvement organizations: statement of work.* (2005). Baltimore: Centers for Medicare and Medicaid Services. Retrieved May 22, 2007 from http://www.cms.hhs.gov/QualityImprovementOrgs/04_9thsow.asp.

Ellis A. (1994). *Reason and emotion in psychotherapy.* New York: Carol Publishing Group.

Fisher R, Ury W, and Patton B. (2003). *Getting to yes: negotiating agreement without giving in.* New York: Random House Business Books.

George B. (2006, Oct 30).Truly authentic leadership. *U.S. News and World Report.* pp. 52, 54.

Goleman D, Boyatzis R, and McKee A. (2002). *Primal leadership: realizing the power of emotional intelligence.* Boston: Harvard Business School Publishing.

Gonzalez C. *Diffusing discords.* (2007, May 28). Advance Online Edition for Nurses. Retrieved June 13, 2007 from http://nursing.advanceweb.com/Common/Editorial/PrintFriendly.as.

Herzberg F. (1993). *The motivation to work.* New Brunswick, NJ: Transaction Pubs.

Hirschy B. (2006, Jan). Like it or not—nurses are leaders. *Nursingmatters*, 18(1):4–5.

Howlett H. (1989, Nov; amended 2007). The Howlett theory of management for nursing instructors (unpublished paper).

Huber, D. *Leadership and nursing care management.* St Louis: Elsevier, 2006.

Lencioni P. (2005). *Overcoming the five dysfunctions of a team: a field guide for leaders, managers, and facilitators.* San Francisco: Jossey-Bass.

Maslow A. (1998). *Maslow on management.* New York: John Wiley and Sons.

Sorrentino S, Gorek B. (2007). *Mosby's textbook for long-term care assistants.* St Louis: Mosby.

Thomas K. (2003). *Intrinsic motivation at work: building energy and commitment.* San Francisco: Berrett-Koehler Publications.

Vision and expertise: nursing education and the future. (1995). Seminar presented by Venner Farley, RN, Lake Geneva, WI, April 24–25, 1995.

Wendt A. (2007). *2006 LPN/VN practice analysis: linking the NCLEX-PN examination to practice* (Research Brief Vol. 28). Chicago: National Council of State Boards of Nursing.

Wywialowski E. (2004). *Managing patient care*. St Louis: Mosby.

Yoder-Wise P. (2007). *Leading and managing in nursing*. St Louis: Mosby.

Chapter 16

Bauer B, and Hill S. (2000). *Mental health nursing: an introductory text*. Philadelphia: WB Saunders.

Blanchard K, Oncken W, and Burrows H. (1989). *The one minute manager meets the monkey*. New York: William Morrow.

Darrah J. (2007, Feb 26). Changing with the times. *ADVANCE for LPNs*, 7(2):19–20, 23–24.

deWit S. (2005). *Fundamental concepts and skills for nursing*. Philadelphia: Elsevier.

Grumet B. Personal communication, April 20, 2005.

Hansten R, and Jackson M. (2004). *Clinical delegation skills: a handbook for professional practice*. Boston: James and Bartlett.

Hansten R, and Washburn M. (2001, March 12). Delegating to UAPs—making it work. *NurseWeek*, 2:3, 21–22.

Howlett H. (1989, Nov; amended 2007). The Howlett theory of management for nursing instructors (unpublished paper).

LaCharity L, Kumagai C, and Bartz B. (2006). *Prioritization, delegation, assignment*, St Louis: Elsevier/Mosby.

Linton A. (2007). *Introduction to medical-surgical nursing*. St Louis: Elsevier.

McVay S. (2007, March/April). Conflict resolution: turning a negative into a positive. *LPN2007*, 3(2):9–10.

National Council of State Boards of Nursing. (1995). *Acceptable use of the authority to delegate: delegation: concepts and decision-making process*. Chicago: NCSBN.

Nightingale F. (1946). *Notes on nursing. What it is, and what it is not*. Philadelphia: Edward Stern and Co.

Rachels M. (1994, Aug 24). President of the National Council of State Boards of Nursing. Letter.

Reynolds J. (2007, March). Negativity in the workplace. *AJN*, 107(3):72D–72F.

Romero S. (2005, April 13). Creating a caring culture. *ADVANCE for LPNs*. Retrieved April 19, 2005 from http://LPN.advanceweb.com/common/Editorial/PrintFriendly.aspx?CC=51987.

Romero S. Taking control. (2006, Jan 25). *ADVANCE for LPNs*. Retrieved January 27, 2006 from http://LPN.advanceweb.com/common/editorial/PrintFriendly.aspx?CC=66192.

Schaeffer, N. (2007, Feb 26). Leading a Diverse Staff. *ADVANCE for LPNs*, 7(2):17, 18.

Schroeder, S. (2007, March/April). Improving Intershift Handoff—and Patient Safety. *LPN2007*, 3(2):22–23.

The Joint Commission. *2007 National patient safety goals*. Retrieved June 1, 2007 from http://www.jcrinc.com/13474/.

Ulrich B. (1992). *Leadership and management according to Florence Nightingale*. Norwalk, CT: Appleton and Lange.

Wendt A. (2006). *2005 Job analysis of nurse aides* (Research Brief Vol. 23). Chicago: National Council of State Boards of Nursing.

Wendt A. (2007). *Report of findings from the 2006 LPN/VN practice analysis: linking the NCLEX-PN examination to practice* (Research Brief Vol. 28). Chicago: National Council of State Boards of Nursing. Retrieved from www.ncsbn.org/359.htm.

Wisconsin Association of Licensed Practical Nurses. *Neumann Update on legal matters in the State of Wisconsin*. (1995, Nov 3). *Fall Conference of WALPN*, Wisconsin Dells, WI.

Working with others: a position paper. Attachment A of the NCSBN 2005 Annual Meeting. *Mission impossible: building a safer workforce through regulatory excellence*. Retrieved from ncsbn.org under delegation.

Wywialowski E. (2004). *Managing patient care*. St Louis: Mosby.

Yoder-Wise P. (2007. *Leading and managing in nursing*. St Louis: Mosby.

Chapter 17

AHCA. *Alternatives to nursing homes, nursing home guide*. Retrieved April 4, 2007 from http://ahcaxnet.fdhc.state.fl.us/nhcguide/alternatives.shtml.

BUPA Care Homes. *Types of care*. Retrieved April 4, 2007 from http://www.bupacarehomes.co.uk/asp/guidance/typesofcare.asp.

CAPC Manual. *Financing subacute and skilled care*. Retrieved May 14, 2003 from http://64.85.16.230/educate/content/elements/financingsubacutecare.html.

Christensen BL. (2006). Home health nursing. In Christensen BL, and Kockrow (eds.). *Foundations of nursing* (5th ed.). St Louis: Mosby.

Gliem V. (2000, Nov 6). History of Detroit's black hospitals detailed in project. *The University Record*. Retrieved April 30, 2003 from http://www.umich.edu/~urecord/0001/Nov06_00/10.htm.

Health pages. *All hospitals are not created equal*. Retrieved April 30, 2003 from www.thehealthpages.com/articles/ar-hosps.html.

Health Scope. *Types of hospitals*. Retrieved April 30, 2003 from www.healthscope.org/Interface/hospitals/types_of_hospitals.asp.

Helpguide. *Nursing homes (skilled nursing facilities)*. Retrieved April 4, 2007 from http://www.helpguide.org/elder/nursing_homes_skilled_nursing_facilities.htm.

Linton AD, Matteson, MA, and Maebius NK. (2000). Patient care settings. In *Nursing care of adults*, (2nd ed, ch 2). Philadelphia: WB Saunders.

Nursing homes–how to compare. In *Helping your aging parent*. Boomer Books. Retrieved April 4, 2007 from http://www.boomer-books.com/nursing_homes/how-to-find-a%20nursing-home.htm.

Strong health. Seniors. Retrieved April 4, 2007 from http://www.stronghealth.com/services/seniors/Caring/levelsofcare.cfm.

U.S. Department of Health and Human Services. *Glossary of terms*. Retrieved May 14, 2003 from http://aspe.hhs.gov/dalcp/diction.shml.

U.S. Department of Health and Human Services. *Medicare*. Retrieved April 4, 2007 from http://www.medicare.gov/LongTermCare/Static/typesoverview.asp.

Chapter 18

$4 Prescriptions. WalMart.com, 2007. Retrieved July 30, 2007 from http://www.walmart.com/catalog/catalog.gsp?cat=546834

Barry P. (2003, June). Why drugs cost less up north. *AARP Bull*, 44:6, 8, 10.

Cherry B, and Jacob S. (2007). *Contemporary nursing: issues, trends, and management*. St Louis: Mosby.

Chitty K, and Black, B. (2007). *Professional nursing: concepts and challenges*. St Louis: Elsevier/Saunders.

DeBack, V. (2007, March). The U.S. health care system: the best or just the most expensive? *Nursingmatters*, 18(3):6, 13.

e-Alert. *The Commonwealth Fund*. (2007, Aug 28). Retrieved August 28, 2007 from www.amwf.org.

e-Alert. *The Commonwealth Fund*. (2008). Retrieved May 30, 2008 from www.amwf.org.

Electronic health records: useful tools or high-tech headache? (2007, March). *AJN*, 107(3):25–26.

England M. (2007). Diagnosing the U.S. health care system. *America*, 197(18): 9–13.

Falling into the doughnet hole. (2006, Oct 6). *The New York Times*. Retrieved October 2, 2006 from http://www.nytimes.com.

Freudenheim M. (2006, Sept 27). Health care costs rise twice as much as inflation. *The New York Times*. Retrieved September 30, 2007 from http://www.nytimes.com.

Freudenheim M. (2007, April 6). New urgency in debating health care. *The New York Times*. Retrieved April 7, 2007 from http://select.nytimes.com/mem/tnt.html?tntget=2007/04/06/business.

Gawande A. (2007, May 10). Curing the system. *The New York Times*. Retrieved May 10, 2007 from nytimes.com.

Gawande A. (2007). The Obama health plan. *The New York Times*. Retrieved May 31, 2007 from nytimes.com.

Gerber M. Hospitals are beyond compare. (2007). *Washington Post*. Retrieved July 3, 2007 from http://www.washingtonpost.com/wp-dyn/content/article/2007/06/2.

Graham J. (2007 8). Should age determine who gets a kidney transplant? *Chicago Tribune*. Retrieved February 8, 2007 from http://www.chicagotribune.com.

Hacker J. (2007). Healing our sicko health care system. *N Engl J Med*, 357(8):733–735. Retrieved August 25, 2007 from http://content.nejm.org/cgi/content/full/357/8/733?query=TOC.

Hadley J, and Holahan J. (2004) *The cost of care for the uninsured: what do we spend, who pays, and what would full coverage add to medical spending?* Washington, DC: The Kaiser Commission on Medicaid and the Uninsured. Retrieved August 7, 2007 from http://covertheuninsured.org/media/research/KaiserReport.pdf.

Hall E. (2003, Oct 3). *U.S. national debt clock FAQ*. Retrieved September 26, 2003 from www.brillig.com/debt_clock/faq.html.

Health care reform in the United States: arguments for a single-payer system. (2006, Aug). *Public Citizen Health Research Group Health Letter* 22(8):1–3.

Hoffman C, and Tolbert J. (2006, Oct). *Health savings accounts and high deductible health plans: are they an option for low-income families?* Kaiser Family Foundation. Retrieved August 20, 2007 from http://www.kff.org.

Insuring America's health: principles and recommendations (report brief). (2004). Institute of Medicine of the National Academies. Retrieved August 7, 2007 from http://www.iom.edu/?id=19175.

Japsen B. (2006). America bails out on HMOs. *Chicago Tribune*. Retrieved November 19, 2006 from http://www.chicagotribune.com/features/lifestyle/health/chi-0611190266nov.19.1.6215594story?coll=chi-health-hed.

Kaiser Family Foundation. (2006). *Medicaid and the uninsured: health savings accounts and high deductible health plans: are they an option for low-income families?*. Retrieved August 7, 2006 from http://www.kff.org.

Kaiser Family Foundation (2007). *2007 Benchmark study finds health insurance premiums continue to rise faster than wages*. Retrieved September 11, 2007 from www.kff.org.

Kaiser Family Foundation. *Fast Facts* (2008). Retrieved on May 29, 2008 from http://www.kff.org.

Kaiser Family Foundation. (2007, Aug). *Health care costs: a primer*. Retrieved August 8, 2007 from www.kff.org.

Kaiser Family Foundation. (2007). *New report compares health spending in U.S. to other countries*. Retrieved January 4, 2007 from http://www.kff.org.

Kaiser Family Foundation. (2007, March). *Medicaid: a primer*. Retrieved March 27, 2007 from http://www.kff.org.

Kaiser Family Foundation. (2007). *Medicare advantage*. Retrieved August 7, 2007 from http://www.kff.org.

Kaiser Family Foundation. (2007). *Medicare prescription drug benefit fact sheet*. Retrieved July 15, 2007 from http://www.kff.org.

Kaiser Family Foundation. (2007, Aug 20). *Medicare will not pay for preventable conditions acquired at hospitals*. Retrieved August 20, 2007 from http://www.kaisernetwork.org/daily_reports/print_report.cfm?DR_I.

Kolata G. (2007). Some chronically ill adults wait for Medicare. *The New York Times*. Retrieved July 12, 2007 from http://www.nytimes.com/2007/07/12/us/12medicare.html?th=andemc.

Krauss C. (2006, Feb. 26). As Canada's slow-motion public health system falters, private medical care is surging. *The New York Times*. Retrieved July 22, 2007 from http://www.nytimes.com/2006/02/26/international/americas/26canad.

Kristof N. A short American life. (2007). *The New York Times*. Retrieved May 21, 2007 from http://select.nytimes.com/mem/tnt.html?tntget=2007/05/21/opinion.

Krugman P. (2006). Death by insurance. *The New York Times*. Retrieved May 1, 2006 from http://www.nytimes.com.

Lee J. (2006). For insurance, adult children ride piggyback. *The New York Times*. Retrieved September 18, 2007 from www.nytimes.com.

Lillesand K. (2007). "Sicko:" a must-see for anyone interested in health care. *Nursingmatters*, 18(8):2.

Many eligible for child health plan have no idea. (2007). *The New York Times*. Retrieved August 22, 2007 from http://select.nytimes.com/mem/tnt.html?emc=tntandtntget=2007/08/2.

Mason D. EDs in crisis. (2007). *Am J Nurs*, 107(1):40–47.

Massachusetts Nurses Association. *Definition of single-payer terms*. Retrieved August 12, 2007 from http://www.massnurses.org/single_payer/definitions.htm.

Pear R. (2007). Democrats press house to expand health care bill. *The New York Times*. Retrieved August 24, 2007 from www.nytimes.com.

Pear R. (2003). New study finds 60 million uninsured during a year. *The New York Times*. Retrieved May 13, 2003 from http://www.nytimes.com/2003/05/13/health/13HEAL.html?th=andpagewanted=printandposition.

Pear R. (2006). Medicare links doctor's pay to practices. *The New York Times*. Retrieved December 13, 2006 from www.nytimes.com.

Povich E. (2006). Medical nest egg. *AARP Bull*, 47(4):22.

Public vs private health care. (2006). *CBC news*. Retrieved July 22, 2007 from http://www.cbc.ca/news/background/healthcare/public_vs_private.html.

Pulcini J. (2007). The State Children's Health Insurance Program. *AJN*, 107(3):29–30, 32.

Retail health clinics on the rise. (2007). *Am J Nurs*, 107(7):25–26.

Reuters, (December 31, 2007). *Bush signs child health extension into law*. Retrieved January 9, 2008 from http://www.medscape.com/viewarticle/568112_print.

Shuman J. (1995). Navigating the white waters of change. *Am J Nurs*, 95(pt 1 of 2):15–17.

Slavin S. (1999). *Economics: a self-teaching guide*. New York: John Wiley and Sons.

Steinbrook R. (2006). Private health care in Canada. *N Engl J Med*. Retrieved July 18, 2007 from http://www.nejm.org.

The Commonwealth Fund Commission on a High Performance Health System. (2006). *Why not the best? Results from a national scorecard on U.S. health system performance*. Vol. 34. Retrieved July 28, 2007 from http://www.commonwealthfund.org/publications/publications_show.

The Joint Commission. (2007). *Facts about The Joint Commission*. Retrieved May 22, 2007 from http://www.jointcommission.org/AboutUs/joint_commission_facts.htm.

The Pew Research Center, (January 24, 2005). *An even more partisan agenda for 2008*. Retrieved January 30, 2008 from http://people-press.org/reports/display.php3?Report ID=388.

The President's risky health plan. (2007). *The New York Times*. Retrieved January 26, 2007 from http://www.nytimes.com.

Toner R. (2007). 2008 Candidates vow to overhaul U.S. health care. *The New York Times*. Retrieved July 6, 2007 from http://www.nytimes.com.

U.S. Department of Health and Human Services (January 2008). *Medicare and you*. CMS publication number 10050. Retrieved from http://www.cms.hhs.gov/apps/media/press/factsheet.asp?Counter=361.

Understanding the Medicare program. (2007). *AgeWISE*. Madison, WI: WEA Trust.

Washington Health Policy Week in Review. (2007). *The Commonwealth Fund*. Retrieved August 20, 2007 from http://www.commonwealthfund.org/healthpolicyweek/healthpolicyw.

World's best medical care? (2007, Aug 12). *The New York Times*. Retrieved August 12, 2007 from http://select.nytimes.com/mem/tnt.html?tntget=2007/08/12/opinion.

World Health Organization (2007). *World Health Organization assesses the world's health systems*. Retrieved July 28, 2007 from http://www.who.int/whr/2000/media_centre/press_release/en/index.html.

Yi D. Report criticizes high deductibles. (2006, Dec 8). *latimes.com* Retrieved November 10, 2007 from http://www.latimes.com/business/la-fi-health8dec08,0,4362137,story?coll=la-headlines-business.

Zimmerman M, and Huffstutter P. (2007). Health costs to top auto talks. *Baltimore Sun*. Retrieved July 13, 2007 from http://www.baltimoresun.com/business/bal-bz.automakers11jul,1,2731076,print.story?coll=bal-businessheadlinesandctrack=1andcset=true

Chapter 19

Armstrong RM. (2003). *Turning to Islam: African-American conversion stories*. Chicago: Christian Century.

Brent N. (2001). Ethics and nursing practice. In *Nursing and the law: a guide to principles and applications*. Philadelphia: WB Saunders.

Carpenter, A. (2007). Ethical suspicion and Katrina's nurses. *AJN*, 107(3):15.

deWit S. (2005). *Fundamental concepts and skills for nursing* (Ch. 3). Elsevier/Saunders: Philadelphia.

Haddad A. (2005). Ethics in action. *RN*, 68(5).

Ham K. (2000). Legal/ethical components of nursing. In *From LPN to RN role transitions* (Ch. 10). Philadelphia: WB Saunders.

Health workers can refuse to participate in procedures. (2003). In *Midwest/Heartland NurseWeek*, 4:3.

O'Keefe M. (2001). Ethics in nursing. In *Nursing practice and the law* (Ch. 4). Philadelphia: FA Davis.

Parker-Feliciono K. (2003). Legal and ethical aspects of nursing. In Christensen B, and Kokrow E. *Foundations of nursing* (Ch. 2). St Louis: Mosby.

Rumbold G. (2002). *Ethics in nursing practice* (Ch. 1, 3, 13, 14, 15, 16). Edinburgh: Elsevier Science Ltd.

Shannon J. (2003). *Legal and ethical issues in counseling: a primer for mental health and substance abuse professionals*. Duluth, MN: Workshop.

Soglin B. (2005). *Teaching medical students to examine ethics.* Spectator: University of Iowa.

Tyson S. (2002). Ethical issues with age. In *Gerontological nursing care* (Ch. 3). Philadelphia: WB Saunders.

Venes, D (Ed.) (2005). *Taber Cyclopedic Medical Dictionary.* (20th ed.). Philadelphia: FA Davis, pp. 679–680.

Chapter 20

2001 Partnership in Caring, Inc. (2003). *Choice in dying honoring a legacy.* Retrieved August 11, 2003 from www. partnershipforcaring.org/Aboutus/choice_content. html.

Alfaro-LeFevre R. (2009). *Critical thinking and clinical judgment: a practical approach* (4th ed.). Philadelphia: WB Saunders.

American Hospital Association. (2003). *The patient care partnership: understanding expectations, rights and responsibilities.*

Anderson F. (2007, February). *AJN,* 107(2):66–72.

Bioethics. *Policy on do not resuscitate.* Retrieved May 25, 2007 from http://www.clevelandclinic.org/bioethics/policies/dnr.html.

Brent N. (2001). *Nurses and the law* (2nd ed.). Philadelphia: WB Saunders.

Brown SM. (1999). Good Samaritan laws: protection and limits. *RN,* 62(11):65–68.

Charting Checkup. (2006). Making it clear with an incident report. *LPN2006,* 2(3)17–19.

Christensen E, and Kockrow E. (2006). *Foundations and adult health nursing* (5th ed., Ch. 2). St Louis: Elsevier: Mosby.

Cox R, and Parkman C. (2002, March/April). The end of life movement. *Contin Care,* 23:2.

Daly BJ, Berry D, Fitzpatrick JJ, et al. (1997). Assisted suicide: implications for nurses and nursing. *Nurs Outlook,* 45:209–214.

Dempski K. (2000). If you have to give a deposition. *RN,* 63(1):59–60.

deWit, S. (2005). *Fundamental concepts and skills for nursing* (2nd ed., Ch. 3). Philadelphia: Elsevier Saunders.

DHS Oregon Department of Human Services. (2003). *Physician-assisted suicide: Oregon's Death with Dignity Act.* Retrieved August 11, 2003 from www.dhs.state. or.us/publichealth/chs/pas/pas.cfm.

Earll C. The courts have no constitutional right to assisted suicide. Retrieved from Citizen Link at www.family.org/cforum/research/papers/a0001018. html.

Ecker M. (2003). Protecting patient privacy: understanding the new federal HIPAA standards. Midwest/Heartland *NurseWeek,* pp. 20–21.

Ethics in Medicine. *Physician-assisted suicide.* Retrieved May 25, 2007 from http://depts.washington.edu/bioethx/topics/pas.html.

FamilyDoctor. *Advance directives and do not resuscitate orders.* Retrieved May 25, 2007 from http://familydoctor.org/online/famdocen/home/patadvocacy/endoflife/003.html.

Fest G. (2003). *Legislation would define scope of LVN practice.* Retrieved April 2, 2003 from www.nurseweek. com/news/features/03–02/legislation.asp..

Glazer G. *Legislative and policy issues related to interstate practice.* Retrieved May 17, 2007 from http://www. nursingworld.org/ojin/tpclg/leg_7.htm.

Glazer G. *Multistate licensure: overview and summary.* Retrieved May 17, 2007 from http://www. nursingworld.org/ojin/topic9/tpc.htm.

Goodman M. (2002). *How should incident reports be handled?* Retrieved November 11, 2002 from http://nurses.medscape.com/Medscape/Nurses/AskExperts/2002/01/NP-ae93.html..

Hanawalt A. (2001). End of life issues advanced directives-a health professional's guide to their use. *NFLPN,* 1(1):8–11.

Helm A, and Kihm N. (2006). Liability insurance: is it for you? *LPN2006,* 2(3):14–15.

HIPAA Information. Retrieved May 23, 2007 from http:// www.hipaacompliancebiz/?googadandgclid=CNm7ouS7plwCFQ5cUAodiDxE3g.

HIPAA Rules 101. *Frequently asked questions on HIPAA.* Retrieved May 23, 2007 from http://www. hipaarules101.com/hipaa-faq.htm.

HIPAA Updates (January 2007). Retrieved May 23, 2007 from www.hipaa.com.

Ignatavicius D, and Workman L. (2006). *Medical surgical nursing* (5th ed., Ch. 9). Philadelphia: Elsevier Saunders.

Kirkpatrick C. (2003, March 24). *Safety first: the JCAHO introduces new patient safety goals* (pp. 1–7). Retrieved April 2, 2003 from www.nurseweek.com/ce/ce680a. asp.

Listen up! How to take verbal and telephone orders. (2005). *LPN2005,* 1(2):44–45.

Main A, and Todd, F. (2005, Oct 7) *Depositions 101.* Louisville, KY: American Bar Association Young Lawyers Division.

McNeil D. (2003). *First study on patients who fast to end their lives.* Retrieved Aug 2, 2003 from www.nytimes. com/2003/0731/sciences/31DIE.html..

MedlinePlus. *Advance directives.* Retrieved May 25, 2007 from http://www.nlm.nih.gov/medlineplus/advancedirectives.html.

Minnesota Board of Nursing (2002, 2003). *FYI.* Spring/Summer 2002, 18(2):2, 5; Spring/Summer 2003, 19(1):1–12.

Mosby (2007). *Mosby's surefire documentation* (2006, 2nd ed., pp. 5–7). St Louis: Mosby Elsevier

National Association of Practical Nurse Education and Service. (2003). *NAPNES standards of practice for licensed practical/vocational nurses.* Silver Spring, MD: NAPNES.

National Council of State Boards of Nursing. *Complaints.* Retrieved May 18, 2007 from https://www.ncsbn. org/163.htm.

NCLA: *Participating states in the NCL.* (2007). NCSBN. Retrieved February 15, 2008 from http://www.ncsbn. org.

NFLPN. (2001). *Licensed practical/vocational nurse practice standards*. Raleigh, NC: NFLPN.

O'Keefe M. (2001). *Nursing practice and the law: avoiding malpractice and other legal risks*. Philadelphia: FA Davis.

Oregon. *Death With Dignity Act*. Retrieved May 25, 2007 from http://www.oregon.gov/DHS/ph/pas/faqs.stml.

Oregon's Death With Dignity Law. Retrieved May 25, 2007 from http://theocracywatch.org/oregon_death_dignity.htm.

Phillipsen N, and Haynes D. (2007, March 8). *The multi-state licensure compact: making nurses mobile*. Retrieved May 17, 2007 from http://www.medscape.com/viewarticle/551037.

Potter P, and Perry A. (2003). *Basic nursing: essentials for practice* (5th ed., Ch. 3). St Louis: Mosby.

Quickinfo. (2007, March 16). *National Practitioner Data Bank*. Retrieved May 18, 2007 from info at acnm.org.

Rafter R, and Keown S. (2006). Aim high: achieving JCAHO's National Safety Goals. *LPN*, 2(6):18–20.

Rubinger H, and Gardner R. (2003, March/April). The road to compliance: where are you? *Contin Care*.

Ryan B, Sullivan G, Mackay T, et al. (2007, January). *RN*, 70(1):26–31.

Sloan A. (2001). The national data bank nurses need to know about. *RN*, 64:7, 65–66.

Sullivan GH. (1998). Getting informed consent. *RN*, 61(4):59–62.

Tammelleo AD. (2000). Protecting patients' end-of-life choices. *RN*, 63:8, 75–78.

The Joint Commission. *Facts about the 2007 national patient safety goals*. Retrieved February 16, 2007 from http://www.jointcommission.org/PatientSafety/NationalPatientSafetyGoals/07.

The Joint Commission. *FAQs about the 2007 National Patient Safety Goals*. (Updated 1/07). Retrieved June 29, 2008 from http://www.jointcommission.org/PatientSafetyGoals/07_npsg_faqs.htm.

The Joint Commission. *Introduction to the national patient safety goals*. Retrieved February 19, 2007 from http://www.jointcommission.org/PatientSafety/NationalPatientSafetyGoals/npsg_intro.htm.

The Joint Commission. *National patient safety goals: implementation tips for eliminating dangerous abbreviations*. Retrieved February 19, 2007 from http://www.jointcommission.org/Patient Safety/.

The Joint Commission. *2007 National patient safety goals*. Retrieved February 16, 2007 from http://www.jointcommission.org/PatientSafety/NationalPatientSafetyGoals/.

Tyson S. (1999). *Gerontological nursing care* (Ch. 4). Philadelphia: WB Saunders.

UMHS. *Advance directives/living wills*. Retrieved May 25, 2007 from http://www.med.umich.edi/1libr/aha/umadvdir.htm.

U.S. Department of Health and Human Services. (2003). *OCR privacy brief: summary of the HIPAA privacy rule*. Retrieved June 29, 2008 from www.hhs.gov/ocr/privacysummary.pdf.

U.S. Department of Health and Human Services. Office for Civil Rights-HIPAA. *National standards to protect privacy of personal health information*. Retrieved June 29, 2008 from www.hhs.gov/ocr/hipaa.

Ventura MJ. (1999). Report tracks impact of Oregon's assisted suicide law. *RN*, 62(5):16.

Ventura MJ. (1999). When information must be revealed. *RN*, 62(2):61–64.

Wolfe S. (1998). When care givers endanger patients. *RN*, 61(12):28–32.

You're on trial: how to protect yourself. (2007, March/April). *LPN2007*, 3(2):16–18.

Zittel B. Profession update in teaching techniques. (2007, May 21). *ADVANCE for LPNs*. New York Tri-State Area. 7(5).

Chapter 21

Anderson M. (1997). *Employment process in nursing leadership; management and professional practice for the LPN/LVN*. Philadelphia, PA Davis, p.64.

Anderson M. (2007). *10 Tips for a powerful voice*. Entrepreneur.com. Retrieved September 17, 2007 from www.entrepreneur.com/article/183472.html.

Appold K. (2006, April 19). Networking: how to make a connection; Networking is a skill-it takes knowledge, desire and practice to perfect. *ADVANCE for LPNs* (online).

Block J, and Betrus M. (2004). *Great answers! For your job interview*. New York: McGraw-Hill, pp. 91–151.

Criscito P. (2006) *Designing the perfect resume* (3rd ed., pp. 15, 114.). Hauppauge, NY: Barrons Educational Series, Inc.

Darrah J. (2006) To blog, or not to blog! How it will affect your professional life is the answer to this question. *ADVANCE for LPNs*, 6(13):7A–8A.

Gryskiewicz E. (2003, April 8) Talent management representative. *Corporate employee background checks: personal interview*. St. Paul, MN: 3M Company.

Krumri M. (2003). Employee background checks. *Star Tribune*, Sect. W-1.

Mahan P. (2003). LPN Interviews. Retrieved August 13, 2003 from www.nurse-recruiter.com..

Mercer M. (2005). *7 Tips to make a fantastic impression*. ExpertMagazine.com. Retrieved September 16, 2007 from Dr. Mercer's Human Resources Management and Leadership Expert Blog.

Occupational Outlook Handbook 2006–2007 Edition. (2006). Indianapolis: JIST Publishing. pp. 330–331.

What to ask during your interview. (2003). Retrieved August 12, 2003 from www.travelnursedepot.com.

Yeager N, and Hough L. (1990). *Power interviews: job-winning tactics from Fortune 500 recruiters*. New York: John Wiley and Sons.

Zurlinden J. (2003). *Women: What's your interview wardrobe IQ?* Retrieved August 13, 2003 from www.nursingspectrum.com/MagazineArticles/index.cfm.

Chapter 22*

Gebhardt M, Clifford B, and Bates T. (2006, Oct). What's an educator to do? *AJN*, 106(10):13.

NAPNES. (2005). *NCSBN convenes panels of experts to study continued competence in nursing.* www.napnes.org.

National Council of State Boards of Nursing. *Candidates who ran out of time on the NCLEX examination.* Testing Services, Chicago: NCSBN. Retrieved June 29, 2008 from www.ncsbn.org/pass_fail_rules.pdf

National Council of State Boards of Nursing. *Computerized Adaptive Testing (CAT) overview.* (2003). *NCLEX using CAT brochure.* Chicago: NCSBN. Retrieved January 5, 2003 from www.ncsbn.org/1216.htm

National Council of State Boards of Nursing. (2003, March). *Facts about alternate item formats.* www.ncsbn.org.

National Council of State Boards of Nursing. *Fact versus fiction.* (2003). Testing Services, Chicago: NCSBN. Retrieved January 3, 2003 from www.ncsbn.org.

National Council of State Boards of Nursing. *Frequently asked questions.* (2003, Oct–Dec). NCLEX Candidate Bulletin, Chicago: NCSBN. Retrieved January 5, 2003 from www.ncsbn.org/public/testing/candidate_pre.htm.

National Council of State Boards of Nursing. (2004). *Important information regarding the National Licensure Examinations (the NCLEX-RN and NCLEX-PN).* www.ncsbn.org.

National Council of State Boards of Nursing. *NCLEX Examination Candidate Bulletin.* (2007). NCSBN. www.ncsbn.org.

National Council of State Boards of Nursing. *NCLEX Examination Candidate Bulletin.* (2003). NCSBN. Retrieved January 1, 2003 from www.ncsbn.org.

National Council of State Boards of Nursing. (2004, June 1). *NCSBN selects first three countries to offer NCLEX-RN abroad.* www.ncsbn.org.

National Council of State Boards of Nursing. (2004, Dec 15). NCLEX-PN examination passing standard revised for public safety. *News and Views.* www.ncsbn.org.

National Council of State Boards of Nursing. 2008 *NCLEX-PN test plan.* Chicago: NCSBN.

National Council of State Boards of Nursing. (2006, Fall). *Panel of experts completes 2006 practice analysis for the NCLEX-PN examination in Leader to Leader.* www.ncsbn.org.

National Council of State Boards of Nursing. (2006, May). *Q and A. Ask NCSBN in Leader to Leader.* www.ncsbn.org.

National Council of State Boards of Nursing. (2004). *Quarterly Examination statistics: volume, pass rates and first-time foreign educated candidates' countries.* www.ncsbn.org.

National Council of State Boards of Nursing. 2007 *Test Plan for the National Council of Licensure Examination for Practical/Vocational Nurses.* Chicago: NCSBN.

NLN. (2005). *NLN Pre-NCLEX Readiness Tests available now online: NLN launches readiness tests for RN/PN on Web-based platform.* www.nln.org.

Silvestri LQ. (2007). *Q and A review for the NCLEX-PN Examination.* St Louis: Elsevier/Saunders.

Smith J, Crawford L, and Gawel S. (2001). *Linking the NCLEX-PN national licensure to practice: 2000 practice analysis of newly licensed practical/vocational nurses in the U.S.* Chicago: National Council of State Boards of Nursing.

Stuart G. (2006). Guest editorial. What is the NCLEX really testing? *Nurs Outlook*, 54: 1–2.

Wendt A. (2007). *Report of findings from the 2006 LPN/LVN Practice Analysis: linking the NCLEX-PN Examination to practice.* Chicago: NCSBN

Chapter 23

ABMCN. *What is the American Board of Managed Care Nursing?* Retrieved August 16, 2007 from http://www.abmcn.org/right_pageframe.htm.

Adams N. *Features from ADVANCE for LPNs eNewsletter.* www.AdvanceforLPNs.com.

Advance for LPNs. *Your certificate connection: NAPNES certification.* Retrieved August 2, 2007 from http://lpn.advanceweb.com/common/editorial/editorial.aspx?CTIID=1520.

Ahl ME. (1975). In Lemburg C (Ed.). *Open learning and career mobility in nursing.* St Louis: Mosby.

An internet presentation of the Occupational Outlook Handbook plus related career guidance information. Licensed practical and licensed vocational nurses. (2005, May). http://www.ocouha.com/oesi/i292061.htm.

British Columbia Occupational Outlook, Occupational Profile. Licensed Practical Nurses. (NOC 3233) Retrieved July 30, 2007 from http://www.workfutures.bc.ca/link.cfm?print=trueandlang=enandnoc3233.

Canadian Institute for Health Information. *Numbers of nurses in Canada increasing slightly.* Retrieved July 30, 2007 from http://www.cihi.ca/cihiweb/dispPage.jsp?cw_page=media_18oct2006_e.

Canadian Institute of Health Information. (2005). *B.C. and Ontario attract greatest number of foreign trained nurses.* Retrieved July 30, 2007 from http://www.cihi.ca/cihiweb/disPage.jsp?cw_page=media_26oct2005_e.

Career description: licensed practical nurses. (2003). Retrieved from www.iseeksolutions.com.

CD-ROM is coming to NAPNES long-term care certification. (2002, Summer). *J Pract Nurs*, 52:2, 5–7.

Changes in nursing education. Retrieved August 6, 2007 from http://www.nurseuniverse.com/Nursing-Job/2454.html.

Enhancing end-of-life care in nursing homes: palliative care educational resource team)(PERT) Program. (2005). *AAHPM J Palliat Med*, 8(3):556–566. Retrieved

---

*Information on NCLEX-PN and CAT is based directly on these resources.

July 4, 2007 from http://www.liebertonline.com/doi/abs/10.1089/jpm.2005.8.556?cookieSet=1andjournalCode=.

Excelsior College: School of Nursing. Retrieved August 18, 2007 from http://www.excelsior.edu/portal/page?_pageid=57,53097and_dad=port.

Farr M. (2003). *America's fastest growing jobs* (7th ed., p. 195). Indianapolis: Jist Publishing.

Folger J. (2002). *Team players*. Retrieved November 20, 2002 from www.nurseweek.com/news/features/02–10/lvn.asp.

HRSA. *Supply, demand, and use of licensed practical nurses: executive summary*. http://bhpr.hrsa.gov/healthworkforce/reports/nursing/lpn/default.htm.

HRSA. *Supply, demand, and use of licensed practical nurses: scope of practice and nurse practice acts*. Retrieved July 30, 2007 from http://bhpr.hrsa.gov/healthworkforce/reports/nursing/lpn/c3.htm.

iSeek. *Program: Practical Nursing. Minneapolis Community and Technical College*. 51. 161300. Retrieved August 17, 2007 from http://www.iseek.org/sv/ProgramOpt;jsessionid=878A8829451E7151E0133523B671FF0F.

Joint Commission on Administrative Rules: Administrative Code, Part 300. *Skilled Nursing and Intermediate Care Facilities Code*. Retrieved July 31, 2007 from http://www.ilga.gov/commission/jcar/admincode/077077003000F1200R.html.

Lefer G, and Moss H. (2007). *The LPN: a practical way to alleviate the nursing shortage: a report prepared for the United Nurses of America, AFSCME, AFL-CIO*. Portland, OR: University of Oregon: Education and Research Center.

Licensed practical nurses: current utilization. (2003). Burnaby, BC: Hospital Employee's Union.

Licensed practical nurse job description, career as a licensed practical nurse, salary, employment-definition and nature of the work, education and training requirement, getting a job. Retrieved July 29, 2007 from http://careers.stateuniversity.com/pages/454/Licensed-Practical-Nurse.html.

Licensed Practical Nurses. (2003). Retrieved April 29, 2003 from www.setforlifeincome.com/freereport-196.html.

Mahan P. (2007), Is it worth the price? *Jrnl of Pract Nurs*, 57(4), 22 and 25.

McGregor R, and Romkes T. (2003). *Canada's nursing crisis: perceptions and realities*. Retrieved September 11, 2003 from www.canadasnursingconference.com/session-17.html.

MedHunters. *Job details: licensed practical nurse—community sector–AV-41368-cc*. Retrieved July 31, 2007 from http://www.medhunters.com/job/684071.html.

Minnesota health and medical careers. 2:20 and 2:28. Retrieved from www.usmedicalcareers.com.

Moore S. No place like it. (2006). *ADVANCE for LPNs*, New York Tri-State Area. 7(17).

NAPNES. *eJournal of Practical Nursing*, 1(4). Retrieved July 27, 2006 from www.NAPNES.org.

NAPNES. *Long-term care certification*. Retrieved August 13, 2007 from http://www.napnes.org/certifications/ltc.htm.

NAPNES. *Pharmacology certification*. Retrieved August 3, 2007 from http://www.napnes.org/certifications/pharmacology.htm.

NAPNES. *Welcome to the virtual home of the world's oldest LPN/LVN association*. Retrieved August 14, 2007 from http://www.napnes.net/.

National Council of State Boards of Nursing. NCLEX Statistics from NCSBN. *Quarterly examination statistics, volume, pass rates and first-time foreign-educated candidates' countries*. Retrieved July 2007 from www.ncsbn.org.

National news in ADVANCE for LPNs. Retrieved February 3, 2005 from www.AdvanceforLPNs.com.

NFLPN. Retrieved August 13, 2007 from www.iStudySmart.com.

NFLPN. *IV Certification, training and exam testing*. Retrieved August 13, 2007 from http://www.nflpn/org/ecertification.html.

NLN. *About the NLN*. http://www.nln.org/aboutnln/index.htm.

NurseUniverse.com. *National League for Nursing calls for evidence-based standards*.

NurseWeek. *Travel. How or where can I get detailed information about travel nursing as a career?* Retrieved February 27, 2004 from http://www.nurseweek.com/travel/amswerZ_rnnetwork.asp.

PayScale. *Salary survey report for job: Licensed Practical Nurse (LPN)*. Retrieved July 4, 2007 from http://www.payscale.com/research/US/Job=Licensed_Practical_Nurse_(LPN)/Salary.

Polick T. (2007). *Nursing voices in cyberspace in ADVANCE online editions for nurses*. www.advanceweb.com.

Progress in scope of practice issues in Atlantic, Canada, in nursing environments: knowledge to action. Retrieved August 2007 from http://cord.aacadiau.ca/neka.

Regulating U.S. nursing homes: are we learning from experience? *Health Affairs*, 20(6).

RUE Education NFLPN. (2005, Spring). *Visions*, 11(2).

RUE Education NFLPN. (2006, Winter).*Visions*, 12(1).

Sabatini J. *Starting out in ADVANCE for LPNs*. Retrieved August 14, 2005 from http://lpnadvANCEWEB.COM/COMMON/EDITORIAL/EDITORIAL.ASPX?cc=51490.

Schaefer N. *Does wound certification make a difference?* ADVANCE for LPNs. Retrieved August 2, 2007 from http://lpn.advanceweb.com/common/Editorial/Search/Aviewer.aspx?AN=LW_06nov13_lpn.

Scudder S, Yox S. (2006). *A daily dose of continuing education: good news for nurses*. Medscape from WEBMD. Retrieved February 19, 2007 from mpmailings@webmd.net.

Skilled nursing facility ("SNF") services. Center for Medicare Advocacy, Inc. http://www.medicareadvocacy.org/FAQ_SNF.htm.

Starks P. Student involvement. (2006, May 22). *ADVANCE for LPNs*, New York tri state area.

Story D. (1974). *Career mobility*. St Louis: Mosby.

Summary report for licensed practical and licensed vocational nurses. O-NET OnLine. Retrieved July 30, 2007 from http://online.onecenter.org/link/summary/29–2061.00.

U.S. Department of Labor Bureau of Labor Statistics. *Occupational outlook handbook. licensed practical and licensed vocational nurses*. http://www.bls.gov/oco/ocos102.htm.

U.S. Department of Veterans Affairs. *Nursing—licensed practical/vocational nurse*. Retrieved July 29, 2007 from http://www.vacareers.va.gov/lpn.cfm.

Wendt A. *Report on findings from the 2006 LPN/LVN Practice Analysis: Linking NCLEX-PN Examination to Practice*. Chicago: NCSBN.

Work-at-home: job report: licensed practical nurses. Retrieved June 29, 2007 from www.work-at-home.org/sreport/career/62.htm.

Yox S. *MedPulse, CE Edition*. Retrieved December 25, 2004 from mpmailings@webmd.net.

Illustration Credits List

Chapter 7

Figure **7-1:** Nursing Mirror Photograph. From Dolan JA, Fitzpatrick, MK., Herrmann EK. (1983) *Nursing in society: A historical perspective.* (15th ed.). Philadelphia: WB Saunders.

Figure **7-2:** Courtesy of Yale Medical Library. From Dolan JA, Fitzpatrick, MK., Herrmann EK. (1983) *Nursing in society: A historical perspective.* (15th ed.). Philadelphia: WB Saunders.

Figures **7-3 and 7-4:** From Dolan JA, Fitzpatrick, MK., Herrmann EK. (1983) *Nursing in society: A historical perspective.* (15th ed.). Philadelphia: WB Saunders.

Chapter 10

Figures **10-1 and 10-2:** From U.S. Department of Agriculture. (2006). Center for Nutrition Policy and Promotion, Washington, DC, www.mypyramid.gov.

Chapter 11

Figure **11-1:** Graybel K, Marion RN, Brown M, Patch P, Kruckenberg D. Courtesy of Good Samaritan Hospital, Pullayup, WA. In Ignatavicius DD, Workman ML, and Misherler, MS (1999). *Medical-surgical nursing: A nursing process approach.* (3rd ed.). Philadelphia: Saunders.

Index

A

Abandonment, legal concerns regarding, 381
Abbreviations, use in charting, 365
Abnormal observations, recording, 366
Abuse, 360, 361
    requirement to disclose, 369b
Accessories, for job interviews, 410
Accountability
    of charge nurses, 288
    as ethical responsibility of nurses, 344
    legal responsibility and, 367
Accounting, patient access to, in Notice of Privacy
    Practices, 371
Acronyms
    as aids to memory, 54–55
    as memory aids, 54
Active euthanasia, 376, 377b, 377t
Active learning, 7–8
Active listening, 44, 44b
    during class time, 65–66
Activities of daily living (ADLs), assistance with,
    312, 313
Acute care
    delivery of nursing care in, 172–176
    role of LPN/LVNs in, 170
Acute care skilled nursing facility, 311
Adaptive testing, 424–425
Administrative responsibility, employment opportunities
    with, 430
Administrative simplification under HIPAA, 369–370
Adult ADD, 22–23
Adult care homes, 312
Adult day care centers, 313–314
Adult learners
    challenges for nursing students, 6
    defined, 1–2
    with English as additional language, challenges for, 6
    formal educational experiences of, 2
    informal educational experiences of, 2
    liabilities and pitfalls for, 3–5
    recycled, 2
    responsibilities of, 6–12
    returning, 1–2
    rights of, 6
    traditional, 1
Adults, communicating with, 133
Advance directives, 375
Advance for LPNs, 64, 441
Advance for Nurses, 443
Advanced practice registered nurses, 167
    Doctor of Nursing Practice degree as future requirement
        for, 168

Advice
    legal implications of, 380–381
    unsolicited, giving, blocking communication, 127
Affective communication, 123, 125
African Americans
    communication styles of, 128–129
    diversity profiles of, 196b
Aggressive behavior, 228–229
    by patients' families, 284–285
    work-related issues and, 239–244
Aging
    of nursing workforce, 177b
    of population, nursing shortage and, 176
Agnostics, beliefs of, 209
Alaskan natives, diversity profiles of, 197b
Alcohol
    abuse of
        versus alcoholism, 150–151
        disciplinary action for, 356b
    use of, among nurses, 149–151
Alcohol, Drug Abuse, and Mental Health
    Administration, 306
Alcoholics Anonymous, 151, 307t
Alexian Brothers, 92
All-or-none thinking, 77
Allah, 217
Alliances, health care, 334
Almshouses, 92
ALS Society of America, 307t
Alternate format items, in NCLEX-PN® examination, 83,
    419–420
Ambulance staff, employment opportunities in, 439
Ambulatory care centers, 310, 336
    LPN/LVNs in, 170
Ambulatory services, 309–310
Ambulatory surgery centers, 310
Amendments to medical records, in Notice of Privacy
    Practices, 371
American Board of Managed Care Nursing Certification in
    Managed Care Nursing, 446
American Cancer Society, 307t
American Diabetes Association, 307t
American Heart Association, 307t
American Indians
    communication styles of, 129
    diversity profiles of, 197b
American Journal of Nursing, 64
American Licensed Practical Nurses Association (ALPNA), 90t
American Lung Association, 307t
American Nurses Credentialing Center (ANCC),
    Open Door policy of, 166
American Red Cross, 98

Page numbers followed by f indicate figures; t, tables; b, boxes.

American Stroke Association, 307t
Analysis
  NCLEX-PN® and, 83
  in NCLEX-PN® examination, 76
Ancient Egypt, nursing in, *90–91*
Ancient Greece, nursing in, 91
Ancient Hebrews, nursing among, 91
Anesthesiologists, 161
Anesthetist, functions of, 161
Anger management, 268–269
Answers, pat, blocking communication, 127
Anthropologist
  definition of, 182
  perspective of, on culture, 182–183
Antiseptic methods, historical development of, 93
Anxiety, critical thinking ability and, 82
Apartment management, shortcuts to, 38–39
Application, NCLEX-PN® and, 83
Applied critical thinking, 76–77
Appointment to test, for NCLEX-PN®
  examination, 421, 423
Arab Americans, diversity profiles of, 197b
Aristotle, 91
Artful vagueness, in making impression, 386–387
Articles, in learning resource center, 64
Assault, 239–241, 360
  counseling victims of, 244
  filing charges after, 244
Assertiveness, 226–246
  examples of, 229–231
  filing charges after assault a, 244
  moving toward
    guidelines for, 233–238
    problem-solving in, 233–238. *See also* Problem-solving
      process
  in women's health issues, 350–351
Assigning residents, 300
Assigning tasks, 285–289
  criteria for, 292–298
  defined, 286
  delegation differentiated from, 286–288, 288t
  planning for, 290–298
  refusal by nursing assistants, 205–296
Assignments, completion of, evaluating, 39
Assimilation, cultural, 183
Assisted living facilities, employment opportunities in,
  439–440
Assisted living programs, 312
Associate degree nursing (ADN) program, 165
Atheists, beliefs of, 209
Attention deficit disorder (ADD), adult, 22–23
Attention span, in planning, 35
Attitude
  critical thinking and, 80
  nonjudgmental, in home health nursing, 435
Attitude problems, by nursing assistants, 296
Audiovisual materials, as learning resources, 69
Auditory learners, 16, 17
Aurora Health Care system, 333
Authority to delegate, 285–286
Authorization to test (ATT), in NCLEX-PN®
  examination, 421, 423

Authorized consent, 374
Autocratic leadership style, 252, 253b
Autonomy
  as ethical principle, 347–348
  patient, support of, 343
Autotutorial method, of training for unlicensed assistive
  personnel, 171

B

Baby Boomers, as returning adult learners, 1
Babylonia, ancient, nursing in, 91
Baccalaureate nurses, training of, 161
Baccalaureate nursing programs, 165
Bachelor of science in nursing (BSN)
  programs for, for registered nurses, 166
  RN with, as anesthetist, 161
Back injuries in nursing, 144–145
Back pain, relieving, stretching in, 143
Back stretches, 143
Background checks, pre-employment, 413
Background noise, managing, to optimize concentration, 42
Bad debt, in health care costs, 329
Baha'i patients, 221b
Balanced brain, 21
Balanced Budget Act of 1997, 323–324
Baptism, in Christianity, 213, 213b
Barriers to learning
  illiteracy as, 24–25
  racial bias in textbooks as, 23–24
Barton, Clara, 88t, 98
Basic daily needs, cross-cultural view of, 185–187
Basic nursing care, 354
Basic patient situation, 354
Battery, 360
Beans, in MyPyramid, 141f
Behavior
  aggressive, 228–229
  assertive, 229–231
  nonassertive (passive), 227–228
  styles of, 227–231
Belittling communication, blocking communication, 127
Beneficence, as ethical principle, 344–347
Beneficent paternalism, 349–351
Bible, 212–213
Biomedicine, 193
Blue Cross/Blue Shield, 320
Board and care homes, 312
Bodily/kinesthetic learner, 18
Body alignment and activity, as basic daily need, 186
Body language, 124
Borrowed servant doctrine, 366
Bound periodical indexes, 71–72, 72f
Brain
  balanced, 21
  empathizer, 21
  systemizing, 21
Brain development
  adult ADD and, 22–23
  E-S theory of, 21
  emotional mind and, 19
  fight-flight responses and, 19
  gender-based developmental differences, 21

Brain development (*Continued*)
  learning and, 19–22
  learning process and, 22
  right and left hemispheres in, 20–21, 20t
  thinking mind and, 19
Brain hemispheres, 20–21, 20t
Breach of duty, 363b
Breathing, deep, stretching in, 143
Brief relaxation, as stress prevention, 155, 155b
Bubonic plague, nursing during, 92
Bucket theory of education, 64–65
Buddhism, 221, 222–223t, 223
  nursing interventions for patients, 222–223t, 223–224
Buddy, discussion, as learning strategy, 65, 65b
Burnout
  prevention of, 146–147
  stress differentiated from, 146–148, 147t

C

Calendars, in time management, 32–33
Call number, in locating materials, 63
Canada
  health insurance system of, 317–318
  LPN employment opportunities and salaries in, 431
Capability in nursing, critical thinking and, 82
Capitation, 318, 319t
Captain of the ship doctrine, 366
Care managers, RNs as, 169t
Care pair, 171
Care plan(s), 116
  documenting, 116–117
  implementation of, 118
  student assignment sheet and, 114t
Care planning
  adapting for culturally diverse patients, 201–202
  for culturally diverse patients, 199–201
Care plan(s)
  and charge nurse delegation, 292
  developing, 110, 113, 336
Career advancement, noncredit RN programs in, 449
Career changes, 1
Career growth, 429–450
  2006 job analysis and, 430–431
  in assisted living facilities, 439–440
  in chiropractic offices, 437
  in coroners' offices, 439
  in doctors' offices, 437
  in extended care facilities, 432–323
  in health insurance companies, 438
  in home health nursing, 434–435
  in hospice care, 438
  in hospital nursing, 436
  job outlook for LPN/LVNs and, 430–431
  in mental health nursing, 435–436
  in military services, 436
  in operating room nursing, 437
  in outpatient clinics, 437
  in parish nursing, 439
  personal attributes and, 432
  in pharmaceutical and medical equipment sales, 438
  in private duty nursing, 439
  professional organizations in, 440–442

Career growth (*Continued*)
  in temporary help agencies, 439
  in travel nursing, 438
  in Veterans Administration Hospitals and homes, 438
  in veterinary clinics and hospitals, 438
  wages for LPN/LVNs and, 430–431
  work sites and nursing characteristics for, 432–440
Career ladder programs, 447–449
Caring, in NCLEX-PN® examination, 421
Case management, 173–174, 175t
  employment opportunities in, 439
Case method, of nursing care delivery in acute care
    setting, 172
Case scenarios, as learning resources, 71
Catalog, library, online, 63
Catholicism, 213, 214–215b, 216
CD-ROM databases, as learning resources, 73
Cell phones, 135
Centers for Disease Control (CDC), 306
Centers for Medicare and Medicaid Services (CMS), 263
Centers of Excellence in Nursing Education, 440
Cerebrum, hemispheres of, 20, 20t
Certification
  in gerontology, 445–446
  in IV Therapy, 445
  long-term, development of, 103
  in long-term care, 444
  in managed care, 446
  in pharmacology, 433, 444–445
  of RNs, 166–167
  as State Board of Nursing function, 355b
Certified nurse-midwives, 167
Certified nursing assistants assisting with ADLs, 313
Certified Registered Nurse Anesthetists (CRNAs), 167
Change of condition
  in end-of-shift reporting, 301
  reporting of, to physicians, 281–282
Change-of-shift report, 280, 289–290
  in task/duty allocation, 292
Charge nurse(s)
  assignment and delegation by, 285–289
  change-of-shift report and, 280
  collecting data as, 280–282
  common problems of, 282–285
  duties of, in job description, 276
  end-of-shift reporting for, 300–302
  in extended-care facilities, practical/vocational
    nurses as, 169
  job description for, 275–277
  nursing process guidelines for assignment/delegation,
    289–300
  in organizational hierarchy, 248f, 249f
  preparation time for, 277
  skills of, 274–303
  stress management skills for, 261
Charge nurse skills
  documentation related, 279
  equipment related, 279
  facility organization-related, 278
  housekeeping, maintenance, supply related, 279
  medication related, 279
  miscellaneous, 280

Charge nurse skills (*Continued*)
 nursing care procedures and, 279
 personnel policies and, 278
 for physician assistance, 279
 policies, regulations, routines included in, 278–279
 records and unit routines and, 278
 regulations related to, 278
 resident food service related, 279
 safety policies and, 278–279
 in special areas, 279–280
 unit administration and, 278
Charting
 of care plan, 116–117
 computer, 135
 by exception, 337
 general legal guidelines for, 365–366
 late entries in, 379
 subjective vs. objective, 262–263
Chemical dependency among nurses, 149–151
Chemical restraint, 361
Chiding behaviors blocking communication, 127
Children, delegating tasks to, 33, 34b
Children's Health Insurance Program (CHIP),
 324, 331
Chiropractic offices, employment opportunities in, 437
Cholera epidemic, 93
Christian Scientists, 220b
Christianity, 212–217
 baptism in, 213, 213b
 communion in, 213
 general beliefs in, 212–213
 major divisions of, 213–217
Circulation, improving, stretching in, 143
Circulation desk, 63
Civil action, 359–331, 360t
Civil War, nursing developments during, 97
Clarification, as active listening skill, 125
Class participation, evaluating, 39
Classroom learning strategies, 64–67
Clerk receptionists, 161, 171–172
Clinical application, of theory, 5
Clinical competency, 373
Clinical nurse specialists, 167
Clinical pathways
 as multidisciplinary plan, 116
 in nursing case management, 173–174
 oncology example, 175f
Clinical performance evaluations, 9–10
Clinical problem-solving, in NCLEX-PN® examination,
 420–421
Clinical rotations, 9
 requesting reference letter commitment before
  completion of, 387
Closed-ended questions, in therapeutic
 communication, 126
Clothing
 in nonverbal communication, 124
 nosocomial infections and, 146
 recommendations on
  for job interviews, 409–410
  for NCLEX-PN® examination, 426
Clustering, in mapping method of note making, 45, 48f
Codependency in nurses, 151–152

Coinsurance
 definition of, 319
 in fee-for-service plans, 319
Collaboration, critical thinking and, 82
Collaborative care plans, 116
Color
 as aid in focusing attention, 23
 in enhancing understanding, 52
Commitment, in patient/staff communication,
 131–132
Common law, 358–359
Communicable disease, requirement to disclose,
 369b
Communication, 122–137
 blocks to, 127
 confidential, in Notice of Privacy Practices, 371
 in conflict resolution, 134–135
 coverage in NCLEX-PN® examination, 421
 cultural differences in, 128–129
 cultural diversity in, 190–191
 in delegation of duties, 296–297
 electronic, 135
 improving effectiveness among caregivers, 373b
 male/female differences in, 127–128
 nurse/patient, evaluation, 126
 with patients, instructors, staff, 131–132
 poor, lawsuits based on, 362b
 types of, 123–125
Communication process
 factors affecting, 135
Communication skills
 affective communication as, 123, 125
 applying as LPN/LVN leader, 256–257
 critical thinking and, 81
 excluding formal interview process, 110
 for home health nursing, 434
 needed by health care team members, 164
 nonverbal, 124
 by patient age, 132–134
 in reporting patient findings, 119
 verbal, 123, 124
Communication strategies, 125–127
 aggressive behavior and, 228–229
 assertive behavior and, 227
 passive behavior and, 227–228
Communion, in Christianity, 213
Community health nursing services, 312–313
Community resources, 73
Compensation mechanisms, 233
Competence
 evaluating before delegating duties, 294–295
 requirement to demonstrate, 337
Competency, patient, 373
Complaining families, dealing with, 284–285
Complementary and alternative medicine, 193
Complex nursing situations, 354–355
Compliment, giving, in making impression, 387
Comprehension
 NCLEX-PN® and, 82–83
 phases of, 24–25
 problems with, 24–25
 of reading assignments, 47, 49–52
 visual strategies to enhance, 52–53

Computer-aided instruction (CAI), 70–71
Computer simulation, as learning resource, 71
Computerized adaptive testing (CAT), for NCLEX-PN®
  Examination, 418, 424–425
Computerized care plans, 116
Concentration, improving, 42–44
Concept map
  as multidisciplinary plan, 116
  in note making, 45–46
Conditional job offers, 412–414
Confidential communication, in Notice of Privacy
  Practices, 371
Confidentiality
  cultural diversity in, 190
  fidelity and, 349
  legal issues relating to, 368
  patient's right to, 368
Conflict resolution, 134–135
Conflict resolution skills, 266–267
Congressional Budget Office (CBO), Medicare and, 330b
Connecticut Training School, 98f
Consent
  authorized, 374
  general, 374
  implied, 360, 374
  informed, 374
    as common law, 359
    underage children and, 348
  patient's right to, 373–374
Conservative Judaism, 212
Consolidated Omnibus Reconciliation Act
  (COBRA), 317
Consolidated systems of health care, 333
Constructive criticism/evaluation, 9–10
Context, affecting communication, 123
Continuing education, 442–443
  certification opportunities in, 443–446
  CEUs for, 442–443
  in-service training as, 442
  Internet resources for, 443
  orientation to facility as, 442
  workshops for, 442
Continuing Education Record Keeping System
  (CERKS), 441
Continuing education units (CEUs), 442–443
Continuous care retirement community, 312
Continuous quality improvement (CQI), 265–266, 336
Conversation patterns
  cultural diversity in, 191
  male/female differences in, 127–128
Cool-downs, 142
Cooperative learning, suggestions for, 66
Copayments
  definition of, 319
  in fee-for-service plans, 318
Coping mechanisms, 153–157, 231–233
  compensation as, 233
  denial as, 232–233
  projection as, 231
  rationalization as, 231
Copyright laws, for articles, photocopying and, *64*
Coroner's office, employment opportunities in, 439
Corpus callosum, 21

Cost issues
  in Canadian health care system, 318
  health care cost containment as, 325
Counseling, of assault victim, 244
Counselor, referral to, 11
Course outlines, as learning resources, 68
Courtesy
  during job interviews, 411
  resignation, 415
Courtesy letter, requesting reference letter, 387, 388b
Cover letter
  for employment, 393b, 395–396, 401b, 402b
  for newspaper ad response, 401b
  regarding unsolicited phone call, 400b
Covered entity under HIPAA, 370b
Cramming, 5, 55
Crimean War, development of nursing in, 95
Criminal action, 336–338
  requirement to disclose, 369b
Criminal activity, disciplinary action and, 356b
Crisis situations, inadvisability of delegating in, 294
Critical pathways
  in health care delivery, 337
  in nursing case management, 173–174, 175f
Critical thinking, 75–85
  applied, 76–77
  definition of, 76, 77
  overview of, 75–76
  principles of, 78
  questions in, 78
Critical thinking skills
  charge nurses and, 277
  comprehending information as, 47, 49–53
  development of, instructors encouraging, 8
  factors influencing, 80–82
  general hints for learners, 42–47
  NCLEX-PN® and, 82–83
  practical/vocational nursing and, 78–79
  prerequisites for, 79
  remembering and forgetting as, 53–55
  test-taking skills as, 55–59
Criticism, constructive, 9
Cross-training, 176
  future trends in, 335
Cultural bias, 182
Cultural characteristics, affecting communication, 123
Cultural competence, 181
  in health care situations, developing, 197–198
Cultural differences, in communication, 128–129
Cultural diversity, 187–197
  areas of, 188–195
  in communication styles, 190–191
  in concepts of mental illness, 193
  in concepts of modesty, 193
  in concepts of time, 190
  in economic status, 192–193
  in educational backgrounds, 191
  in family structure, 188–189
  in food preferences, 189
  importance of, 187–188
  learning about, 188
  in manipulation, 238–239
  modifying work settings for, 198, 198b

Cultural diversity (*Continued*)
    in pregnancy and birth beliefs and practices, 194
    in religious beliefs, 189
    in terminal illness and death beliefs, 194
    in wellness/illness beliefs, 193–194
Cultural groups
    in area, identifying, 198
    diversity profiles of, 196–197b
Cultural sensitivity, 181
Cultural uniqueness, 183
Culturally competent care, 181
Culture
    characteristics of, 181–182
    critical thinking and, 80
    definition of, 181
    medical ethics and, 348
Cumulative Index to Nursing and Allied Health Literature
    (CINAHL®), 72, 72f
Cupping, 99
Curing illness, cultural diversity in beliefs about, 193
Curriculum, organized, learner's right to, 6
Custodial care, 310, 312
Customs, 181

D

Daily planning, 36
Damages, 363b
Danger, requirement to disclose, 369b
Dark Ages, nursing in, 92
Data collection
    for charge nurses, 280–282
    communicating information to health care team
        members in, 111
    for Hmong patients, 199b
    in leadership scenario, 258
    in NCLEX-PN® examination, 420
    in nursing process, 108, 109, 110–112
        accuracy in, 111–112
        barriers in, 112
        evaluation phase, 118, 118t
        examples of practical/vocational nurse, 111b
        questioning in, 112
    for religious beliefs and practices of patients, 211b
    reporting by charge nurses, 289–290
    for spiritual issues, 207
    systematic method of, 110
    in time management, 31
    verification in, 110–111
Databases, CD-ROM, as learning resources, 73
Day care centers, employment opportunities in, 439, 440
Day supervisors, in extended-care units, 163
Daydreaming, as distraction from study, 43
Death
    Buddhist/Hindu patients and, 223t
    cultural diversity in beliefs and practices related to, 194
    Jewish patients and, 212b
Deceit, disciplinary action and, 356b
Decentralizing service departments, 176
Deductibles
    definition of, 319
    in fee-for-service plans, 318
    under Medicare, 320
Deep breathing, stretching in, 143

Defamation, 360, 361
Deficit spending, health care entitlement programs and, 326
Dehydration, learning impairment from, 22
Delegated medical act, 355
Delegated nursing act, 355
Delegating duties, 33–35
    assignment differentiated from, 286–288, 288t
    authority for, 285–286
    by charge nurses, 285–289
    criteria for, 292–298
    defined, 287–288
    importance of, 288
    legal aspects of, 288–289
    planning for, 290–298
    refusal by nursing assistants, 295–296, 298
Delegation, of duties, beyond scope of practice/experience,
    response to, 367–368, 368b
Delegation decision-making tree, 301t
Demanding families, dealing with, 284–285
Democratic leadership style, 253b
Denial, as coping mechanism, 232–233
Denial system, in chemical dependency, 151
Denomination, religious, definition of, 209
Department of Health and Human Services (DHHS),
    306, 371
Dependent role
    of LPN to RN, 108
    of nurses to physicians, 108
Depositions, 363–364
Detail-focused interpersonal style, 387b
Developmental differences in brain, gender and, 21
Dewey decimal system, 63
Diagnosis
    medical, in multidisciplinary care plans, 116
    nursing. *See* Nursing diagnosis
Diagnosis-related groups (DRGs), Medicare and, 322–323
Diagnostic tests, Medicare Part B provision for, 321b
Diagrams, as study aids, 52
Dickens, Charles, reflection of nursing in, 93
Dietary rules, Jewish patients and, 212b
Dietitians, 163
Difficulty levels, of NCLEX-PN® examination
    questions, 425
Diploma programs
    for nurses, 165
    for surgical technicians, 161
Direct supervision, 355
Directed thinking, 77
Directions, following, in test taking, 56
Discharge instructions, legal implications of, 381–382
Disciplinary action
    against LPN/LVN licenses, 289
    by other jurisdictions, 356b
    process of, 357–358
    responsibility of nurse regulatory boards for, 356–357,
        356b
    steps in, 357b
Disciplined attention, 125
Disclosure of required information, legal issues relating to,
    368, 369b
Discrimination, dangers of, 182
Discussion buddy, as learning strategy, 65, 65b
Disorganization, reasons for, 28–29

Distance learning
   hints for success in, 66–67
   registered nursing degree via, 449
Distracters, in multiple choice question, 57
Distractions, avoiding/managing, 42–43
Diversion and recreation, as basic daily need, 186
Divide-and-conquer manipulator, 239
Division of labor, in functional nursing, 172
Dix, Dorothea Lynde, 88t, 97
Do-not-resuscitate (DNR) order, 376
Doctoral degree nursing programs, 167–168
Doctors' offices, employment opportunities in, 437
Documentation
   of care plan, 116–117
   charge nurse responsibilities for, 279
   coverage in NCLEX-PN® examination, 421
   forgotten entry in, 379
   of handling of illegible physician's order, 379–380
   of illegal alteration of patient's record, 379
   in nurse leadership, 262–263
   of someone else's care, 379
   of telephone orders, 380
   of UAP care, 379
   of verbal orders, 380
Doers, learning styles of, 16
Domain names, 69
Dress codes, 124
Drug abuse, disciplinary action and, 356b
Drug screening, pre-employment, 412
Due process, as applied to learners, 6
Durable medical power of attorney, 375
Duty(ies)
   breach of, 363b
   delegating, 287–288
   legal definition of, 363b

E

E-mail, 135, 135b
   in Notice of Privacy Practices, 371
E-S theory of brain development, 21
Earnings ability, for LPN/LVNs, 430–431
Easter Seals National Headquarters, 307t
Eastern religions
   Buddhism as, 221, 222–223t, 223
   Hinduism, 219, 221
   nursing interventions for, 219, 221–223
Economic status, cultural diversity in, 192–193
Economy, national, health care and, 327–328
Education
   bucket theory of, 64–65
   continuing, 442–443
   patient. *See* Patient education
Educational backgrounds
   cultural diversity in, 191
   in résumé, 398b
Educational experiences, formal *vs.* informal, 2
Educational mobility for LPN/LVNs, 446–449
   distance learning nursing program at Excelsior College
     in, 448
   Itasca Nursing Education Consortium program in,
     447
   Minneapolis Community and Technical College
     Mobility Program in, 448

Educational mobility for LPN/LVNs (*Continued*)
   NFLPN's iStudySmart.com program in, 448–449
   noncredit RN programs in, 449
   Sheridan College School of Nursing Associate degree
     program in, 447–448
Educational standards, Nurse regulatory boards and, 355b
Effective study habits, 30
Efficiency, in study habits, 30
Egypt, ancient, nursing in, 90–91
Eighteenth century, nursing in, 92–93
eJournal of Practical Nursing, 441
Elderly
   abuse and neglect of, requirement to disclose, 369b
   communicating with, 133–134
Electronic communication, 135
Electronic format, for journal articles, 64
Electronic medical records, 337
Electronic résumés, 395, 396b
Electronic simulations, as learning resources, 71
Elimination, as basic daily need, 186
Emergency, ability to deal with, in home health nursing, 435
Emergency care
   employment opportunities in, 439
   health care teams in, 160–161
   Medicare Part B provisions for, 321b
Emergency data, communication of, 111
Emergency medical technicians (EMTs), 160
Emergency room (ER), care in, 160
Emotional abuse, 361
Emotional and spiritual support, as basic daily need, 186
Emotional expression, cultural diversity in, 190
Emotional mind, 19
Emotional needs, 206
Empathizer brain, 21
Empathy
   in patient/staff communication, 131
   vs. sympathy in burnout prevention, 146–147
Employed uninsured, 328
Employee violence, 241–242
Employment, as distraction for adult learners, 4
Employment opportunities. *See* Career growth
Employment Verification Firms, 413
Empowering team members, 271
Enculturation, 181–182
End-of-life issues, 375–378
   advance directives as, 375
   do-not-resuscitate orders as, 376
   durable medical powers of attorney as, 375
   end-of-life movement organizations and, 378
   life support removal as, 376
   living wills as, 375
   organ donation as, 377–378
   Patient Self-Determination Act and, 375
   physician-assisted suicide and euthanasia as, 376–377
End-of-shift reporting, 300–302
Endorsements, interstate, 357, 418
Enriched housing, 312
Entitlement program, Medicare as, 321
Environment
   as basic daily need, 186
   study, reducing distractions in, 42
Environmental factors, affecting concerns upon
   hospitalization, 130

Equipment
    charge nurse responsibilities for, 279
    injuries related to, requirement to disclose, 369b
Ethical expectations, for cultural sensitivity, 181
Ethics, 339–352
    beneficent paternalism and, 349–351
    and decisions in health care, 343–344
    description and scope of, 340
    legal aspects of nursing and, 340, 340t
    nurses' responsibilities and, 344
    nursing, 341
        roots of, 342–343
    personal code of, 342
    principles of, 344–349
        autonomy as, 347–348
        beneficence as, 346–347
        fidelity as, 348–349
        justice as, 349
        nonmaleficence as, 345–346
Ethics committees, 343
Ethnicity, concept of, 187
Ethnocentrism, dangers of, 182
Euthanasia, 376–377, 377t
Evaluation
    in delegation by charge nurses, 299–300
    in leadership scenario, 258–259
    in learning process, 8–10
    in NCLEX-PN® examination, 421
    of nurse-patient communication, 126
    in nursing process, 108, 109, 118–119
    in problem-solving process, 237–238
    of self with detachment, 147
Exam candidates, 417
Examination results, reporting, 424
Examination security, for NCLEX-PN® examination, 423–424
Excelsior College, distance learning nursing program at, 448
Exercise equipment, using, 142
Experience, functioning beyond, liability and, 367–368, 368b
Extended care facilities
    care in, 163
    employment opportunities in, 432–434
    Medicare provisions for, 321b
    nursing assistants in, 171
External distractions, 42–43
Extroversion, learning and, 14–15
Eye wear, for job interviews, 410–411
Eyestrain, avoiding, 42

F

Fabiola, in nursing in ancient Rome, 92
Facilitators of learning, instructors as, 7
Facility organization, charge nurses and, 278
Facility policy, on delegation of nursing duties, 286
Failure, fear of, as liability for adult learners, 3–4
Failure to intervene, as source of malpractice, 362b
False imprisonment, 361
False-positive testing, pre-employment, 412
False reassurance blocking communication, 127
Family
    demanding/complaining, dealing with, 284–285
    structure of
        cultural diversity in, 188–189
        diversity profiles of, for U.S. cultural groups, 197b

Family practice physicians, 160, 308
Fasting, as means of patient suicide, 377
Fatigue
    mental, as distraction, 43
    nurses', consequences of, 336
Fax machines, 135
Faxes, HIPAA and, 371
Fear
    of failure, as liability for adult learners, 3–4
    of unknown, patient, 130
Federal health care agencies, 306
Federal privacy standards, 208
Federal regulations
    charge nurses and, 278
    of health care facilities, 263
Fee-for-service, 318, 319t
Fee setting as State Board of Nursing function, 355b
Feedback, in communication, 123
Feelings, expression of, cultural diversity in, 190
Felonies, 359
Female brain, 21
FICA withholding, 326b
Fidelity, as ethical principle, 348–349
Fight-flight mine, 19
Fill-in-the-blank items, in NCLEX-PN® examination, hints for, 57, 58
Fingernails, nosocomial infections and, 146
First Amendment rights, 6
First-line leaders, practical/vocational nurses as, 248
Flexibility, for home health nursing, 434
Float duty, legal implications of, 381
Fluids, as basic daily need, 185–186
Focus, in active listening, 125
Focused questions, in therapeutic communication, 126
Follow-up, after interview, 413–414
Following directions, in test taking, 56
Food and Drug Administrations (FDA), 306
Food preferences
    cultural diversity in, 189
    diversity profiles of, for U.S. cultural groups, 197b
Food service, charge nurse responsibilities for, 279
Forgetting, possible causes of, 53
Formal educational experiences, 2
Fourteenth Amendment rights, 6
Fragmentation
    as bias in textbooks, 24
    of care, in functional nursing, 172
Fraud, disciplinary action and, 356b
Free care, 329
Free clinics, 310
Free-standing ambulatory centers, 309
Frequent study periods, in storing information in long-term memory, 53–54
Friendly-focused interpersonal style, 387b
Friends, delegating tasks to, 34b
Fruits, in MyPyramid, 141f
Functional nursing, in acute care setting, 172
Fundamentalism, 217

G

Gallows humor, 131
Gamp, Sairy, 93

Gender differences
    in brain development, 21
    in communication styles, 127–128
General supervision, 355
Generalizations
    about adult learners, 2
    avoiding, 182
Generation Xers, as returning adult learners, 1
Gerontology vertification, 445–446
Goals
    in leadership scenarios, 258
    long-term, setting, 30
    and outcomes, 115
    in problem solving, deciding on, 236–237
    resident, formulating, in charge nurse delegation, 291
    short-term, setting, 30
Good Samaritan acts, 378
Google, 70
Gossip, dangers of, 233
Government health care agencies, 305, 306
Government-sponsored health insurance, 321–325
    Medicaid as, 323–324
    Medicare as, 320–323
    revenue sources for, 325, 326b
Grade inflation, dangers of, 4
Gradual improvement, in MyPyramid, 140f
Grains, in MyPyramid, 141f
Graphic information, organizing via mapping, 45–46, 47b, 48f
Great Depression, nursing in, 100
Greece, ancient, nursing in, 91
Greeting forms, cultural diversity in, 190
Gretter, Lystra, 96
Gross domestic product (GDP), percentage of, spent on health care, 318
Group homes, 312
Guest speakers, as learning resources, 73

H

Habit(s)
    definition of, 30
    personal, during job interview, 411
    time management and, 32
Habitual thinking, 77
Hand hygiene, nosocomial infections and, 145
Handling tasks
    most stressful, 144b
    preventing injuries during, 144–145
Head movements
    head roll exercises, 143
    male/female differences in, 128
Health belief systems
    adapting care plans based on culturally diverse, 201
    major, categories of, 195–196
Health care
    HIPAA definition of, 370b
    methods of delivering, 336–337
    national economy and, 327–328
    patient-focused, 336–337
    retail, 333
Health care agencies, comparing public and private, 305–306, 306t
Health care alliances/networks, 333

Health care costs
    fee-for-service vs. capitation, 318, 319t
    financing of, 318, 319t
    lack of insurance and, 328–329
    payroll deductions and, 326b
    single-payer system for, 333
    trends and issues in, 324–328
Health care crisis, 317
Health care financing, issues and trends in, 324–328
Health care providers
    capitation plans and, 318
    defined, 319
Health care settings, 304–305
    adult day care centers as, 313–314
    ambulatory services, 309–310
    assisted living programs as, 312
    board and care homes as, 312
    community health nursing services as, 312–313
    free clinic as, 310
    home health agencies as, 313
    hospice care as, 314
    hospitals as, 308–309
    intermediate care facilities as, 311
    long-term care facilities as, 311–312
    nursing homes as, 311
    one-day surgical care centers as, 310
    outpatient clinics as, 309–310
    post-acute care, 311
    private health care agencies as, 308
    public health care agencies as, 305–306
    rehabilitation services as, 311
    residential care facilities as, 312
    skilled nursing facilities as, 311
    urgent care centers as, 310
    voluntary health care agencies as, 307–308
    wellness centers as, 314
Health care system
    change in, handling, 337–338
    financing of
        issues and trends in, 324–328
        methods for, 318, 319t
    patient payment methods for, 319–324
    quality improvement in, 337
    rankings of, 317–318
    repair of, 331–333
        comprehensive changes in, 333–334
        incremental changes in, 332–333
    restructuring of, 333–336
    uncompensated care in, 329–331
Health care team(s), 159–179
    members of, 164–172
        empowering, 271
    nursing assistants on, 171
    nursing's place on, 165
    practical/vocational nurses on, 168–170. *See also* Practical/vocational nurses (LPN/LVNs).
    registered nurses on, 165–168. *See also* Registered nurses (RNs).
    student nurses on, 170–171
Health information, protected, restrictions on use of, in Notice of Privacy Practices, 371
Health insurance, 319–324
    alternatives in coverage, 333–330, 334b4

Health insurance (*Continued*)
   basic terms pertaining to, 319
   Canadian system, 318–319
   coinsurance and, 319
   copayments and, 319
   costs of, 327–328
   deductibles and, 319
   federal changes to, 331
   government-sponsored, 321–325
      Medicaid as, 324–325, 325t
      Medicare as, 321–324, 322b, 323b, 324b, 325t
      revenue sources for, 325, 326b
   group, 319–320
   issues and trends in, 328b
   lack of, cost of, 329–330
   Medicaid as, 323–324
   Medicare as, 320–323
   nongroup, private, 321
   payroll deductions for, 326b
   portability of, under HIPAA, 369, 370b
   premiums and, 319
   private, 320–321
Health Insurance companies, employment opportunities in, 438
Health Insurance Portability and Accountability Act (HIPAA)
   health provisions of, 331b
   legal implications of, 369–372
Health maintenance organizations (HMOs), 309, 321, 334, 334b
   reactions to, 334
Health promotion, 138–158
   chemical dependency in nurses and, 149–151
   coping with negative stress in, 153–157
   fingernail length and safety issues in, 146
   in NCLEX-PN® examination, 420
   nutrition and, 138–140
   preventing back injuries in nursing in, 144–145
   preventing burnout in, 146–148
   secondary traumatic stress issues in, 148–149
Health Resources Administration (HRA), 306
Health savings accounts, 333–334
Health Services Administration (HSA), 306
Health unit clerks, 171–172
Health unit coordinators, 171–172
Hebrews, ancient, nursing among, 91
Henry Street Settlement, 88t, 99
Highlighting, as study aid, 44
Hinduism, 219, 221, 222–223t
Hippocratic oath, applicability to nursing, 91
Hispanic Americans, diversity profiles of, 196–197b
Hmong Americans
   communication styles of, 129
   diversity profiles of, 196b
   sample data gathering sheet for, 199b
Home health care agencies, 313
   employment opportunities in, 430–431
   LPN/LVNs in, 170
   Medicare provision for, 321b
   nursing assistants in, 171
Home health nursing, employment opportunities in, 434–435
Home management, shortcuts to, 38–39

Home nursing care, 307–308
   history of, 98–99
Honesty
   assertiveness as, 229
   in patient/staff communication, 131
   vs. nonassertive (passive) behavior, 227
Hospice care, 314
   employment opportunities in, 438
   Medicare provision for, 321b
Hospital insurance, in Medicare Part A, 320, 321b
Hospital jobs, employment opportunities in, 430
Hospital nursing, employment opportunities in, 436
Hospitals, 308–309
Housekeepers, 163
   charge nurses and, 279
Howlett hierarchy of work motivators, 254–255, 255f
Human needs, understanding, in leadership roles, 254–256
Human relationship skills
   for first-line LPN/LVN leaders, 267–271
   resources for, 272
Humor
   in burnout prevention, 147–148
   in patient/staff communication, 131
Hygiene
   hand, nosocomial infections and, 145
   personal
      as basic daily need, 185
      for job interview, 405–406, 409

Idea sketches, as study aids, 52, 52f
Identification, for NCLEX-PN® examination, 423
Illegal questions, in application, answering, 398, 406b
Illegible physician's orders, 379–380
Illiteracy, as barrier to learning, 24–25
Illness, preventing, 318
Illness belief systems, diversity profiles of, for U.S. cultural groups, 197b
Illness beliefs, cultural diversity in, 196–197b
Imagery, as stress prevention, 154–155, 155b
Imbalance, as bias in textbooks, 24
Implementation
   in NCLEX-PN® examination, 421
   in nursing process, 108, 109
   of task assignment/delegation, 298–299
   of time management program, 36–39
Implied consent, 360, 374
Imprisonment, false, 361
In-service training, 442
Inactive status lists maintenance, as State Board of Nursing function, 355b
Incident report on personal criticism in patient's record, 379
Incompetence
   disciplinary action and, 356b
   requirement to disclose, 369b
Incomplete toolbox, communication of, 111
Independence
   as goal of occupational therapy, 163
   of registered nurses on health care teams, 166
Independent living apartments, 312
Index cards, as planning aids, 33
Indigent care, 329

Individual worth, philosophy of, 187
Individualistic learners, 19
Industrial age, nursing in, 93
Industry, LPN/LVNs in, 170
Infants, communicating with, 132
Inflation, health care spending and, 319
Informal educational experiences, 2
Information
    health, protected, restrictions on use of, in Notice of
        Privacy Practices, 371
    patient, requiring disclosure, 368, 369b
    subjective *vs.* objective, 110
Informational interview, 390–394
    follow-up letter after, 392b
Informed consent, 374
    as common law, 359
    underage children and, 348
Injuries, preventing, 144–145
Inpatient hospital care, under Medicare, 320
Institutional liability, 366
Instructors
    as facilitators of learning, 7
    legal liability of, 367
    responsible, learner's right to, 6
    as sources of references, 387
Insurance
    health, 320–325. *See also* Health insurance.
    malpractice, 362–363, 363b
Intelligence, multiple types of, 18–19
Intensive care units (ICUs), care in, 161–162
Intentional torts, 359
Interdependence
    of LPN/LVNs on health care team, 168–169
    of RNs with other health care team members, 166
Interlibrary loan services, 64
Intermediate care facilities, 311
Intermediate nursing facilities, OBRA and, 432
Internal distractions, 43
International health care agencies, 306
Internet
    career sites on, 389b
    as distraction from study, 43
    guidelines for gathering information from, 70b
    in job hunt, 389
    as learning resource, 69–70
Internet registration for NCLEX-PN® examination, 422
Internship, for physician, 160
Interpersonal learners, 18–19
Interpersonal styles, by prospective employers, 386,
    387b
Interpreters, use of, 192b
Interstate endorsements, 357, 418
Interventions. *See* Nursing interventions.
Interview, informational, 390–394
    follow-up letter after, 392b
Interview process, 110. *See also* Job interview(s).
Intrapersonal learners, 19
Introductions, 129–130
Introversion, learning and, 15
Invasion of privacy, autonomy and, 347
Invisibility, as bias in textbooks, 24
Irrational thinking, avoiding, in stress management, 261
Islam, 217–218, 218–219b

Isolation, as bias in textbooks, 24
Itasca Nursing Education Consortium program, 447
IV Therapy certification, 445

J

Jehovah's Witnesses, 220b
Job Analysis of Newly Licensed Practical Nurses,
    430–431
Job application questions
    answering expertly, 396–398
    examples of, 402–405b
Job descriptions
    for charge nurses, 275–277
    reviewing prior to delegation of duties, 294–295
Job interview(s), 399–401
    accessories during, 410
    answering illegal questions during, 398, 406b
    clothing for, 410
    courtesy during, 411
    differences between interviewer and you in,
        handling, 406b
    discussing pregnancy during, 411–412
    eye wear during, 410–411
    follow-up after, 413–414
    make-up for, 410
    manner during, 411
    personal habits and, 411
    posture recommendations, 411
    preparing for, 399–400
    questions and answers during, 400–401, 407–409b
    sample questions to ask interviewer during, 406b
Job outlook, for LPN/LVNs, 430–431
Job search
    attending professional conferences for, 389–390
    career choices in nursing, 385–386
    conducting informational interviews in, 390–394
    hidden job market in, 393
    Internet sites for careers in, 389b
    interpersonal styles of prospective employers
        and, 386, 387b
    interview preparation tips, 399–400
    interview questions and answers in, 400–401,
        407–409b
    job application questions and answers, 396–398,
        402–405b
    networking in, 387–390
    personal hygiene during, 405–406, 409
    references in, 387–388
    résumés in, 393, 395, 396b
    searching for employment openings in, 392–394
    use of cover letters in, 393b, 395–396, 401b, 402b
Joint Commission, The (TJC), 101
    in accreditation of health care facilities, 264, 336
    National Patient Safety Goals of, 372, 373b
    verification of licensure and, 358
Journal of Practical Nursing, 64, 89t, 441
Judaism, religious beliefs and practices of, 211–212, 212b
Justice, as ethical principle, 349

K

Key, in multiple choice question, 57
Kinesthetic learners, 16, 17
Knights Hospitalers, 92

Knowledge
  NCLEX-PN® and, 82
  in patient/staff communication, 131
Koran, 217

L

La Leche League, 307t
Laboratory personnel, 161
Lady with the Lamp, 95
Laissez-faire leadership style, 253b
Last Acts, 378
Late entries in charting, 379
Latinos. *See* Hispanic Americans.
Leadership
  anger management techniques in, 268–269
  applying communication skills for, 256–257
  conflict resolution in, 266–267
  documentation in, 262–263
  in empowering team members, 271
  in encouraging personal growth in nursing assistants, 271
  human relationship skills in, 267–271
  knowledge and skills needed for
    core, 253–262
    specific, 262–272
  legal aspects of, 263–264
  occupational skills for, 262–264
  organizational skills for, 264–267
  stress management in, 260–262
  team building in, 259–260
  understanding motivation and human needs for, 254–256
  using mission statements in, 259
Leadership activities
  discovering personal leadership style as, 251–252
  examining organizational charts as, 249
  identifying signs of stress as, 261
  performance evaluations as, 269–271
  state requirements for LPN/LVN charge nurse as, 249–250
Leadership continuum, 253
Leadership hints
  on applying nursing process to conflict resolution, 266–267
  for avoiding irrational thinking, 261
  on communication of practical/vocational charge nurse, 256–257
  on continuous quality improvement skills, 266
  for creating less stressful workplaces, 260
  on encouraging participation in evaluation process, 270
  in encouraging self-confidence in nursing assistants, 271
  on final evaluation interview, 270–271
  for life skills to control stress, 250
  OBRA provisions for nursing assistants as, 263
  in preventing anger in nursing assistants, 268
  in preventing workplace violence, 268–269
  problem-solving decision tree as, 258f
  on providing feedback to nursing assistants, 269
  on sources of learning skills, 272
  on using nursing process to organize shifts, 264–265
Leadership roles
  applying problem-solving skills for, 257–259
  management roles differentiated from, 250–251
  preparing for, 250
Leadership skills, 246–273

Leadership styles, 252–253, 253b
  autocratic, 252, 253b
  benefits and disadvantages of, 252
  democratic, 253b
  laissez-faire, 253b
  personal, discovering, 251–252
  situational, 252
Learned behavior, culture as, 181
Learners
  left-brained, 20–21
  left-handed, 20
  right-brained, 20
Learning
  barriers to, 23–25
  brain development and, 19–22
  instructors as facilitators of, 7
  lifetime ability for, 8
  methods and skills used in, 41–59
  in NCLEX-PN® examination, 421
  responsibility for, 6–12
  vs. teaching, 7–8
  water intake and, 22
Learning preferences, 16–17
Learning process, 22
Learning resource center (LRC), 61–64
  holdings of, 63
  investigating, 62–63
  resources of
    general information about, 63
    student skill levels and, 61, 62b
Learning resources
  audiovisual materials as, 69
  CD-ROM databases as, 73
  community resources as, 73
  computer-aided instruction as, 70–71
  computer simulations as, 71
  course outlines as, 68
  guest speakers as, 73
  Internet as, 69–70
  learning resource center (LRC) as, 61–64
  nursing skills lab as, 68–69
  periodicals as, 71–73
  study groups as, 68
  study skills lab as, 69
  syllabi as, 67
  tutoring as, 68
Learning strategies
  classroom, 64–67
  cooperative learning as, 66
  distance learning as, 66–67
  for lecture-discussions, 66
  for lectures, 64–66
Learning style(s), 15–17
  auditory, 16, 17
  bodily/kinesthetic learners, 18
  interpersonal learners, 18–19
  intrapersonal learners, 19
  kinesthetic, 16, 17
  linguistic learners, 18
  logical/mathematical learners, 18
  musical learners, 18
  perceptual, 15–17

Learning style(s) (*Continued*)
  personality patterns affecting, 14–15
  self-evaluation of, 15–16
  spatial learners, 18
  successful, developing, 14–27
  visual, 16–17
Lecture-discussion strategy, for instruction, 66
Lectures
  brief, to enhance learning, 65
  classroom learning strategies for, 64–66
Leeches, 99
Left-brain thinking, time-management skills
  and, 31
Left-brained learners, 20–21
  outlining method of note making for, 45
Left-handed learners, 20
Left hemisphere of cerebrum, 20, 20t
Legal action, steps for bringing, 363–364, 364b
Legal aspects, of nursing, ethics and, 340, 340t
Legal competency, 373
Legal issues, 353–384
  advance directives as, 375
  charting guidelines as, 365–366
  common law vs. statutory law as, 358–359
  confidentiality as, 368
  criminal vs. civil action as, 359–331, 360t
  disciplinary process and action as, 357–358
  disclosure of required information as, 368, 369b
  do-not-resuscitate order as, 376
  end-of-life, 375–378
  end-of-life organizations and, 378
  Good Samaritan acts as, 378
  HIPAA laws as, 369–372
  liability as, 366–368
  life support removal as, 376
  National Patient Safety Goals of The Joint
    Commission as, 372, 373b
  negligence as, 361–362
  for nurse leaders, 263–264
  nursing standard of care as, 358
  organ donation as, 377–378
  patient competency as, 373
  patient's right to consent as, 373–374
  patient's rights as, 368–369, 369b
  physician-assisted suicide and euthanasia as,
    376–377
  privacy as, 368
  State Board of Nursing and, 356–357, 356b
  steps for bringing legal action as, 363–364, 364b
Legal liability, for charge nurse delegation, 292
Legal precedents, 358–359
Letter
  cover. *See* Cover letter.
  follow-up, after informational interview, 392b
  of reference, sample, 389b
  resignation, sample, 415b
  thank you, after interview, 413, 414b
Liability, 366–368
  legal, for charge nurse delegation, 292
Libel, 360, 361
Librarians, 62, 63
Library of Congress classification system, *63*

Licensed practical nurse (LPN). *See also* Practical/
  vocational nurses (LPN/LVNs).
  development of title, 101
  role differentiation from RNs, 109, 166, 168–169, 169t
Licensing requirements
  mandatory, development of, 100
  as State Board of Nursing function, 355b
Licensure, 357
  multi-state, 357
  verification of, 358
Life span communication issues, 132–134
Life support systems, removal of, 376
Life-threatening situations, charge nurse delegation and, 291
Lighting, for study, optimizing, 42
Linguistic bias, in textbooks, 24
Linguistic learners, 18
Listeners, 16
Listening skills
  active listening behaviors as, 125–126
  active *vs.* passive, 44
  note making *vs.* note taking, 44–46, 46f, 47b
Literacy, phases of, 24–25
Living wills, 375
Local public health care agencies, 306
Logical/mathematical learners, 18
Long-term care facilities, 311–312
  assigning residents in, 300
  certification in, 444
  job opportunities in, 430
  LPN/LVNs in, 170
Long-term certification, 103
Long-term goals, 30
Long-term memory, aids for storing information in, 53–55
Long-term skilled nursing facility, 311
Loose-leaf notebooks, 45
LPN 2008, 64
LRC. *See* Learning resource center (LRC).

M

Magazines, 64
Mail registration for NCLEX-PN® examination, 422
Make-up, for job interviews, 410
Male brain, 21
Male/female differences, in communication styles, 127–128
Malpractice insurance, 362–363, 363b
Managed care, 333–334, 334b
  certification in, 446
  reaction to, 335–336
Management roles, . leadership roles differentiated from,
  250–251
Management skills, for reviewing policies and routines, 280
Management tools/hints, 277
  on assigning tasks, 287
  on communicating assigned tasks and delegated
    duties, 296–297
  on communication responsibilities of charge nurse
    in delegation, 297
  on criteria for delegating duties, 293
  on delegating duties, 287–288
  on demanding/complaining families, 284–285
  on duties not to delegate, 294
  on end-of-shift reporting, 302

Management tools/hints (*Continued*)
on evaluation and feedback, 299
on handling refusal of assignment by nursing assistants, 288, 295–296
on impracticality of listing duties to delegate, 294
on legal soundness in delegation, 289
on nursing assistants bringing problems to work, 283
on nursing group/employer positions on delegation, 286
onr encouraging personal responsibility in nursing assistants, 283
on reporting change of condition to physician, 281–282
on reviewing policies and routines, 280
on specific tasks for nursing assistant assignment, 292–293
on supervision and feedback, 298–299
Mandatory law, HIPAA definition of, 370b
Manipulation, cultural differences in, 238–239
Mapping method of note making, 45–46, 47b, 48f
Maslow's Hierarchy of Needs, 113, 254–255, 254f
Master of Nursing programs, 166
Matures, as returning adult learners, 1
Maturity, critical thinking and, 81
Meat, in MyPyramid, 141f
Medi-Van, 163
Medicaid, 323–324, 324t
Medical diagnosis, in multidisciplinary care plane, 116
Medical equipment sales, employment opportunities in, 438
Medical insurance, Medicare provisions for, 320, 321b
Medical jargon, 124, 130
Medical Leave Act, 411
Medical management companies, employment opportunities in, 439
Medical Practice Acts, 308
Medical records
amendments to, in Notice of Privacy Practices, 371
electronic, 337
patient access to, in Notice of Privacy Practices, 370–371
Medical records department, 161
Medical technologists, 161
Medicare, 320–323, 321b, 322b, 323b, 324b
basic components of, 321
health care plans under, 322–323
issues and trends in, 330b
Medicare Advantage Plan, 322, 323b
Medication errors, as source of malpractice, 362b
Medications
charge nurses and, 279
side effects of, in end-of-shift reporting, 301
Meditation, as stress prevention, 154
Medscape, for continuing education, 443
Memorization, rote, insufficiency of, 50
Memory
enhancing, 52–53, 53b
mnemonic devices for, 54–55
undependable, 22
Men in Nursing, 64
Mental fatigue, as distraction, 43
Mental health nursing, employment opportunities in, 435–436
Mental hygiene, as basic daily need, 186
Mental illness, cultural diversity in beliefs about, 193

Mental imagery, as study aid, 52–53, 53b
Mentors, critical thinking ability and, 82
Mexican Americans, communication styles of, 129
Middle Ages, nursing in, 92
Middle managers, 249
Midwives. *See* Certified nurse-midwives.
Military services, employment opportunities in, 436
Military time, use in charting, 365
Milk, in MyPyramid, 141f
Minilectures, to enhance learning, 65
Minimal encouraging, as active listening skill, 126
Minimum necessary rule in Notice of Privacy Practices, 371
Minimum nurse-to-patient ratios, 336
Minitasking, 37–38
Minneapolis Community and Technical College Mobility Program, 448
Minnesota border recognition agreement, 358
Misdemeanors, 359
Mission statements, in team building, 259
Mississippi, origins of licensing laws in, 88t, 100
Mnemonic devices, 54–55
Moderate physical activity, 141, 142t
Moderation, in MyPyramid, 140f
Moderation Management, 151
Modesty, cultural diversity in, 193
"Monkey trap," 283
Moral development, critical thinking and, 81
Morals, 340
Mormons, 220b
Motivation
critical thinking and, 80
Howlett hierarchy of work motivators and, 254–255, 255f
for study, lack of, in traditional learners, 4
understanding, in leadership role, 254
Movers as learners, 18
Multi-state licensure, 357
Multidisciplinary care plans, 116
Multiple-choice items
hints for, 57–58, 57b
in NCLEX-PN® examination, 83, 419
Multiple intelligences, 18–19
Multiskilled workers, 171
Muscle cramps, preventing, stretching in, 143
Musical learners, 18
Mutual recognition compacts, 357

N

NANDA-I. *See* North American Nursing Diagnosis Associatio-I (NANDA-I).
NAPNES. *See* National Association for Practical Nurse Education and Service, Inc. (NAPNES).
Narcotics Anonymous, 151
NAs. *See* Nursing assistants (NAs).
National Association for Practical Nurse Education and Service, Inc. (NAPNES), 89t, 440–441
critical thinking guided by, 76
ethical codes of, 341
postgraduate programs offered by, 433, 444
professional guidelines of, 356
National Committee for Quality Assurance (NCQA), 335

National Council for the State Boards of Nursing (NCSBN), critical thinking guided by, 76
National Council Licensing Examination for Practical/Vocational Nursing. *See* NCLEX-PN® Examination.
National Council of State Boards of Nursing Disciplinary Data Bank (NCSBNDB), 356b
National Council of State Boards of Nursing (NCSBN), 108, 109
   on delegation issue, 285
   practice analysis by, 250
National Federation of Licensed Practical Nurses (NFLPN), 441–442
   critical thinking guided by, 76
   ethical codes of, 341
   iStudySmart.com program of, 448–449
   postgraduate programs offered by, 433, 445–446
National League for Nursing (NLN), 99, 440
   NCLEX-PN® Readiness Tests by, 426–427
National Patient Safety Goals, 372, 373b
National Practitioner Data Bank (NPDB), 356b
Naturalistic system of health beliefs, 195, 196b
NCLEX® Examination Candidate Bulletin, 421
NCLEX-PN® Examination, 417–428
   application process for, 421–424
   before computerized adaptive testing, 417–418
   computerized adaptive testing in, 418, 424–425
   core content of, 419
   critical thinking skills for, 82–83
   description of, 418
   development of, 76
   as first computerized adaptive test, 90t
   integration of nursing concepts and processes in, 420–421
   mental health nursing coverage in, 435
   mock examinations for, 426–427
   overview of, 424–425
   patient needs focus in, 420–391
   as resource for standard of care, 359b
   results of, reporting, 424
   review books for, 426–427
   security measures for, 423–424
   test fees for, 422
   test question types in, 419–420
   test-taking procedure for, 56
   time limit for taking, 424
   updating content of, 419
   validity dates for, 423
Negative interactions
   coping mechanisms and, 231–233
   manipulative, 238–239
Negative stress, coping with, 153–157
Negative thinking, 77
Neglect, requirement to disclose, 369b
Negligence, 361–362
   disciplinary action and, 356b
   possible, documentation of, 381
   professional, 362–363
   proof of, 363, 363b
Net Generation/Millennials, as traditional adult learners, 1
Networking
   in health care system, 333
   in job search process, 387–390
   for references, 387–388
   through professional organizations, 440

Neural traces, in storing information in long-term memory, 53–54
Newspaper articles, 64
NFLPN. *See* National Federation of Licensed Practical Nurses (NFLPN).
Nightingale, Florence, 88t, 94–95
   core belief of, about nursing, 96
   drop in death rate due to, 96
   school of nursing established by, in Englant, 96
Nightingale Museum, 97
Nightingale Pledge, 88t, 96, 97
Nineteenth century, nursing development in, 93
Noise, background, managing, to optimize concentration, 42
Nonassertive behavior, 227–228
Nonfocused thinking, 77
Nonjudgmental attitude, in home health nursing, 435
Nonmaleficence, as ethical principle, 345–346
Nonverbal communication, 124
   smiling as, 128
North American Nursing Diagnosis Association-I (NANDA-I), 120
   spiritual distress and, 205
Nosocomial infections
   fingernails as source of, 146
   hand hygiene and, 145
Note making, 44–46, 46f, 47b
Note taking, 44, 45
Notes, making and reviewing, methods of, 45–46, 47b
Notice
   giving, 415
   of privacy practices under HIPAA, 370–371, 370b
NPA. *See* Nurse Practice Act (NPA).
Nurse(s)
   baccalaureate, training of, 161
   ethical responsibilities of, 344
   practical. *See* Practical/vocational nurses (LPN/LVNs).
   private practice, 308
   registered. *See* Registered nurses (RNs).
   self-proclaimed, 86
   student, 170–171
Nurse anesthetists, 167
Nurse extenders, 171
Nurse managers, 162
Nurse Practice Act (NPA), 108, 354–355
   assignment and delegation in, 285–286
   charge nurse prerequisites in, 277
   content of, 355
   ethical issues and, 341–342
   requirements for charge nurse in, 249
   as resource for standard of care, 359b
   violation of, 356b
Nurse practitioners, 167
Nurse-to-patient ratios, minimum, 336
Nurse's aide, 163
Nursing
   capability in, critical thinking and, 82
   career opportunities available in, 429–430
   definition of, 164–165
   place of, on health care team, 165
Nursing, 64

Nursing action, in implementation phase of nursing process, 117
Nursing assistants (NAs), 163, 171
  bringing problems from home, 283
  criteria for assigning/delegating to, 292–298
  encouraging personal responsibility in, 283
  OBRA provisions specific to, 263
  performance evaluations of, 269–271
  refusal of assignments by, 295–296, 298
Nursing brotherhoods, 92
Nursing care
  basic, 354
  delivery of, in acute care settings, 172–176
  procedures for charge nurses related to, 279
Nursing care plans. *See* Care plan(s).
Nursing case management, in acute care setting, 173–174, 175f
Nursing diagnosis
  added to nursing process, 108
  assisting RN to develop, 112–113
  explanation of, 109
  spiritual distress as, 205
Nursing duties, delegating, 287–288
Nursing experience, critical thinking ability and, 82
Nursing history, 86–106
  important influence in, 103–104t
Nursing Home Reform Ace, 263
Nursing homes, 311. *See also* Extended care facilities.
  alternatives to, 311–312
  employment opportunities in, 430
  nursing assistants in, 171
Nursing interventions
  assisting RN to develop, 115–117, 116t
  for Baha'i patients, 221b
  for Buddhist and Hindu patients, 222–223t, 223–224
  for Catholic patients, 214–215b
  for Christian Scientists, 220b
  for demanding/complaining families, 284
  for Eastern religions, 219, 221–223
  for Jehovah's Witnesses, 220b
  for Jewish patients, 212b
  in leadership scenario, 258
  for Mormon patients, 220b
  for Muslim patients, 218–219b
  in nursing process, 108, 117–118
Nursing Interventions Classification (NIC), 119
Nursing jargon, inappropriate use of, 130
Nursing journals, 64
Nursing liability, 366–368
Nursing organizations
  American Nurses Association as, 440
  as learning resources, 73
  National Association for Practical Nurse Education and Service, Inc. as, 440–441
  National Federation of Licensed Practical Nurses (NFLPN) as, 441–442
  National League for Nursing as, 440
  standards of, on delegation of nursing duties, 286
Nursing Outcomes Classification (NOC), 119–120
Nursing problems, 116
Nursing process, 107–121
  data collection phase of, 110–112

Nursing process (*Continued*)
  evaluation phase of, 118–119
  five-step, 108
  four-step, 108, 110–119
  getting organized with, 31–39
  as guide for assigning tasks and delegating duties, 289–300
  implementation phase of, 117–118
  importance of, for leaders, 262
  in NCLEX-PN® examination, 421
  1950s developments in, 108
  organizing shifts using, 264–265
  planning phase of, 112–117
  role of critical evaluation in, 9–10
Nursing regulatory boards, 355–357
Nursing schools
  founded by Florence Nightingale, 96
  historical development of, 94
Nursing shortages, 176–177
  action by AMA to reduce, 102
  after World War I, 100·
  causes of, 177b
  concerns for patient safety, 102
  legal implications of, 381
  solutions for, 178b
Nursing situation, complex, 354–355
Nursing skills, burnout prevention and, 148
Nursing skills lab, as learning resource, 68–69
Nursing standard of care, 358
  resources for, 359b
Nursing students, special challenges for, 6
Nutrition
  adequate, planning for, 36
  as basic daily need, 185–186
  in health promotion, 138–140
  USDA MyPyramid and, 139–140, 140–141f

O

Obesity, as health risk, 138–139
Objective charting, subjective charting versus, 262–263
Objective information, 110
Objective statements, in résumés, 368
Objective tests, hints for, 57, 57b
Observers, 16
Occupational skills
  for first-line LPN/LVN leaders, 262–264
  resources for, 272
Occupational therapists (OTs), 163
  Medicare provision for, 321b
Occupational therapy assistants (OTAs), 163
Occurrence coverage, 363
Official health care agencies, 305, 306
Oils, in MyPyramid, 141f
Omnibus Budget Reconciliation Act (OBRA), 171, 263
  skilled and intermediate nursing facilities and, 432
One-day surgical care centers, 310
One-way communication, 123
Online catalogs, 63
Open-ended questions, in therapeutic communication, 126
Operating room nursing, employment opportunities in, 437
Operating room technicians, 437
Oregon Death With Dignity Act, 377

Organ donation, 377–378
Organizational charts, 248–249, 248f, 249f
Organizational skills
  in continuous quality improvement, 265–266
  for first-line LPN/LVN leaders, 264–267
  resources for developing, 272
  time management, 264–265
Orthodox Eastern churches, 214b, 216–217
Orthodox Judaism, 212
Orthopedic surgeons, 160
Outcomes. *See* Patient outcomes.
Outlining method, of note making, 45, 46f, 47b
Outpatient clinics, 309–310
  employment opportunities in, 437
Outpatient hospital services, Medicare provisions for, 321b
Outside responsibilities, as dangers for returning adult
  learners, 5
Overtime, voluntary *vs.* mandatory, 336

P

Pain expressions, cultural diversity in, 190–191
Pamphlet files, 64
Paradigm shift, 7
Paraphrasing, as active listening skill, 125–126
Parish nurses, 207
  employment opportunities for, 439
Partnership for Caring: America's Voices for the Dying, 378
Party-focused interpersonal style, 387b
Party mentality, 4
Passive-aggressive manipulator, 239
Passive behavior, 227–228
  by patients' families, 284
Passive euthanasia, 376, 377t
Passive learners, 7
Passive listening, 44
Pastoral care team, 161, 208
Pat answers blocking communication, 127
Paternalism
  beneficent, 349–351
  women's health and, 350–351
Patience, in patient/staff communication, 131
Patient(s)
  competency of, 373
  identification of, improving accuracy of, 373b
  needs of, as basis for NCLEX-PN® examination, 420
  rights of, 368–369, 369b
    to consent, 373–374
Patient advocacy
  as ethical responsibility of nurses, 344
  women's health issues and, 350–351
Patient care
  responsibility for
    in emergency room, 160–161
    on extended care unit, 163
    in intensive care, 161–162
    in postanesthesia care unit, 161
    during surgery, 161
    on surgical floor, 162–163
  standards of, 166
Patient care assistant, 163
Patient care associate, 171
"Patient Care Partnership,", 368, 369b

Patient care plans. *See* Care plan(s).
Patient care technician, 171
Patient care technologists (PCTs), 163
Patient charting. *See* Charting.
Patient-controlled analgesia (PCA), 162
Patient education
  coverage in NCLEX-PN® examination, 421
  inadvisability of delegating, 294
  legal and ethical implications of, 381–382
Patient-focused care, 336–337
  as delivery system, 174, 176
Patient outcomes
  assisting RN to develop, 113, 115
  documentation of, 262
  in evaluation phase of nursing process, 119
  as indication of quality of care, 265
Patient payment methods
  government-sponsored health insurance as, 320–324
  health insurance, 319–324
  health insurance as. *See also* Health insurance.
  Medicaid as, 323–324
  Medicare as, 320–323
  private pay, 319
Patient records
  illegal alteration of, 379
  personal criticism in, 379
Patient safety
  back injury prevention and, 144–145
  Joint Commission National Patient Safety Goals for,
    372, 373b
  maintaining in nursing process, 116, 117
  in NCLEX-PN® examination, 420
Patient Self-Determination Act, 375
Patient situation, basic, 354
Patient/staff communications, 131–132
Payroll deductions, for funding health care, 336b
Peace Corps, employment opportunities in, 440
Pearson Professional Centers, 421
Peer reporting, as ethical responsibility of nurses, 344
Peers, as distraction from study, 43
Perceptual learning styles, 15–17
Performance evaluations, 8
  of nursing assistants, 269–271
Periodical indexes, 71–72, 72f
Periodical listings, 72
Periodicals
  as learning resources, 71–73
  nursing, 64
Personal care, 310
  as basic daily need, 185
  and hygiene, as basic daily need, 185
Personal characteristics
  affecting communication, 123
  self-evaluation of, 126
Personal criticism, documented in patient records, 379
Personal digital assistants (PDAs), as planning aids, 33
Personal distractions, 43
Personal factors, affecting concerns upon hospitalization,
  130
Personal goals, reviewing, importance of, 30
Personal habits, during job interviews, 411
Personal health information (PHI), HIPAA and, 371

Personal hygiene, for job interview, 405–406, 409
Personal liability, 366
Personal responsibility, in nursing assistants, encouraging, 283
Personal Responsibility and Work Opportunity Reconciliation Act, 323
Personal study area, reducing distractions in, 42
Personal support system, 33
Personalistic system of health beliefs, 195, 195b
Personality, learning and, 14–15
Personalization, in MyPyramid, 140f
Personnel policies, charge nurses and, 278
Pharmaceutical sales, employment opportunities in, 438
Pharmacists, 161
Pharmacology, certification in, 433, 445–446
Phoebe, as first visiting nurse, 92
Physical abuse, 361
Physical activity
    as aid in focusing attention, 23
    as aid in information retention, 54
    making time for, 140–144
    moderate, 141, 142t
    in MyPyramid, 140f
    vigorous, 142
Physical assessment, 110
Physical challenges, for returning adult learners, 5
Physical examination, prior to hiring, 412
Physical therapists (PTs)
    in extended-care facility, 163
    Medicare provision for, 321b
    on surgical floor, 162
Physical therapy assistants (PTAs)
    in extended-care facility, 163
    on surgical floor, 162
Physician-assisted suicide, 376–377
Physicians
    family practice, 308
    offices of, LPN/LVNs in, 170
    orders of, illegible, handling of, 379–380
    reporting change of condition to, 281–282
Physiological integrity, in NCLEX-PN® examination, 420
Physiological needs, 108
Plague, bubonic, nursing during, 92
Plain-text résumés, 395, 396b
Planning
    arguments against, 32
    by charge nurses for assigning/delegating, 290–298
    in NCLEX-PN® examination, 420
    in nursing process, 108, 109, 112–117
        assisting RN in developing nursing diagnosis, 112–117
        assisting RN in developing outcomes, 113, 115
    in time management, 32–36
PMA. *See* Positive mental attitude (PMA).
Podcasts, for continuing education, 443
Policies, related to charge nurses, 278–279
Policy manuals for facilities, review of, in job search, 392
Portability of insurance under HIPAA, 369, 370b
Positive mental attitude (PMA), 4
    as factor in learning, 54
    in test taking, 56
Post-acute care facilities, 311
Post-it notes, as planning aids, 33

Postanesthesia care units, care in, 161
Postgraduate certification programs, 433, 443–446
Posture
    male/female differences in, 128
    poor, correcting , stretching in, 143
    recommendations on, for job interviews, 411
Power of attorney, durable medical, 375
PQRST method of study
    for distance learning, 67
    for professional journal articles, 64
    for textbooks, 49–51
Practical Nurse training programs
    American history of, 98–99
    early history of, 86–87
Practical Nursing Today, 89t
Practical/vocational nurses (LPN/LVNs)
    in age of industrialization, 93
    during American Civil War, 97
    among ancient Hebrews, 91
    in ancient Egypt, 90–91
    in ancient Greece, 91
    in early Christian age, 91–92
    early training programs for, 86–87
    education of, 168
    in 1887, job description for, 105b
    evolution of, 86–106
    in extended-care units, 163
    as first-line leaders, 248
    first school of nursing for, 94
    Florence Nightingale in history of, 94–95
    formal training programs for, 98–99
    independent roles of, 109
    interdependence of, with RNs, 109
    in Middle Ages, 92
    modern, 87
    in nineteenth century, 93
    nursing history milestones, 87–90t
    outline of duties of, 101
    relevance of Hippocratic oath to, 91
    during Renaissance, 92
    role differentiation from registered nurses, 166, 169t
    role of
        expanded, 169–170, 249–250
        on health care teams, 168–169
    self-proclaimed nurses in, 86
    in seventeenth and eighteenth centuries, 92–93
    sites of employment of, 170
    on surgical floor, 162
    tasks differentiated from RN tasks, 101–102
    twentieth-century developments in, 99–103
    in twenty-first century, 103
Practical/vocational nursing students (SPNs/SVNs), role differentiation from LPN/LVN, 118
Prayer, 210
Pre-employment hurdles, 412–414
Precedents, legal, 358–359
Preferred provider organizations (PPOs), 334b
Pregnancy and birth
    cultural diversity in beliefs and practices related to, 194
    discussing during job interviews, 411–412
Pregnancy Discrimination Act, 411
Prejudice, dangers of, 182

Premiums, definition of, 319
Preponderance of evidence in civil action, 360
Preschoolers, communicating with, 133
Prescription drugs
    buying from foreign sources, 328
    cost of, 327–328
    under Medicare, 321–322
    Medicare coverage for, 322–323, 323b
Preventing illness, cultural diversity in beliefs about, 193
Previewing information, 49
Prig, Betsy, 93
Primary care nursing, in acute care setting, 173
Priorities
    honoring, 35, 37–38
    setting, 30, 33
        in charge nurse delegation, 291
Prison systems, employment opportunities in, 439
Privacy
    HIPAA and, 208, 331
    lack in health care settings, 130
    legal issues relating to, 368
    protection of, under HIPAA, 369, 370b
    role of, in patient autonomy, 347
    violations of, complaints about, in Notice of Privacy
        Practices, 371
Privacy officers under HIPAA, 370b
Private agency regulations, charge nurses and, 278
Private duty nursing, employment opportunities in, 439
Private health care agencies, 308
Private practice nurses, 308
Probing blocking communication, 127
Problem, in leadership scenario, 258
Problem-oriented thinking, 77
Problem solving, 231, 232f
Problem-solving process, 233–238
    clinical, in NCLEX-PN® examination, 420–421
    defining problem in, 235–236
    evaluating effectiveness of approach in, 237–238
    implementing alternatives in, 237
    repeating process in, 238
Problem-solving skills
    applying as LPN/LVN leader, 257–259
    charge nurses and, 277
    choosing alternatives in, 237
    deciding on goals in, 236–237
    development of, instructors encouraging, 8
Procrastination, 37
Professional conferences, attending, for job networking,
    389–390
Professional journals, 64
Professional nursing organizations, 440–442
Progressive relaxation, 155–156, 156b
Projection mechanism, 231
Proportionality, in MyPyramid, 140f
Prospective payment system, 322
Protestant churches, 215–216b, 217
Proximate cause, 363b
Psychological needs, 108
Psychosocial integrity, in NCLEX-PN® examination, 420
Public health care agencies, 305–307
    examples of, 306

Public health nursing, 99
Public hospitals, 309
Public Law 911, 102
Purpose, in active listening, 125

Q

Quality control, in U.S. health care system, 334
Quality improvement, 337
Quality Improvement Organization Program, 266
Questionable orders, documentation of, 380
Questioners as learners, 18
Questioning method, in textbook study, 49–50
Questions, in therapeutic communication, types of, 126
Qur'an (Koran), 217

R

Race, categorization by, 187
Racial bias, in textbooks, 23–24
Radiologists, 160
Random thoughts, 77
Rationalization, 231
Reader's Guide to Periodical Literature, 71–72
Reading
    effective, 51–52
    in textbook study, 50
Reading assignments, 47, 49–52
Reasonable doubt, in criminal action, 359
Reasoning model of nursing process, 108
Receiver, in communication, 123
Recordkeeping, charge nurses and, 278
Recreation
    as basic daily need, 186
    in stress prevention, 153–154
Recycled adult learners, 2
    attributes of, for success, 3
    dangers for, 5
    prior educational experiences of, 2
Red Cross, introduction to U.S, 98
Reference materials, locating, 63–64
References
    in job hunt, 387–388, 394–395
        hierarchy of, 394
        networking for, 387–388
    networking for, 387–388
Referrals, to school counselors, 11
Reflection, as active listening skill, 125
Reflective thinking, in PQRST method, 51
Reform Judaism, 212
Registered Care Technologist (RCT) initiative, 102
Registered nurses (RNs)
    certification of, 166–167
    education for, 165
        beyond basic nursing programs, 166–168
    historical differentiation of practical nurses from, 101–102
    independent functioning of, 109
    interdependence of, with LPN/LVNs, 109
    noncredit programs to advance as, 449
    role differentiation from LPNs, 109, 166, 168–169 169t
    role in health care teams, 160
    role of, 165–166
    staff, as sources of references, 387
    teaching role of, 117–118

Registration, for NCLEX-PN® examination, 422
Regression during illness, 113
Regulations, related to charge nurses, 278
Rehabilitation services, 311
Reincarnation, Hinduism and, *221*
Relatives, delegating tasks to, 34b
Relaxation techniques
    for adult ADD, 23
    brief relaxation as, 155, 155b
    overcoming test anxiety with, 426
    progressive relaxation as, 155–156, 156b
    as stress prevention, 149
Religion
    Eastern religions in North America, 219–223
    medical ethics and, 348
    patients and, 209
    in U.S, 210–211
    vs. spirituality, 206
Religious beliefs
    cultural diversity in, 189
    diversity profiles of, for U.S. cultural groups, 197b
Religious denomination, definition of, 209
Religious practices, value of, 209
Renaissance, nursing in, 92
Repatterning harmful health practices, 202, 203b
Reporting
    guidelines for, 297
    oncoming shift reporting, 290, 289–290
    peer, as ethical responsibility of nurses, 344
    timely, lack of, lawsuits based on, 362b
Res ipsa loquitur, 362
Research, role of LPN/LVN *vs.* RN in, 169t
Research hospitals, 309
Residency programs, for physicians, 160
Resident goals, in charge nurse delegation, 291
Residential care facilities, 312
    employment opportunities in, 439
Resignation, 414–415
Resignation letter, 415b
Respect, in patient/staff communication, 131
Respiratory therapists, 162
Respondeat superior, 366
Responsibility, legal accountability and, 367
Rest
    as basic daily need, 185
    periods of, in storing information in long-term
        memory, 54
Restatement
    as active listening skill, 125
    as study aid, 50
Results-focused interpersonal style, 387b
Résumés, 393, 395, 396b
    electronic, plain-text, sample, 399b
    typed
        starting with education, sample, 398b
        starting with work experience, sample, 397b
Retail health care, 333
Retention
    ensuring recall, 47
    of learned material, review of notes in, 45
    via oral rehearsal of material, 68

Returning adult learners, 1–2
    attributes of, for success, 3
    dangers for, 5
    formal educational experiences of, 2
Review, periodic, for tests, 55
Revocation of license, as State Board of Nursing function,
    355b
Rhymes
    as aids to memory, 54
    auditory learners and, 17
Right-brain thinking, time management skills and, 31–32
Right-brained learners, 20
Right hemisphere of cerebrum, 20t, 220
Rights
    of adult learners, 6
    patients', ethical health care decisions supporting, 344
Rituals, value of, 209
RN, 64
Role changes, patient, 129–130
Roles, life, identification of, 183–184
Rote memorization, insufficiency of, 50
Ruminative thinking, 77

S

Safety, patient
    maintaining, in nursing process, 116, 117
    nurse fatigue and, 336
Safety policies
    charge nurse delegation and, 292, 296
    charge nurses and, 278–279
    Joint Commission National Patient Safety Goals as, 372,
        373b
St. Vincent de Paul, 92
Sarcasm, by patients' families, 284
Savings accounts, health, 333–334
Scannable résumés, 395, 396b
Schedules, aids to organizing, 33
School-age children, communicating with, 133
School placement personnel, as sources of references, 387
Scolding behaviors, blocking communication, 127
Scope of practice
    functioning beyond, liability and, 367–368, 368b
    for LPN/LVNs, 289
Seacole, Mary, 95
Seamless systems, health care alliances as, 334
Search engines, 70
Second-career learners, 2
Secondary traumatic stress, 148–149
Secular institutions, nursing in, 93
Security standards, addressed by HIPAA, 370
Seducer, in negative manipulative interactions, 238–239
Selectivity, as bias in textbooks, 24
Self-confidence
    encouraging in employees, 271
    for home health nursing, 435
    required for critical thinking, 81
Self-directed learners, 3, 7
Self-discipline, 430
    in distance learning, 67
Self-esteem, in patient/staff communication, 132
Self-evaluation, 9, 10

Self-knowledge, 183–184
Self-paced instruction, 19
Self-proclaimed nurses, 86
Semester planning, 35
Semmelweis, Ignaz Philipp, 93
Sender, in communication, 123
Sensitivity
    in patient/staff communication, 131
    to physical and emotional changes in home health
        nursing, 435
Service issues, in Canadian health care system, 318
Seventeenth century, nursing in, 92–93
Sexual harassment, 243–244
Sheridan College School of Nursing Associate degree
    program, 447–448
Short-answer questions, hints for, 57, 57b, 58
Short study periods, in storing information in long-term
    memory, 54
Short-term goals, 30
Short-term skilled nursing facility, 311
Shorthand, disadvantages of note-taking in, 45
Side effects, in end-or-shift reporting, 301
Signs and symptoms, in charge nurse data collection, 281
Silence
    as active listening skill, 126
    cultural diversity in meaning of, 191
    as tool in job interview, 410
Simulations, as learning resources, 71
Single-parent families, 188
Single parents, challenges for, 6
Single-payer system, for health care costs, 333
Sisters of Charity, 92, 93, 95
Sisters of Mercy, 95
Situational influences, affecting communication, 123
Situational leadership style, 252
Skill mix, for health care team, 176
Skilled nursing care, 310
Skilled nursing facilities, 311
    Medicare coverage for, 321b
    OBRA and, 432
Skipping class, 65
Slander, 360, 361
Slang, 124
Sleep
    adequate, planning for, 36
    as basic daily need, 185
    before NCLEX-PN® examination, 426
    in stress prevention, 156–157
Smiling, gender differences in, 128
Smith Hughes Act of 1917, 89t, 100
Social activities, hidden dangers of, 4
Social needs, 108
Social responsibilities, as dangers for returning adult
    learners, 5
Social service agencies, employment opportunities in, 439
Social workers, 162
Socialization, 182
Socializers as learners, 18–19
Songs, auditory learners and, 17
Spatial learners, 18
Special care units, 172

Speech therapists, Medicare provisions for, 321b
Spiral-bound notebooks, disadvantages of, 45
Spiritual care
    importance of, 206
    interventions for, 208b
    need for, 206–207
Spiritual dimension, of person, 206
Spiritual distress, 205, 209
Spiritual needs, 108, 205–225
    of patients and families, 206
    meeting, 207–208, 208b
Spiritual practices, by patients, 209
Spiritual support, as basic daily need, 186
Spirituality, religion vs., 206
Spouse-only time, 34–35
Spouses, delegating tasks to, 33–35, 34b
Stacks, 63
Staff nurses, 161
Staffing limitations, delegation and, 296
Standardized care plans, 116
Standards of care, 166, 358
    resources for, 359b
Standing orders, documentation of, 381
State Boards of Nursing, 355–357, 417
    in application for NCLEX-PN® examination, 421
    locating approved RN programs through, 449
State health departments, 306
State regulations
    charge nurses and, 278
    of health care facilities, 263–264
Static simulations, as learning resources, 71
Stating in textbook study, 50
Statutory law, 359
Stem, in multiple choice question, 57
Stereotypes, religious, avoiding, 211
Stereotyping
    avoiding in workplace, 182
    of culturally diverse patients, avoiding, 200b
    racial, as bias in textbooks, 24
Sterile technique procedures, inadvisability of
    delegating, 294
Stoic behavior, cultural diversity in, 191
Stress
    burnout differentiated from, 146–148, 147t
    traumatic, secondary, 148–149
Stress management, 153–157
    by LPN/LVN leader, 260–262
Stretching, 142–143
    health benefits of, 143–144
Structured activities, in planning, 31
Student nurses
    liability of, 367
    role on health care teams, 170–171
Study buddies, auditory learners and, 17
Study group, as learning resource, 68
Study skills
    lack of, school failure and, 41
    PQRST method of textbook study as, 49–51
Study skills lab, 69
Studying, motivation for, lack of, in traditional learners, 4
Subjective charting, objective charting versus, 262–263

Subjective information, 110
Subjective tests, hints for, 57, 57b
Subungual zone, pathogens in, 146
Suicide, risk of, for nurses, 235
Summarizing, as active listening skill, 126
Supervision
  direct, 355
Supervision (*Continued*)
  failed, consequences of, 299
  general, 355
  of nursing assistant with delegated duty, 298–299
Supervisors, as sources of references, 387
Supplemental insurance for Medicare, 322
Surgical floor, care on, 162–163
Surgical health care teams, 161
Surgical technicians, 161
Suspension of license, as State Board of Nursing function, 355b
Syllabi as learning resource, 67
Sympathy vs. empathy in burnout prevention, 146–147
Systemizing brain, 21

T

Talmud, 211–212
Tasks, delegating, 33–35
Teaching
  in NCLEX-PN® examination, 421
  role of LPN *vs.* RN in, 117–118
  vs. learning, 7–8
Teaching and research hospitals, 309
Team, health care. *See* Health care team.
Team building, leadership in, 259–260
Team leaders, 162
  as sources of references, 387
Team nursing, in acute care setting, 173
Teenagers, communicating with, 133
Telephone logs, 382
Telephone orders, documentation of, 380
Telephone registration, for NCLEX-PN® examination, 422
Telephone requests, for protected health information in Notice of Privacy Practices, 371
Temporary help agencies, employment opportunities in, 439
Temporary permits, 357
  applying for, 425
Terminal illness, cultural diversity in beliefs and practices related to, 194
Test(s)
  content and form of, clarifying, 55
  periodic review for, 55
  preparation for, 55
  reviewing, 57
Test anxiety, 426
  overcoming, 425–426
Test fees, 422
Test framework, of NCLEX-PN® examination, 420
Test Plan for the National Council Licensure Examination for Practical Nurses, 419
Test questions, types of, in NCLEX-PN® examination, 419–420
Test-taking, 55–57
  following directions in, 56
  successful, hints for, 55–59

Test-taking skills, of traditional learners, 3
Testimony, 364
Testing in textbook study, 50–51
Testing time, for NCLEX-PN® examination, 424
Text messaging, 135
Thank-you letters, for interview, 413, 414b
Theory, clinical application of, 5
Theory tests, 8
Therapeutic communication, 126
Thinking mind, 19
Third-party coverage, 320
Time, scheduling, 32–33
Time concepts, cultural diversity in, 190
Time limit, for NCLEX-PN® examination, 424
Time line as planning aid, 33
Time long, in time management, 31
Time management, 28–40, 430
  benefits of, 30
  burnout prevention and, 147
  data collection in, 31
  implementing, 36–39
  planning in, 32–36
  program for, evaluation of, 39
  skills in
    for distance learning, 67
    lack of, in traditional learners, 4
    for leadership, 264–265
    self-test in, 29–30
    for test preparation, 55
  in test preparation, 55
Torah, 211–212
Tort law, 359, 360–363
Total care nursing, 172
Total quality management, 337
Traditional adult learners, 1
  attributes of, for success, 3
  formal educational experiences of, 2
  hidden dangers for, 4
  test-taking skills of, 3
Training sessions, attending, for job networking, 389–390
Transport aides, 161, 162
Traumatic stress, secondary, 148–149
Travel Nurses, 438
Treatment plans, negotiating with culturally diverse patients, 201b
Trust, in patient/staff communication, 131
Tutoring, as learning resource, 68
Two-way communication, 123

U

UAP. *See* Unlicensed assistive personnel (UAP).
Uncompensated care, 329–331
Underachievement, past, dangers of, 3
Underlining, as study aid, 44
Understaffed units, legal implications of, 381
Understanding
  reading with, 47, 80–81
  visual strategies to enhance, 52–53
Unethical conduct, disciplinary action and, 356b
Uniforms, nosocomial infections and, 146
Uninsured persons, 328
  state-level solutions for, 332
  as unsolved problem, 333–334

Unintentional torts, 359–360, 361–363
Uniqueness
   celebrating, 187–188
   exploring your, 183
Unit administration, charge nurses and, 278
Unit managers, 172
   as sources of references, 387
Unit routines, charge nurses and, 278
United Nations (UN), 306
United Ostomy Association, 307t
Universal coverage, 332
Unknown, patient fears of, 130
Unlicensed assistive personnel (UAP), 163, 171
   documenting care by, 379
   future trends in, 336
   legal issues pertaining to, 358
Unprofessional acts, requirement to disclose, 369b
Unreality, as bias in textbooks, 24
Upbringing, critical thinking and, 80
Upward mobility, 446–449
Urgent care centers, 310
URLs, 69
U.S. Department of Vocational Education, 101
U.S. Public Health Service (USPHS), 306
USDA MyPyramid, 2005, 139–140, 140–141f
Utilization review system in managed care, 334

V

Vaccine-related adverse reactions, requirement to disclose, 369b
Validation, as active listening skill, 126
Validity dates, for NCLEX-PN® examination, 423
Values, 340
   personal, medical ethics and, 348
Variety, in MyPyramid, 140f
Vegetables, in MyPyramid, 141f
Verbal communication, 123–124
Verbal cues, in minilectures and discussions, 65–66, 65b
Verbal orders, documentation of, 380
Verification of licensure, 358
Vertical files, 64
Veterans Administration Hospitals and veterans retirement homes, employment opportunities in, 438
Veterinary clinics and hospitals, employment opportunities in, 438
Vicarious liability, 366
Violations of privacy, complaints about, in Notice of Privacy Practices, 371
Violence
   employee, 241–242
   factors contributing to, 240–241
   sexual harassment as, 243–244
   workplace, prevention of, 242–243b, 268–269
Virtual clinical excursions, as learning resources, 71
Virtual reference programs, 63
Visiting Nurses Association, 307–308
VISTA, employment opportunities in, 440
Visual learners, 16–27
Visualizers as learners, 18
Vocational nurses. *See* Practical/vocational nurses (LPN/LVNs).
Voice, powerful, steps in developing, 391
Voluntary community hospitals, 309

Voluntary health care agencies, 305–306, 307–308
   examples of, 307t

W

Wage expectations, for LPN/LVNs, 431
Wald, Lillian, 99
Ward clerks, 162, 171–172
Warm-ups, 142
Water, intake of, learning and, 22
Weekly planning, 35–36
Weight-loss clinics
   employment opportunities in, 439
   LPN/LVNs in, 170
Wellness centers, 314
Western secular belief system, ethical health care decisions and, 343–344
White American communication styles, 128
Wills
   living, 375
   signing of, witnessing of, by nurse, 381
Word players, 18
Work experience, in résumé, 397b
Work sites
   assisted living facilities as, 439
   chiropractic offices as, 437
   coroner's office as, 439
   doctors' offices as, 437
   extended care facilities as, 432–434
   health insurance companies as, 438
   home health nursing as, 434–435
   hospice care as, 438
   hospital nursing as, 436
   mental health nursing as, 435–436
   military services as, 436
   operating room nursing as, 437
   outpatient clinics as, 437
   parish nursing as, 439
   pharmaceutical/medical equipment sales as, 438
   private duty nursing as, 439
   residential treatment centers as, 439
   temporary help agencies as, 439
   for travel nursing, 438
   Veterans Administration Hospitals and veterans retirement homes as, 438
   veterinary clinics and hospitals as, 438
Working the room in job search, 389–390
Workouts, parts of, 14
Workplace violence, 241–242
   prevention of, 242–243b, 268–269
Workshops, 442
World Health Organization (WHO), 306
   ranking of U.S. health care system, 317
World War I/II, nurses in, 100
World Wide Web (www), as learning resource, 69
Worldview, from enculturation, 181–182
Written policies
   on delegation of nursing duties, 286
   as resource for nursing standard of care, 359b
Written tests, 8

X

X-ray technicians, 160

ANSWERS TO REVIEW ITEMS

Chapter 1
1. 1
2. 3
3. 1
4. 4
AFI: **1 and 4**

Chapter 2
1. 1
2. 2
3. 3
4. 4
AFI: **1 and 3**

Chapter 3
1. 1
2. 2
3. 3
4. 2
AFI: **1, 3, 4, and 5**

Chapter 4
1. 4
2. 1
3. 3
4. 1
AFI: **1, 2, 3, and 4**

Chapter 5
1. 3
2. 4
3. 1
4. 1
AFI: **1 and 4**

Chapter 6
1. 4
2. 2
3. 4
4. 2
AFI: **1 and 2**

Chapter 7
1. 1
2. 4
3. 3
4. 1
AFI: **1**

Chapter 8
1. 3
2. 2
3. 1
4. 1
AFI: **2 and 4**

Chapter 9
1. 4
2. 1
3. 3
4. 2
AFI: **1, 2, 3, and 4**

Chapter 10
1. 3
2. 2
3. 1
4. 4
AFI: **4**

Chapter 11
1. 4
2. 2
3. 4
4. 4
AFI: **2 and 4**

Chapter 12
1. 1
2. 1
3. 4
4. 3
AFI: **1 and 4**

Chapter 13
1. 3
2. 2
3. 4
4. 1
AFI: **5**

Chapter 14
1. 4
2. 4
3. 3
4. 1
AFI: **1 and 2**

Chapter 15
1. 1
2. 4
3. 3
4. 1
AFI: **3, 4, and 5**

Chapter 16
1. 1
2. 2
3. 4
4. 4
AFI: **1 and 4**

Chapter 17
1. 1
2. 4
3. 2
4. 3
AFI: **1, 2, 3, and 4**

Chapter 18
1. 1
2. 3
3. 2
4. 2
AFI: **1, 2, 4, and 5**

Chapter 19
1. 3
2. 1
3. 4
4. 2
AFI: **1 and 4**

Chapter 20
1. 2
2. 4
3. 1
4. 4
AFI: **1, 3, and 5**

Chapter 21
1. 3
2. 3
3. 1
4. 2
AFI: **2, 3, 4, and 5**

Chapter 22
1. 4
2. 3
3. 2
4. 2
AFI: **1, 2, 4, and 5**

Chapter 23
1. 2
2. 1
3. 4
4. 2
AFI: **1, 3, and 4**